Developing Practical Nursing Skills

Developing Practical Nursing Skills helps you learn and perfect the practical skills required to become a qualified nurse. Adopting a patient-focused and caring approach, this essential text helps you integrate nursing values alongside physical skills in your daily practice.

Now in its fifth edition, the text takes into account the NMC standards of proficiency and is relevant to nurses across all fields. Key features of the book include: i) New chapters on mental health assessment and end-of-life care, along with expanded content on sleep, pain and medication management. ii) Full-colour text design with clear illustrations and clinical photographs to aid visual learning. iii) Reader-friendly style with learning outcomes, activities and reflection points to help you link theory to practice. iv) Scenarios from a range of settings, including community, mental health and learning disabilities nursing. v) A focus on adults and young people, and with 'pointers' on caring for children and pregnant mothers to promote a lifespan approach.

This is a complete clinical skills resource for all pre-registration nursing students. It is also a useful text for nursing associate and healthcare support workers.

Nicola Neale is currently an Associate Lecturer with Bucks New University, was trained at St Thomas' Hospital and has since worked extensively in the NHS in medicine and in higher education as a Senior Lecturer. She has an MA in Education and a PG Diploma in Cancer Care. Her main areas of interest are cancer care, long-term conditions and psychological care within an adult setting. In 2011, Nicola set up a Macmillan Cancer Information Centre for an NHS Foundation Trust and managed this for seven years and was awarded The Henry Garnett Award as a Macmillan Professional for outreach activities to local communities.

Joanne Sale is a registered nurse primarily of working-age adults with mental health needs, both in-patient and community settings. Jo also has an interest in psychology, holding a BSc and an MSc in this subject and enjoys applying this knowledge to the nursing arena. She is particularly interested in service user recovery and co-production in education. Along with colleagues in her local trust and the partner university, she was instrumental in the setting up of the Recovery College, which now forms a major pathway in an individual's recovery from mental ill health. Jo has recently retired but continues to offer her support and input to the University of Bedfordshire.

Both Nicola and Joanne have co-authored all previous editions of the communication chapter in this book. However, following the retirement of Lesley Baillie, Nicola and Joanne were very happy to be asked to co-edit this fifth edition.

Developing Practical Nursing Skills

Foundations for Nursing and Healthcare Students

Fifth edition

Edited by

Nicola Neale and Joanne Sale

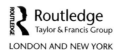

Routledge
Taylor & Francis Group

LONDON AND NEW YORK

Cover image: © Shutterstock

Fifth edition published 2022
by Routledge
4 Park Square, Milton Park, Abingdon, Oxon, OX14 4RN

and by Routledge
605 Third Avenue, New York, NY 10158

Routledge is an imprint of the Taylor & Francis Group, an informa business

© 2022 selection and editorial matter, Nicola Neale and Joanne Sale; individual chapters, the contributors

First edition published by Taylor & Francis 2001
Fourth edition published by Routledge 2014

British Library Cataloguing-in-Publication Data
A catalogue record for this book is available from the British Library

Library of Congress Cataloging-in-Publication Data
A catalog record has been requested for this book

ISBN: 978-0-367-89660-7 (hbk)
ISBN: 978-0-367-89661-4 (pbk)
ISBN: 978-1-003-02066-0 (ebk)

DOI: 10.4324/9781003020660

Typeset in Bembo
by codeMantra

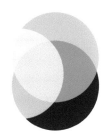

Contents

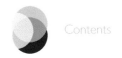

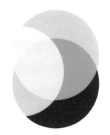

Figures

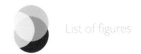

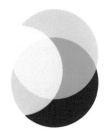

Tables

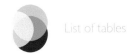

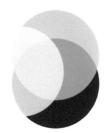

Boxes

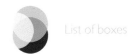

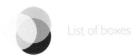

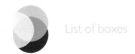

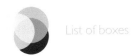

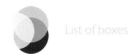

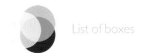

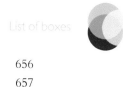

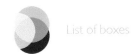

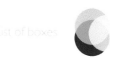

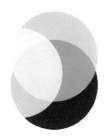

Contributors

Kirsty Andrews is a Course Leader in Adult Nursing at Anglia Ruskin University, UK.

Lesley Baillie is a Visiting Professor at London South Bank University.

Harriet Barker is a Lead Nurse with Senior Adult Medical Services (SAMS) and Frailty team at Ashford and St Peter's Hospitals NHS Foundation Trust.

Rachel Busuttil Leaver was a Lecturer and Practitioner of Urological Care at London South Bank University, UK.

Skye Capolucci is a Mental Health Nurse with the Community Mental Health Team at Central and North West London NHS Foundation Trust.

Scott Elbourne is a District Nurse Clinical Lead with Berkshire Healthcare NHS Foundation Trust.

Katherine Hopkinson is a Senior Lecturer of Adult Nursing at the University of Bedfordshire, UK.

Sue Maddex is a Senior Lecturer in Adult Nursing at London South Bank University, UK.

Aby Mitchell is a Senior Lecturer in Adult Nursing at the University of West London, UK.

Nicola Neale is an Associate Lecturer in Adult Nursing at Buckinghamshire New University, UK.

Martina O'Brien is the Head of Division/Associate Professor in Adult Nursing at London South Bank University, UK.

Lindsey Pollard is a Clinical Nurse Specialist in Pain Management at the University Hospitals Plymouth NHS Trust.

Joanne Sale is Formally Senior Lecturer in Mental Health Nursing at the University of Bedfordshire, UK.

Rowena Slope is a Senior Lecturer in Adult Nursing at the University of Bedfordshire, UK.

Gavin Walker works for the Institute of Vocational Learning at London South Bank University, UK.

Moira Walker is Senior Lecturer in Adult Nursing at the University of Gloucestershire, UK.

Jennifer Wyeth is an Infection Prevention and Control Specialist Nurse, Independent Advisor and Member of the Infection Prevention Society.

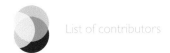
Consultants

Child

Dr Sue Higham is a children's nurse and nurse teacher, currently Head of Nursing at Buckinghamshire New University.

Learning Disability

David Roberts is a Learning Disability Nurse and Practice Experience Manager at the East London NHS Foundation Trust.

Pregnancy and Birth

Andrea Stebbings is a Midwifery Lecturer at the University of Plymouth, UK and Professional Midwifery Advocate.

Foreword

As nurses, we deliver skilled and compassionate care to promote comfort and dignity to people when they are at their most vulnerable. The impression a nurse makes on a person is central to that person's experiences of healthcare, recovery and well-being.

During recent years, we've seen major changes to access points and routes into the professions. For example, the Nursing Associate role, introduced in 2019, is a new pipeline into the workforce, and in 2021, we have seen the highest ever increase in applications to nursing degrees. 2020 was designated the International Year of the Nurse and Midwife, a year to celebrate, thank and respect our professions for the difference they make to the lives of so many people, every day. However, as we know, 2020 became the year of the Covid-19 pandemic. Nurses were seen on the global stage, leading colleagues and those in their care during the pandemic response, and this put a new spotlight on the changing, expanding and vital role of our professions. Across all of health and care, the public saw nurses as clear leaders, in care, in research and in safe staffing.

This fifth edition of *Developing Practical Nursing Skills* retains the caring, person-centred and holistic approach to carrying out practical nursing skills, which the earlier editions established. It is a valuable guide for student nurses, student nursing associates and other care staff, as it will support them in developing their practical skills for nursing care, underpinned by core nursing values. The interactive approach of the book will encourage readers to engage with their own learning and reflect on, and learn from, their practice experiences.

This book provides essential guidance, not only for students and care staff but also for educators and others, in delivering skilled, compassionate and dignified care for all.

Ruth May
Chief Nursing Officer for England

Preface

This book, fully updated and expanded from the fourth edition, aims to assist readers in developing the practical skills necessary to care for adults in varied healthcare settings. Practical nursing skills, when carried out by nurses and nurse associates with competence and compassion, are highly valued by those who need care and their families. Healthcare professionals make an essential contribution towards promoting health, recovery, dignity and comfort, and this enhances a positive healthcare experience.

In 2018, the Nursing and Midwifery Council (NMC 2018a, 2018b) published new standards of proficiencies for registered nurses and nursing associates. These proficiencies outline the skills and underpinning knowledge required by the nurse or nurse associate to provide person-centred care for people of all ages across any setting. In some environments, nurses and nursing associates are more likely to supervise or support others than directly carry out these practical skills. To supervise others in providing quality fundamental care requires leadership, a sound knowledge and understanding of these skills and a commitment to their importance and value.

In this book, practical skills are applied through scenarios to adults with physical health needs, adults with mental health needs and adults with learning disabilities. However, the NMC's (2018a and b) standards of proficiencies include generic competencies and recognise that all nurses should be able to provide essential care across a person's life span; therefore, each chapter of this book includes boxes with practice points for caring for children and young people, and mothers who are pregnant, or after childbirth. These boxes highlight key points that all nurses should be aware of and include recommended further reading and suggested resources. Skills and knowledge related to learning disability and mental health are integrated throughout the chapters. This fifth edition includes a chapter dedicated to mental health assessment and a chapter focusing on end-of-life care skills. It has also increased content about caring for people with dementia in response to reports highlighting the high proportion of people with dementia needing healthcare and the needs to improve their care, particularly in a hospital setting (Alzheimer's Society 2018; Royal College of Psychiatrists 2017).

The first chapter explains the caring context for skills, emphasising the importance of the underpinning knowledge and attitudes of the caregiver, as well as the practical components of skills and safe practice. Chapter 1 also provides guidance to help students maximise learning from their practical experiences. Dignity in care is explored, and subsequent chapters address how to promote the dignity of people when undertaking specific skills in practice. Skills are discussed with application to

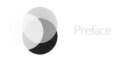

the scenarios, incorporating a problem-solving and caring approach. The book is evidence-based and promotes theory–practice links with a range of activities that help to apply the learning in a reflective way.

This fifth edition is particularly applicable to undergraduate nursing students and associate nurse apprentices following the adult, mental health and learning disability fields of nursing. However, it is also relevant to people who are studying for qualifications in care and healthcare-related programmes and to all those involved in the teaching of practical skills, including university and college lecturers, and practitioners.

Nurses care for people in a wide range of settings in different circumstances, and hence no single term is appropriate to be used in every situation. In the majority of this book, the terms 'person', 'people' and 'individual' are used to refer to those receiving care, and this is in line with the terminology in the NMC proficiencies (2018a, 2018b).

We hope that this book will be really helpful to you as you are developing new skills and knowledge to care with competence and compassion, and we hope that all those using this book have a very successful and rewarding nursing career.

Joanne Sale and Nicola Neale

References

Alzheimer's Society. 2018. *Dementia-the True Cost. Fixing the Care Crisis.* London. Alzheimer's Society. Available from: *https://www.alzheimers.org.uk/about-us/policy-and-influencing/dementia-true-cost-fixing-care-crisis* (Accessed on 10 May 2021).

Nursing and Midwifery Council (NMC). 2018a. *Standards of Proficiency for Registered Nurses.* London: NMC.

Nursing and Midwifery Council (NMC). 2018b. *Standards of Proficiency for Nursing Associates.* London: NMC.

Royal College of Psychiatrists (RCP). 2017. *Report of the National Audit of Dementia Care in General Hospitals.* London: Healthcare Quality Improvement Partnership.

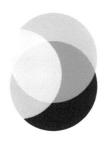

Acknowledgements

Joanne and Nicola would like to thank the following people for their support during the writing and editing processes.

We are enormously grateful to all the contributors and consultants, for their hard work during what has been a hugely challenging 18 months for all practitioners and educators.

We'd like to acknowledge the care and patience of our respective families and friends.

Last but not least, we'd like to thank Evie and the publishing team at Taylor and Francis for their tolerance and guidance in the face of adversity.

This book is dedicated to the memory of Rachel Busuttil Leaver, acknowledging her contribution and commitment to nursing and nurse education.

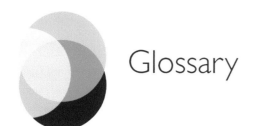

Glossary

Abscess   A localised collection of pus. Pus is a thick fluid containing leucocytes, bacteria and cellular debris, and it indicates infection.

Anaemia   Reduced haemoglobin concentration in the blood or abnormal haemoglobin resulting in reduced oxygen-carrying capacity.

Bacteraemia   An infection in the blood caused by bacteria.

Best interests   Under the MCA 2005 (Great Britain 2005), if a person has been assessed as lacking capacity, then any action or decision must be made in their 'best interests'. This is principle 4 of the MCA, and the person who will make the decision is known as the 'decision maker'. They should ensure that the decision takes into account a number of factors; for example, not to make assumptions about the person's interests based on age, appearance or condition alone, they should take account of all relevant circumstances, they should consider if the decision could wait (if the person may regain capacity), they should involve the person as fully as possible, if they are aware of previous and present wishes and feelings, these must be taken into account, and they should also consult as widely as possible before making the decision.

Bipolar Affective Disorder   This was previously called manic depression. As the phrase suggests, a person with this illness experiences severe mood swings that can last several weeks or months. These are much more than the emotional ups and downs that most of us experience.

Body Mass Index (BMI)   Measurement of body fat based on height and weight.

Care bundle   A care bundle is a set of evidence-based interventions which, when used together, improve patient outcomes.

Clozapine   Clozapine is an atypical antipsychotic drug used to treat schizophrenia in persons who are unresponsive to, or intolerant of, conventional antipsychotic drugs (NICE, 2020). Clozapine can have significant side effects which can impact on wound healing (Kilroy-Findley, 2017).

Dementia   The term 'dementia' is used to describe the symptoms that occur when the brain is affected by specific diseases and conditions. Dementia is progressive; its symptoms include loss of memory, confusion and problems with speech and understanding. See http://alzheimers.org.uk for more information.

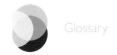

Health Action Plan   A personal action plan should be developed for each individual with a learning disability, which details the actions needed to maintain and improve the person's health and any help needed to accomplish these (Department of Health, 2002). A Health Action Plan contains important information such as lifestyle advice, where to get help and how to stay safe (Mencap, 2016).

Health facilitator   The role focuses on an individual's health outcomes and can be undertaken by a range of people including support workers, family carers, friends and advocates as well as health professionals, see *Health Action Planning and Health Facilitation for people with learning disabilities: good practice guidance* (DH, 2009) and *People with learning disabilities in England* (DH, 2019).

Ileostomy   The end of the small intestine, the ileum, is surgically brought out through an opening (stoma) in the abdomen.

Infection   The successful invasion, establishment and growth of microorganisms within the tissues of the host.

Methicillin-resistant *Staphylococcus aureus* **(MRSA)**   A strain of *Staphylococcus aureus* that is resistant to methicillin★ and other penicillin and cephalosporin antibiotics (Health Protection Agency, 2012, p. 77). ★Also referred to as 'methicillin'.

Multiple sclerosis   Multiple sclerosis (MS) is an autoimmune condition where the immune system attacks the central nervous system including the brain and spinal cord. It is not clear what causes MS, but inherited genes are thought to be partly responsible. The immune system attacks the fatty substance or myelin that protects nerve fibres in the central nervous system. This can make it difficult for the nerves to send signals to each other. Symptoms of MS include problems with vision, balance, cognition, emotions, fatigue, tingling, numbness, spasm and weakness. There is no cure for MS, but medication can bring symptomatic relief and flare ups can be treated with steroids.

Rheumatoid arthritis   A chronic, progressive and disabling autoimmune disease that can affect any joint causing pain, swelling and disability. It is a systemic disease and can affect the whole body, including the lungs, heart and eyes.

Stoma   An artificial permanent opening on the body such as those made in the abdominal wall during a surgical procedure to form a colostomy, ileostomy or urinary conduit.

Stroke   Cerebral damage caused either by decreased blood flow or by haemorrhage. Effects vary, but a stroke often causes paralysis down one side of the body (hemiplegia), and speech and swallowing difficulty.

Suprapubic catheter   A suprapubic catheter is sometimes used to manage urinary elimination in persons who are unable to void the bladder normally. This may be the result of trauma, obstruction or neurological problems. The device has to be inserted surgically by a urology specialist. It consists of a balloon, which is inserted into the

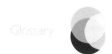

bladder, and then inflated, and connected to a thin hollow tube. The suprapubic catheter is connected to a collecting device and managed by the individual and/or healthcare provider. Suprapubic catheters have a lower risk of infection than indwelling catheters, although infection at the wound site is still possible especially following surgery.

Type 2 diabetes   Type 2 diabetes develops when the body makes insufficient insulin, or when the insulin that is produced does not work effectively (known as insulin resistance). See www.diabetes.org.uk.

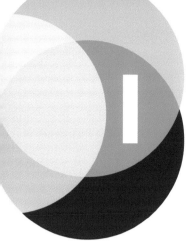

Practical nursing skills: a caring approach

Lesley Baillie

INTRODUCTION

Nursing care should be delivered compassionately and competently in a way that promotes the dignity of the people being cared for. All student nurses need to learn to perform a range of practical skills safely, with a caring and person-centred approach (Nursing and Midwifery Council [NMC] 2018a). Healthcare support workers, assistant practitioners and nursing associates also need to develop practical skills, as they work within nursing teams. This book aims to assist readers in developing a caring and person-centred approach to a range of practical nursing skills, for application with people across different healthcare settings. Practical nursing skills comprise not only the hands-on (psychomotor) element but also an underpinning evidence-based knowledge, effective communication skills, an ethical approach, critical and reflective thinking, and an appropriate professional, caring attitude. These elements are considered throughout the chapters in this book.

This chapter discusses the nature and context of practical skills in nursing and how this book can help you in developing your nursing skills. There is an emphasis on developing and valuing these practical skills as holistic, caring skills that contribute to people's healthcare experiences in a positive way, promote their dignity and support their comfort and well-being.

This chapter includes the following topics:

- The nature of practical nursing skills
- The context for practical nursing skills
- A person-centred approach to practical nursing skills
- A caring and compassionate approach to practical nursing skills
- Cultural competence and practical nursing skills
- Dignity and practical nursing skills
- Learning practical nursing skills

THE NATURE OF PRACTICAL NURSING SKILLS

Nurses need to develop a range of competencies, including skills in practical nursing, communication and management. Practical nursing skills are the hands-on skills that nurses use in their care of people; some of these skills are performed by other

DOI: 10.4324/9781003020660-1

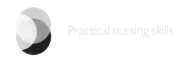

professionals in caring roles too. Healthcare support workers, assistant practitioners and nursing associates carry out many of these skills, and hence, this book is relevant for them too. The NMC's standards for registered nurses and nursing associates include detailed annexes of practical nursing skills (referred to as nursing procedures) (NMC 2018a, 2018b).

Practical nursing skills are used during assessment and interventions to promote comfort and maintain health for people who, due to acute or long-term physical or mental health conditions, cannot care for themselves independently or need help to maintain their health.

Box 1.1 Activity: healthy activities

Reflect on all the activities you carry out to keep yourself comfortable and healthy each day. What would happen if you could not carry out these activities?

You might have reflected that you carry out these activities, often referred to as 'activities of daily living' (Roper et al. 2000) with little thought much of the time: sleeping, eating and drinking, going to the toilet, moving about, and carrying out personal hygiene. You might take medication for one or more health conditions or if you have pain, take painkilling medicines or manage your pain another way. However, any mental or physical health condition can affect these self-care activities; without help, people would quickly become debilitated and uncomfortable, with their health and well-being at risk. There are around 6.5 million unpaid carers in the United Kingdom (UK) who help family, friends or neighbours with care due to health issues (Carers UK 2019). Many nurses are involved in supporting people and their carers at home, for example, teaching them to keep their skin healthy when they lack mobility; to manage medication; to cope with mental health issues; to deal with altered elimination, such as a urinary catheter; or to deliver care at end of life. When people are admitted to hospital, nursing teams must support the individual with activities that they cannot manage themselves as part of their holistic care.

Practical nursing skills are also carried out when assessing a person's condition and delivering interventions to improve or maintain their health; these skills are carried out in acute situations, for people with long-term conditions and people with multiple health needs, in a range of settings. When we feel unwell, we self-assess; for example, we might measure our body temperature. Some people are unable to self-assess or communicate that they feel unwell, for example, a person with advanced dementia or a person with a severe learning disability. Nurses need to be highly skilled in using a range of assessment skills for people with different health needs, and they must be able to interpret and act on the results appropriately and often speedily. People who are acutely ill or who have long-term health conditions that fluctuate in severity, need careful and skilful monitoring. Nurses must also be able to use a wide range of practical skills to promote comfort, safety and well-being, including administration of medication.

Box 1.2 Activity: immunisations

Almost everyone has had an injection at some stage, and you may have had recent immunisations before starting your studies. You probably took it for granted that the skill would be performed competently. What are the different elements of carrying out this skill? List all you can think of.

You probably considered technical aspects such as preparing the correct medicine accurately and safely. You might have identified that the nurse required underlying knowledge of the drug's actions and potential side effects and that the nurse should use a calm and friendly approach to relax you and relieve anxiety. This example illustrates that effective practical nursing skills require a skilled motor performance (the doing element) and a sound knowledge based on best evidence (the cognitive aspect), with both accompanied by an appropriate attitude (the affective aspect).

Oermann (1990) suggested that the motor (doing) element of a practical (psychomotor) skill is often emphasised to the exclusion of the cognitive and affective components. She highlighted the importance of the cognitive base (the scientific principles underlying the performance of the skill) and the affective domain, which reflects the nurse's values and concern for the person while performing the skill. These three aspects are now explored further.

The affective domain

The affective domain is underpinned by values, which can be defined as 'core beliefs that guide and motivate attitudes and actions' (see https://www.ethics.org/resources/free-toolkit/definition-values/). Nurses bring their own personal values into nursing; these values are influenced by a range of factors (e.g. family, education) and hopefully include integrity, compassion, dignity and kindness. Nurses must also embrace professional values, directed by the National Health Service (NHS) and the NMC. Values are important as they influence attitudes and behaviour. For example, Nåden and Eriksson (2004) found that nurses who promoted dignity had a strong moral attitude, underpinned by values such as respect, honesty and responsibility; such nurses had a 'genuine interest and desire to help patients' (p. 90).

The cognitive domain

The cognitive domain reflects the thinking element behind the skill, including the application of best evidence in practice and problem-solving. Being able to adapt a skill in practice requires a sound underlying knowledge of why it is being performed and the rationale for each stage. For example, understanding the principles behind oxygen therapy enables nurses to choose an administration method that is safe and acceptable for people in specific healthcare situations. Practical skills should be based on best available evidence, which may be derived from research, but could be based on experience, and from reflection on practice (see the 'Learning from experience and reflection' section).

Nurses are accountable for their actions, so they must be able to explain the knowledge base underpinning their practice. Benner (1984) explored how expert nurses develop knowledge from their practice, learning to recognise, for example, subtle changes in people's conditions. Not all nursing skills have a firm evidence base on which to implement practice, but in many areas research-based knowledge is available. Within this book, the authors have searched for up-to-date evidence to underpin practical skills, and they refer to evidence-based guidelines where available. These guidelines include the National Institute for Health and Care Excellence (NICE) evidence-based guidelines and quality standards (see www.nice.org.uk) and the Cochrane Library systematic reviews of research. Be aware: these guidelines are regularly reviewed, so check the websites for updates. Often, NHS Trusts and other healthcare organisations have their own clinical guidelines, based on best evidence, to assist nurses and other healthcare professionals to implement evidence-based practice in the local context. You should always work with your employer's guidelines, if available.

The motor domain

Learning the motor dimension of a skill is important for an effective outcome as lack of a skilled motor performance jeopardises both safety and comfort. Knowing how to conduct a practical skill can be termed know-how type of knowledge – practical expertise and skill that is really acquired through practice and experience (Manley 1997). Nursing skills are performed in a changing clinical environment and varied settings, with people who respond and react in different ways. Therefore, nurses need to adapt skills accordingly, so practical nursing skills can never be wholly automatic in nature.

The importance of practical nursing skills for quality care

The importance of high-quality nursing care cannot be overstated, and the application of practical nursing skills is central to people's experiences. The National Nursing Research Unit (2008) identified that from individuals' perspectives, the features of high-quality care are as follows:

- A holistic approach to physical, mental and emotional needs, person-centred and continuous care
- Efficiency and effectiveness combined with humanity and compassion
- Professional, high-quality evidence-based practice
- Safe, effective and prompt nursing interventions
- Empowerment, support and advocacy
- Seamless care through effective teamwork with other professions

Nurses valued being able to make a difference to peoples' lives, having close contact with them, delivering excellent care, working in a team and being a role model to others and continually developing through learning and improving.

However, over the past decade or so, there have been concerns about fundamental care being neglected in healthcare settings, with media headlines about poor attention to nutrition and continence, and reports from the Patients Association (2011), the Health Service Ombudsman (2011) and the inquiry into care standards in Mid Staffordshire (Mid Staffordshire NHS Foundation Trust Inquiry 2013), all revealing a lack of care with poor care experiences and outcomes. Nurses should deliver high-quality fundamental care, and they have a professional and ethical duty to do so. People who are cared for and their families should be confident that nurses will deliver care in a compassionate and competent way and promote comfort and dignity when people are at their most vulnerable. Technology is integral to the application of many practical nursing skills, but its use should be accompanied by a caring and humanistic approach.

This book emphasises that practical skills should be person-centred and delivered within the context of a caring philosophy, with value attached to fundamental as well as technical care. For example, there is great skill involved in helping an older person regain the ability to wash and dress after a stroke, or in assisting a person with confusion to maintain continence.

THE CONTEXT FOR PRACTICAL NURSING SKILLS

Practical nursing skills must be applied within the context of the individual person and the nurse–individual relationship. The wider context for skills application is also relevant: the legal, professional and health policy context.

Legislation

Nursing practice takes place in the context of legislation; some Acts of Parliament with particular relevance to practical skills are briefly presented here. The Human Rights Act (Great Britain 1998) recognised that all individuals have minimal and fundamental human rights including the right to dignity and privacy; dignity and privacy are important principles during delivery of care and are discussed in relation to practical skills throughout this book. Mental capacity legislation is also particularly relevant to practical nursing skills and is considered further in relation to consent in Chapter 2. The relevant acts are the Mental Capacity Act 2005 for England and Wales (Great Britain 2005), the Adults With Incapacity (Scotland) Act 2000 (Scottish Parliament 2000) and the Mental Capacity Act (Northern Ireland) 2016 (Northern Ireland Assembly 2016).

The Equality Act (Great Britain 2010) aims to protect all people against discrimination. The act established protected characteristics that cannot be used as a reason to treat people unfairly and include the following: age, disability, gender reassignment, marriage and civil partnership, pregnancy and maternity, race, religion and belief, sex and sexual orientation. The Nursing and Midwifery Council (NMC 2018b) Code requires all registrants to ensure that people's rights are upheld and to challenge any discriminatory attitudes and behaviours towards those receiving care. Unfortunately, there is evidence that discrimination in healthcare exists and that discriminatory behaviour diminishes the dignity of people being cared for (Baillie and Matiti 2013). For example, a UK Commission to investigate dignified care for older people highlighted that older people continue to experience discrimination despite being the major group of health service users (Commission on Dignity in Care 2012). Mencap (2012), a UK charity campaigning for equal rights for children and adults with a learning disability, highlighted the legal requirement to provide equality in healthcare, so nurses must give the same quality of care and treatment to all individuals, including those with a learning disability. Mencap (2012) suggested that discrimination occurs due to the lack of value afforded to the life of a person with a learning disability, indicating that, despite the Equality Act 2010 and professional codes of practice, some healthcare workers do not recognise the human dignity of people with learning disabilities. The 2012 Mencap report revealed cases where nurses failed to provide even basic care to people with learning disabilities, neglecting nutrition, hydration and pain relief. Unfortunately, the Care Quality Commission's (2020) report again found care for people with learning disabilities, in hospital and other settings, which contravened human rights set out in the Human Rights Act and Equality Act.

Professional requirements

The NMC is the regulator for nursing and midwifery in England, Wales, Scotland and Northern Ireland. The NMC maintains a register of nurses, midwives and nursing associates and provides the standards for nursing and midwifery education and a Code that sets out the professional standards the public can expect of NMC registrants. The NMC requirements are an important context for the development of practical nursing skills, so you should become familiar with the Code (NMC 2018c) and with the education standards for registered nurses (or the standards for nursing associates, if applicable to you).

The Code sets out that registrants must:

- Prioritise people;
- Practise effectively;
- Preserve safety; and
- Promote professionalism and trust.

The section 'Prioritise people' includes the requirement to make people's 'care and safety your main concern and make sure that their dignity is preserved and their needs are recognised, assessed and responded to', and to 'make sure you deliver the fundamentals of care effectively' (p. 6).

The NMC's (2018a) *Standards of proficiency for registered nurses* includes a list of communication and management skills and a separate list of nursing procedures, that all nurses must demonstrate. For nursing associates, there are similar lists provided in the *Standards of proficiency for nursing associates* (NMC 2018b). You will find that this book addresses these required skills across the various chapters.

Each chapter begins with scenarios of adults in physical healthcare, learning disability and mental healthcare settings, and the chapter links the skills back to these scenarios, thus encouraging theory–practice links and a person-centred approach.

The book aims to include a selection of scenarios, from a variety of settings, but it is not intended that all possible situations are represented. All scenarios have been developed from experience with similar people with health needs. Any identifying details have been changed or omitted, and pseudonyms were allocated at random.

As the NMC (2018a) standards expect registered nurses to care for people across the life span, with specialist skills in their own field of practice, the book includes 'Practice points' boxes for care of children, pregnant mothers and birth application while Learning Disability and Mental Health application is integrated within the text. These are supported by references to further reading and resources.

Nurses encountering pregnant mothers in different settings should remember that they are adapting to a life-changing event that may make them feel vulnerable: physically, emotionally and socially. Pregnant mothers may access healthcare in many different healthcare settings and should be partners in their care choices. Contemporaneous, evidence-based information should always be provided to women and families to support this partnership.

All healthcare staff should be able to assess a collapsed person and administer basic life support (BLS). These procedures are updated regularly by the Resuscitation Council (UK) and outlined in detail on their website (http://www.resus.org. uk). Therefore, these procedures, although referred to where appropriate, are not reproduced in detail here. The Resuscitation Council's (UK) very informative website includes other useful sections as well as guidelines, for example, information about legal aspects of resuscitation and decisions relating to cardiopulmonary resuscitation. You must undergo supervised BLS practice in the skills laboratory with a trained instructor, and it is mandatory for all healthcare staff to regularly update their skills. Chapter 11 covers some principles underpinning moving and handling skills. These skills are frequently updated and you must attend the training sessions provided for you, both as a student and as a registered nurse or nursing associate, so that you can practise and update your skills under supervision.

Health policy and guidelines

There are many UK Health and Social Care policy documents that provide context and guidance relevant to nursing practice. As Health and Social Care services are devolved to each UK nation, you should be familiar with the relevant documents for where you are based and also ensure you access the most up-to-date versions, as there are regular policy updates.

All UK nations set out core principles and values for Health and Social Care with an expectation that all Health and Social Care staff will follow these in their practice (see Table 1.1). As you can see, there are close similarities between the nations' expectations although they are stated differently.

In 2012, NICE produced a quality standard for the person's experience in adult NHS services in England, so these standards apply to all nursing practice with adults, in both inpatient and other healthcare settings. These standards recommend that people are 'treated with dignity, kindness, compassion, courtesy, respect, understanding and honesty'. The standards also include that the individual should have regular assessment

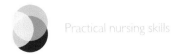
Table 1.1: Core principles and values for healthcare

Nation	Core principles and values
England	Working together for people; Respect and dignity, Commitment to quality of care, Compassion, Improving lives, and Everyone counts; these values apply to all NHS staff (Department of Health and Social Care 2015)
Scotland	Care and compassion; Dignity and respect; Quality and teamwork, openness, honesty and responsibility (NHS Scotland 2013)
Wales	We put people and users of our services first; We seek to improve our care; We focus on well-being and prevention; We reflect on our experiences and learn; We work in partnership and as a team; We value all who work in the NHS (NHS Wales 2016)
Northern Ireland	Empowerment, involvement, respect, partnership, learning, continuity, equity and equality (Department of Health, Social Services and Public Safety 2011)

of their physical and psychological needs, which include nutrition, hydration, pain relief, personal hygiene and anxiety. The standards highlight the importance of meeting both emotional support and fundamental needs such as pain management and nutrition, and of respecting confidentiality, listening in a sensitive and empathetic way and establishing trusting relationships.

Many health policies aim to set out strategy and guidance for particular areas of healthcare, and many of these approaches are applicable to nursing practice. Some key documents are reviewed next, in relation to care of people with learning disabilities, people with mental health problems and people with dementia.

Healthcare for people with learning disabilities

Nurses in all fields of practice care for people with learning disabilities across varying healthcare settings and must ensure the delivery of high-quality, safe care that addresses individuals' needs in a dignified manner. Many people with a learning disability do not have family and carers to advocate for them (Mencap 2012), increasing their vulnerability when accessing healthcare. In 2001, the Department of Health (DH) published *Valuing People: A New Strategy for Learning Disability for the 21st Century*, which stressed that people with learning disabilities are people first and there should be a focus on what they can do rather than what they cannot. This document set out that all people with learning disabilities should have a health facilitator – who may be a keyworker, relative or health or social care professional – appointed to ensure they get the healthcare they need, and a Health Action Plan. An individual's **Health Action Plan** includes details of health interventions, oral health and dental care, fitness and mobility, continence, vision, hearing, nutrition, emotional needs, medication and records of screening. Any nurse carrying out practical skills with people with learning disabilities, or supporting their carers, should refer to the person's Health Action Plan and the person who is acting as their health facilitator.

Since 2001, the DH has carried out progress reviews. In *Good Practice in Learning Disability Nursing*, the DH (2007) emphasised that learning disability nurses are essential for making the 'Valuing People' vision happen and that they can help people with learning disabilities to stay healthy as long as possible. The DH (2009) then published *Valuing People Now: A New Three-Year Strategy for Learning Disabilities*, stating that the key objective for all people with learning disabilities is to get the healthcare and the support they need to live healthy lives. The report again acknowledged that better health for people with learning disabilities is a key priority, as there is clear evidence that most people with learning disabilities have poorer health than the rest of the population.

Despite these various reports, there have continued to be concerns about standards of care and failures in meeting the care needs of people with learning disabilities. An inquiry into premature deaths of people with learning disabilities highlighted that in relation to Health and Social Care needs, people with learning disabilities were very vulnerable (Norah Fry Research Centre 2013). The report noted that nearly all people with learning disabilities had at least one long-term health condition and yet the majority were not accessing health checks. Significantly more were underweight than the general population, two-thirds lacked independent mobility, half had problems with vision, a quarter had problems with hearing, over a fifth had problems with both vision and hearing, and many had limited verbal communication, with over a fifth not communicating verbally at all.

NHS England (2019) acknowledged the significant failings in care that continue, highlighting various initiatives to reduce the inequalities in care for people with learning disabilities, and steps to address them. However, recently, the Care Quality Commission (2020) found many examples of undignified and inhumane care in hospital and care settings, with poor physical healthcare and people not seen as individuals. There are also recognised health inequalities with people with learning disabilities dying, on average, 16 years earlier than people in the general population (Mencap 2016).

NICE (2018) provides a useful guideline for the 'Care and support of people growing older with learning disabilities', which includes quality standards. The Royal College of Nursing's (2017) professional resource 'Dignity in healthcare for people with learning disabilities' identifies the following key components of dignity from the perspective of people with learning disabilities: understanding my health; respect me; get to know me; having choices and making decisions; feeling safe. The document highlights how people with learning disabilities have often not been cared for with dignity while also providing many examples of good practice too, and resources available.

Healthcare for people with mental health problems

At least one in four people will experience a mental health problem at some point in their life, and one in six adults has a mental health problem at any one time (McManus et al. 2009). The DH (2011) published the strategy *No Health without Mental Health* that highlighted the importance of mental health for all ages. One of the objectives is that 'more people with mental health problems will have good physical health' and that 'fewer people with mental health problems will die prematurely, and more people with physical ill health will have better mental health' (p. 6). The strategy highlights that having a mental health problem increases the risk of physical health problems; all nurses should understand the links between mental and physical health and be able

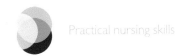

to recognise and address the physical health needs of people who have mental health problems. Chapter 3 addresses the fundamentals of mental health.

The NICE (2011) guidelines *Service User Experience in Adult Mental Health: Improving the Experience of Care for People Using Adult NHS Mental Health Services* presents the components of a good experience in mental health services, with the aim that all adults using NHS mental health services have the best possible experience of care. These guidelines highlight that healthcare professionals who demonstrated support and qualities of empathy and respect could facilitate service users' access to healthcare. The guidelines set out that Health and Social Care professionals should have the knowledge, skills and attitude to assess service users in a sensitive and professional manner and endeavour to build trusting, respectful and empowering therapeutic relationships with service users. The guidelines also highlight that service users want to feel valued and listened to during the process, and for professionals to treat them with dignity, respect and genuine concern. Service users expressed that the most productive relationship with professionals was when it was collaborative, when staff were non-judgemental and caring, and respectful.

Healthcare for people with dementia

In the UK, there are an estimated 850,000 people living with dementia, a figure expected to increase to over 1 million by 2025 (Prince et al. 2014). Dementia primarily affects older people, so many people with dementia have other conditions common to old age that precipitate healthcare use, including hospital admission. In relation to learning disability, people with Down's syndrome have an increased risk of developing dementia due to Alzheimer's disease in middle age (Stanton and Coetzee 2004). An estimated third of hospital inpatients in high-income countries, such as the UK, have dementia (Alzheimer's Disease International [ADI] 2016). Therefore, people with dementia are key service users for whom nurses should be providing high-quality, dignified and compassionate care.

Healthcare for people with dementia should be person-centred and holistic and consider the person's unique context, values and preferences (ADI 2016). Person-centred care approaches originated with Kitwood (1997) and are considered to promote best-quality care for people with dementia (Edvardsson et al. 2010). Brooker (2004, 2007) recommended the VIPS framework for describing person-centred care: V – valuing people with dementia and carers; I – treating people as individuals; P – using the perspective of the person with dementia; S – a positive social environment. However, hospital care has been found to be task-orientated with a lack of focus on the individual (Reilly and Houghton 2019). Furthermore, Boddington and Featherstone (2018) revealed threats to the personhood of people with dementia who were in hospital and were incontinent. Improved care for people with dementia in general hospitals has become a 'policy and practice imperative'; staff need to recognise the benefits of person-centred care and have the ability to deliver person-centred care in practice (Turner et al. 2017). Prato et al. (2019) highlighted the importance of involving relatives of people with cognitive impairment in the hospital setting.

The Alzheimer's Society has produced a personal information document, 'This is me', with spaces for photos and information, to support people with dementia, so that nurses and other healthcare staff can better understand the person's perspectives and take into account their preferences. When caring for people with dementia, be proactive about using 'This is me' (downloadable from the website; https://www.alzheimers.org.uk/get-support/publications-factsheets/this-is-me) and getting to know the person and their family. Baillie and Thomas (2020) found that nurses could use personal information documents to support person-centred care for people with dementia in hospital. Alzheimer's Society's website also contains many other useful resources for nurses and carers who are caring for people who are living with dementia. For example, there is helpful information about mobility, sleep, communication, and support with daily living needs such as bathing, eating and drinking, and continence.

A PERSON-CENTRED APPROACH TO PRACTICAL NURSING SKILLS

The NMC sets out clear expectations that nursing care must be person-centred: registered nurses must 'be able to meet the person-centred, holistic care needs of the people they encounter in their practice' (NMC 2018a, p. 6). Similarly, for nursing associates, the NMC (2018b) sets out that nursing care must be person-centred, safe and compassionate. The NMC (2018a, 2018b) also highlighted that communication skills and nursing procedures are essential for providing safe and compassionate person-centred care. Andersson et al. (2015) found that nurses considered person-centred care, which they viewed as seeing the person instead of the illness, as being integral to caring. Van Belle et al. (2020) argued that effective person-centred care is at the heart of fundamental nursing care.

> **Box 1.3 Activity: person-centred care**
>
> Reflect on what person-centred care means and what would help you to provide person-centred care? How does this contrast with care that is not person-centred?

Person-centred care is broadly interpreted as treating people as individuals (McCance et al. 2008). You could have reflected that this would mean getting to know the person and understanding their individual needs and preferences, while, care that is not person-centred, would be given in a routine way without taking individual needs or preferences into account. McCormack and McCance (2016) developed the person-centred nursing (PCN) framework, which they present in detail in their textbook *Person-Centred Nursing: Theory and Practice*. The framework comprises four constructs:

* pre-requisites (the attributes of the nurse, e.g. professional competence);
* the care environment (the context for care delivery, including systems and staffing);

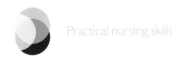

- person-centred processes (how PCN is delivered, e.g. shared decision-making, holistic care);
- expected outcomes (e.g. involvement in care, satisfaction with care).

This framework highlights how the context of care delivery affects person-centredness, as well as the nurse's approach and how they carry out care in practice. Van der Cingel et al. (2016) used this framework to further examine the concepts of PCN, identifying the following elements:

- Nurses know the unique characteristics of the person they care for and what is important to them, and act accordingly;
- Nurses use values such as trust, involvement and humour in their care practice;
- Nurses acknowledge that emotions and compassion create mutuality in the caring relationship.

From a professional perspective, the NMC's (2018c) Code requires nurses to deliver care in a person-centred way:

> You must treat people as individuals. You must listen to the people in your care and respond to their concerns and preferences.

(p. 3)

Some people in your care might not be able to easily communicate their preferences, but you can involve families so that you can get to know them as a person and understand their individual needs and preferences better. In the previous section, you read about the document 'This is me', which enables staff caring for a person with dementia to know about them as an individual, to promote person-centred care. In the chapters that follow, you will be introduced to a range of individual people in scenarios and through these, you will learn about person-centred approaches to practical skills.

McCormack (2004) highlighted that while person-centred care has often been applied to specific contexts (notably older people, particularly those with dementia), as a concept, it is applicable much more generally. In a study based in an acute setting, Ross et al. (2014) found that the nurses appreciated the value of person-centred care although in practice it could be challenging to deliver. However, when care was focused on the person's unique needs, nurses believed there was a positive effect upon the person receiving care, their family and the job satisfaction of nursing staff. Van Belle et al. (2020) found that nurses who approached people in a person-centred manner during fundamental care were able to integrate physical, psychosocial and relational elements of care in practice. For example, they observed a nurse who was helping a person with a wash, and noted her encouraging manner, how she communicated with the person throughout, and picked up on and explored the person's anxiety. However, van Belle et al. (2020) also observed that many nurses worked and communicated in a task-focused manner, focusing on physical care, and this way of working hindered a person-centred approach and effective fundamental care delivery.

For children's nursing, family-centred care models are considered to be a central tenet (Corlett and Twycross 2006). Shields et al. (2006) defined family-centred care as:

a way of caring for children and their families within health services which ensures that care is planned around the whole family, not just the individual child-person, and in which all the family members are *recognized* as care recipients.

(p. 1318)

Family-centred care approaches acknowledge that when a child is admitted, the whole family is affected and so staff must consider the impact of the child's admission on the whole family (Shields et al. 2012). When nursing adults, person-centred care approaches should also encompass involvement of families and others important to each individual.

A CARING AND COMPASSIONATE APPROACH TO PRACTICAL NURSING SKILLS

UK student nurses have expressed enthusiasm about wanting to care for people and to make a difference to people and their families (Phillips et al. 2015). When asked your reasons for wanting to be a nurse, you might well have responded similarly, that you wanted to care for people. Many nursing theorists have recognised that caring and nursing are interrelated. For example, Watson (1979) stated that 'the practice of caring is central to nursing' (p. 9), while Roach (2002) identified caring both as a natural attribute of being human and as the core of nursing. Roach (2002) made a study of caring in relation to nursing and developed the '6Cs' framework: compassion, competence, confidence, conscience, commitment and comportment. Benner and Wrubel (1989) asserted that the 'nature of the caring relationship is central to most nursing interventions' (p. 5). They identified that the same act done in a non-caring way, as opposed to a caring way, has very different consequences so that 'nursing can never be reduced to mere technique' (p. 4).

Cheruiyot and Brysiewicz (2019) revealed the difference between caring and non-caring nursing encounters, as perceived by people in a rehabilitation setting. Features of caring encounters included noticing and acting, and being there for the person. These encounters made them feel they were important and not alone, and gave nurses an opportunity to notice vulnerability and empower the individual. In contrast, non-caring encounters included people being ignored and feeling a burden, unimportant and troublesome to the nurses. The uncaring nursing encounters also led to individual's feeling devalued and depersonalised, which discouraged them in their rehabilitation. As mentioned, in the UK media and other reports, concerns have been expressed about some nurses lacking compassion with a negative impact on the individual's care experiences (Mid Staffordshire NHS Foundation Trust Public Inquiry 2013).

In 2012, the DH in England introduced the '6Cs' as values for practice within a new nursing strategy (Cummings and Bennett 2012). In 2016, the 6Cs were included

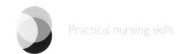

in the new framework for nursing (NHS England 2016). The 6Cs framework places care at the centre with the values of compassion, competence, communication, courage and commitment around them (for a summary, see Box 1.5). The vision aims to embed these values in all nursing, midwifery and caregiving settings across the NHS and social care, to improve care for everyone.

Box 1.4 The 6 Cs

ACTIVITY

Read through Box 1.5. Now reflect on the 6Cs and how you can apply these values in your everyday nursing practice

Box 1.5 The 6 Cs of caring

Care

Care is our core business and that of our organisations, and the care we deliver helps the individual person and improves the health of the whole community. Caring defines us and our work. People receiving care expect it to be right for them, consistently, throughout every stage of their life.

Compassion

Compassion is how care is given through relationships based on empathy, respect and dignity – it can also be described as intelligent kindness and is central to how people perceive their care.

Competence

Competence means all those in caring roles must have the ability to understand an individual's health and social needs and the expertise, clinical and technical knowledge to deliver effective care and treatments based on research and evidence.

Communication

Communication is central to successful caring relationships and to effective teamworking. Listening is as important as what we say and do and essential for 'no decision about me without me'. Communication is the key to a good workplace with benefits for those in our care and staff alike.

Courage

Courage enables us to do the right thing for the people we care for, to speak up when we have concerns and to have the personal strength and vision to innovate and to embrace new ways of working.

Commitment

A commitment to everyone in our care and the general population is a cornerstone of what we do. We need to build on our commitment to improve the care and experience of those we care for; to take action to make this vision and strategy a reality for all; and to meet the health, care and support challenges ahead.

Source: Department of Health (DH). 2012. *Compassion in Practice: Nursing, Midwifery and Care Staff: Our Vision and Strategy.* Gateway reference 18479. London: DH, p. 13.

All the values are important for people being cared for by nurses to have positive experiences. Roach (2002) argued that compassion is needed more than ever to humanise the ever-increasing cold and impersonal technology used within healthcare. Box 1.6 illustrates this need with a nurse's act of compassion that occurred in the highly technical environment of the intensive therapy unit. Communication is essential for portraying compassion and building relationships and is discussed in detail in Chapter 2. Hudacek (2008) found that compassion requires nurses to be present for the person both emotionally and physically and to focus on alleviating suffering and pain through empathic concern. In a study of compassion within the relationship between nurses and older people with a chronic disease, van der Cingel (2011) revealed seven dimensions of compassion: attentiveness, listening, confronting, involvement, helping, presence and understanding.

Box 1.6 Compassion: an illustrative example from an intensive therapy unit

James was in the final stages of heart and lung failure, and his nurse, about to go home after a 12-hour shift and knowing that she would not see him again, asked him if there was anything she could get him before she left. He replied, 'Oh, a port and brandy please!' Phone calls around the hospital were unsuccessful in locating any, and the nurse went off shift. She returned half an hour later with a small glass of port and brandy brought from home. As James was unable to swallow she dipped sponge mouth sticks into the drink and put them in his mouth for him to suck. James grinned and said it was 'wonderful'. This act of compassion brought tenderness to this person's final hours and made an immeasurable difference to his relatives' feelings about his death.

Competence is a commonly used term in nursing and is frequently interpreted as being about a skilled performance (Bing-Jonsson et al. 2015; Garside and Nhemachena 2013). Practical skills must be carried out competently to ensure safe, effective care. Indeed, Roach (2002) stated that 'while competence without compassion can be brutal and inhumane, compassion without competence may be no more than a meaningless, if not harmful, intrusion into the life of a person or persons needing help' (p. 54). Bing-Jonsson et al. (2015) considered competence to encompass knowledge, skills and personal attributes but also recognised contextual aspects of competence, including political, technical and structural factors. Competence should also include cultural competence, with nurses providing care in a culturally appropriate manner for each person and their family (Baillie 2017) (see the later section 'Cultural competence').

Courage is an important value in caring, as nurses must raise any concerns about people who may be at risk and speak out if they feel that care is compromised. The NMC Code (2018c) requires that registrants use their professional 'duty of candour' and raise 'concerns immediately whenever you come across situations that put patients or public safety at risk' (p. 13). It is really important as a student that you know how to raise any concerns you might have about practice. The NMC

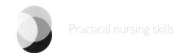

(2019) provides guidance on raising concerns, to supplement the Code: 'Raising concerns: guidance for nurses, midwives and nursing associates'. Raising concerns may include a practice known as 'whistleblowing', which is defined as being where a person identifies 'an incompetent, unethical or illegal situation in the workplace and reports it to someone who has the power to stop the wrong' (Ahern and McDonald 2002, p. 303). The NMC (2019) guidance includes information about the legislation to protect 'whistle-blowers' and the organisations that can support whistle-blowers or people who raise concerns. Your university will also have information about how you can raise concerns, so make sure you are aware of how to access this.

Commitment as part of care requires that nurses will carry out necessary care in a consistent, reliable and timely way, regardless of barriers and constraints. Henderson et al. (2007) found that nurses needed to respond to the persons' needs in a timely manner to be perceived as caring; people were dissatisfied when nurses apparently forgot them and their needs. In Box 1.6, the nurse's action exemplified compassion and also demonstrated commitment to James, by bringing the drink from home despite just finishing a 12-hour shift. In a study of caring for people dying in an intensive care unit, Borhani et al. (2014) identified commitment to care as a dominant theme in interviews with nurses who were caring for those who were dying.

CULTURAL COMPETENCE AND PRACTICAL NURSING SKILLS

Nursing care should be carried out in a culturally competent manner, taking into account the values, culture and health beliefs of the individual (Papadopoulos et al. 2016). The American nurse and anthropologist Madeleine Leininger (1981) studied transcultural caring over many years and identified how acts of caring such as comforting and physical care, and the meaning attached to them, can vary between cultures. Leininger suggested that culture and caring cannot be separated within nursing actions and decision-making.

Papadopoulos (2006a) presented the Papadopoulos–Tilki–Taylor model for transcultural nursing and health, consisting of four linked elements: cultural awareness, cultural knowledge, cultural sensitivity and cultural competence.

- **Cultural awareness** includes examining and questioning one's personal value-base and beliefs. Chapter 2 of this book will help you to develop self-awareness.
- **Cultural knowledge** may be drawn from sources such as sociology, anthropology and research, and from experience of people. Where appropriate to specific practical skills, cultural variations (particularly related to religious beliefs) are considered in this book. However, there are often individual and regional variations, so it is important to avoid stereotyping and making ethnocentric judgements that serve as barriers to cultural sensitivity. In Cioffi's (2005) Australian study, the nurses used experiences of caring for culturally diverse individuals to develop their knowledge;

sources were bilingual health workers and colleagues, people they cared for, their families and support persons. Some nurses used stereotypical views of the person's cultural group to give care, but others used the individual's perspective: 'You actually have to ask the person. You can't assume they're going to be the traditional Chinese or Arabic lady' (Cioffi 2005, p. 81).

- **Cultural sensitivity** can be achieved by nurses working with people as partners, offering choices in care. In Cioffi's study, one nurse said that when caring for culturally diverse people, 'If I am not sure, I just say to the patient "What is the right thing for me to do?", "Can I do this?" or "Would you mind if I do this?"'. Another nurse said, 'It's just finding out what they believe and what they don't believe in and then you can work it out from there with them and individualise their care'. Communication skills, respect and empathy are all very important for cultural sensitivity (see Chapter 2).

- **Cultural competence** requires the application of cultural awareness, knowledge and sensitivity to achieve effective healthcare, which addresses people's cultural beliefs, behaviour and needs. The culturally competent nurse also challenges prejudice, discrimination and inequality. Leishman (2006) highlighted the importance of mental health nurses developing cultural competence in an increasingly culturally diverse UK society. A concept analysis defined cultural competence as being 'the ability to provide effective, safe, and quality care to patients from different cultures and to consider the different aspects of their cultures in care provision' (Sharifi et al. 2019, p. 6).

In Cortis's (2000) UK study, Pakistani adults provided some examples of good healthcare experiences where staff were sensitive to their rights for privacy, provided for their need to pray and offered opportunities to maintain cultural practices in the hospital environment. However, nurses were generally perceived as seriously lacking cultural knowledge about this community; they lacked awareness of appropriate support systems, hygiene practices, the significance of Halal food and practices associated with caring and spiritual needs. One participant said, 'Nurses are not particularly interested to find out about our way of life. I feel that it is [the] nurses' duty to get to know some things about our customs or at least learn from us. This will be a great help to nurses as well, but they do not ask us anything either' (Cortis 2000, p. 114). This comment indicated the willingness of the participant to share cultural knowledge but their perception that nurses were not interested in learning.

In contrast to Cortis's (2000) study, Leever (2011) reports examples of nurses who took time to listen to individuals so that they could understand their perspectives and be able to adjust care delivery so that it was culturally comfortable and acceptable. Forssa et al. (2019) highlighted that student nurses emphasised the challenges of caring for people from different cultural backgrounds, and suggested that students instead needed caring curiosity and a strong cultural readiness to care for people from different cultural backgrounds, when entering their clinical placements.

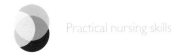

Box 1.7 Activity: cultural competence

Reflect on your own cultural competence at this stage. Jot down a few notes about your personal values and beliefs, your cultural knowledge and your skills that will aid you to demonstrate cultural sensitivity

Several models have been proposed for assessment with diverse groups (Higginbottom et al. 2011). Narayanasamy and Narayanasamy (2012) suggested using the 'ACCESS model' as a framework for responding to diversity in healthcare:

- **A**ssessment,
- **C**ommunication,
- **C**ultural negotiation and compromise,
- **E**stablishing respect and rapport,
- **S**ensitivity,
- **S**afety.

Assessment using the ACCESS model will provide a cultural awareness that is a deliberate, cognitive process in which health professionals appreciate and become sensitive to the values, beliefs, practices and problems of each individual person, as the basis for enhancing involvement in decision-making.

Papadopoulos' (2006b) textbook *Transcultural Health and Social Care: Development of Culturally Competent Practitioners* provides a comprehensive guide to this important dimension of practice and is recommended further reading.

DIGNITY AND PRACTICAL NURSING SKILLS

The NMC Code (2018c) requires registrants to: 'Treat people as individuals and uphold their dignity' (p. 6). However, dignity can be difficult to define, and people may have different interpretations of its meaning.

Box 1.8 Activity: dignity

Spend a few minutes reflecting on the following:

- What is dignity?
- How does it feel to have your dignity?
- How does it feel to lose your dignity?

Now ask someone else for their views and compare these with your own. The Royal College of Nursing (RCN) (2008) developed a working definition to guide nursing practice (Box 1.9). How does this definition compare with your ideas? Whether people are treated with dignity in healthcare affects perceptions of their whole experience and their satisfaction with care (Beach et al. 2005; Valentine et al. 2008).

Box 1.9 Definition of dignity

Dignity is concerned with how people feel, think and behave in relation to the worth or value of themselves and others. To treat someone with dignity is to treat them as being of worth, in a way that is respectful of them as valued individuals.

In care situations dignity may be promoted or diminished by: the physical environment; organisational culture; the attitudes and behaviour of nurses and others; and the way in which care activities are carried out. When dignity is present, people feel in control, valued, confident, comfortable and able to make decisions for themselves. When dignity is absent, people feel devalued, lacking control and comfort. They may lack confidence and be unable to make decisions for themselves. They may feel humiliated, embarrassed or ashamed.

Dignity applies equally to those who have capacity and to those who lack it. Everyone has equal worth as human beings and must be treated as if they are able to feel, think and behave in relation to their own worth or value. Dignity applies equally to those who have capacity and to those who lack it.

Source: Royal College of Nursing (RCN). 2008. *Defending Dignity: Challenges and Opportunities for Nurses*. London: RCN, p. 8. Reproduced with kind permission from the Royal College of Nursing.

Although government health policies have often focused on dignity of older people, studies have indicated that people across the life span are concerned about their dignity and can be vulnerable to a loss of dignity in healthcare (Matiti and Baillie 2011). A survey of the nursing workforce illuminated how three key areas affected dignity:

- **Place:** the physical environment and organisational culture
- **People:** the attitudes and behaviour of nurses and others
- **Processes:** care activities and how they are carried out (RCN 2008)

The RCN's (2008) survey highlighted many care activities during which people were vulnerable to a loss of dignity, but nurses described in detail the actions they took to prevent dignity being lost, which related to privacy, communication and physical actions (Table 1.2). When carrying out skills with people in practice, you need to ensure that your behaviour promotes their dignity. Chapter 2 focuses in detail on your communication, and how it can portray care and compassion. Other chapters highlight dignity in relation to specific skills.

In a study of UK nurses' strategies to promote dignity, Baillie and Gallagher (2011) found that treating people as valued individuals was the core factor. The nurses recognised the vulnerability of people to dignity loss in their specific care settings. The nurses were proactive in promoting dignity through enhancing privacy, improving communication with individuals and their families and building relationships, enhancing the care environment and addressing issues that mattered to individuals. From the perspective of care homes, having opportunities to be involved (as a human being, as a person one is and strives to be and as a member of society) was found to be crucial for residents' dignity (Høy et al. 2016). People who are nearing the end of their lives are also vulnerable, particularly in an acute hospital setting,

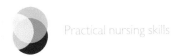

Table 1.2: How nurses protect dignity during care activities

Privacy	Communication	Physical care actions
Physical environment • Side rooms • Quiet/private room/area • Bathroom/toilet use • Curtains/blinds • Curtain clips/pegs/signs • Managing smells • Auditory privacy	**Interactions that make people feel comfortable** • Sensitivity • Empathy • Developing relationships • Non-verbal communication • Conversation • Reassurance • Professionalism • Family involvement	**Preparation** • Procedure • Environment • Timeliness • Equipment
Staff behaviour • Discretion • Prevent/manage interruptions • Sensitivity to culture/religion • Respect for personal space	**Interactions that make people feel in control** • Explanations and information giving • Choices and negotiation • Gaining consent	**Staff management** • Promoting independence • Physical comfort
Managing people in the environment • Staff: number present, gender • Other people • Family • Ward visitors/public	**Interactions that make people feel valued** • Giving time • Concern for people as individuals • Courteousness	
Bodily privacy • Covering body • Minimising time exposed • Privacy during undressing • Clothing		

Source: Royal College of Nursing (RCN) 2008. Defending Dignity: Challenges and Opportunities for Nurses. London: RCN, p. 8. Reproduced with kind permission from Royal College of Nursing.

and dignified and person-centred care is essential (Pringle et al. 2015). Chapter 15 explores the care of people at end of life in detail.

LEARNING PRACTICAL NURSING SKILLS

To make the most of opportunities to learn practical skills, it is helpful to think about how skills are learned.

Box 1.10 Activity: learning practical skills

Reflect back on a practical skill that you have learned, for example, learning to drive. How did you learn this skill?

ACTIVITY

You may recall that you built up the skill in step-by-step stages, learning each subskill one at a time. You could probably focus only on the skill and found that it was difficult to do anything else (e.g. have a conversation) at the same time. Benner (1984) identified that when learning any new skill, the performance is initially 'halting and rigid' (p. 37) and that one must pay careful attention to the explicit rules relating to the skill.

As a student, you are not expected to be an expert in your practical skills; expertise develops through substantial experience. Benner's research adapted a skill acquisition model by Dreyfus and Dreyfus to describe different levels of performance in nurses. She conducted paired interviews with beginners and experienced nurses and also used participant observation to study nurses with various levels of experience. The five stages of performance are as follows:

- **Stage 1 – Novice.** Novice nurses have no experience on which to draw; this lack of experience applies not only to new students but also to experienced nurses moving to an unfamiliar area of practice. Benner describes the novice as being 'rule-governed' in behaviour; that is, the novice needs explicit guidelines about what to do and in which sequence. However, these guidelines need to be adapted to the actual situation, and novice nurses need help and guidance to make these adaptions.
- **Stage 2 – Advanced beginner.** Advanced beginners can use previous experience and apply it in practice but continue to need adequate support, particularly with aspects that are situational, such as prioritising. They have difficulty seeing a situation as a whole and focus on the specific skill to be carried out, regardless of additional situational factors.
- **Stage 3 – Competent.** Competent nurses are able to carry out conscious and deliberate planning and prioritise and manage their work. However, they lack the flexibility and speed of proficient nurses.
- **Stage 4 – Proficient.** Proficient nurses perceive situations holistically, recognise important and less important elements and make decisions quickly. Benner found proficiency in nurses who have worked in an area for some time.
- **Stage 5 – Expert.** Expert nurses have a deep understanding and an intuitive grasp of situations, gained from substantial experience in the practice setting. You may observe this level in some practitioners with whom you work. In her book, Benner gives many examples of expert nurses' care for clients. Such nurses may be excellent and inspirational role models, but it is important not to feel inadequate or overawed by such expertise.

Developing the affective, cognitive and motor dimensions of a skill

The affective dimension

This book includes activities that focus on the affective dimension, asking you to think about, for example, how a person might feel in a particular care situation. Chapter 2 concentrates on the affective dimension of practical skills and will help you to understand the concept of self-awareness and how your values might affect how you carry out your care.

The cognitive dimension

Learning the cognitive elements of skills involves you acquiring and understanding the underpinning knowledge and rationale. Throughout this book, the evidence base for practical skills is discussed, but there are also activities encouraging you to draw on other sources of knowledge, such as undertaking further reading and reflecting on your experience. These activities will help you to develop an enquiring and problem-solving approach to your nursing practice.

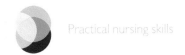

Practical nursing skills

The motor dimension

Learning the motor dimension of a psychomotor skill requires practice – the opportunity to try out and repeat performance. It is only with practice that movement becomes refined and a smooth, coordinated performance can develop. The amount of practice needed varies according to motivation to learn the skill, previous related skills learning, familiarity with equipment, level of anxiety, the physical resources and the learner's coordination (Oermann 1990). More complex skills need more practice. Motivation affects mastery as many skills are initially difficult, but highly motivated students will persevere. If you have had previous experience of a related skill, some of the skill's component parts will be familiar, so then your practice can focus on parts of the skill not already learned. Familiarity with equipment also eases the learning of a new skill. This book will help by explaining what type of equipment is used for the skills and includes illustrations of equipment. There is also advice about where you can access equipment with which to become familiar.

Support for learning skills

There are key points a facilitator can do to help when you are learning a new skill Box 1.11). You can be active about promoting these conditions. For example, the best time to ask a nurse to supervise you drawing up an injection for the first time is not in the middle of an emergency situation, as the stress and anxiety in the environment are unlikely to be conducive to learning. Thus, when asking to be supervised carrying out a skill, pick the right moment! Be open about your prior knowledge, saying explicitly that you have, for example, practised injection technique in the skills laboratory, have observed injection administration in practice and now feel ready to prepare and administer an injection under supervision. Supervisors should avoid the temptation to take over, but they will need to do so if safety is compromised. Learning practical skills requires the opportunity to practise and gain feedback (Quinn and Hughes 2007) to reinforce correct behaviour and eliminate error.

Box 1.11 How a facilitator can help a student learn a practical skill

- Provide an atmosphere conducive to learning.
- Carry out a skills analysis.
- Determine the procedure sequence.
- Assess the student's prior knowledge.
- Demonstrate the skill at normal speed.
- Teach the procedure sequence.
- Teach the skill by either whole learning or part learning.
- Allocate sufficient time to practise.
- Provide feedback on performance.
- Prompt student to self-evaluate.
- Encourage transfer of skills.

Source: Adapted from Quinn, F. and Hughes, S.J. 2007. *Quinn's Principles and Practice of Nurse Education*, 5th edn. Cheltenham: Nelson-Thornes.

The importance of obtaining feedback

Gaining feedback when you are developing skills is important for your learning. Staff supervising you can give you feedback; it is more helpful if the comments are specific rather than a general comment such as 'very good' or 'you need to be quicker'. It will help your supervisor if you identify any aspects for which you particularly want feedback. For example, you might say that when performing the skill last time, you were told that you need to give clearer explanations to the person, so ask that the supervisor gives you feedback on this specific aspect. The people you are caring for can give you feedback too. They may make spontaneous comments, such as that they feel 'much more comfortable now' or 'thank you for your kindness', but you can also seek feedback specifically, by asking how they feel at different stages. If you are approachable in the way you seek feedback, people are more likely to give honest responses. Your observation of people while you are carrying out practical skills will also give you feedback; for example, you can observe for facial expressions that might indicate fear or discomfort.

The sources of feedback outlined so far will provide *extrinsic* feedback. Combined with *intrinsic* feedback, you get a balanced view of your performance. Intrinsic feedback involves you reflecting on your performance and asking yourself about the strengths and weaknesses and how you could improve your performance next time.

Learning from experience and reflection

Carrying out practical nursing skills with different individuals in different circumstances provides rich opportunities for learning from practical experience. Developing your reflective skills will help you learn and develop your practice so that you optimise your learning. Dewey (1929), an educational theorist, argued that we do not 'learn by doing' but by 'doing and realizing what came of what we did' (p. 367). Dewey's theories were developed further by Kolb and Fry (1975) and then more fully by Kolb (1984). The theory of how we learn from experience is often referred to as *experiential learning* and is portrayed as a cycle. The process starts at the point of a concrete experience or event, after which observations and reflections occur, followed by abstract conceptualisation, where new ideas are developed, linked to other knowledge and experience, and then the new knowledge arising from the experience is tested out in a new situation. This new experience then starts the experiential learning cycle once again.

Reflection enables you to consider what you did and why, and it provides opportunities to develop knowledge from experience and link theory and practice. Knowledge gained from reflection on practice has been termed *practical knowledge* (Schön 1987), and reflection can help uncover the knowledge embedded in practice (Lawler 1991). Reflecting on your practice helps you to examine your experience and consider other explanations for what happened and alternative ways of doing things (Howartson-Jones 2010). Reflection may occur during the experience (reflection-in-action) or following the experience (reflection-on-action) (Schön 1991). There are various models and frameworks to provide a structure for reflection;

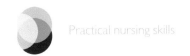

you will be introduced to these models during your studies, and you should pursue further reading from the many texts on reflective practice available.

To help you develop your reflective skills, you could write reflective accounts that you may include in your portfolio, recording significant events that you experience in your nursing practice. This activity can assist you in developing analytical skills and help you to learn from your experience, linking theory and practice. *Remember:* You must not identify people (either by name or by other identifying material) in your reflective writing, to maintain confidentiality. You may take part in reflective activities within the classroom setting where you will be encouraged to reflect on specific incidents from practice.

Skills laboratories and simulation

As students need opportunities to rehearse skills in a safe environment, most universities have simulation facilities: skills laboratories or centres where you can practise skills. In simulation, students learn in a realistic clinical environment where they practise a range of skills without the risk of harming anyone and then apply these skills in the clinical setting (Wilford and Doyle 2006). Learning in the skills laboratory can help to reduce anxiety about clinical placement experience and develop confidence. Skills laboratories provide a more controlled environment for familiarisation with skills than do practice settings. Practice in simulation also provides opportunities for reflection in and on practice.

Skills laboratories vary in complexity and resources, but they usually contain clinical equipment for practising technical procedures. Some skills, such as blood pressure measurement, can be practised safely on your peers, and there will be simulation models for practising other skills. Some skills laboratories organise volunteers for students' practice. Universities have different systems for learning in skills laboratories, which you should become familiar with. There may be compulsory sessions, optional workshops and formal or informal sessions. There may be a behaviour and dress code; for example, you may be expected to wear uniform and will certainly be expected to behave in a professional and considerate manner, maintaining safety at all times. Activities within the chapters of this book often suggest that you access equipment to practise with, if possible. You will need to find out about your local policies and procedures for use of equipment in the skills laboratory, and there may be a code of behaviour for users to ensure safety. Your placement provider or employing organisation may have simulation facilities for skills learning too.

Learning in the practice setting

Skills laboratory practice does not replace skills practice within clinical placements; practising skills with people in the healthcare environment is essential to develop competent, caring skills. You should take every opportunity to develop new skills, but not within a task-orientated framework that is dehumanising and objectifies people. Practical skills development and practice should take place as part of holistic care, within the total care required for each individual.

When starting a new clinical placement, you may well feel anxious or even fearful, but be reassured that you are not alone in these feelings. Starting a new practice placement has been likened to starting a new job! You will need to familiarise yourself with the environment and staff. Some practice settings send you information before your placement to help you feel welcome and reduce anxiety, and they may encourage a preplacement visit. Alternatively, this information may be available to you on the Intranet; do make sure you access it and make good use of this facility.

When students enter a new practice setting, they can sometimes feel overwhelmed by the range of learning opportunities. Placement areas often identify what specific learning opportunities are available, and these opportunities will include learning practical skills. Your practice assessment document will include the skills and competencies expected of you at each level, to meet the NMC's requirements. In each year, you will have a designated practice assessor, to verify you have met the standard of practice required, and supervisors, who will supervise your development on a day-to-day process. Your role should be an active role throughout the learning process.

Identifying your learning needs

When identifying your learning needs, you should take into account the following:

- Learning outcomes for your stage of the course
- Your prior learning, from previous practice placements, and any relevant experience before entering nursing education
- Any learning needs that were identified during any previous practice placements
- Specific learning opportunities identified by the current practice placement.

Your assessor and supervisors will discuss these learning needs with you and can advise of the learning opportunities in the practice area that can assist you, but you must be honest about your strengths and areas needing improvement. Your learning needs are likely to include practical skills, but they will address other needs too.

Addressing your learning needs

The 'Learning from experience and reflection' section provides ideas on how you can benefit the most from your clinical experience. You need to be active in seeking out your learning opportunities. Being aware of how to learn practical skills will help you to make the best use of opportunities available, ensuring that you observe a skill first, and ask for supervised practice until you feel confident to practise the skill independently. Although some skills need minimal practice, others are much more complex and need repeated practice. You should not attempt a skill unsupervised unless you are confident of your ability. You will be given feedback during practice placements to guide your learning. As mentioned, the practical skills you develop should be considered within the holistic care of people and not as isolated tasks that you have learned to perform.

You can be more proactive about learning in the practice setting if you are aware of different learning methods. There is much you can learn from observing others in the practice setting, but you need to distinguish between good professional role models

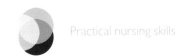

and poor models. In some practice settings, there may be formal teaching sessions organised. This approach might be particularly appropriate when there are several students in a placement area, and where workload is predictable so that a specific time can be set aside for teaching sessions. Formal teaching sessions enable you to prepare, by pre-reading for example. Informal teaching occurs more spontaneously, that is, on the spot. Such sessions can be particularly meaningful as they are likely to be linked with the clinical practice occurring at that time. Sometimes, a critical incident can be used as a basis for reflection in the practice setting. This incident might be a situation that has occurred, which was difficult or challenging, such as where a relative has raised a concern. Critical incident analysis can aid reflection and learning from such situations.

Here is an example of how you might use different learning methods in the practice setting. When taking part in medicine administration, you can actively observe a qualified nurse, either asking questions at the time (if appropriate) or making a note of questions for later or of specific medicines you want to find out about. The nurse you are with might ask you questions to check your understanding and encourage you to think about what is happening. You may be able to take part in practical elements such as dispensing of tablets or preparing a nebuliser. If a difficult situation occurs, for example, a person declines their tablets, you could use this incident to reflect on afterwards and develop knowledge from this experience. You could consider, for example, whether a different approach to the individual would have made any difference, or whether an adequate explanation about the tablets was given. You could also follow up later by looking up information about medicines that you encountered and were not familiar with.

RECOMMENDED READING

As stated, the remit of this book is to help you to develop your practical nursing skills. For guidance about reading material and for other aspects, you should refer to the recommended reading list for your course.

Many practical nursing skills require an underlying biological knowledge base. For example, when taking and recording blood pressure, you need to understand what blood pressure is and how it is maintained. However, a foundation in biology is not within the scope of this book, and you should gain your biological knowledge from the biology texts available, many of which are aimed specifically at student nurses. When working through each chapter of this book, it is sensible to have an understanding of the related biology, so each chapter includes biology questions. Use your recommended text to check your biological knowledge by finding out the answers to the questions posed. Studying the relevant biology and then working through the chapter can help to make the biology more comprehensible and memorable, as you can see its immediate relevance and applicability to nursing practice.

Your recommended reading list is likely to include ethics, sociology and psychology texts, all of which also provide underpinning knowledge for nursing skills, assisting you to care for people holistically.

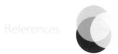

CHAPTER SUMMARY

All nurses must be competent in a range of practical nursing skills and apply these in practice in a compassionate manner. This book addresses skills that are generally applicable to nurses working with adults in a range of settings, and they address the annexes of skills identified in the NMC Standards (NMC 2018a, 2018b). Skills should be carried out within the context of a caring relationship and within the wider legal, professional and health policy context. Nurses need to develop cultural competence and must ensure that they promote people's dignity while carrying out care.

To develop competent, compassionate caring skills, you need practice and experience, which should include gaining feedback and reflection, thus maximising learning from experience. Through classroom preparation in a skills laboratory or equivalent setting, you can develop familiarity with equipment and the sequential steps of a skill, and the cognitive and affective domains can also be introduced. Carrying out practical skills in the dynamic and variable environment of practice settings is affected by many factors. You will need repeated practice to become competent and confident in practical skills, and you need to be proactive in seeking out opportunities for learning.

REFERENCES

Ahern, K. and McDonald, S. 2002. The beliefs of nurses who were involved in a whistle-blowing event. *Journal of Advanced Nursing* 38: 303–9.

Alzheimer's Disease International. 2016. *World Alzheimer Report 2016: Improving Healthcare for People Living with Dementia Coverage, Quality and Costs Now and in the Future*. London: Alzheimer's Disease International. Available from: https://www.alz.co.uk/research/WorldAlzheimerReport2016.pdf (Accessed on 5 June 2020).

Andersson, E.K., Willman, A., Sjöström-Strand, A. and Borglin, G. 2015. Registered nurses' descriptions of caring: A phenomenographic interview study. *BMC Nursing* 14: 16.

Baillie, L. 2017. An exploration of the 6Cs as a set of values for nursing practice. *British Journal of Nursing* 26(10): 558–63.

Baillie, L. and Gallagher, A. 2011. Respecting dignity in care in diverse care settings: Strategies of UK nurses. *International Journal of Nursing Practice* 17: 336–41.

Baillie, L. and Matiti, M. 2013. Dignity, equality and diversity: An exploration of how discriminatory behaviour of healthcare workers affects patient dignity. *Diversity and Equality in Health Care* 10: 5–12.

Baillie, L. and Thomas, N. 2020. Personal information documents for people with dementia: healthcare staff's perceptions and experiences. *Dementia: The International Journal of Social Research and Practice* 19(3): 574–89.

Beach, C., Sugarman, J., Johnson, R., et al. 2005. Do patients treated with dignity report higher satisfaction, adherence and receipt of preventive care. *The Annals of Family Medicine* 3: 331–8.

Benner, P. 1984. *From Novice to Expert*. Boston, MA: Addison-Wesley.

Benner, P. and Wrubel, J. 1989. *The Primacy of Caring*. Boston, MA: Addison-Wesley.

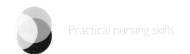

Bing-Jonsson, P.C., Bjørk, I.T., Hofoss, D., Kirkevold, M. and Foss, C. 2015. Competence in advanced older people nursing: Development of 'nursing older people—competence evaluation tool'. *International Journal of Older People Nursing* 10(1): 59–72.

Boddington, P. and Featherstone, K. 2018. The canary in the coal mine: Continence care for people with dementia in acute hospital wards as a crisis of dehumanization. *Bioethics* 32: 251–60.

Borhani, F., Hosseini, S.H. and Abbaszadeh, A. 2014. Commitment to care: A qualitative study of intensive care nurses' perspectives of end-of-life care in an Islamic context. *International Nursing Review* 61(1): 140–7.

Brooker, D. 2004. What is person-centred care in dementia? *Reviews in Clinical Gerontology* 13: 215–22.

Brooker, D. 2007. *Person Centred Dementia Care: Making Services Better.* London: Jessica Kingsley.

Care Quality Commission. 2020. *Out of Sight: Who Cares? A Review of Restraint, Seclusion and Segregation for Autistic People, and People with a Learning Disability and/or Mental Health Condition.* Available from: https://www.cqc.org.uk/sites/default/files/20201023_rssreview_report.pdf (Accessed on 27 October 2020).

Carers UK. 2019. *Facts about Careers: Policy Briefing August 2019.* Available from: https://www.carersuk.org/images/Facts_about_Carers_2019.pdf (Accessed on 28 October 2020).

Cheruiyot, J.C. and Brysiewicz, P. 2019. Patients' perceptions of caring and uncaring nursing encounters in inpatient rehabilitation settings. *Africa Journal of Nursing and Midwifery* 21(2): 18 pages.

Cioffi, J. 2005. Nurses' experiences of caring for culturally diverse patients in an acute care setting. *Contemporary Nurse* 20(1): 78–96.

Commission on Dignity in Care. 2012. *Delivering Dignity: Securing Dignity in Care for Older People in Hospitals and Care Homes.* Available from: https://www.nhsconfed.org/resources/2012/06/delivering-dignity-securing-dignity-in-care-for-older-people-in-hospitals-and-care (Accessed on 28 October 2020).

Corlett, J. and Twycross, A. 2006. Negotiation of parental roles within family-centred care: A review of the research. *Journal of Clinical Nursing* 15(10): 1308–16.

Cortis, J.D. 2000. Perceptions and experiences with nursing care: A study of Pakistani (Urdu) Communities in the United Kingdom. *Journal of Transcultural Nursing* 11: 111–18.

Cummings, J. and Bennett, V. for the Department of Health. 2012. *Compassion in Practice: Nursing, Midwifery and Care Staff: Our Vision and Strategy.* Available from: https://www.england.nhs.uk/wp-content/uploads/2012/12/compassion-in-practice.pdf (Accessed on 28 October 2020).

Department of Health (DH). 2001. *Valuing People: A New Strategy for Learning Disability for the 21st Century.* London: DH.

Department of Health (DH). 2007. *Good Practice in Learning Disability Nursing.* London: DH.

Department of Health (DH). 2009. *Valuing People Now: A New Three-Year Strategy for Learning Disabilities.* London: DH.

Department of Health (DH). 2011. *No Health without Mental Health: A Cross-Government Mental Health Outcomes Strategy for People of All Ages.* Gateway Reference 14679. London: DH.

Department of Health and Social Care. 2015. *The NHS Constitution for England.* Available from: https://www.gov.uk/government/publications/the-nhs-constitution-for-england/the-nhs-constitution-for-england (Accessed on 28 October 2020).

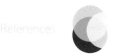

Department of Health, Social Services and Public Safety. 2011. *Quality 2020: A Ten Year Strategy to Protect and Improve Quality in Health and Social Care in Northern Ireland*. Available from: https://www.health-ni.gov.uk/sites/default/files/publications/dhssps/q2020-strategy.pdf (Accessed on 28 October 2020).

Dewey, J. 1929. *Experience and Nature*. New York: Grove Press.

Edvardsson, D., Fetherstonhaugh, D. and Nay, R. 2010. Promoting a continuation of self and normality: Person-centred care as described by people with dementia, their family members and aged care staff. *Journal of Clinical Nursing* 19: 2611–18.

Forssa, K.S., Perssona, K. and Borglin, G. 2019. Nursing students' experiences of caring for ethnically and culturally diverse patients. A scoping review. *Nurse Education in Practice* 37: 97–104.

Garside, J.R. and Nhemachena, J.Z.Z. 2013. A concept analysis of competence and its transition in nursing. *Nurse Education Today* 33(5): 541–5.

Great Britain. 1998. *Human Rights Act c. 42*. London: HMSO. Available from: http://www.legislation.gov.uk/ukpga/1998/42/contents (Accessed on 28 October 2020).

Great Britain. 2005. *Mental Capacity Act*. Available from: http://www.legislation.gov.uk/ukpga/2005/9/pdfs/ukpga_20050009_en.pdf (Accessed on 28 October 2020).

Great Britain. 2010. *The Equality Act*. Available from: http://www.legislation.gov.uk/ukpga/2010/15/contents (Accessed on 23 May 2020).

Health Service Ombudsman. 2011. *Care and Compassion? Report of the Health Service Ombudsman on Ten Investigations into NHS Care of Older People*. Available from: http://www.ombudsman.org.uk/care-and-compassion/home (Accessed on 28 October 2020).

Henderson, A., van Eps, M.A., Pearson, K., James, C., Henderson, P. and Osborne, Y. 2007. 'Caring for' behaviours that indicate to patients that nurses 'care about' them. *Journal of Advanced Nursing* 60(2): 146–53.

Higginbottom, G.M.A., Richter, M.S., Mogale, R.S., Ortiz, L., Young, S. and Mollel, O. 2011. Identification of nursing assessment models/tools validated in clinical practice for use with diverse ethno-cultural groups: An integrative review of the literature. *BMC Nursing* 10(16). doi:10.1186/1472-6955-10-16.

Howartson-Jones, L. 2010. *Reflective Practice in Nursing*. Exeter: Learning Matters.

Høy, B., Lillestø, B., Slettebø, A. Sæteren, B., Heggestad, A.K.T., Caspari, S., Aasgaard, T., Lohne, V., Rehnsfeldt, A., Råholm, M.-B., Lindwall, L. and Nåden, D. 2016. Maintaining dignity in vulnerability: A qualitative study of the residents' perspective on dignity in nursing homes. *International Journal of Nursing Studies* 60: 91–8.

Hudacek, S. 2008. Dimensions of caring: A qualitative analysis of nurses' stories. *Journal of Nursing Education* 47(3): 124–9.

Kitwood, T. 1997. *Dementia Reconsidered: The Person Comes First*. Buckingham: Open University Press.

Kolb, D.A. 1984. *Experiential Learning: Experience as the Source of Learning and Development*. London: Prentice Hall International.

Kolb, D.A. and Fry, R. 1975. Towards an applied theory of experiential learning. In: Cooper, C.L. (ed.) *Theories of Group Processes*. London: John Wiley, 33–57.

Lawler, J. 1991. *Behind the Screens: Nursing Somology and the Problem of the Body*. London: Churchill Livingstone.

Leever, M.G. 2011. Cultural competence: Reflections on patient autonomy and patient good. *Nursing Ethics* 18(4): 560–57.

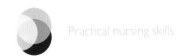
Leininger, M. 1981. Transcultural nursing: Its progress and its future. *Nursing and Health Care* 2: 365–71.

Leishman, J.L. 2006. Culturally sensitive mental health care: A module for 21st century education and practice. *International Journal of Psychiatric Nursing Research* 11(3): 1310–21.

Manley, K. 1997. Knowledge for nursing practice. In: Perry, A. and Jolley, M. (eds.) *Nursing: A Knowledge Base for Practice*, 2nd edn. London: Arnold, 301–33.

Matiti, M. and Baillie, L. (eds.) 2011. *Dignity in Healthcare: A Practical Approach for Nurses and Midwives*. London: Radcliffe Publishers.

McCance, T., Slater, P. and McCormack, B. 2008. Using the caring dimensions inventory as an indicator of person-centred Nursing. *Journal of Clinical Nursing* 18: 409–17.

McCormack, B. 2004. Person-centredness in gerontological nursing: An overview of the literature. *International Journal of Older People Nursing (in association with the Journal of Clinical Nursing)* 13: 31–8.

McCormack, B. and McCance, T. (eds.) 2016. *Person-Centred Practice in Nursing and Health Care: Theory and Practice*, 2nd edn. Chichester, UK: Wiley and Sons.

McManus, S., Meltzer, H., Brugha, T., Bebbington, P. and Jenkins, R. 2009. *Adult Psychiatric Morbidity in England, 2007: Results of a Household Survey*. Leeds: NHS Information Centre for Health and Social Care.

Mencap. 2012. *Death by Indifference: 74 Deaths and Counting: A Progress Report 5 Years On*. London: Mencap.

Mencap. 2016. *Health Vision Statement*. Available from: https://www.mencap.org.uk/sites/default/files/2019-09/2019.093%20Health%20vision%20vision%20statement.pdf (Accessed on 5 June 2020).

Mid Staffordshire NHS Foundation Trust Public Inquiry. 2013. *Report of the Mid Staffordshire NHS Foundation Trust Public Inquiry*. Available from: https://www.gov.uk/government/publications/report-of-the-mid-staffordshire-nhs-foundation-trust-public-inquiry (Accessed on 28 October 2020).

Nåden, D. and Eriksson, K. 2004. Understanding the importance of values and moral attitudes in nursing care and preserving human dignity. *Nursing Science Quarterly* 17(1): 86–91.

Narayanasamy, A. and Narayanasamy, G. 2012. Diversity in caring. In: McSherry, W., McSherry, R. and Watson, R. (eds.) *Care in Nursing: Principles, Values and Skills*. Oxford: Oxford University Press, 61–77.

National Institute for Health and Care Excellence (NICE). 2011. *Service User Experience in Adult Mental Health: Improving the Experience of Care for People Using Adult NHS Mental Health Services*. Clinical Guidelines 136. Available from: https://www.nice.org.uk/guidance/cg136 (Accessed on 28 October 2020).

National Institute for Health and Care Excellence (NICE). 2012. *Patient Experience in Adult NHS Services: Improving the Experience of Care for People Using Adult NHS Services*. Clinical Guidelines 138. Available from: https://www.nice.org.uk/guidance/cg138 (Accessed on 23 May, 28 October 2020).

National Institute for Health and Care Excellence (NICE). 2018. Care and support for people growing older with learning disabilities. *NICE guideline NG96*. Available from: https://www.nice.org.uk/guidance/ng96 (Accessed on 28 October 2020).

National Nursing Research Unit. 2008. *What Matters to Patients: The Nursing Contribution*. Policy + Issue 9. London: Kings College London. Available from: https://www.kcl.ac.uk/nmpc/research/nnru/policy/policy-plus-issues-by-theme/impactofnursingcare/policyissue13.pdf (Accessed on 28 October 2020).

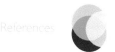

NHS England. 2016. *Leading Change, Adding Value. A Framework for Nursing, Midwifery and Care Staff.* Available from: https://www.england.nhs.uk/wp-content/uploads/2016/05/nursing-framework.pdf (Accessed on 28 October 2020).

NHS England and NHS Improvement. 2019. *The NHS Patient Safety Strategy: Safer Culture, Safer Systems, Safer Patients.* Available from: https://www.england.nhs.uk/wp-content/uploads/2020/08/190708_Patient_Safety_Strategy_for_website_v4.pdf (Accessed on 28 October 2020).

NHS Scotland. 2013. *Everyone Matters: 2020 Workforce Vision. Implementation Framework and Plan 2014–15.* Available from: https://www.gov.scot/publications/everyone-matters-2020-workforce-vision-implementation-framework-plan-2014-15/ (Accessed on 28 October 2020).

NHS Wales. 2016. *The Core Principles of NHS Wales.* Available from: https://www.wales.nhs.uk/nhswalesaboutus/thecoreprinciplesofnhswales (Accessed on 28 October 2020).

Norah Fry Research Centre. 2013. *The Confidential Inquiry into Premature Deaths of People with Learning Disabilities (CIPOLD).* Available from: http://www.bristol.ac.uk/media-library/sites/cipold/migrated/documents/fullfinalreport.pdf (Accessed on 28 October 2020).

Northern Ireland Assembly. 2016. *Mental Capacity Act (Northern Ireland).* Available from: http://www.legislation.gov.uk/nia/2016/18/contents/enacted (Accessed on 28 October 2020).

Nursing and Midwifery Council (NMC). 2018a. *Future Nurse: Standards of Proficiency for Registered Nurses.* London: NMC.

Nursing and Midwifery Council (NMC). 2018b. *Standards of Proficiency for Nursing Associates.* London: NMC.

Nursing and Midwifery Council (NMC). 2018c. *The Code: Professional Standards of Practice and Behaviour for Nurses, Midwives and Nursing Associates.* London: NMC.

Nursing and Midwifery Council (NMC). 2019 *Raising Concerns: Guidance for Nurses, Midwives and Nursing Associates.* Available from: https://www.nmc.org.uk/globalassets/blocks/media-block/raising-concerns-v2.pdf (Accessed on 28 October 2020).

Oermann, M.H. 1990. Psychomotor skill development. *Journal of Continuing Education in Nursing* 21: 202–4.

Papadopoulos, I. 2006a. The Papadopoulos, Tilki and Taylor model of developing cultural competence. In: Papadopoulos, I. (ed.) *Transcultural Health and Social Care: Development of Culturally Competent Practitioners.* Edinburgh: Churchill Livingstone, 7–24.

Papadopoulos, I. (ed.). 2006b. *Transcultural Health and Social Care: Development of Culturally Competent Practitioners.* Edinburgh: Churchill Livingstone.

Papadopoulos, I., Shea, S., Taylor, G., Pezzella, A. and Foley, L. 2016. Developing tools to promote culturally competent compassion, courage, and intercultural communication in healthcare. *Journal of Compassionate Healthcare* 3(2): 1–10.

Patients Association. 2011. *We've Been Listening, Have You Been Learning?* London: Patients Association.

Phillips, J., Cooper, K., Rosser, E., Scammell, J., Heaslip, V., White, S., Donaldson, I., Jack, E., Hemingway, A. and Harding, A. 2015. An exploration of the perceptions of caring held by students entering nursing programmes in the United Kingdom: A longitudinal qualitative study phase 1. *Nurse Education in Practice* 15: 403e408.

Prato, P., Lindley, L., Boyles, M., Robinson, L., Abley, C. 2019. Empowerment, environment and person-centred care: A qualitative study exploring the hospital experience for adults with cognitive impairment. *Dementia* 18(7–8): 2710–30.

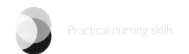

Prince, M., Knapp, M., Guerchet, M., McCrone, P., Prina, M., Comas-Herrera, A., Wittenberg, R. and Salimkumar, D. 2014. *Dementia UK: Update*. London: Alzheimer's Society. Available from: https://www.alzheimers.org.uk/download/downloads/id/2323/dementia_uk_update.pdf (Accessed on 28 October 2020).

Pringle, J., Johnston, B. and Buchanan, D. 2015. Dignity and patient-centred care for people with palliative care needs in the acute hospital setting: A systematic review. *Palliative Medicine* 29(8): 675–94.

Quinn, F. and Hughes, S.J. 2007. *Quinn's Principles and Practice of Nurse Education*, 5th edn. Cheltenham: Nelson-Thornes.

Reilly, J.C. and Houghton, C. 2019. The experiences and perceptions of care in acute settings for patients living with dementia: A qualitative evidence synthesis. *International Journal of Nursing Studies* 96: 82–90.

Roach, M.S. 2002. *Caring, the Human Mode of Being: A Blueprint for the Health Professions*, 2nd rev. edn. Ottawa, ON: Canadian Hospital Association Press.

Roper, N., Logan, W.W. and Tierney, A.J. 2000. *The Roper–Logan–Tierney Model of Nursing: Based on Activities of Living*. Edinburgh: Elsevier Health Sciences.

Ross, H., Tod, A.M. and Clarke, A. 2014. Understanding and achieving person-centred care: the nurse perspective. *Journal of Clinical Nursing* 24: 1223–33.

Royal College of Nursing (RCN). 2008. *Defending Dignity: Challenges and Opportunities for Nurses*. London. Available from: https://www.dignityincare.org.uk/_assets/RCN_Digntiy_at_the_heart_of_everything_we_do.pdf (Accessed on 28 October 2020).

Royal College of Nursing (RCN). 2017. *Dignity in Healthcare for People with Learning Disabilities*, 3rd edn. London: RCN.

Schön, D. 1987. *Educating the Reflective Practitioner*. San Francisco, CA: Jossey-Bass.

Schön, D. 1991. *The Reflective Practitioner*. Aldershot: Ashgate Publishing Ltd.

Scottish Parliament. 2000. *The Adults with Incapacity (Scotland) Act 2000*. Available from: http://www.legislation.gov.uk/asp/2000/4/contents (Accessed on 28 October 2020).

Sharifi, N., Adib-Hajbaghery, M. and Najafi, M. 2019. Cultural competence in nursing: A concept analysis. *International Journal of Nursing Studies* 99: 103386.

Shields, L., Pratt, J. and Hunter, J. 2006. Family centred care: A review of qualitative studies. *Journal of Clinical Nursing* 15: 1317–23.

Shields, L., Zhou, H., Pratt, J., Taylor, M., Hunter, J. and Pascoe, E. 2012. Family-centred care for hospitalised children aged 0–12 years. *Cochrane Database System Review* 17: 10.

Stanton, L.R. and Coetzee, R.H. 2004. Down's syndrome and dementia. *Advances in Psychiatric Treatment* 10: 50–8.

Turner, A., Eccles, F.J., Elvish, R., Simpson, J. and Keady, J. 2017. The experience of caring for patients with dementia within a general hospital setting: A meta-synthesis of the qualitative literature. *Aging and Mental Health* 21(1): 66–76.

Valentine, N., Darby, C. and Bonsel, G.J. 2008. Which aspects of quality of care are most important? Results from WHO's general population surveys of 'health system responsiveness' in 41 countries. *Social Science & Medicine* 66: 1939–50.

van Belle, E., Giesen, J., Conroy, T., van Mierlo, M., Vermeulen, H., Huisman-de Waal, G. and Heinen, M. 2020. Exploring person-centred fundamental nursing care in hospital wards: A multi-site ethnography. *Journal of Clinical Nursing* 29(11–12): 1933–44.

van der Cingel, M. 2011. Compassion in care: A qualitative study of older people with a chronic disease and nurses. *Nursing Ethics* 18(5): 672–85.

van der Cingel, M., Brandsma, L., van Dam, M., van Dorst, M., Verkaart, C. and van der Velde, C. 2016. Concepts of person-centred care: A framework analysis of five studies in daily care practices. *International Practice Development Journal* 6(2): 1–17.

Watson, J. 1979. *Nursing: The Philosophy and Science of Caring.* Boston, MA: Little Brown.

Wilford, A. and Doyle, T.J. 2006. Integrating simulation training into the nursing curriculum. *British Journal of Nursing* 15(11): 604–7.

USEFUL WEBSITES AND RESOURCES

Alzheimer's Society: http://www.alzheimers.org.uk/

Care Quality Commission: http://www.cqc.org.uk

Dignity in Care: http://www.dignityincare.org.uk

Dignity toolkit for care homes: http://dignitytoolkitsurrey.org/

Evidence Search: Health and Social Care: http://www.evidence.nhs.uk

Mencap: http://www.mencap.org.uk

National Institute for Health and Clinical Excellence: www.nice.org.uk

Nursing and Midwifery Council: www.nmc-uk.org

Resuscitation Council (UK): www.resus.org.uk

Royal College of Nursing: http://www.rcn.org.uk

Social Care Institute for Excellence: www.scie.org.uk.

MULTIPLE CHOICE QUESTIONS

1. The three dimensions of practical nursing skills are:
    a. Cognitive, functional, affective
    b. Cognitive, motor, affective
    c. Motor, affective, technical
    d. Cognitive, technical, motor

Answer: b

2. The Nursing and Midwifery Council Code's (NMC) 4Ps stand for:
    a. Plan care; Prioritise people; Promote safety; Preserve dignity and trust
    b. Prioritise people; Preserve dignity; Practise safely; Promote health
    c. Preserve safety; Practise professionally; Promote dignity; Prioritise people
    d. Prioritise people; Practise effectively; Preserve safety; Promote professionalism and trust

Answer: d

3. At any one time, what proportion of the population have a mental health problem?
    a. 1 in 3
    b. 1 in 4
    c. 1 in 5
    d. 1 in 6

Answer: d

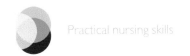
4. The 6Cs from the Department of Health comprise:
    a. Care, compassion, competence, communication, courage, and commitment
    b. Compassion, competence, care, cleanliness, courage, and commitment
    c. Care, communication, commitment, connection, courage, compassion
    d. Care, competence, compassion, confidence, calmness, courage

Answer: a

5. According to Benner (1984), what are the stages in developing a skilled performance:
    a. Beginner, Advanced beginner, Competent, Expert
    b. Novice, Competent, Proficient, Specialist, Expert
    c. Novice, Advanced beginner, Competent, Proficient, Expert
    d. Novice, Advanced Beginner, Competent, Specialist, Expert

Answer: c

6. What is the right order for the elements of Kolb's (1984) experiential cycle of learning:
    a. Reflection; experience or event; conceptualisation (developing new ideas); testing out new knowledge in a new situation
    b. Experience or event; reflection; conceptualisation (developing new ideas); testing out new knowledge in a new situation
    c. Experience or event; conceptualisation (developing new ideas); testing out new knowledge in a new situation; reflection
    d. Conceptualisation (developing new ideas); experience or event; testing out new knowledge in a new situation; reflection

Answer: a

QUESTION AND ANSWER

1. Name three Acts of Parliament relevant to carrying out practical nursing skills

Answer:

Any of these: Human Rights Act 1998, Mental Capacity Act 2005, or the Adults With Incapacity (Scotland) Act 2000, or the Mental Capacity Act (Northern Ireland) 2016

2. When carrying out mouthcare for a person, how would you demonstrate the cognitive, affective and motor aspects of the skill?

Answer:

Cognitive: know the evidence base for mouthcare and rationale; Affective: a caring approach to the person that makes them feel comfortable and upholds dignity; Motor: carry out mouthcare skilfully and safely

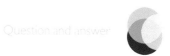

3. Identify four of the stated values for healthcare, for the UK nation in which you are based:

Answer:

- *England*: Working together for patients; Respect and dignity, Commitment to quality of care, Compassion, Improving lives, and Everyone counts; these values apply to all NHS staff;
- *Scotland*: Care and compassion; Dignity and respect; Quality and teamwork, openness, honesty and responsibility;
- *Wales*: We put patients and users of our services first; We seek to improve our care; We focus on well-being and prevention; We reflect on our experiences and learn; We work in partnership and as a team; We value all who work in the NHS;
- *Northern Ireland*: Empowerment, involvement, respect, partnership, learning, continuity, equity and equality.

4. People with learning disabilities have poorer physical health than the general population: True or False?

Answer:

True

5. What is the purpose of the 'This is me' tool, produced for people living with dementia, by Alzheimer's Society?

Answer:

The main purpose is as a communication tool so that carers, nursing staff and others will know more about the person and their preferences, thus supporting person-centred care

6. What are key aspects of person-centred care?

Answer:

Getting to know the person and understanding their individual needs and preferences

7. When might you use whistleblowing as a student nurse?

Answer:

To raise your concerns about poor practice you have witnessed with someone who can act

8. When caring for someone from a different culture from yourself, what could you do to develop cultural competence in your practice?

Answer:

Ask the person (or family) about how they would like their care delivered and really listen to their responses, so you understand their preferences. Avoid stereotyping and making assumptions.

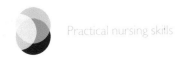

9. Write down a few key phrases to describe dignity.

Answer:

Check your notes against the RCN's (2008) definition: Dignity is concerned with how people feel, think and behave in relation to the worth or value of themselves and others. To treat someone with dignity is to treat them as being of worth, in a way that is respectful of them as valued individuals. When dignity is present, people feel in control, valued, confident, comfortable and able to make decisions for themselves.

10. Feedback is essential for learning practical nursing skills. How can you obtain feedback?

Answer:

Extrinsic (from supervisor and patient) and intrinsic (through reflection)

Communication: a person-centred approach

Nicola Neale and Joanne Sale

When we communicate with others, they are inevitably influenced by our behaviour and responses. Our actions and those of others do not happen in isolation; they are a reflection of the internal and external environment of all involved in the interaction. Any interaction is a two-way process; therefore, nurses must be aware that their approach to people in any setting affects the outcome. It is important that as professionals, we develop good relationships with individuals to collect information, assess behaviours and provide feedback to others including team members – so how we communicate is vital in these processes (McCorry and Mason 2019).

This book focuses on practical nursing skills, and in this chapter, we explore interactions between nurses and people while carrying out skills. The chapter addresses aspects of the Standards of Proficiency for registered nurses and nursing associates (Nursing and Midwifery Council [NMC] 2018a, 2018b), which outline expectations of nurse associates, nursing students and newly qualified nurses.

This chapter includes the following topics:

- Understanding what influences the nurse's approach to care
- The communication process
- Developing and maintaining therapeutic relationships
- Communication in challenging situations.

PRACTICE SCENARIOS

The following scenarios, taken from later chapters, are referred to in the text. Definitions of medical terms in these scenarios can be found in the chapters in which they appear or the glossary of terms at the end of the book.

Adult

William Newton, who likes to be called Bill, is a retired accountant aged 73. He is terminally ill with a history of oesophageal cancer and metastases in his lungs. He is cared for by his wife at home with the support of the community nurses and the Macmillan nurse. He is taking regular oral morphine for pain control. He has very low haemoglobin and has been admitted for a blood transfusion. He is weak and breathless, and his general condition is poor. He has a body mass index of 16. He can swallow only very small amounts of liquidised food and drink. He has some of his

DOI: 10.4324/9781003020660-2

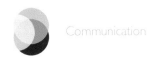

own teeth but also has a partial denture, which he likes to wear although it is now ill-fitting. His tongue appears coated, and his mouth is dry.

Learning disability

Maria is a 58-year-old woman with a moderate learning disability who has been living in a group home for the past five years. She has long-standing **diabetes mellitus** treated with insulin and has recently developed painful diabetic neuropathy. She has pain in both legs below the knees, which she finds particularly distressing when she is walking and during the night; her sleep is disturbed. She is in the care of both her general practitioner and the diabetic team at her local hospital. Maria's mother, who is 85 years old and recently widowed, visits weekly and is concerned about Maria's distress. Her community learning disability nurse would like to understand more about how he can support Maria, her mother and the group home staff on how to manage Maria's pain and increase her comfort.

Mental health

Natalie Turney is 21 years old. She has been admitted as a voluntary person to an acute mental health ward with severe depression. After going home for a day, she returns, appearing unsteady on her feet and she has a strong smell of alcohol. Her speech is very slurred, and she is quite uncommunicative. When the staff asks her if she has taken any tablets, she mentions some 'little yellow pills' and paracetamol. However, she does not give details about the quantity or when she took them.

Violet Davies, aged 76, has moderate Alzheimer's disease. She has been admitted to a care home for respite as her husband is physically and emotionally exhausted and needs a break. He has refused help in the past as he has been determined to look after his wife, but he has now agreed to take a holiday visiting friends. Violet is physically well, but she is also known to have osteoarthritis in her right hip. She looks permanently worried and is agitated; she keeps repeating the same phrase over and over. Mr Davies looks shaky and tearful at the thought of leaving his wife for a week.

UNDERSTANDING WHAT INFLUENCES THE NURSE'S APPROACH TO CARE

Box 2.1 Learning outcomes

By the end of this section, you will be able to:

1 explain the terms *self-awareness* and *self-concept* and apply them in a reflective manner within a caring context;
2 reflect on how personality may be important in nurse–client relationships;
3 discuss attitudes, values and beliefs and their impact in the care environment;
4 explain the terms *stereotyping* and *labelling* and discuss their significance to the care environment.

Learning outcome 1: Explain the terms self-awareness and self-concept and apply them in a reflective manner within a caring context

Self-awareness includes focusing on self and recognising, knowing and being accepting of self. It is a skill that nurses need to develop and comprises three components: how we think, how we feel and how we behave. There is a dynamic relationship between these components, and an awareness of self is essential to inform supportive therapeutic relationships. Stein-Parbury (2018) suggests that it is important to be aware of how these *cognitive*, *affective* and *behavioural* elements impact upon our approach to individuals. So, for example, you need to be aware of what you think about a client who has an alcohol problem and how this perception may affect your feelings and behaviour towards that client. Your behaviour will include verbal and non-verbal aspects, and these are the observable part of our interaction with others. How an individual has been discussed in a handover may influence whether you feel negatively or positively towards them. What you think about the person may be influenced by a personal experience and it is important to be aware that this may affect how we interact in the clinical situation.

Webb (2020) also suggests that self-awareness is an important part of developing effective communication and a skill that healthcare professionals need to develop to inform supportive therapeutic relationships. As such, our thoughts, feelings and emotions, and how we behave are generally considered to be important aspects to consider.

One way of developing self-awareness is to use a model such as the Johari window (Luft and Ingram 1955) (Figure 2.1), a model developed to help individuals identify aspects of self. This model suggests that self-disclosure and receiving feedback — that is, telling others about yourself and seeking feedback from them — help increase your awareness of self. Improved self-awareness will mean that the public area increases in relation to the other three areas as your understanding of your own strengths and weaknesses grows.

Consider how being self-aware might be important for you when carrying out practical skills. For example, if you have had an argument at home, you may understand why you feel impatient with a person who appears to lack motivation to assist with their hygiene needs. Acknowledging your emotional state will help you to understand your feelings and the subsequent effects on your caregiving. This increased awareness may highlight a need to adapt your behaviour and it is through

	You know	You do not know
Others know	Public area	Blind area
Others do not know	Hidden area	Unknown area

Figure 2.1: Johari window. (From Luft, J. and Ingram, H. 1955. *The Johari Window: A Graphic Model of Interpersonal Relations*. Los Angeles, CA: University of Los Angeles Press.)

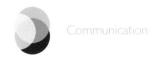

being self-aware that you may realise that you could be making a situation worse. Healthcare professionals should develop an understanding of how and why they behave in certain circumstances because, the crucial point about self-awareness is its impact on our communication with others, and how it can help us recognise the effects of our behaviour (Rasheed et al. 2019).

Nurses also need to be mindful that they may not be fully aware of aspects of their behaviour – this is called the 'unconscious bias'. This is important because as health professionals we may make decisions or communicate not fully appreciating the effects on another. For example, considering Maria, you may make a decision about her care based on your beliefs about someone who has a learning difficulty. This may have a detrimental impact on the developing relationship between you and Maria. Webb (2020) suggests that self-awareness helps professionals to understand those aspects of their own behaviour and attitudes that may hinder effective two-way communication (Rasheed 2015).

ACTIVITY

Box 2.2 Activity: assumptions

Think about some situations where you may have made assumptions regarding gender, sexuality, role, ethnicity, age or ability/disability.

You may have considered whether someone's culture affected your perception – do you treat someone from a different culture to yourself in a different way to others? You may have assumed that someone's partner was the opposite sex, then had to apologise when you realised your mistake. Or you may have assumed someone's religion based on their ethnicity.

One of the authors had an experience with her elderly father who was being admitted to hospital via ambulance. The admitting nurse did not seem to believe that a gentleman of 88 could have all his own teeth, to the extent that he asked his age, date of birth and to confirm that he had no caps, false teeth at least five times. Even a placid gentleman was driven to distraction by the nurse's fixed assumptions.

In Chapter 1, reflection was identified as being a conscious activity that usually involves a change in behaviour. Reflection, therefore, should help to increase awareness of how psychological, sociological, physical and contextual factors influence relationships with others.

ACTIVITY

Box 2.3 Activity: feelings and emotions, and how they affect relationships

Think about a recent situation where your behaviour might have had an impact upon the interaction. Recall your thoughts, feelings and emotions related to this incident and whether these affected your actions, choice of words or your relationship with others.

For example, you may have considered the following:

- If you were angry at the time, did you shout?
- Did you say things that you regretted? Did you storm off?
- If you were sad, did you cry? Were you too emotional to speak?
- Were you able to listen effectively or were you distracted?

Now consider how your behaviour might have influenced the situation, either positively or negatively:

- If you raised your voice, did the other person also raise their voice or did they withdraw and become quiet?
- Did they become angry, aggressive or cry?

It is helpful for nurses to reflect upon their own behaviour because it will *always* affect the response of others to a lesser or greater degree. A lack of self-awareness can lead to serious problems in professional relationships, and Eckroth-Bucher (2010) suggests that understanding another person begins with understanding self and this is emphasised in the proficiencies for nurses and nurse associates (NMC 2018a, 2018b). The qualities of emotional intelligence (EI), resilience and the ability to reflect on practice are highlighted in these proficiencies. Raghubir (2018) suggests that while there is still lack of clarity regarding the concept of EI, it is an important aspect of nursing because being sensitive to a person's mood and emotional state is integral to good nursing care. She suggests that it has the potential to influence not only care but also the professional in terms of their decision-making and well-being. Nicol and Hollowood (2019) outline aspects of EI to include self-awareness, empathy, motivation, self-regulation and social skills. For example, thinking about the scenarios, Natalie, may frustrate you by her reluctance to help herself by telling you what drugs she has taken. Your frustration may lead to your being short tempered with her. However, a good level of self-awareness/regulation along with EI and empathy would mean that you would be more likely to accept her decision and try to work effectively with her. This is more likely to lead to a positive relationship with Natalie.

Self-concept can be defined as the information and beliefs that individuals have about their own nature, qualities and behaviour (Rogers 1961). However, Gross and Kinnison (2014) suggest that it is a 'hypothetical construct' that each of us develops about ourselves: this construct is dynamic, never complete and helps us to understand not only who we are but also how we fit into society. Our sense of who we are is influenced and affected by how other people act towards us (Pearce 2011), and this supports Schaffer's (2004) suggestion that self-concept is *always* affected by how other people evaluate us.

It is generally accepted that there are three components to self-concept (Gross and Kinnison 2014): self-image, self-esteem and the ideal self.

Self-image

Self-image is the way in which we would describe ourselves, and this description may include social roles, physical characteristics and personality traits.

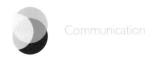

Self-esteem

Self-esteem is the extent to which we value and approve of ourselves and relates to how much we like ourselves.

Ideal self

The ideal self is the person we would like to be.

Box 2.4 Activity: comparing descriptions

Describe yourself, including your strengths and weaknesses. Spend five minutes writing down the aspects of yourself that you would like a stranger to know. Then ask one of your friends to describe you and compare as follows:

- Does their view match yours?
- Were there things that you did not know about yourself?
- What do any differences tell you about yourself?
- Were there any aspects about yourself that you would choose to keep hidden?

When you have analysed your responses, identify how these responses reflect the three components: self-image, self-esteem and ideal self. Now link this information back to the Johari window.

Self-image

Related to self-image, you may have thought about your social roles, physical characteristics and personality traits (Figure 2.2). In relation to your social roles, did you consider the different roles you have in your life: student, friend, nurse, parent, lover, partner, sibling and child? Did you consider your lifestyle and how it might affect choices you make? Did you consider whether your religious or spiritual beliefs and how your sexuality may affect your sense of who you are? For example, looking at the scenarios, Mr Davies may now consider one of his roles to be 'a carer' and he may perceive a change in his role as husband, lover or partner. You may also have included your physical characteristics, for example, your height, weight and skin colour. How you view your body is referred to as 'body image'.

Body image is the individual's interpretation of their bodily self, and it includes physical characteristics such as being tall, short, fat, thin, brown eyed or blond haired. Price (1990) identifies three aspects of body image:

- **Body ideal** is how we would like to look. This ideal may be guided by society's views and is a dynamic process that is influenced by social norms and cultural variations about what is considered desirable at any specific time.
- **Body presentation** is how we present ourselves, for example, our clothes, hair style and how we sit and walk. Social expectations may influence this presentation; you would probably choose different clothes to wear to a party than for a job interview. The NMC Code (2018c) suggests that nurses should be aware at all

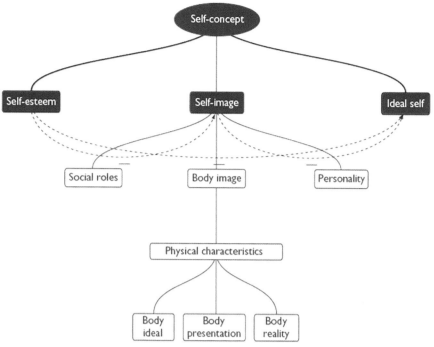

Figure 2.2: Pictorial representation of how self-concept links to other aspects of self.

times of how their behaviour affects and influences the behaviour of other people. Consider the effect of a nurse having dirty nails when about to give an injection; it is unlikely to demonstrate a professional manner and might affect the person's or a relative's confidence in the nurse.

- **Body reality** is the way we are, which may be very far from our body ideal; this reality might be thinner, taller, stronger or weaker than we really are. For example, Bill, as a result of his cancer, may have a completely different body reality having lost substantial weight in a short space of time.

During the earlier activity, you may also have considered aspects of your personality that you consider to be important in how you view yourself and your strengths and weaknesses. For example, do you see yourself as an outgoing person or a shy person? How might your personality characteristics be important in establishing and maintaining communication with your service user? We return to the concept of personality in more detail later in this chapter.

Self-esteem

Self-esteem is also one of the aspects of self-concept, and it can be viewed as a critical, personal evaluation of our own self-worth. It is an essential part of psychological well-being, and childhood and adolescence are especially important periods for the development of our self-esteem. This evaluation of ourselves can be general or specific for example, we might like ourselves generally but might not like a particular aspect, such as how tall we are, or our short temper. Society appears to value certain characteristics more highly than others and culture, gender, age and social

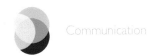
aspects influence the value attached to particular characteristics (Cribb and Haase 2016; Gross and Kinnison 2014). For example, people with healthy physical and psychological attributes are seen positively and as possessing qualities to be attained. However, some health conditions may be seen in more negative terms and these include physical disability, mental illness and certain physical illnesses such as human immunodeficiency virus (HIV) (Jackson-Best and Edwards 2018). If a disfigurement or disability is visible to others, there may be a particularly acute effect on body image and self-esteem; for example, an adolescent with acne or a child with a facial port-wine stain.

Some illnesses may be stigmatising as a result of the way that society views them. Stigma, originally from the Greek, stigmata, stands for a mark, scar or burn. It is now seen as being an attribute that is discrediting and reduces the person or taints them. So it is something that is shameful and may set people apart and can lead to discrimination (Goffman 1990). It is also thought to lead to marginalisation and low self-esteem in children, for example, Keane and Loades's (2017) systematic review suggests that young people with clinical depression and anxiety often have low self-esteem. Someone such as Natalie, who has mental health issues may be treated less favourably than others in society (WHO 2020). The Mental Health Foundation (2015) found that 'Nearly nine out of ten people with mental health problems say that stigma and discrimination have a negative effect on their lives'. This discrimination is not only unlawful and damaging but can potentially have a negative impact upon their view of self. Stigma can affect people at all ages, but for adolescents and young adults, like Natalie, these stages are a particularly important time of their development, and their social skills, identity and psychological well-being are vulnerable to negative attitudes (WHO 2020).

Ideal self

Ideal self relates to our desire to have certain qualities. However, this desire is not just about physical characteristics but also considers wider issues such as personality and relationships. We might want to change some aspects of ourselves, or we might wish we were a different person altogether, perhaps kinder or more intelligent. In relation to your nursing, you may yearn to feel more confident when starting a new placement, wish that you could remember people's names better, or perhaps wish you could perform more confidently when calculating medication for injection. Sometimes, through illness, people undergo changes in their ideal self; these changes may be sudden as in surgery or might progress slowly such as the changes that occur in rheumatoid arthritis. For example, Bill has lost weight and feelings related to this loss may contribute to how he responds and copes with his illness.

ACTIVITY

Box 2.5 Activity: perceptions of self

Consider the scenarios at the beginning of this chapter. How might Maria and Mrs Davies's perceptions of self be influenced by what they are experiencing?

Maria may have difficulty understanding what is happening to her due to her moderate learning disability. Her diagnosis, her increasing lack of mobility and pain could also affect her body image and contribute to a low self-esteem. Mrs Davies's Alzheimer's disease might affect her sense of self from any or all perspectives – physical, psychological and social. It is possible that she might have periods of insight into her loss of intellectual functioning and that she might be aware of other people's reactions and a change in their attitude and approach towards her.

Many people in different care settings have changes to their self-concept due to their illness experiences; therefore, it is vital that nurses are aware that their approach, while carrying out practical skills, can negatively or positively affect a person's self-image, self-esteem and potentially acceptance of their health conditions.

The concept of self is complex, and all of the above aspects are interrelated and dynamic. They are influenced by individual, family, society, culture and expectations throughout the life span. Self-esteem and self-image are connected, and as Rogers (1961) suggests, the greater the gap between your self-image and your ideal self, the lower your self-esteem, thus reiterating the importance for health professionals to have an awareness and understanding about how an illness may impact upon the sense of self.

Learning outcome 2: reflect on how personality may be important in nurse–client relationships

Personality is part of what makes people unique but at the same time allows people to be compared with each other. Personality is seen in psychological theories as being either a relatively stable component of the self or as varying depending on an individual's situation. There have been many approaches to the study of personality and how personality may be relevant within healthcare settings. Eysenck (1965) proposed one approach to explaining personality, identifying two principal dimensions: introversion–extroversion and neuroticism–stability. For example, an introverted nurse may find communicating with individuals or colleagues in groups more stressful than an extroverted nurse. However, on a one-to-one basis, introvert nurses might be comfortable in this situation and thus may be more effective in their communication.

The behaviour that you observe may give small, but important, insights into a person's personality; however, inappropriate interpretation of personality traits can be unhelpful as it may lead to the perception that the person is not responsive to change (Walker et al. 2012). For example, Natalie may be quiet and uncommunicative. What conclusions could you draw from this behaviour? You might decide that Natalie is introverted and shy, or that she is thoughtful and polite. These views might indicate to you something about her personality from your viewpoint, but how can you be assured as to the accuracy of these views? Although it is important to be cautious when judging personality traits, an awareness of personality can help nurses understand individuals and their illnesses and, therefore, may enhance the delivery of person-centred care.

Stein-Parbury (2018) cite Liaschenko and Fisher (1999) who highlight the importance of 'patient' and 'person' knowledge alongside case knowledge. This entails

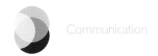
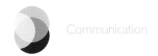

understanding not only physical and medical aspects but also how the individual responds to their illness and their unique characteristics and background. They argue that therapeutic relationships may vary depending upon the clinical context; however, nurses always need 'patient knowledge' in relation to how the person is responding to their health and healthcare.

Nichols (2003, 2005) suggests that patient-centred psychological care, of which communication is a key area, is often unsystematic and arbitrary, leading to unmet needs that can affect recovery, their concordance with interventions and their response to illness.

Concordance

A partnership process between people and healthcare professionals to agree on treatment (Chapter 10 discusses concordance further in relation to medicines).

Box 2.6 Activity: psychological care of people

ACTIVITY

When you are next on an adult medical or surgical ward, randomly choose one person on the ward and ask their named nurse 'who is handling this patient's psychological care and how is it going?' (Nichols 2005).

- Although Nichols was writing more than 15 years ago, he was still finding that the psychological care for adults in a hospital setting remained hit and miss leaving some people distressed and with unmet needs. These failings continue as seen in examples from both Winterbourne Vale (DH 2012a) and Mid Staffordshire Trust (Mid Staffordshire NHS Foundation Trust Inquiry 2010; Mid Staffordshire NHS Foundation Trust Public Inquiry 2013). Nichols (2005) suggests that unless hospitals and health centres 'develop psychological care as part of the thinking, culture and routines then this situation will continue to affect patients' responses and thus their recovery' (p. 26). The recent report about midwifery services at Shrewsbury and Telford Hospital NHS Trust found that the lack of kindness and compassion from some staff members caused great distress to parents, and bereavement support for those whose baby had died in some cases was severely lacking and, in some cases non-existent (Ockenden 2020). The NMC (2018d), when responding to the Gosport Independent Panel Report, highlights the importance of facilitating the care and treatment of individuals and families as many families felt not listened to when they raised concerns.

Learning outcome 3: discuss attitudes, values and beliefs and their impact on the care environment

The NMC (2018a, 2018b) recommends that nurses and nursing associates should provide and promote non-discriminatory, person-centred and sensitive care, while being able to understand other values, beliefs, preferences, diversity and needs to respond accordingly.

First, some definitions (Gross and Kinnison 2014):

* **Value** – the person's sense of desirability, worth or utility of obtaining some outcome.
* **Belief** – an opinion held about something: the information, knowledge or thoughts about a particular thing.

Our values and beliefs underpin our attitudes and affect how we behave with others. Attitudes have been described as feelings that give order and shape to our lives, but defining attitudes is difficult. For example, what is your opinion about smokers receiving healthcare? You may value life but believe in the right to freedom of choice; therefore, your attitude might be ambivalent.

Rosenberg and Hovland (1960, cited in Gross and Kinnison 2014) suggested that there are three components to attitudes:

* **Affective** – how we feel about a person, object or situation.
* **Cognitive** – our thoughts and perceptions about the person, object or situation.
* **Behavioural** – how we act towards the person, object or situation.

Box 2.7 Activity: dementia related to alcohol abuse

Consider the scenario concerning Mrs Davies. Would you feel any differently about her if you found out that her dementia was related to alcohol or drug abuse? Be as honest with yourself as possible.

You might feel less keen to care for Mrs Davies because you believe her condition to be her own fault, or you might even openly criticise her behaviour. The Royal College of Nursing (RCN) Review carried out by The Evidence Centre (2013) found that individuals' opinions often reflected on the nurse's attitude and/or their behaviour, with some nurses being heard to say uncomplimentary things about the person or families or appearing to see the person or families as an inconvenience. However, the NMC (2018c) states that nurses should treat people with kindness, respect and compassion.

Box 2.8 Activity: illnesses where lifestyle is responsible

Are there other illnesses where health professionals may decide that the individual or their lifestyle is responsible for the health problem?

While the authors do not want to stereotype in the examples they use below, it is however useful to consider our own beliefs therefore you may have thought of or encountered the following:

* A person who is HIV positive as a result of unsafe sex (in contrast to someone infected due to a contaminated blood transfusion).
* A person who has deliberately taken an overdose (in contrast to someone who has mistakenly taken an overdose).

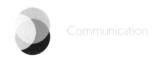

- A cocaine addict who is experiencing hallucinations (in contrast to someone who is experiencing hallucinations either because of their treatment or due to an infection).

These examples are linked to diagnosis. However, in reality, there are many subtle, social factors that influence our judgements in client-centred relationships (Johnson and Webb 1995, Price 2015). It is therefore important to be aware that values, beliefs and attitudes are central to how we behave, and to examine whether these affect the quality of our communication, how we care and our compassion for individuals and their circumstances. Pope (2012), citing McCormack and McCance's (2010) person-centred framework, suggests that amongst the prerequisites of the nurse are clarity of personal beliefs and values, and self-knowledge. These qualities are seen as a necessity for nurses and nursing associates who must 'avoid making assumptions and recognise diversity and individual choice' (NMC 2018c, p. 6).

Learning outcome 4: explain the terms stereotyping and labelling and discuss their significance to the care environment

Stereotyping is the belief that attributes of an individual are based on their membership of a particular group (Gross and Kinnison 2014). Stein-Parbury (2018), when discussing cultural stereotypes, suggests that if nurses rely on stereotypes, then they may miss aspects related to individual care and fail to identify specific care needs and this can be a barrier to effective communication (Arnold and Boggs 2020). **Labelling** is a form of stereotyping where we categorise people by, for example, aspects such as their behaviour or their age.

ACTIVITY

Box 2.9 Activity: are judgements being made?

When next in the practice setting, listen carefully to how nurses and other healthcare professionals speak about service user and their families. Are value judgements being made, and if so, do these judgements affect caring relationships? Are people labelled according to their diagnosis? If so, how?

What did you notice about the words used to describe the person being cared for and their behaviour? Examples that we have heard include 'difficult', 'attention-seeking', 'lovely', 'a pain in the neck', 'demanding' and 'bless him.' You might also have observed body language that reflects attitude: sighing, raising eyes to the ceiling and shrugging shoulders. What kind of labels may be used about the people in the scenarios from any of the chapters? Are you aware of any times where you have used labels that could have influenced other people's views and as a result the care given? Handover offers a powerful opportunity for nurses to state their own subjective beliefs in regard to those in their care. These may influence and reinforce other nurses' beliefs about or attitudes to the individual (Sarvestani et al. 2013).

The words nurses use in describing a family during shift report can affect how other nurses approach a family. Although the goal of shift report is to exchange objective data, value judgements and labels often accompany these data. These labels can limit the opportunity of families to learn the skills needed to manage the problems and meet their essential needs and decrease their involvement.

High-profile cases such as Winterbourne Vale (DH 2012a) and Mid Staffordshire (Mid Staffordshire NHS Foundation Trust Inquiry 2010; Mid Staffordshire NHS Foundation Trust Public Inquiry 2013) demonstrate the devastating effect upon individuals and their families when nurses lose sight of the core elements of their role. As recently as 2019, a BBC investigation into care at a specialist hospital for learning disability, autism and child and adolescent mental health issues, found that people were seen 'as a condition or a collection of negative behaviours' (Care Quality Commission [CQC], 2020). Although all nurses need knowledge to perform skills within the clinical setting, these skills must also be practised in a manner that continually demonstrates an awareness of the person and their needs at each stage of the care experience. The Evidence Centre (2013, p. 3) found that

the things most commented on were non-technical skills such as communication, bedside manner and information provision rather than clinical skills or patient safety or hygiene. In fact, the issue that people most commonly commented upon about was the nurses' overall manner such as being friendly and smiling versus appearing rude and brusque.

Compassion in practice (DH 2012b) was a response to the failings that have been highlighted and analysed in the earlier high-profile reports. As discussed in Chapter 1, the 6Cs identified should underpin the caring professions: care, compassion, communication, commitment, courage and competence. Two of the 6Cs defined in this report confirm the importance of effective communication and compassion as fundamental within the caring environment. The report Out of Sight – Who Cares? (CQC 2020), however, demonstrates that there is still a need for vigilance for those vulnerable clients who depend upon professional staff for their care needs.

As discussed, the judgements we make of others may affect the care that we give. Sometimes, we make these judgements as a result of personal bias, thus failing to see the individual as a unique human being and leading to prejudice in the care provided. The word *prejudice* means 'to prejudge', and it is a constant challenge in our interpersonal relationships to remain as non-judgemental as possible. Arnold and Boggs (2020) suggest that prejudices are stereotypes based upon strong emotions – we often have strong emotions around aspects of culture, illness and religion so when caring for people, we need a heightened awareness of how this may interfere with communication and therefore our care.

Gross and Kinnison (2014) suggest that prejudice – an extreme attitude – also has cognitive, affective and behavioural components. According to Pettigrew and Meertens (1995), direct or open prejudice is blatant and obvious, for example, an individual refusing to be looked after by a nurse who is a person of colour. Indirect

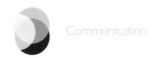

or closed prejudice is more subtle; for example, a nurse who does not approve of an individual who has acquired HIV through their choice of lifestyle might provide the minimum acceptable level of care and not talk to them or make eye contact. However, there is a debate as to the nature of prejudice with theorists suggesting that there are various dimensions that include determinants and the consequences (see Coenders et al. 2001; Pettigrew and Meertens 2001).

Box 2.10 Activity: direct and indirect prejudice

Consider the practice scenarios. How might both direct and indirect prejudice manifest itself?

If Maria is judged as a result of her learning disability, staff may not explain what they are doing or what is happening to her, assuming that she will not understand. However, Transforming Care for People with Learning Disabilities: Next Steps (NHS England et al. 2015) suggests that people with learning difficulties have rights about choice and rights to inclusion. Therefore, Maria should be included, and careful thought should be given to the use of appropriate communication skills to enable her to contribute to any decisions about her care. Mrs Davies may be avoided by staff if she is agitated, as they might consider her difficult, resulting in her physical needs not being met.

We make attempts at ordering the world around us in an effort to understand what is happening, but this can lead to erroneous perceptions that can affect care delivery. Our communication with people can reflect our underlying prejudices. At one time, labelling of people was considered fairly fixed in nature, so that once labelled, this label would remain. (Stockwell 1972). However, Johnson and Webb (1995) found that labels were more flexible and transient, changing with time and experience. When approaching individual care, you should be aware of your behaviour and if it is affected by any labels or stereotypical views.

Parson's seminal work (1951 cited in Price 2013) describing the sick role, suggested that individuals needed to conform to expected behaviours when in hospital, for example, accepting that healthcare staff know how to treat them and the need to cooperate with staff.

Box 2.11 Activity: expectations of people in hospital care

Do you feel that people in hospital care are expected to behave in certain ways?

Make a list of the positive and negative attributes that are assigned to individuals in, for example, handover. What factors may affect these?

Suggestions have been that those who have a shorter stay in hospital, people with multi-comorbidities and those who are acutely ill have an increased chance of being labelled negatively – and especially the elderly and those with dementia (Price 2013). He also describes how disadvantaged individuals may change their behaviour and expect less from healthcare interactions, for example, by not adhering to treatments. Baillie and Matiti (2013) suggest healthcare professionals can be influenced in labelling people, particularly the elderly who may be viewed less favourably as they can be seen as non-productive and potentially less valuable in society and less worthy of investment. Recent reports regarding attitudes to the most vulnerable to COVID-19 have questioned whether society puts less value on the elderly. Early in the pandemic, elderly care home residents were discharged from hospital without due care given to whether this was safe for them or other residents, and Oliver (2015) writes powerfully about professional and societal attitudes to the elderly and the language used around their care. For example, he reports that the elderly are described as 'bed-blockers', 'poor historians', or 'waiting for Geris' (geriatricians), and he suggests these terms undermine the individuals and the teams looking after them. The Panorama programme 'Behind Closed Doors' (2014) highlighted neglectful, indifferent and, in some cases, abusive behaviour in care homes that were supposed to be a place of safety for the vulnerable elderly (Oliver 2015). For example, even if Violet's constant repeating of the same phrase is annoying, it is the healthcare professional's responsibility to treat her with care, dignity and respect however frustrating they may find the situation.

Within an adult care setting, nurses need to be aware that individuals who have a mental illness or learning disability are vulnerable to disadvantage and exclusion (Mental Health & Joseph Rowntree Foundation 2016; While and Clark 2010). Nurses in any sector may care for people with learning disabilities or with a history of mental health problems; if nurses hold stereotypical or prejudiced views, such views could affect their approach to care and their interactions. These points are emphasised by NMC (2018a, 2018b) and, in summary, underline that nurses and nurse associates always need to promote person-centred care and act in a non-discriminatory manner. They should also ensure that personal judgements, prejudices, values, attitudes and beliefs do not compromise, even subtly, care provision.

Summary

- An understanding of self-concept and related aspects informs and enhances professional relationships.
- Developing self-awareness improves nurses' approach to individuals in their care.
- Personality and attitudes are influential in affecting relationships.
- Awareness of attitudes, prejudices and labelling – and responding to these appropriately – helps to reduce negative effects.

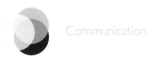

THE COMMUNICATION PROCESS

Box 2.12 Learning outcomes

By the end of this section, you will be able to:

1. explain appropriate verbal and non-verbal communication skills;
2. identify barriers to communication and reflect on how these barriers can be addressed;
3. discuss elements of effective written communication;
4. outline elements of appropriate telephone communication;
5. appreciate the importance of effective communication between members of the multi-disciplinary team (MDT).

Communication involves the successful transfer of a message and also the meaning of that message from one person or group to another (McCorry and Mason 2019).

Learning outcome 1: explain appropriate verbal and non-verbal communication skills

In everyday life, we constantly communicate, either verbally, or through the written word, or by our gestures or body language. Communication involves transmitting information and messages from one individual to another, but it is also one of the fundamental ways of demonstrating care and compassion. It is therefore important for nurses to have an understanding of the different aspects of communication to maximise positive effects within the nurse–patient relationship. Communication is essential for initiating, forming and maintaining relationships.

Box 2.13 Activity: ways to send a message

ACTIVITY

Write down as many different ways that you can think of to send a message.

You may have thought of speaking to someone either face to face individually or in a group. You may have considered the telephone, writing a note, sending a text message or an e-mail or participating in an online forum. Did you think of sign language too? In 2003, the United Kingdom (UK) Government Department of Work and Pensions recognised British Sign Language as a language in its own right (British Deaf Association 2021). However, their report highlights the many issues still faced by the deaf community for example, deaf people still do not have access to the same information and services that are available to the hearing population. Deaf people are forced to rely on inadequate disability discrimination legislation to access information in their own language (bda.org.uk/bslactnow/).

There are two aspects of interpersonal communication: *verbal* and *non-verbal*.

Box 2.14 Activity: 'verbal' and 'non-verbal' communication

ACTIVITY

List under the headings 'verbal' and 'non-verbal' as many aspects of communication you can think of.

The verbal aspects you may have thought of include tone of voice, pitch (or loudness), use of silence and pauses. These verbal components express our emotions and communicate information about our interpersonal attitudes. Sometimes, a person's speed of speech indicates their emotional state – someone who is depressed may speak in a slow, flat, monotone voice. Mrs Davies, who is increasingly agitated, keeps repeating the same phrase over and over again and her speech may become faster and louder. Sometimes, the way we use communication alters the meaning of the words used. For example, consider the different ways 'What do you want?' can be said. The way this is said may convey exasperation or compassion. Non-verbal aspects include proximity, posture, body movements, touch, eye contact, facial expression and gesture. Both verbal and non-verbal behaviour are culturally determined and interpretation of messages may be influenced by individual experience and background (Arnold and Boggs 2020). (See also Learning outcome 2.)

Several authors have developed models or frameworks of the communication process to portray the complexity of interpersonal interactions. Most authors now recognise that communication involves processes where there is continual receiving, responding and interacting and frameworks incorporate wider aspects in relation to communication. The framework in Figure 2.3 has been developed from reviewing several previous models published in the literature: steps in the communication process (Porritt 1984, adapted from Berlo 1960), a conceptual model of message transmission and reception (Minardi and Riley 1997), and a skill model of interpersonal communication (Hargie 2017).

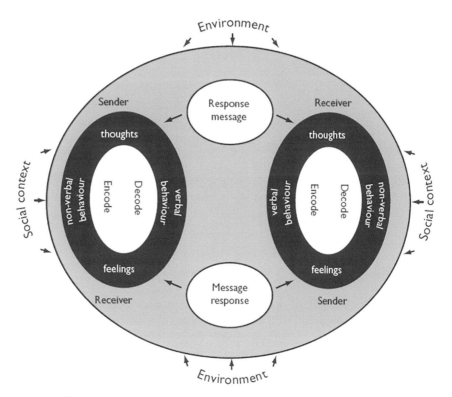

Figure 2.3: Framework for communication.

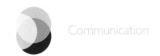
The framework in Figure 2.3 illustrates that the social context and environment encompass and influence all areas of the interaction process. It also shows that, at any given moment, the sender of a message is also the receiver of messages. Our thoughts, feelings and behaviour (verbal and non-verbal) influence our interpretation and, therefore, our response to the message and its perceived meaning. *Encoding* entails turning our thoughts and feelings into a recognisable message that is in many cases reflected in our responses. *Decoding* is about how we interpret a message we have received, to make sense of it. Therefore, we are continually receiving and sending messages in this dynamic process of interaction.

Listening is an essential part of the communication process, and there are many different definitions of listening emphasising the aural (hearing), oral (spoken) and environmental aspects. Stein-Parbury (2018) underlines the importance of recognising that listening is a complex, active process that requires concentration and effort to enable appropriate skills development.

REFLECTION POINT

Reflect on a recent occasion when you were speaking to a friend, a colleague or a client. What can you recall about the following?

* Verbal ways that you showed that you were listening
* Body positions: yours and theirs
* Eye contact
* Facial expressions
* Other non-verbal communication, for example, gestures
* Were their distractions in the environment?

What can you remember about the content of your discussion?

How we select, perceive and retain messages is influenced by our values and beliefs and by our cultural upbringing. How are these aspects relevant to your reflections in the activity above? Was it easier to remember what you discussed with your friend rather than a colleague? This exercise may demonstrate how important attention and memory are within the listening process, as well as context.

Egan (2010) uses the acronym SOLER to help us remember how to use our body position when listening:

* **Sit** squarely in relation to the client.
* Maintain an **Open** position.
* **Lean** slightly towards the client.
* Maintain reasonable **Eye** contact.
* **Relax**.

Did you identify these aspects of body language? You may also have reflected on the use of space, silence, touch and gestures, such as nodding in agreement or using facial expression to show interest or understanding. You or others may have used verbal signals to indicate that you were listening – for example, 'umm', 'aah', 'uh-huh', 'oh' or 'I see'. Sometimes, when we are supposed to be actively listening, we can slip into automatic pilot and are not really fully responsive to the message. Stein-Parbury (2018) suggests that there are many barriers to effective listening, both external and internal, such as our own thoughts, value judgements and feelings.

When we are with individuals, we need to demonstrate that we have heard and understood both the emotional and factual content of their message. This acknowledgement can be done by paraphrasing important statements that the person has said, allowing both individual and carer to seek clarification. We must also be alert to any non-verbal messages, as this information may reflect the person's feelings and help to achieve a true understanding of their needs. For example, Natalie may say that she is 'OK', but you determine from her non-verbal cues that she is anxious. A recognition of this discrepancy may be important in her therapeutic care.

To recognise incongruence between the verbal and non-verbal message, sensitive observational skills and an empathetic approach are required. Empathy can be described as being emotionally attuned to a person's perspective of a situation as well as its reality, or the ability to be sensitive to and communicate understanding of an individual's feelings or the ability to put yourself in another's position (Arnold and Boggs 2020). Cuff et al. (2016) reviewing the concept of empathy outline the cognitive and affective aspects and it is suggested that empathetic communication is essential to nursing practice (Grant and Goodman 2019). Being empathetic involves understanding and interpreting a person's meaning and situation in a compassionate manner. For example, recognising that Maria may be feeling embarrassed, upset or angry and then listening, clarifying and reflecting will all be important aspects of supporting her. Exploring Mr Davies's thoughts in relation to his carer's role would help you to understand and respond to his feelings in his situation and gain insight into what some writers call someone's 'inner life'.

Being empathetic requires the appropriate use of skills mentioned earlier – touch, eye contact and use of voice. Vocal features may encompass not only the words we use but also, just as importantly, the tone and manner. An example would be using a calm and soothing voice. It has been suggested that self-aware nurses are more likely to be empathetic (Moss 2020).

Learning outcome 2: identify barriers to communication and reflect on how these barriers can be addressed

The NMC (2018a, 2018b) stressed the importance of nurses acquiring effective communication skills, including verbal and non-verbal aspects and making any adjustments to enhance communication as necessary.

ACTIVITY

Box 2.15 Activity: factors that may act as barriers to communication

Identify factors that may act as barriers to your communication and relationships with the service user.

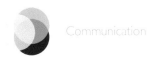

Barriers to communication can be physical, psychological or social, although the distinction between these types is not always clear-cut.

- **Physical barriers** could include visual, auditory or speech impairment, pain, or how the surrounding environment is organised (a desk between two participants, one person sitting and the other standing, or background noise).
- **Psychological barriers** may relate to personality (e.g. if someone is very shy), attitudes, beliefs and labelling (either the caregiver's or the client's), the emotional state of either party (e.g. anxiety), and cognition or thought processes, which may affect language, understanding or both. For example, Maria, who has a learning disability, might understand what is said to her, but she may be unable to express herself verbally.
- **Social barriers** may include social status, culture, religious and spiritual beliefs. Social status may affect how we interact with others due to our place in the hierarchy or the context of the relationship. Is there a difference in how you would communicate with a doctor or a healthcare assistant?

The influence of an individual's culture and their religious and spiritual beliefs are important factors that are often overlooked in nurse–client interactions. The NMC (2018c) requires that nurses be aware of cultural sensitivities (see Chapter 1 for an explanation on cultural competence). Napier et al. (2017) suggest that culture is a shared meaning based on beliefs, values, and lifestyles (and much more), that help us to make decisions and act. It informs our self-perception, our perception of others and our place in the world.

Vydelingum's (2000) study, which included Hindu, Sikh and Muslim service users, highlighted how communication difficulties led to people feeling isolated due to language barriers. For example, nurses did not provide sufficient information in relation to diagnosis or medication. Furthermore, language barriers may disadvantage the person because it is more difficult to develop a rapport, to obtain relevant clinical information and to emotionally engage. The person is also less able to convey their concerns and needs (McCorry and Mason 2019). Perceptions about causation of illness are also important because they affect how the person explains to themselves and others what is happening and why it is happening. For example, beliefs about possession by spirits have been demonstrated in some cultures; in Malaysia, 53% of those diagnosed with a mental health problem attributed the problem to supernatural agents such as witchcraft (Stefanovics et al. 2016). Therefore, an understanding of the individual's cultural background will help to ensure that their needs are fully addressed.

There are differences in the use of eye contact, gesture, proximity and touch that may affect communication. For example, looking directly into the other person's eyes can be considered disrespectful or a sign of honesty, depending on the culture. The unspoken conventions that accompany language in different cultures, such as politeness, degrees of directness, pace and the use of silence, may also cause misunderstandings. Arnold and Boggs (2020) suggest ways to facilitate communication with individuals from different ethnic groups and stresses using clear simple language and avoiding complexity – for example, keeping an even tone, maintaining a consistent speed of delivery and avoiding shouting. Frequent checks of understanding are also important and an awareness of differences in non-verbal aspects of communication.

Communication can be aided by using pictures, photos and mime, and these strategies may help to ascertain and enhance understanding. Translators and interpreters may be necessary, but where possible, professional interpreters should be used rather than untrained personnel or family members. Zendedel et al. (2015) found that different perspectives of the informal interpreter's role, the power dynamic and trust between parties could lead to miscommunication and even conflict. They propose that a better understanding of the role and appropriateness of the employment of informal interpreters is needed along with training for professional staff in how and when to use both informal and formal interpreters.

The year 2020 was a very difficult time for those who had impaired senses. People who had difficulty hearing and seeing were further disadvantaged in communication interactions due to social distancing and mask wearing. Being able to comfort a person by the use of appropriate instrumental touch has also been affected. Mitchell and Hill (2020) suggest a number of practices to overcome some of the difficulties of communicating while wearing a mask. The use of a clear mouth window in a mask will be especially important for those who lip read – which can include those who have hearing loss and some older people. Making sure you have the person's attention and giving consideration to vocal aspects of your speech as well as use of body language are all important aspects. Eliminating background noise and distraction and asking the person if there are any strategies that will enhance communication for them are also important to be aware of. People who are deaf and those with dementia are often skilled at reading facial expression and rely on this to help their understanding therefore we need to make particular efforts to be aware of verbal and non-verbal aspects of our interactions (Carter 2020). Carter also suggests making use of apps that turn speech into text as they can be helpful for some. If an individual uses sign language, learning some signs can help the person feel less isolated and to feel valued.

Box 2.16 Activity: reflecting on recent clinical experience

ACTIVITY

Looking at the section above, reflect on a recent clinical experience and list some of the factors that may have affected your ability to deliver culturally sensitive care and the effect upon the communication process.

You may have included whether

- individuals' food preferences were addressed (e.g. halal meat or vegetarian);
- provisions were made for particular religious beliefs or practices;
- the number of visitors was limited, making it difficult for extended families to visit;
- eye contact, personal space and touch were adjusted appropriately;
- adjustments were made in the interaction if an individual's English language skills were limited.

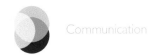

The above-mentioned points all highlight the importance of recognising a range of influences within the communication experience and the potential barriers to the supportive nurse–client relationship.

Learning outcome 3: discuss elements of effective written communication

Written communication is an important but often neglected area in nursing and is increasingly emphasised in relation to documentation and record-keeping and includes electronic record-keeping. The NMC (2018c, p. 11) states that nurses and nurse associates should 'keep clear and accurate records relevant to your practice.'

Good record-keeping helps to protect an individual's welfare by promoting high standards of continuity and clinical care and provides evidence of the care and treatments a person has received (Beach and Oates 2014). It also ensures effective and accurate communication and dissemination of information between healthcare team members. The Francis Report (2013 cited in Brooks 2021) found incomplete records that also lacked consistency and accuracy.

The NMC Code (2018c) outlines principles of good record-keeping. Some of these principles are considered below, with application to the scenarios. The individual's records should:

- be completed accurately and without any falsification, taking immediate and appropriate action if you become aware that someone has not kept to these requirements. Mrs Davies's behaviour should be documented in an unbiased and non-judgemental way. The RCN (2019a) suggests that jargon and speculation should be avoided.
- all records should be completed at the time or as soon as possible after an event, recording if the notes are written sometime after the event. When Bill, who is terminally ill, is at home, he will be cared for by various community and specialist nurses. Therefore, his care must be documented immediately and in sufficient detail so that the team can interpret easily.
- attribute any entries you make in any paper or electronic records to yourself, making sure they are clearly written, dated and timed, and do not include unnecessary abbreviations, jargon or speculation. If any changes have to be made, you must write your name and job title, and sign and date the original documentation. Think carefully about the words you use in any written reports and ensure everything is legible and others can understand easily – for example, recording aspects of Violet's needs to be in enough detail so that care staff have a clear picture of the best way to communicate with her and to help her anxiety.
- ensure that all steps have been taken to make sure that all records are kept securely, and collect, treat and store all data and research findings appropriately. This is especially important in the community where a number of people both lay and professional may have access.
- identify any risks or problems that have arisen and the steps taken to deal with them, so that colleagues who use the records have all the information they need.

For example, it will be important to ensure changes to Natalie's physical condition are clearly recorded and therefore improvements and deterioration recognised and acted upon.

RCN (2019a) also emphasises the importance of secure storage and to follow local and national policies with regard to destroying any records.

Carry out the activity below and see how confusing and potentially dangerous using abbreviations can be.

Box 2.17 Activity: abbreviations in healthcare settings

What do the following abbreviations mean: CF, CPA, PID, TPR, BP, OE, RXT, ABC, ETA, TTA, DNA, DOA, GCS? All of these abbreviations can be applicable in healthcare settings. Discuss them with a friend or colleague.

How many of these abbreviations did you know without further investigation? (see definitions at the end of this chapter). Were there any that could have more than one meaning? One example is that PID can mean either 'prolapsed intervertebral disc' or 'pelvic inflammatory disease'. Other examples are that BP could mean 'blood pressure' or 'bedpan' and DOA might mean 'dead on arrival' or 'date of admission'. You might think DNA is to do only with genetics, but it is often used to abbreviate the phrase 'did not attend (an appointment)'.

The context of the clinical environment may influence your interpretation of an abbreviation. Generally, although abbreviations are part of everyday life, there are few that are acceptable in healthcare practice, especially in written records.

When completing nursing records, nurses must have a comprehensive awareness of all the pertinent issues contained in the NMC proficiencies (2018a, 2018b) as these are professional standards for practice. Nurses who have a diagnosis of dyslexia may have particular need for support when completing written records and should be supported appropriately by colleagues and the organisation.

The Internet now plays a vital role in healthcare communications. Nurses should be aware of issues relating to the use of e-mail. For example:

- Be concise.
- Do not include confidential information unless appropriate encryption is used.
- Check spelling and grammar.
- Avoid abbreviations and acronyms.
- Reply quickly.

In relation to the last point, it is also important to remember the immediacy of e-mail messages and the possibility that a hurried, ill-thought-through response may be a source of regret in the future. Therefore, although responding in a timely manner is important, there is also the need to think carefully about any response. It may be more appropriate that some issues are dealt with either by a formal written response or by a telephone conversation.

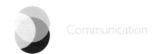

Terez Malka et al. (2015) suggest a formal set of evidence-based guidelines for the use of e-mail in a professional setting:

These include, for example:

- Ensuring you have proofread each e-mail for spelling, grammar and punctuation.
- Having a clear subject line relevant to the content.
- Avoiding capitals, unusual fonts and ensure a professional look.
- Checking that you are sending to the right person and do not reply to all unless necessary.
- Thinking carefully whether it may be better to speak in person if the e-mail contains sensitive information.
- Always ensure personal and confidential data are forwarded according to local and national data protection policies.

Grenon (2010) also includes specific guidelines for nurse–patient e-mail communication and the importance of consent. As face-to-face meetings may continue to be reduced due to airborne infections such as COVID-19, the use of e-mail may be increasingly important.

Most employers will have policy documents concerning information governance and data protection, and it is vital that nurses are aware of local as well as national requirements. Information governance (IG) involves how information or data is managed and shared appropriately and this also includes information about the person that may be collected digitally. It is important to understand how to treat information about people, and if and when you should share that information with others who are involved in that care. IG also relates to the use of data for other purposes such as research or evaluating the quality of care. In the UK, the main legislation related to IG is the EU General Data Protection Regulation (GDPR) (2018) and the UK Data Protection Act 2018. For nurses and nurse associates, the key aspects of IG are consent, confidentiality and information sharing (Beach and Oates 2014).

The NMC Code (2018c, p. 8) states that a nurse, midwife or nursing associate… 'owe a duty of confidentiality to all those who are receiving care. This includes making sure that they are informed about their care and that information about them is shared appropriately'. This also extends to after someone's death. Confidentiality applies to all communications whether oral, written or digital and team members should share information when it is essential for the person's safe, effective care (Health and Social Care Information Centre [HSCIC] 2013).

While consideration needs to be given to the mental capacity of everyone – it is particularly important for children and young people, someone with dementia or a mental health issue, and anyone where there are concerns regarding their understanding and ability to consent. This is discussed more fully in Learning outcome 4: Explain key features of gaining informed consent.

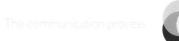

Learning outcome 4: outline elements of appropriate telephone communication

Box 2.18 Activity: making appointments

Reflect on the last time you telephoned someone to make an appointment or to clarify something. Did you know who you were speaking to? Did they give you the information you wanted? How did it feel if your needs were met or not met; for example, you ended up being directed to a message box or a queue?

Increasingly, telephones are an important mode of communication within healthcare settings; however, there is little guidance about using them appropriately. Organisations provide their own corporate guidance about telephone use; therefore, you must ensure that you are aware of local policy.

- **Answering the telephone.** It is important that you clearly state where you are and who you are.
- **Maintaining confidentiality.** It is essential that you ensure confidentiality. You need to know who you are talking to at the other end of the telephone. If someone asks about a client by name, you must ensure that the client is happy for information to be passed on. If possible, and the client has access to a telephone, they should be encouraged to make contact independently.
- **Acknowledging your level of competence.** For example, if you were asked to take down a message or a set of laboratory results and you did not understand what you were being told, you should explain to the caller that you need to get someone else to take the details.
- **Documenting and disseminating the information.** Make sure that messages are documented accurately and clearly and that they are promptly passed on to the relevant individuals. This dissemination includes passing messages to the person; knowing that others are thinking of them is good for their sense of belonging and self-esteem.

How we communicate with people we are caring for in 2020–21 has had to change significantly, and these changes include social distancing, the wearing of personal protective equipment and the increased use of telephone calls to families when people are in hospital. All these changes have impacted upon how nurses relate to those they are caring for. The Maguire Communication Skills Training Unit (Trueland 2020), however, suggests that the main principles in relation to compassionate communication are the same whether speaking face to face or over the telephone.

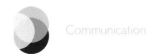

The RCN (2020a, 2020b) offers several guidelines for remote consultations that may have to be conducted for example by general practitioners, for out-patient appointments or by specialist nurses. These include clear introductions and considering any adjustments that may be needed. They also suggest making sure you are telephoning from a quiet private space and that any conversations will need to be documented clearly in line with professional guidance.

Social distancing has given further challenges to communication, and while these measures are constantly under review (and will hopefully become redundant), it has caused great distress to those in care environments and relatives unable to visit their loved ones either in hospital or in care homes. Based on the SPIKES model (see also Chapter 15 Managing care at the end of life), the Maguire Communication Skills Training Unit suggests the following principles:

* Elicit worries and ensure you acknowledge these
* If you are giving bad news – try to give a warning for example 'sadly' or 'unfortunately'
* Check the pace of delivery
* Ensure empathetic responses such as 'this must be hard for you to hear'
* Acknowledge emotion (Trueland 2020).

Lowe and Jones (2020) emphasise treating telephone and video communications similarly to face to face in terms of prearrangement and timing and ensuring a clear agenda

Learning outcome 5: appreciate the importance of effective communication between members of the MDT

Effective communication within the MDT is important in all areas of nursing, both in hospital and community settings, and it is essential for maintaining a high standard of care management. Afriyie (2020) suggests that communication with colleagues is one of the most important areas for ensuring that we are working in the persons' best interests – it is vital that health professionals coordinate and share verbal and written information so that communication with individuals about their care is clear and relevant. If you look back at the scenarios at the start of this chapter, you can see that nurses would need to communicate with a wide range of healthcare professionals. Some upcoming chapters explore the MDT and their work necessary for the effective care of these individuals.

ACTIVITY

Box 2.19 Activity: looking at Maria's scenario

Look at Maria's scenario. Identify members of the MDT between whom communication would be necessary to address her ongoing care needs. What form of communication would be used?

You might have identified that effective communication must occur between Maria, her mother, and the community and specialist health and social care staff including: the pain specialist nurse, group home staff, diabetes team, medical staff, pharmacist, social worker and community learning disability nurse. Other staff might be involved, too, depending on her assessed needs (e.g. dietician, chaplain, physiotherapist, occupational therapist, voluntary organisations). Communication will be verbal (including telephone) and written (including documentation, e-mail and fax).

In relation to skills, nurses must ensure that information is recorded accurately and communicated unambiguously and concisely to other team members, for example, communicating with medical staff about changes to observations that may require medication adjustment, or communicating with the physiotherapist to ensure analgesics are given if needed before exercise. The key principles relating to effective communication discussed in this chapter also apply to communication within the MDT.

Box 2.20 Children and young people: practice points for communication

Communicating with children and young people in any healthcare setting must take into account their cognitive ability and understanding. Communication is undertaken in partnership with parents/carers to ensure their needs are met and appropriately supported. Parents/carers are in the best position to understand their young child's communication. They may be anxious or frightened when their child is ill or injured, so appropriate communication will reduce this anxiety. Play is often used as a means to communicate effectively with children.

For a review of communication with children and families, see:

Lambert, V., Long, T. and Kelleher, D. (eds.). 2012. *Communication Skills for Children's Nurses*. Maidenhead Open University Press.

Summary

- Communication can be both verbal and non-verbal.
- Identifying barriers to communication and having an awareness of how these barriers might be overcome are important.
- Effective written communication skills are an essential component of nursing practice.
- Telephone communication is an important method of sharing information and must be conducted in a professional manner.
- Remote consultations should follow guidelines that encompass usual good practice.
- Effective communication within the MDT is essential for people's well-being and safety.

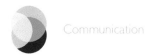

DEVELOPING AND MAINTAINING THERAPEUTIC RELATIONSHIPS

Box 2.21 Learning outcomes

By the end of this section, you will be able to:

1 Appreciate important aspects of initiating successful interactions.
2 Identify how to give clear explanations.
3 Demonstrate an awareness of a range of questioning styles.
4 Explain key features of gaining informed consent.
5 Reflect on the features of appropriate professional behaviour.

Learning outcome 1: appreciate important aspects of initiating successful interactions

Stein-Parbury (2018) suggests that the initial phase of a nurse–patient relationship is full of uncertainty and that there is a need to reduce this uncertainty. Therefore, gaining trust is essential and can be achieved through learning about each other. For nurses and nurse associates, this trust should be within the boundaries of the professional role (NMC 2018c).

Box 2.22 Activity: meeting people from the scenarios of the chapter

ACTIVITY

Imagine you are meeting people in different scenarios (refer to the beginning of the chapter). Write down how you think you would introduce yourself to each of them.

You might introduce yourself by giving your first name: for example, 'Hello, I'm Jane' or 'I'm Jane Smith', or perhaps 'Hello, I'm student nurse Smith'.

In 2011, Dr Kate Granger was diagnosed with a rare cancer – she noticed that nurses and doctors frequently did not introduce themselves. She felt that '…It's not just about an introduction. It's about being decent to another human being and ensuring the person is not 'lost' as he or she passes through the system.' The '# hellomynameis' is an initiative that she introduced, and it has been adopted by many trusts and care environments and is a reminder of the importance of introductions when meeting people in your care. (www.hellomynameis.org.uk/)

If you offer your first name, you may make it difficult for the service user not to give you their first name. Some people prefer to be called by their formal titles, for example, Mrs Davies rather than Violet. Usually, if the person wants you to call them by their first name, they will give you permission sometime in the relationship. Using a formal title is a sign of respect, whereas first names imply intimacy or familiarity. A recent study into the nature of healthcare communication with people who have dementia found that 'the phrasing, tone and question construction used by professionals could make refusal more or less likely' (National Institute for Health

Research, [NIHR] 2020). Think back to the first time you met the practitioner in charge of a recent placement – how did you address them? It is likely that you adopted a formal approach until told otherwise.

Here again, cultural aspects should be considered. For example, it would be disrespectful for a nurse to call a Sikh man by his first name or to ask him for his 'Christian' name. As highlighted earlier, cultural norms determine all aspects of the communication process including the verbal and non-verbal.

ACTIVITY

Box 2.23 Activity: Natalie's blood pressure

Imagine that you have been asked to measure Natalie's blood pressure. You are meeting her for the first time. How would you establish rapport?

Opening introductions often involve some small talk. You might, for example, see that Natalie is wearing a scarf of a local football team. You could comment, 'I see you are wearing City's colours, how do you think they're doing this season?' Any introductory conversation should focus on putting the client at ease, thus enabling assessment to be more accurate. Trust can be achieved only if the client experiences the nurse as consistent in approach, be it in attitude, behaviour or communication. Therefore, how we initiate interactions is important for developing therapeutic relationships.

Learning outcome 2: identify how to give clear explanations

Explanations are only effective if they are given clearly and help individuals to remember what has been said to them.

ACTIVITY

Box 2.24 Activity: Bill's blood transfusion

Imagine you are looking after Bill, and you need to explain to him about his blood transfusion. What principles should you remember when giving him an explanation?

- Did you think about identifying his *understanding* about his anaemia and the need for a transfusion?
- Did you think about the importance of the *language* you used?
- Did you think about the need to check his *understanding throughout?*
- Did you consider the *order* in which you would give information – for example, important aspects first?
- Did you acknowledge that you need to give *specific rather than general or vague* information?
- Did you consider the need to *emphasise certain information, repeating it* where necessary?

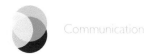

Box 2.25 Activity: explaining practical skills

Consider the principles highlighted above. How might you explain to any of the people in the scenarios what practical skill you are about to carry out?

You might have thought about how you would ensure Maria understands you when assessing her pain. You should use clear, short questions, and communication methods could include interpreting non-verbal cues, using pictures and signing. The nurse should work closely with Maria and her carers to explain things in an understandable manner. NHS England (2017) emphasised that people with learning disabilities and their families should be empowered and supported to be listened to and should be equal partners in their own care and treatment pathway. The onus is on staff to adapt and use different approaches to meet individuals' needs. When discussing Bill's pain management, you should check and recheck that he understands what you are saying, as his deteriorating condition may lead to confusion and an inability to concentrate. Having completed an explanation, you should check that the person understands the information accurately, therefore minimising any misunderstanding or mistakes (NMC 2018c). Swann (2021) highlights that the words people use to describe their pain may have a bearing on the care provided. For example, she suggests that words such as pain and discomfort are sometimes used interchangeably, which may be misleading, if we are enquiring about pain by asking if a person is 'comfortable'. There may be other environmental factors that are causing discomfort, and, therefore, appropriate comfort measures may not be implemented.

An important part of giving explanations relates to the *words* that we use. Thompson (2015) suggests language can reinforce social and cultural divisions and expectations. It can also reinforce power structures and we must be constantly aware of the potential for the way we use words with the people in our care to be oppressive rather than positive and therapeutic. Imagine that Bill needed to wear an incontinence pad and the nurse said, 'Let's put your nappy on'. How do you think he would feel even if this was said kindly? How would you feel if someone spoke to your father or grandfather in this way? Thompson (2015) suggests several ways we can avoid treating older people in a demeaning way – for example,

- Avoid patronising language – sweetie/ dearie/luvie/addressing older people by their first name without having checked this with them.
- Encourage participation in decisions that affect them.
- Value their experiences and recognise they still may have much to offer.

Corwin (2018) citing several authors and studies describes 'elderspeak' as including baby talk and includes aspects such as speaking slowly, an exaggerated tone, high pitch, using simple vocabulary and using we instead of you i.e., 'Shall we get up now'? instead of e.g., 'Would you like to get up now'? Corwin also highlights that elderspeak is detrimental to well-being, which is dependent upon interactions that are stimulating. Elderspeak is generally seen as patronising and lacking in respect and as professionals, we must treat all individuals and their families with respect and dignity. McLaughlin (2020) suggests elderspeak can be described as overadjusting communication without meeting needs and highlights some of the detrimental effects upon the person. These include lowering mood, feeling misunderstood, feeling undervalued and feeling incompetent and a burden. Think about how Violet and Bill may feel if just because of their age it is assumed they cannot understand and contribute to decisions about their care.

Learning outcome 3: demonstrate an awareness of a range of questioning styles

There are many different types of questions that may be utilised within the therapeutic relationship. It is important for nurses to be aware of how these questions may enhance (or detract from) the quality of information gathered, specifically within the assessment process in relation to ascertaining important and relevant aspects of the person's thoughts, feelings and attitudes to their situation.

Consider the following:

- **Closed questions** (e.g. 'Would you like a cup of tea?' 'Have you got pain?'). Closed questions can gain factual information, but they do not allow further exploration. They frequently require a yes/no answer and are helpful for gaining information from individuals who can only respond briefly (e.g. in acute breathlessness). Often, closed questions are used in initial individual assessments and lead to the second major type of question.
- **Open questions** (e.g. 'What symptoms have you experienced in the last week?' 'How would you describe your pain?'). Open questions allow a fuller response, enabling people to reply in their own manner. Sometimes, open questions precipitate a long and not necessarily relevant response, and a closed question can refocus the conversation. Thus, both closed and open questions are valuable when interviewing.
- **Probing questions** (e.g. 'You say that the pain is worse in the mornings. Tell me when else it is particularly bad?'). Probes or prompts can assist people in talking about their thoughts and feelings and express their concerns.
- **Leading questions** (e.g. 'You don't look as if you are in pain. Are you?'). Leading questions are best avoided as they can pressure people to respond in a particular way. However, nurses are often unaware of using them.
- **Affective questions.** Affective questions specifically address people's emotions and indicate concern. For example, if Natalie is quiet and uncommunicative, she could be asked how she feels about being in hospital. We need to have established a good rapport before asking this kind of question and should ensure that we can give time for responses. We should also know our own limitations in terms of helping responses.

Learning outcome 4: explain key features of gaining informed consent

Nurses must ensure that they gain consent before any care or treatment is given (NMC 2018c). The Code states that the nurse/nurse associate must 'make sure that you get properly informed consent and document it before carrying out any action'

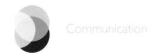

(NMC 2018c, p. 7). Seeking consent is a common courtesy, but people also have a legal and ethical right to determine what happens to them within healthcare settings, so consent, as stated above, is needed before any action is taken with the individual – for example, administering an injection or helping with personal hygiene. Informed consent is an ongoing agreement by a person to receive treatment, undergo procedures or participate in research, after risks, benefits and alternatives have been adequately explained to them. Key features of valid informed consent include being given:

- voluntarily and freely,
- without pressure or undue influence,
- by an appropriately informed person who has the capacity to consent to the intervention in question.

For example, if Mrs Davies were to be asked to consent to having an X-ray of her right hip, informed consent would include ensuring that she understands what an X-ray will show, why she needs it, what would happen when she goes for this X-ray, and the implications of not having the X-ray.

People have different information needs, and these needs should be discussed as early as possible. Some people would choose to have the minimum amount of information and prefer others to make choices. Other people will want to be involved throughout any decision-making process. Assessing and meeting individual information needs minimise undue anxiety and distress. Stein-Parbury (2018) suggests that acknowledging the individual's experience encourages further interaction. Explanations should be high quality and adjusted to meet their needs, and they should receive comprehensive information about all aspects of their care.

Acts of Parliament, the Mental Capacity Act (MCA) (Great Britain 2005) and the Mental Health Act (Great Britain 2007) have strengthened protection for those who lack the mental capacity to consent to the care or treatment they need. The MCA 2005 Code of Practice (Department of Constitutional Affairs [DCA] 2007) provides a detailed guide to the practical implementation of the MCA, including methods of communication and a recommended further reading list. One of the statutory principles of the MCA is that it is important to take all practical and appropriate steps to enable people to make decisions for themselves before deciding that an individual lacks capacity to make a particular decision (DCA 2007). A person's capacity (or lack of capacity) refers specifically to their capacity to make a particular decision at the time it needs to be made, and individual circumstances and needs must be taken into account. For example, someone with a learning disability, such as Maria, may need a different approach, to a person with dementia, such as Mrs Davies.

The DCA's Code of Practice (2007, pp. 29–30) suggests the following good practice in relation to helping someone to make a decision for themselves:

Providing relevant information

- Does the person have all the relevant information they need to make a particular decision?
- If they have a choice, have they been given information on all the alternatives?

Communicating in an appropriate way

- Could the information be explained or presented in a way that is easier for the person to understand (e.g. by using simple language or visual aids)?
- Have different methods of communication been explored if required, including non-verbal communication?
- Could anyone else help with communication (e.g. a family member, support worker, interpreter, speech and language therapist or advocate)?

Making the person feel at ease

- Are there particular times of day when the person's understanding is better?
- Are there particular locations where they may feel more at ease?
- Could the decision be put off to see whether the person can make the decision at a later time when circumstances are right for them?

Supporting the person

- Can anyone else help or support the person to make choices or express a view?

Care home staff should apply the above-mentioned suggestions in the care of Mrs Davies, enabling her to make her own decisions wherever possible; for example, use of pictures may help her to make choices and Mr Davies may be able to help her to express her views. If decisions are made on her behalf, they must be in her best interests and the least restrictive interventions should be used (Great Britain 2005). These interventions would need to be discussed within the MDT and involve her husband too.

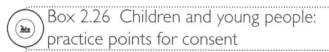

Box 2.26 Children and young people: practice points for consent

Children and young people have the right to be involved in decisions about their care and for their voices to be heard. Children and young people are able independently to consent for procedures or treatments if they are deemed competent; thus, have a cognitive understanding for the rationale, what is involved, outcome, etc. Informed consent must be achieved with the healthcare professional. Consent is usually undertaken in partnership with parents/carers, and if the child is under 18 years of age, a parent/carer who has parental responsibility may give consent, and this can override a child's refusal.

For further information regarding consent in children, see https://www.nhs.uk/conditions/consent-to-treatment/children/

General Medical Council. 2018. 0–18 Guidance for all doctors Manchester, General Medical Council. Available from https://www.gmc-uk.org/-/media/documents/0_18_years_english_0418pdf_48903188.pdf?la=en&hash=3092448DA3A5249B297C4C5EAEF1AD7549EEB5C7 (Accessed on 6 April 21).

Palmer, R. and Gillespie, G. 2014. Consent and capacity in children and young people. *Archives of Disease in Childhood – Education and Practice* 99(1): 2–7.

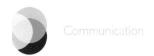

Learning outcome 5: reflect on the features of appropriate professional behaviour

The Code (NMC 2018c) assumes that nurses, in upholding the reputation of the profession, are in positions of trust, and to justify this trust, they must act with integrity and leadership. The Code further highlights some areas of particular concern:

- stay objective and have clear professional boundaries at all times with people in your care (including those who have been in your care in the past), their families and carers
- refuse all but the most trivial gifts, favours or hospitality as accepting them could be interpreted as an attempt to gain preferential treatment
- never ask for or accept loans from anyone in your care or anyone close to them
- act with honesty and integrity in any financial dealings you have with everyone you have a professional relationship with, including people in your care

Other relevant aspects to maintaining appropriate professional boundaries within therapeutic relationships include avoidance of

- being over-friendly;
- inappropriate self-disclosure;
- doing too much for a client at the expense of others;
- taking advantage of a client for one's own needs or gain;
- taking too much interest in the client beyond the confines of the supportive relationship.

ACTIVITY

Box 2.27 Activity: handling personal information

Reflect on the extent to which you would disclose personal information if you were caring for Natalie or Violet.
One of the members of care staff has a good working relationship with Natalie. Natalie asks for their mobile phone number – how might they respond?
Having looked after Violet and her husband for a while – to what extent might one of the care staff talk about their own situation looking after their own mother?

Most people in your care are vulnerable to some extent, including those with short episodes of illness and temporary dependence or individuals with severe and ongoing physical, emotional or cognitive impairments. In reference to the activity above – suppose you are the only person Natalie seems to communicate with, and, therefore, when she asks for your personal mobile number you may be tempted to give her this number. However, this would be an inappropriate response that compromises the professional relationship, potentially making her more dependent in the relationship. However, discussing your own situation with Violet's husband may be comforting to him if dealt with sensitively and empathetically – it may help him to feel less alone.

Summary
- Establishing the initial rapport is an important stage in developing trusting nurse–patient/client relationships.
- Clear explanations are essential to ensure understanding.
- There are different types of question that should be used appropriately for effective interactions.
- Informed consent must be gained. Where the person lacks the mental capacity for consent, what must be conducted in their best interests?
- It is vital to behave in an appropriate professional manner at all times, in accordance with the NMC's Code (2018c).

COMMUNICATION IN CHALLENGING SITUATIONS

Box 2.28 Learning outcomes

By the end of this section, you will be able to:

1. appreciate how anxiety is experienced and managed;
2. discuss how depression is recognised and managed;
3. reflect on how to recognise and manage anger;
4. appreciate ways of communicating with people who are confused;
5. consider communication in relation to sensitive issues, such as sexuality;
6. discuss how to communicate with and support people who are in distress.

The Code (NMC 2018c, p. 1) states that the nurse must '…provide a high standard of care at all times'. This standard would include showing sensitivity and compassion at all times, even in difficult and challenging situations.

Learning outcome 1: appreciate how anxiety is experienced and managed

Anxiety is one of our basic emotions and can range from mild to very severe, serving as a warning and helping us to cope with threatening situations. However, if anxiety is excessive and left untreated, it may be detrimental and interfere with a person's normal day-to-day life and interactions. Excessive anxiety can cause suffering and disability and can be costly at both an individual and societal level. Someone who has unresolved anxiety may have difficulty sustaining relationships, maintaining employment or both. This anxiety could lead to a loss of confidence, loss of role, loss of job/earnings and in the extreme perhaps loss of housing. The National Institute of Health and Clinical Excellence (NICE 2014) asserts that anxiety disorders are a common mental health issue that may present in any care settings.

If you think about the scenarios, Maria may be anxious because she may not understand what is happening or she may be a naturally anxious person. She may be lonely and have more time to worry about what is happening to her.

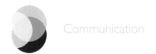
Box 2.29 Activity: Bill's anxiety

- What are the cues that may lead you to think a person is anxious?
- What aspects of Bill's situation may give rise to anxiety?

In answer to the first question, you might have considered facial expression, restlessness, wringing hands and profuse sweating, indicators that an individual is anxious due to a feeling of impending doom. The resulting fear, which can be intense, may also cause some or all of the following: dry mouth, racing heart, butterflies in the stomach, shortness of breath, having to go to the toilet repeatedly, irregular heartbeats (palpitations), cognitive impairment including poor concentration, impatience, irritability, painful or missed periods and difficulty in falling or staying asleep (see NHS Choices: https://www.nhs.uk/mental-health/conditions/generalised-anxiety-disorder/symptoms/).

Anxiety about illness and implications for the future are often linked to fearfulness, uncertainty or both. Bill could have fears for the future and uncertainty about his situation, causing anxiety; for example, how he will cope in a hospital setting as opposed to the home environment. He may also be anxious about whether he will continue to be given his pain medication when he needs it, as he may no longer perceive himself to be in control of when he is able to take this medication.

Other factors that may cause healthcare recipients anxiety include:

- awaiting a life-threatening or life-changing diagnosis;
- fear of an operative procedure;
- fear about treatments;
- fear about the short- and long-term effects of treatments;
- fear of the unknown environment, leading to feelings of vulnerability and insecurity;
- fear of being treated in an uncaring manner.

The pandemic of 2020 has led to increased levels of anxiety, according to the Office for National Statistics (2020) up to 17% of the population are likely to experience some form of anxiety. Issues such as the impact on health and well-being, a lack of independence and freedom, an inability to make plans, the impact on relationships and work have all been seen to have a negative impact on people.

Any or all of the above-mentioned factors may be relevant to individuals, so we should make no assumptions about what may be causing their anxiety. Careful assessment, including observation and information gathering, and the development of trusting relationships can enable nurses to accurately identify causes of anxiety.

Anxiety management techniques include:

- explanation of the process of anxiety and the symptoms experienced;
- breathing control;
- relaxation therapy;

- challenging of cognition (thoughts);
- mindfulness;
- assertiveness training.

Nichols (2003) suggests that effective communication and information-giving skills can reduce anxiety, fear and uncertainty, enabling service user to work in partnership and follow treatment in a more relaxed manner, while positively contributing to recovery. NICE (2021) provides a detailed evidence-based approach to anxiety disorders (see www.nice.org.uk/guidance/conditions-and-diseases/mental-health-and-behavioural-conditions/anxiety/products?ProductType=Pathways).

Learning outcome 2: discuss how depression is recognised and managed

Depression is a common mental disorder characterised by sadness, loss of interest in activities and decreased energy. It is differentiated from normal mood changes by the extent of its severity, the symptoms and the duration of the disorder. It is estimated that 264 million people worldwide experience depression (WHO 2020). According to NICE (2020), 'depression is two to three times more common in people with a chronic physical health problem; for these people, functional impairment is likely to be greater than if a person has depression or the physical health problem alone'. NICE (2019) suggests that in the year 2017–18, over 4.5 million adults had a diagnosis of depression. This is around 10% of all adults registered with a GP, up from around 6% in 2012–13.

A depressed mood is common when a person has a life-threatening illness and is often a stage of adjustment to their illness, and it is estimated that 5–20% of people who are terminally ill can suffer from some degree of depression (Twycross and Wilcock 2018). Depression is the leading cause of disability and premature death for 18–44 year olds (NICE 2021). The impact of this depression may be that having both physical and mental health problems can delay recovery from both. In fact, depression may also have a negative impact on life expectancy (NICE 2009b). During the pandemic, the Office for National Statistics (2020) found that 19% of the population experienced moderate to severe symptoms of depression with similar triggers to those that caused anxiety such as well-being being affected and a lack of freedom and independence.

Depression is difficult to diagnose and can be unrecognised in acute hospital care settings; therefore, it is important to differentiate between someone who is sad, perhaps due to receiving unwelcome news about their prognosis, and someone who is in need of clinical support for depression. NICE guidelines (2009a, 2009b) for managing depression detail the assessment of depression and recommend a stepped care approach. Nurses need to be able to assess individuals accurately to recognise these differences and to ensure appropriate referral for those in need of specialist support (NICE 2009b). Nurses have an important role in identifying depression, and their communication skills can help with the effective assessment and screening of vulnerable people. Assessment can highlight those at risk – for example, those

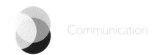

who have a past history of brain pathology, those who have not maintained good relationships with healthcare professionals in the past, or service users who have poor social support. It is recognised that many people with functional illnesses are at high risk of developing depression (NICE 2009a).

Depression has various physical and psychological symptoms, but they may not be identified in the clinical setting for various reasons, including the knowledge and attitudes of healthcare staff or resource and time issues. People may also not complain of depression, or depression may manifest itself in other symptoms–for example, pain that is difficult to control. Nurses are best placed in recognising the physical and psychological changes that may indicate a client is in need of support.

ACTIVITY

Box 2.30 Activity: symptoms of depression

What might indicate to you that a person is depressed? List features that you are aware of. Then, read about symptoms of depression on Mind's website at https://www.mind.org.uk/information-support/types-of-mental-health-problems/depression/about-depression/

Have you seen any assessment tools used in practice to help assess depression?

As detailed on Mind's website, there are many signs and symptoms of depression. People who are depressed may also be anxious, and it is not always clear whether anxiety leads to depression or whether depression causes anxiety. Various assessment tools are used in healthcare settings to assess depression and anxiety – for example, the Hospital Anxiety and Depression Scale (Zigmund and Snaith 1983) and Beck's Depression Inventory (Beck et al. 1961) – so you may have seen these assessments or similar tools. See Chapter 3 that focuses on the assessment of mental health needs.

NICE (2009a) advises that treatment and care should:

- take into account a person's needs;
- take into account a person's preferences;
- provide the opportunity to make informed decisions;
- include the opportunity to make advance decisions and statements;
- be culturally appropriate;
- be accessible to people with additional needs, such as physical, sensory or learning disabilities;
- be accessible to people who do not speak or read English;
- be supported by evidence-based written information tailored to the individual's needs.

The healthcare team should be fully aware of all the above principles, and good communication skills will be essential throughout the person's care experience. It is important to recognise 'normal' responses to adverse events/life-threatening illnesses, as opposed to responses that indicate a person needs further psychological assessment and support.

Learning outcome 3: reflect on how to recognise and manage anger

Anger is a natural response to feeling frustrated, attacked, injured or violated. It is part of being human; it is not necessarily a bad emotion as it can be positive and can even motivate us and help with our focus (MIND 2021). Nurses are sometimes confronted with people who are displaying strong emotions, such as anger and aggression. It is important to use good interpersonal skills at these times to minimise the psychological impact of the emotions. People who are in hospital can become angry for many reasons, and this anger is often related to a loss of control over their circumstances and may be a reaction to the uncertainty around their situation. Anger from both individual's and their relatives is also associated with a lack of effective therapeutic communication. It is important to recognise when a person is becoming angry and to be able to manage this anger is an effective way.

Box 2.31 Activity: dealing with anger

Think back to the last time you were with anyone who was angry. How did you recognise that the person was becoming angry? What can you remember about how you felt and your responses?

Examples that you might remember may include both verbal and non-verbal aspects related to anger. Verbal indications include a raised voice, tense tone, fast speech or using obscenities. Non-verbal indications include changes in body language: the person may display exaggerated movements, clenched fists, pace back and forth or throw or kick objects. There may be changes in facial expression, for example, frowning, and eye contact may be negligible, or it might be extended – glaring. These expressions are just some indications that an individual is becoming angry. In terms of your own reaction, did you feel angry, did you feel that you were able to remain calm? Did the way you respond influence the situation positively or negatively?

A nurse who has recognised these signs should act to disperse the anger by the following means:

- Maintaining a calm, respectful demeanour (McCorry and Mason 2019).
- Listening actively to what the person has to say, thus showing a non-judgemental stance.
- Being aware that prolonged eye contact may be seen as threatening.
- Maintaining adequate space.
- Keeping an open posture (McCorry and Mason 2019).
- Acknowledging the anger, thereby demonstrating empathy with what the person is feeling.
- Encouraging the person to identify the cause of the anger, through use of skilful questioning.
- Where possible, empowering the person to resolve any causes.

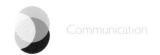

The NMC (2018a, 2018b) states that nurses need to be able to manage and defuse situations effectively and to be able to recognise and respond to verbal and non-verbal cues.

The aim in any situation where a person may become aggressive is a peaceful resolution. Meeting anger with anger – through direct confrontation, defensiveness or questioning of the person's feelings – may lead to an escalation in anger and maybe to aggression, even violence. Appropriate communication skills and good self-awareness can minimise and de-escalate potential points of conflict. Arnold and Boggs (2020) emphasise that individuals and their families who are angry often need understanding and human caring more than anything else and that careful listening is the most effective way of helping to neutralise anger and hostile feelings.

Learning outcome 4: appreciate ways of communicating with people who are confused

Acute *confusion* is usually defined as having a rapid onset and is characterised by changeable levels of consciousness often with an impaired ability to think and concentrate. NHS UK suggests that individuals who have sudden confusion (delirium) may have difficulty thinking or speaking clearly. They may feel disorientated and struggle to attend to their surroundings and some people also have hallucinations – seeing or hearing things that are not there (www.nhs.uk/conditions/confusion). Sudden confusion can be caused by a number of conditions for example low blood sugar, some medications, infection, alcohol or head injury. It is therefore crucial that thorough assessment is carried out and ensuring appropriate communication skills are applied sensitively.

Dementia affects around 850,000 people over the age of 65 across the UK, with some areas having a greater number of people living with dementia than others and costing an estimated 34.7 billion a year. (https://www.dementiastatistics.org/statistics/dementia-maps/) (https://www.alzheimers.org.uk/about-us/policy-and-influencing/dementia-scale-impact-numbers). Two-thirds of those with dementia are women, and there are 700,000 carers of people with dementia (Alzheimer's Society 2021a). Living with dementia and individual experiences of living with this diagnosis vary with the challenges that it poses and Wray (2020) outlines why its effect on communication can be so distressing for the person and their family and emphasises the importance of kindness and compassion.

Box 2.32 Activity: characteristics of someone with dementia

ACTIVITY

Make a list of the possible characteristics of someone with dementia.

You may have thought about the following:

- impairment in memory;
- difficulty with understanding;
- difficulty undertaking certain tasks;
- poor judgement and difficulty reasoning.

A person with dementia can become confused as a result of cognitive impairment, and it can gradually affect the person's ability to communicate. This confusion can result in individuals being excluded from being involved in their care, which can be upsetting and frustrating for the person and their loved ones.

Confusion is often a relatively permanent feature in the later stages of dementia; however, for someone like Mrs Davies who is in the earlier stage of dementia, confusion may be unpredictable, transient and intermittent. However, the nurse and nurse associate must avoid making assumptions about her confusion as it may be due to other factors, as suggested above, such as the physical factors of malnutrition, dehydration, constipation or an acute infection. She may also be disorientated because she is in an unfamiliar environment, and this disorientation would be compounded if she had a visual or hearing impairment. Nicol and Hollowood (2019) emphasise that people with dementia need to have regular eye and hearing tests and that a person-centred approach is vital to focus on the person's abilities and not their inabilities.

Sometimes, despite all attempts to help a person, their confusion makes it difficult to make needs known and for nurses to identify appropriate interventions. In these situations, the person's safety and best interests are paramount, as previously discussed, with reference to the Mental Capacity Act (Great Britain 2005). The Code (NMC 2018c, p. 8) highlights the nurse's responsibility to ensure that they

keep to all relevant laws about mental capacity that apply in the country in which you are practising, and make sure that the rights and best interests of those who lack capacity are still at the centre of the decision-making process.

It is important in these situations to remember to continue to provide person-centred care that promotes respect and dignity in line with benchmarks for best practice (DH 2010) and the proficiencies for undergraduate nursing education and nursing associates (NMC 2018a, 2018b).

Box 2.33 Activity: providing emotional support

Mrs Davies is looking for her husband, who has just said goodbye and told her he is going home, and she is becoming more agitated. Suggest strategies you could use to help her.

Strategies to consider include both verbal and non-verbal aspects:

- use of appropriate physical contact that can show interest and provide reassurance;
- sitting or standing at eye level;
- remember your body language and reduce any sudden movements;
- pay attention to the person's body language;
- help the person orientate to time and place;
- ensure a calm environment;
- use of visual prompts such as memory books, cue cards or pictures. Some apps may be useful;

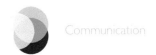

- use of appropriate and understandable language that matches the person's cognitive abilities;
- a calm, clear voice;
- use of active listening skills.

The Alzheimer's Society (2021b).

The Alzheimer's Society (2021b) and Dementia UK (2021) outline other useful tips in relation to communication with someone who has dementia, and these tips include the best way to approach someone with dementia and the importance of minimising distractions. They also give tips about how vital an awareness of non-verbal behaviour is, such as tone of voice, eye contact and learning to recognise what is most helpful for the person. People with dementia often have difficulty processing questions and information; therefore, attention needs to be given to the speed of delivery; careful listening; and not being patronising, arguing and contradicting. They also suggest some things *not* to say to someone with dementia. For example, avoiding saying 'Do you remember when' but perhaps 'I remember when'. The way that you greet someone with dementia is important as is using their preferred name rather than luvie/dearie or other 'elderspeak'.

Whether the individual has an acute confusional state or has dementia, as in the case of Mrs Davies, nurses are in a unique position to ensure accurate assessment and to ensure that person is treated with respect, dignity and compassion at all times. NMC proficiencies (2018a, 2018b) require nurses and nurse associates to act with dignity and respect at all times and to act autonomously to challenge situations or others when someone's dignity may be compromised.

Learning outcome 5: consider communication in relation to sensitive issues such as sexuality

There are various sensitive issues that nurses may need to discuss with people in their care; sexuality is one such area. Sexuality plays an important part in the development of self-concept and who we are as human beings (Lipinska and Heath 2020). The way individuals perceive themselves sexually affects self-image, body image and self-esteem, and it is an important aspect of the quality of life as a human being (Wilschut et al. 2020). Indeed, the nurse's own sexuality may have an impact on their assessment of situations and behaviour. It is important that nurses are aware of the various ways individuals may identify in relation to their sexuality, for example, heterosexual, gay, lesbian or bisexual. Explorations of how illness affects an individual's sexuality is often neglected due to nurses' own inhibitions about discussing intimate issues and other institutional and client-related factors (Evans 2013). Heath (2019) suggests that although sexuality is a fundamental aspect of life, many nurses find it a difficult area to address, and this is particularly so with an older person. WHO (2017) defines sexuality as a central aspect of being human and outlines that it includes sex, gender roles, gender identities and intimacy; however, their definition also emphasises that older people often enjoy active sex lives, an aspect that may not be fully appreciated due to stereotypical views about the elderly?

Gregory (2000) outlines the difference between sexuality (concepts of identity) and sexual functioning (bodily function). Major illnesses such as depression, cancer, stroke and arthritis can affect sexuality either because of the effects of the illness itself or due to hospitalisation, treatments or medication.

> ### Box 2.34 Activity: considering a person's gender or sexuality
>
> Reflect upon situations where a person's gender or sexuality needed to be considered.

Did you think of the following examples?

- How the client identifies in relation to their sexuality.
- After a mastectomy or other surgery that alters body image.
- Where appearance has been altered due to medication (e.g. chemotherapy may cause a loss of hair and steroid therapy may cause weight gain).
- Effects of long-term medication use (e.g. some medications used for hypertension and mental illnesses can cause impotence/sexual dysfunction).
- People with long-term urinary catheters.
- People who are paralysed or have had a stroke.
- People who have had genital or reproductive surgery.

Assessment can help to discover the physical, psychological and relational aspects of an individual's sexual needs, but a sensitive and skilled approach is vital. It is important to adopt a structured approach suggesting that the benefits of including sexuality in individual assessment should include:

- helping individuals understand their situation/condition and possible effects on their sexual functioning;
- helping relieve fear and anxiety;
- helping towards an understanding of treatment options.

The P-LI-SS-IT model (Annon 1976) and the extended P-LI-SS-IT model (Taylor and Davis 2006) is a framework that can help nurses support those who are experiencing difficulties in sexual functioning recognising different levels of expertise

- Permission: Creating an environment that permits discussion relating to sexual issues enables this issue to be integrated into the service. Heath (2019) suggests all healthcare staff should feel confident in creating an ethos of permission.
- Limited information: staff should have the ability to provide general information and guidance and acknowledge the effect of sexual issues on health.
- Specific suggestions: this relates to recognising when individuals need specialist support from, for example, a specialist nurse.
- Intensive therapy: usually undertaken in specialist centres and encompasses physical, psychological and interpersonal and relationship aspects.

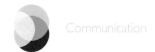

Within a general care setting such as a hospital unit or community, it is important that nurses and nurse associates have an understanding that managing sexual problems is primarily about giving information and allowing the person to respond to options in care and treatment. However, it also involves recognising when more in-depth support is needed. Davis (2006) highlights research that suggests that people often do not voice concerns about their sexuality as they prefer nurses to raise the subject. However, Güdül Öz et al. (2021) suggest that the nurses' own beliefs may hinder their exploration and communication with individuals about sexuality. Nurses might be unsure about when to raise the topic and be concerned that individuals themselves might feel uncomfortable. Price (2010) also highlights the fact that nurses often have difficulty with discussions about sexuality and sexual relationships with individuals but emphasises that it is important to be able to have these sensitive discussions. He suggests that open dialogue will help the person to make sense of how the illness or treatment may impact on their sexuality and intimate relationships. Some suggestions in relation to opening a conversation and 'giving permission' could include saying

- `Some people taking this drug find it affects how they feel about intimacy and relationships – this maybe something that has affected you.
- `Many people are worried about resuming sexual relationships after a heart attack – this maybe something you are worried about.

An active awareness of the person and the issues related to their health can also guide how staff address sexual health needs, and Heath (2019) outlines amongst a number of tips for discussing sexuality, the importance of open questions and listening carefully to language and terminology used.

It is important that nurses are able to discuss sensitive issues because as we have seen, illness often affects sexuality, sexual functioning and relationships and how people may perceive themselves – this in turn can impact upon their coping and recovering from acute and chronic changes to their health.

Learning outcome 6: discuss how to communicate with and support people who are in distress

According to the American Psychological Association 2021 (APA-dictionary.apa. org/psychological-distress), psychological distress is 'a set of painful mental and physical symptoms that are associated with normal fluctuations of mood in most people'. Recognising when someone is in distress is an important part of the nursing role and includes engaging in difficult conversation with compassion and sensitivity for those who are vulnerable emotionally (NMC 2018a, 2018b). Nursing staff are the only health staff who routinely provide the most intimate of care and are therefore provided with many opportunities to be a source of support and to recognise those in distress. Being ill, in hospital or requiring care at home is challenging for both the person and their relatives. The role of the nurse and nursing associate means we are in a privileged position to support the person or their family.

Box 2.35 Activity: supporting distressed individuals

Consider the scenarios of Violet and Maria, they are both distressed at times, how might their behaviour reflect this? What approach would you take in supporting them and why?

Think about Violet – her distress could be partly due to her new environment and confusion caused by it. Her behaviour of repeating the same phrase and becoming agitated may be signs of her distress. Staff would need to approach her gently, speaking slowly and not using jargon. They should not be challenging her as this may cause further upset, they may try to distract her onto something she likes, for example talking about her family, when her husband will be visiting.

Maria's distress could be due to her pain (especially at night) therefore she may become particularly distressed overnight. This will mean that staff have to try to support her in managing her pain and distress, while also being aware of the potential impact on other people in the environment. This would be a fine line to walk, and staff would need to try to prioritise people's needs and minimising Maria's distress would be of paramount importance. Staff should ensure that they communicate clearly with Maria to get a full understanding of her distress. She should receive the relevant analgesia and they should also ensure that pressure relieving equipment be used appropriately. Everything they do should be fully documented and discussed with the MDT and people involved in Maria's care.

Many trusts run or provide access to SAGE and THYME® courses specifically designed to provide concise support using a structured approach and this approach can be helpful for when we recognise that someone is struggling and distressed. SAGE and THYME is a mnemonic that acts as an aid memoire for a structured conversation with a person in distress or with concerns, and is based on the evidence behind effective communication skills. The first part of the model, SAGE, encourages active listening and disclosure of all the person's concerns, without interruption, while the second part THYME addresses problem solving (Griffiths 2017).

Key aspects are:

Setting – it is important to be aware of privacy and dignity especially in a hospital environment, but equally, in someone's home, an awareness of these aspects is important.

Ask – the nurse is encouraged to ask a direct question regarding the person's concerns. This may be, for example, – 'Can you tell me what is distressing you?' 'Can I ask what you are concerned about?'

Gather – rather than accept the first concern, this model suggests that you follow up with 'Is there something else?' Their list of concerns may be long, so seeking permission to write down these is encouraged.

Empathy – empathy and demonstrating that you are listening throughout will encourage the person to continue. However, at this point when all concerns have

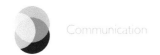

been aired, a sensitive empathetic response such as 'You do seem to have a lot to deal with at the moment' is appropriate.

At this point, it may seem overwhelming, especially if the person is very distressed. The SAGE part of this framework helps the nurse understand the individual's concerns, THYME helps the nurse address the provision of solutions and an exit, and the person has been given the opportunity to talk and will hopefully be calmer.

Talk – this aims to find out who supports the person and who they find helpful. 'Who do you have to talk to?'

Help – 'How do they help?' This may be practical or emotional support from family, friends or perhaps community groups, for example, a religious group.

You – 'What do *you* think would help you?' This helps the person to focus on what may be most beneficial

Me – 'Is there something *I* can do to help?' 'Is there something you would like *me* to do?'

End – summarise and close – for example, 'Can we leave it here?'

Available from: http://www.sageandthymetraining.org.uk/sage-thyme-model-and-benefits-1 (Accessed on 30 May 2021).

The advantage of this short course (usually three hours) is that it provides practitioners with an evidence-based approach that many nurses feel has a very positive influence on how they address and support the distressed person. For further information, see: http://www.sageandthymetraining.org.uk/

Box 2.36 Children and young people: practice points – dealing with distress

Developmentally appropriate explanations and providing a sense of control by giving choices where possible can help the child or young person cope with procedures and investigations. Distraction and play can also help, and the hospital play specialist can be involved to support the younger child, while guided imagery and relaxation techniques may support the older child or young person. However, sometimes children may become distressed about procedures or investigations that are necessary, and then nurses should work with the child and family and try to calm and de-escalate these situations. Brenner and Noctor (2010) explore communication in situations where children may resist procedures, and they suggest four key questions when assessing the situation:

1 What am I feeling now? The nurse's feelings could affect communication and exacerbate the situation.
2 What does this child feel, want or need – try to understand the motivation behind the child's behaviour.
3 How is this environment affecting this child – could the environment be modified? Hospitalisation is always stressful for children.
4 How can I best respond? Respond to the child's distress in a timely and helpful way.

> **For further information, see**
>
> Brenner, M. and Noctor, C. 2010. Clinical holding of children and young people. In: Glasper, A., Aylott, M. and Battrick, C. (eds.) *Developing Practical Skills for Nursing Children and Young People*. London: Hodder Arnold, 18–25.
>
> For guidance on therapeutic holding of children, for example, for procedures, and legal and ethical aspects, see
>
> Hore, S. 2017. The use of restraint in children and young people's nursing chapter. In: Davies, R. and Davies, A. (eds.) *Children and Young People's Nursing: Principles for Practice*, 2nd edn. London: CRC Press, 49–72.
>
> Royal College of Nursing (RCN). 2019. *Restrictive Physical Intervention and Therapeutic Holding for Children and Young People: Guidance for Nursing Staff*, 2nd edn. Available from: https://www.rcn.org.uk/professional-development/publications/pub-007746
>
> Mental health problems, including depression and anxiety, are common in young people. See:
>
> Terry, J. and Davies, A. 2017. Children and Young People's Mental Health. In: Davies, R. and Davies, A. (eds.) *Children and Young People's Nursing: Principles for Practice*, 2nd edn. London: CRC Press, 199–222.

Impact on self and self-care

We have long known that nursing is a stressful profession, in part due to the face-to-face nature of the job and part due to the pressures of the role/s. The RCN (2013) survey of nurses' well-being and stress found that high levels of stress were experienced by respondents, with reasons given such as working long hours, unrealistic time pressures and distress caused due to an inability to give the high standard of care needed.

Compassion fatigue is sometimes seen as being an indication of the impact of the role of the healthcare profession. It is said by Peters (2018) to occur when nurses experience declining empathy as a result of repeated exposure to others' suffering.

In 2019, the proportion of respondents agreeing with the statement 'I feel under too much pressure at work', had risen from 51% in 2009 to 63% in 2019 (RCN 2019b, p. 6). The 2017 American Nurses Association health risk appraisal found that 82% of respondents experienced high levels of workplace stress.

The recent Covid-19 pandemic has further placed pressure on nurses and healthcare workers, who have taken the brunt of the caring role with 76% experiencing more workplace stress (RCN 2021, p. 9). They have often been working even longer hours than normal – 33% reported this (RCN 2021, p. 12), frequently in new environments such as Intensive Care Units and at their own personal risk. Greenberg et al. (2021) found that of those who responded to their survey, 45% had experienced one of the following: severe depression (6%), post-traumatic stress disorder (PTSD; 40%), severe anxiety (11%) or problem drinking (7%). More worryingly, 13% of respondents reported frequent thoughts of being better off dead, or of hurting themselves in the previous two weeks.

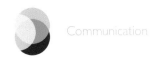

It is not all negative though as Aughterson et al. (2021) found that there were some positive effects of dealing with the pandemic with interviewees reporting that they felt they had developed resilience and coping strategies, some also noted that they had slowed down and non-work relationships had improved. The RCN (2021, p. 14) found that 88% still felt passionate about being a nurse.

> ### Box 2.37 Activity: work/life balance
>
> Reflect on your role as a healthcare worker, is there a time when you have not been able to stop thinking about work when at home? How has this affected you (physically and emotionally) and your home life?

You may have felt unable to sleep, you might have become tearful, angry, agitated. You might have eaten little, or you may have binged or eaten very unhealthy foods. You might have not wanted to see others so isolated yourself from family and friends, and this might have caused arguments or at least tensions.

It is important that we know when we are being affected by our experiences and how to deal with this. The starting point is self-awareness, which we discussed earlier in this chapter. This may be different for us all, but we need to develop the open area of our awareness. Asking for feedback from trusted peers and disclosing your worries to them may help you to understand what is happening.

Recognising that you are struggling is key to your being able to do something about it. There are numerous strategies for us to employ to improve our mental well-being; self-care thus becomes essential to our health. At work, talking to colleagues (debriefing) can be supportive, especially following a particularly stressful situation, seeking counselling from Occupational Health or the GP may help. Maintaining a healthy lifestyle is important, for example, sleeping well, eating healthily, keeping hydrated, exercising, continuing with interests/hobbies and talking to friends and family. For some practising mindfulness or meditation or connecting with nature, going for a walk in the local park/woods will help improve their well-being. These things can be very personal, but part of self-care is knowing what helps you and when you need to employ them.

Sites that may help in relation to mental/psychological self-care:

Royal college of Psychiatrists, Feeling Overwhelmed. Available from: https://www.rcpsych.ac.uk/mental-health/problems-disorders/feelingoverwhelmed?searchTerms=self%20help

Royal College of Nursing, Wellbeing, Self-care and Resilience. Available from: https://www.rcn.org.uk/library/subject-guides/wellbeing-self-care-and-resilience

The Kings Fund. The Courage of Compassion. Available from: https://www.kingsfund.org.uk/publications/courage-compassion-supporting-nurses-midwives

Summary
- This section highlighted and raised awareness on communication with people who are angry, depressed, confused or who have sensitive issues to address or who are distressed.
- Excellent interpersonal communication skills are particularly needed in challenging situations.
- Key aspects of communication in challenging situations are as follows:
  - Be prepared to listen and hear what the person is saying.
  - Give permission to raise their concerns.
  - Ask questions sensitively.
  - Give timely information.
  - Respond and refer appropriately.
  - Be aware of self.

CHAPTER SUMMARY

Understanding influences such as self-awareness, personality, attitudes and stereotyping are important aspects in the provision of sensitive, compassionate communication – and therefore of care. Communication takes many forms and has verbal and non-verbal components. Nurses need to use a range of interpersonal skills effectively. In relation to practical nursing skills, initiating interactions, listening, non-verbal communication, questioning and giving explanations are all of particular importance. There are many situations where communication is challenging and requires nurses to be skilled and empathetic.

In conclusion, this chapter aimed to provide insight into the importance of nurse–patient relationships. It included a discussion about the impact of self within this relationship, and how it affects communication and thus the care of people. The scenarios highlighted how communication principles are applied in a variety of care settings with different individuals and within MDTs. This chapter has emphasised the vital role that communication plays throughout the persons' care experiences. The following chapters focus on specific practical nursing skills and demonstrate the importance of effective communication for all nurses, in all care settings at all times.

ANSWER TO ABBREVIATIONS (activity section 2)

CF: Cystic fibrosis

CPA: Care Programme Approach

PID: Pelvic inflammatory disease or prolapsed intervertebral disc

TPR: Temperature, pulse and respiration

BP: Blood pressure or bedpan

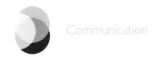

OE: On examination

RXT: Radiotherapy

ETA: Estimated time of arrival

TTA: To take away

DNA: Did not attend or deoxyribonucleic acid

DOA: Dead on arrival or date of admission

GCS: Glasgow Coma Scale

REFERENCES

Afriyie, D. 2020. Effective communication between nurses and patients: an evolutionary concept analysis. *British Journal of Community Nursing* 25(9). doi:org/10.12968/bjcn.2020.25.9.438

Alzheimer's Society. 2021a. How many people have dementia and what is the cost of dementia care. Available from: https://www.alzheimers.org.uk/about-us/policy-and-influencing/dementia-scale-impact-number (Accessed on 30 March 2021).

Alzheimer's Society. 2021b. Tips for communicating with a person with dementia. Available from: https://www.alzheimers.org.uk/about-dementia/symptoms-and-diagnosis/symptoms/tips-for-communicating-dementia#content-start (Accessed on 25 March 2021).

American Nurses Association. 2017. Executive summary health risk appraisal. Available from: https://www.nursingworld.org/~495c56/globalassets/practiceandpolicy/healthy-nurse-healthy-nation/ana-healthriskappraisalsummary_2013-2016.pdf (Accessed 25 March 2021).

American Psychological Association. 2021. APA dictionary of psychology. Available from: APA- dictionary.apa.org/psychological-distress (Accessed on 5 May 2021).

Annon, J.S. 1976. The PLISSIT model: a proposed conceptual scheme for the behavioral treatment of sexual problems. *J Sex Educ Ther* 2: 1–15.

Arnold, E. and Boggs, K. 2020. *Interpersonal Relationships: Professional Communication Skills for Nurses*, 8th edn. St, Louis: Elsevier.

Aughterson, H. et al. 2021. Psychosocial impact on frontline health and social care professionals in the UK during the COVID-19 pandemic: A qualitative interview study. *BMJ Open* 11: e047353. doi:10.1136/bmjopen-2020–047353

Baillie, L. and Matiti, M. 2013. Dignity, equality and diversity: An exploration of how discriminatory behaviour of healthcare workers affects patient dignity. *Diversity and Equality in Health and Care* 10: 5–12.

Beach, J. and Oates, J. 2014. Maintaining best practice in record-keeping and documentation. *Nursing Standard* 28(36): 45–50.

Beck, A.T., Ward, C.H., Mendelssohn, M.J. and Erbaugh, J. 1961. An inventory for measuring depression. *Archives of General Psychiatry* 4: 561–71.

British Deaf Association. 2021. BSL act now. Available from: https://bda.org.uk/bslact-now/ (Accessed on 20 March 2021).

Brooks, N. 2021. How to undertake effective record keeping and documentation. *Nursing Standard*. doi: 10.7748.ns/2021.e11700.

Care Quality Commission. 2020. *Out of sight-Who Cares?* Newcastle: Care Quality Commission.

Carter, L. 2020. Facemasks: How nurses can overcome communication barriers and reassure patients. *Primary Health Care*. Available from: https://rcni.com/nursing-standard/

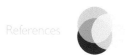

opinion/comment/face-masks-how-nurses-can-overcome-communication-barrier-and-reassure-patients-163116 (Accessed on 20 April 2021).

Coenders, M., Scheepers, P., Sniderman, P.M. and Verberk, G. 2001. Blatant and subtle prejudice: dimensions, determinants, and consequences; some comments on Pettigrew and Meertens. *European Journal of Social Psychology*. Available from: https://onlinelibrary.wiley.com/doi/abs/10.1002/ejsp.44 (Accessed on 26 March 2021).

Corwin, A.I. 2018. Overcoming elderspeak: A qualitative study of three alternatives. *The Gerontologist* 58(4): 724–729.

Cribb, V.L. and Haase, A.M. 2016. Girls feeling good at school: School gender environment, internalization and awareness of socio-cultural attitudes associations with self-esteem in adolescent girls. *Journal of Adolescence* 46: 107–14.

Cuff, B.M.P., Brown, S.J., Taylor, L. and Howat, D.J. 2016. Empathy: A review of the concept. *Emotion Review* 8(2): 144–53.

Data Protection Act. 2018. Available from: https://www.legislation.gov.uk/ukpga/2018/12/contents (Accessed on 20 April 2021).

Davis, T.B. 2006. Using the extended PLISSIT model to address sexual healthcare needs. *Nursing Standard* 21(11): 35–40.

Dementia UK. 2021. Tips for better communication. Available from https://www.dementiauk.org/get-support/understanding-changes-in-behaviour/tips-for-better-communication/ (Accessed on 29 March 2021).

Department for Constitutional Affairs (DCA). 2007. *Mental Capacity Act 2005 Code of Practice*. Norwich: The Stationery Office. Available from: https://assets.publishing.service.gov.uk/government/uploads/system/uploads/attachment_data/file/921428/Mental-capacity-act-code-of-practice.pdf (Accessed on 5 May 2021).

Department of Health (DH). 2010. *Equity and Excellence Liberating the NHS*. London: DH.

Department of Health (DH). 2011. *No Health without Mental Health: A Cross-Government Mental Health Outcomes Strategy for People of All Ages*. London: DH.

Department of Health (DH). 2012a. *Transforming Care: A National Response to Winterbourne View Hospital: Department of Health Review Final Report*. London: DH.

Department of Health (DH). 2012b. *Compassion in Practice: Nursing, Midwifery and Care Staff: Our Vision and Strategy*. London: DH.

Eckroth-Bucher. 2010. Self-awareness: a review and analysis of a basic nursing concept. *Advances in Nursing Science* 33(4): 297–309.

Egan, G. 2010. *The Skilled Helper: A Problem-Management and Opportunity-Development Approach to Helping*, 9th edn. California: Brooks/Cole.

Evans, D.T. (2013) Promoting sexual health and wellbeing: the role of the nurse. *Nursing Standard* 28(10): 53–7.

The Evidence Centre. 2013. Review for the RCN: Content analysis of 'patient opinion' website stories about nurse attitudes and behaviours. Available from: https://www.careopinion.org.uk/resources/site?id=blog-resources/1-files/rcn-professional-attitudes-behaviours-patient-opinion-stories-report.pdf (Accessed on 26 March 2021).

Eysenck, H.J. 1965. *Fact and Fiction in Psychology*. Harmondsworth: Penguin Books.

General Data Protection Regulation. 2018. Available from: https://www.gov.uk/government/publications/guide-to-the-general-data-protection-regulation (Accessed on 12 April 2021).

Goffman, E. 1990. *Stigma: Notes on the Management of a Spoiled Identity*. London: Penguin Books.

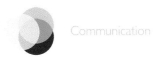
Grant, A. and Goodman, B. 2019. *Communication and Interpersonal Skills in Nursing*, 4th edn. London: Sage.

Great Britain. 2005. *Mental Capacity Act*. Available from: https://www.legislation.gov.uk/ukpga/2005/9/contents (Accessed on 5 May 2021).

Great Britain. 2007. *Mental Health Act*. Available from: https://www.legislation.gov.uk/ukpga/2007/12/contents (Accessed on 5 May 2021).

Greenberg, N. et al. 2021. Mental health of staff working in intensive care during Covid-19. *Occupational Medicine* 71: 62–7. doi:10.1093/occmed/kqaa220 2021.

Gregory, P. 2000. Patient assessment and care planning: sexuality. *Nursing Standard* 15(9): 38–41.

Grenon, J. 2010. Nurse-patient email communication: Comprehensive guidelines. *Canadian Journal of Informatics* 5(4). Available from: https://cjni.net/journal/?p=1009 (Accessed on 15 April 2021).

Griffiths, J. 2017. Person-centred communication for emotional support in district nursing: SAGE and THYME model. *British Journal of Community Nursing* 22(12): 593–7. https://doi.org/10.12968/bjcn.2017.22.12.593

Gross, R. and Kinnison, N. 2014. *Psychology for Nurses and Health Professionals*, 2nd edn. Boca Raton, FL: CRC Press.

Güdül Öz, H., Balci Yangin, H. and Ak Sözer, G. 2021. Attitudes and beliefs of nursing students toward sexual healthcare: A descriptive stud. *Perspectives in Psychiatric Care* 57(4): 1–7.

Hargie, O. 2017. *Skilled Interpersonal Communication*, 6th edn. London: Routledge.

Health and Social Care Information Centre (HSCIC). 2013. A Guide to confidentiality in health and social care: references. Available from: https://digital.nhs.uk/data-and-information/looking-after-information/data-security-and-information-governance/codes-of-practice-for-handling-information-in-health-and-care/a-guide-to-confidentiality-in-health-and-social-care. (Accessed on 5 May 2021).

Heath, H. 2019 Sexuality and sexual intimacy in later life. *Nursing Older People*. doi: 10.7748/nop.2019.e1102.

Jackson-Best, F. and Edwards, N. 2018. Stigma and intersectionality: A systematic review of systematic reviews across HIV/AIDS, mental illness, and physical disability. Available from: *BMC Public Health* 18, 919 (2018). https://doi.org/10.1186/s12889-018-5861-3. (Accessed on 26 March 2021)

Johnson, M. and Webb, C. 1995. Rediscovering unpopular patients: Concept of social judgement. *Journal of Advanced Nursing* 21: 466–75.

Keane, L. and Loades, M.E. 2017. Low self-esteem and internalizing disorders in young people: A systematic review. *Child and Adolescent Mental Health* 22: 4–15. doi:10.1111/camh.12204.

Liaschenko, J. and Fisher, A. 1999. Theorizing the knowledge that nurses use in the conduct of their work. *Sch. Inq. Nurs. Pract. An International Journal* 13(1): 29–41.

Lipinska, D. and Heath, H. 2020. Sexually speaking: person-centred conversations with people living with a dementia. *Nursing Older People*. doi:10.7748/nop.2020.e1207.

Lowe, C. and Jones, C. 2020. How to conduct difficult conversations digitally. *Cancer Nursing Practice* 19(5): 14–15.

Luft, J. and Ingram, H. 1955. *The Johari Window: A Graphic Model of Interpersonal Relations*. Los Angeles, CA: University of Los Angeles Press.

McCormack, B. and McCance, T. 2010. *Person-Centred Nursing Theory and Practice*. Oxford: Wiley-Blackwell.

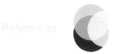

McCorry, L.K. and Mason, J. 2019. *Communication Skills for the Healthcare Professional*, 2nd edn. Baltimore, MD: Lippincott.

McLaughlin, K. 2020. Recognising elderspeak and how to avoid its use with older people. *Mental Health Practice*. doi:10.7748/mhp.2020.e1472.

Mental Health Foundation. 2015. Stigma and discrimination. Available from: https://www.mentalhealth.org.uk/a-to-z/s/stigma-and-discrimination (Accessed on 14 April 2021).

Mental Health & Joseph Rowntree Foundation. 2016. Poverty and mental health. Available from: https://www.mentalhealth.org.uk/sites/default/files/Poverty%20and%20Mental%20Health.pdf (Accessed on 25 March 2021).

Mid Staffordshire NHS Foundation Trust Inquiry. 2010. *Independent Inquiry into Care Provided by Mid Staffordshire NHS Foundation Trust*. January 2005–March 2009, Volume I & 2. Available from: http://www.official-documents.gov.uk/document/hc0910/hc03/0375/0375_ii.pdf (Accessed on 20 March 2021).

Mid Staffordshire NHS Foundation Trust Public Inquiry. 2013. *Report of the Mid Staffordshire NHS Foundation Trust Public Inquiry*. Available from: http://www.midstaffspublicinquiry.com/report (Accessed on 8 March 2021).

Minardi, H.A. and Riley, M.J. 1997. *Communication in Health Care: A Skills Based Approach*. Oxford: Butterworth Heinemann.

Mind. 2021. Managing anger. Available from: https://www.mind.org.uk/information-support/for-children-and-young-people/anger/dealing-with-anger/#ManagingAngerInTheMoment (Accessed on 20 March 2021).

Mitchell, A. and Hill, B. 2020. How to communicate effectively while wearing face masks. *Practice Nursing* 31(12): 84–6.

Moss, B. 2020. *Communication Skills in Nursing, Health and Social Care*, 5th edn. London: Sage.

Napier, A.D. et al. 2017. *Culture Matters: Using a Cultural Contexts of Health Approach to Enhance Policy-Making*. Available from: https://www.euro.who.int/__data/assets/pdf_file/0009/334269/14780_World-Health-Organisation_Context-of-Health_TEXT-AW-WEB.pdf (Accessed on 5 May 2021).

National Institute for Health and Clinical Excellence (NICE). 2009a. Depression in adults: Recognition and management Clinical guideline [CG90]. Available from: https://www.nice.org.uk/guidance/cg90/chapter/Update-information (Accessed 15 March 2021).

National Institute for Health and Clinical Excellence (NICE). 2009b. Depression in adults with a chronic physical health problem: recognition and management Clinical guideline [CG91]. Available from: https://www.nice.org.uk/guidance/cg91 (Accessed on 15 March 2021).

National Institute of Health and Clinical Excellence (NICE). 2014. Anxiety Disorders, Quality standard QS53. Available from: https://www.nice.org.uk/guidance/qs53/chapter/Introduction. (Accessed on 5 May 2021).

National Institute for Health and Clinical Excellence (NICE). 2019. NICE Impact Mental Health. Available from: https://www.nice.org.uk/Media/Default/About/what-we-do/Into-practice/measuring-uptake/NICEimpact-mental-health.pdf (Accessed on 19 April 2021).

National Institute for Health and Clinical Excellence (NICE). 2020. *Depression Overview*. Available from: https://pathways.nice.org.uk/pathways/depression#content=view-info-category%3Aview-about-menu (Accessed on 19 April 2021).

National Institute for Health and Clinical Excellence (NICE). 2021. *Anxiety Products*. Available from: www.nice.org.uk/guidance/conditions-and-diseases/mental-health-and-behavioural-conditions/anxiety/products?ProductType=Pathways. (Accessed on 29 March 2021).

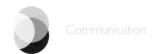

National Institute for Health Research (NIHR). 2020. Careful phrasing of requests by hospital staff could help people with dementia accept care. Available from: https://evidence.nihr.ac.uk/alert/hospital-patients-dementia-careful-phrasing-cut-refusals/ (Accessed on 28 March 2021). doi: 10.3310/alert_43178

NHS England et al. 2015. Transforming care for People with Learning Disabilities: Next steps. Available from: https://www.england.nhs.uk/wp-content/uploads/2015/01/transform-care-nxt-stps.pdf (Accessed 5 May 2021).

NHS England. 2017. Care and Treatment Reviews (CTRs): Policy and Guidance. Available from: https://www.england.nhs.uk/wp-content/uploads/2017/03/ctr-policy-v2.pdf. (Accessed on 29 March 2021).

Nichols, K. 2003. *Psychological Care for Ill and Injured People: A Clinical Guide.* Maidenhead: Open University Press.

Nichols, K. 2005. Why is psychology still failing the average patient? *The Psychologist* 18(1): 26–7.

Nicol, J. and Hollowood, L. 2019. *Nursing Adults with Long Term Conditions.* London: Sage.

Nursing and Midwifery Council (NMC). 2018a. *Future Nurse; Standards of Proficiency for Registered Nurses.* London: NMC.

Nursing and Midwifery Council (NMC). 2018b. *Standards of Proficiency for Nursing Associates.* London: NMC.

Nursing and Midwifery Council (NMC). 2018c. *The Code Professional Standards of Practice and Behaviour for Nurses, Midwives and Nursing Associates.* London: NMC.

Nursing and Midwifery Council (NMC). 2018d. Learnings from Gosport: Communication. Available from: https://www.nmc.org.uk/standards/guidance/learning-from-gosport/learnings-from-gosport-communication/ (Accessed on 7 May 2021).

Ockenden Review of Maternity Services at Shrewsbury and Telford Hospital NHS Trust. 2020. Independent Report. Department of Health and Social Care. Available from: https://assets.publishing.service.gov.uk/government/uploads/system/uploads/attachment_data/file/943011/Independent_review_of_maternity_services_at_Shrewsbury_and_Telford_Hospital_NHS_Trust.pdf (Accessed on 27 March 2021).

Office for National Statistics. 2020. Coronavirus and depression or anxiety in Great Britain. Available from: https://www.ons.gov.uk/peoplepopulationandcommunity/healthandsocialcare/healthandwellbeing/datasets/coronavirusanddepressionoranxietyingreatbritain (Accessed on 16 April 2021).

Oliver, D. 2015. Minding our language around care of older people and why it matters. Available from: http://stg-blogs.bmj.com/bmj/2015/05/07/david-oliver-minding-our-language-around-care-for-older-people/ (Accessed on 19 April 2021).

Pearce, R. 2011. Clarifying your Own Personal Values and Beliefs. In: Docherty, T. Franks, J. Pearce, R. and Trenoweth, S. (eds.) *Nursing and Mental Health Practice: An Introduction for all Fields of Practice.* Exeter: Learning Matters Ltd, 23–38.

Peters, E. 2018. Compassion fatigue in nursing: A concept analysis. *Nurse Forum* Oct 53(4): 466–80. doi: 10.1111/nuf.12274. Epub 2018 Jul 2.

Pettigrew, T.F. and Meertens, R.W. 1995. Subtle and blatant prejudice in Western Europe. *European Journal of Social Psychology* 25: 55–75.

Pettigrew, T.F. and Meertens, R.W. 2001. In defense of the subtle prejudice concept: A retort. *European Journal of Social Psychology* 31: 299–309.

Pope, T. 2012. How person centred care can improve nurses' attitudes to hospitalised older patients. *Nursing Older People* 24(1): 32–6.

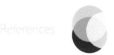

Porritt, L. 1984. *Communication: Choices for Nurses*. London: Churchill Livingston.

Price, B. 1990. *Body Image: Nursing Concepts and Care*. London: Prentice-Hall.

Price, B. 2010. Sexuality: Raising the issue with patients. *Cancer Nursing Practice* 9(5): 29–35.

Price, B. 2013. Countering the stereotype of the unpopular patient. *Nursing Older People* 25(6): 27–34.

Price, B. 2015. Understanding attitudes and their effects on nursing practice. *Nursing Standard* 30(15): 50–7.

Raghubir, A.E. 2018. Emotional Intelligence in professional nursing practice: A concept review using Rodger's evolutionary analysis approach. *International Journal of Nursing Sciences*. doi: 10.1016/j.ijnss.2018.03.004.

Rasheed, S.P. 2015. Self-awareness as a therapeutic tool for nurse/client relationship. *International Journal of Caring Sciences* 8(1): 211–16.

Rasheed, S.P., Younas, A. and Sundus, A. 2019. Self-awareness in Nursing: A scoping review. *Journal of Clinical Nursing* 28(5–6): 762–74.

Rogers, C.R. 1961. *On Becoming a Person*. Boston, MA: Houghton Mifflin.

Royal College of Nursing (RCN). 2013. *Beyond Breaking Point – A Survey Report of RCN Member on Health and Wellbeing and Stress*. London: RCN. Available from: www.rcn.org.uk/publications (Accessed on 8 June 2021).

Royal College of Nursing (RCN). 2019a. Record keeping: The facts. Available from: https://www.rcn.org.uk/professional-development/publications/PUB-006051 (Accessed on 30 March 2021).

Royal College of Nursing (RCN). 2019b. Employment survey. Available from: https://www.rcn.org.uk/professional-development/publications/pub-007927 (Accessed on 8 June 2021).

Royal College of Nursing (RCN). 2020a. Remote consultations guidance under COVID-19 restrictions. Available from: https://www.rcn.org.uk/professional-development/publications/rcn-remote-consultations-guidance-under-covid-19-restrictions-pub-009256 (Accessed on 31 March 2021).

Royal College of Nursing (RCN). 2020b. Consultation guidelines (end of life care): Having Courageous Conversations by telephone or video, during the COVID-19 pandemic. Available from: https://www.rcn.org.uk/professional-development/publications/rcn-courageous-conversations-covid-19-uk-pub-009-236 (Accessed on 31 March 2021).

Royal College of Nursing (RCN). 2021. Building a better future. Available from: https://www.rcn.org.uk/professional-development/publications/rcn-builiding-a-better-future-covid-pub-009366 (Accessed on 8 June 2021).

Sarvestani, R.S. et al. 2013. Challenges of nursing handover: A qualitative study. Available from: https://www.researchgate.net/publication/259155142_Challenges_of_Nursing_Handover_A_Qualitative_Study (Accessed on 26 March 2021).

Schaffer, H.R. 2004. *Introducing Child Psychology*. Oxford: Blackwell.

Stefanovics, E.A. et al. 2016. Witchcraft and biopsychosocial causes of mental illness. *Journal of Nervous &Mental Disease* 204(3): 1.

Stein-Parbury, J. 2018. *Patient and Person: Interpersonal Skills in Nursing*, 6th edn. Australia: Elsevier.

Stockwell, F. 1972. *The Unpopular Patient*. London: Royal College of Nursing.

Swann, M. 2021. Recognizing the importance of language in effective pain assessment. *Nursing Standard*. doi: 10.7748/ns.2021.e11563.

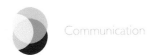
Taylor, B. and Davis, S. (2006) using the extended PLISSIT model to address sexual health-care needs. *Nursing Standard* 21(11): 35–40.

Terez Malka, S., Chad, S., Kessler, C.S. et al. 2015. Professional e-mail communication among health care providers: Proposing evidence based guidelines. *Academic Medicine* 90(1): 25–9.

Thompson, N. 2015. *People Skills*, 4th edn. Hampshire: Palgrave Macmillan.

Trueland, J. 2020. Nurse-patient conversations. *Cancer Nursing Practice* 19(5): 15–18.

Twycross R. and Wilcock, A. 2018. *Introducing Palliative Care*, 5th edn. Nottingham: Palliativedrugs.com.

Vydelingum, V. 2000. South Asian patients' lived experience of acute care in an English hospital. *Journal of Advanced Nursing* 32: 100–7.

Walker, J., Payne, S., Smith, P., Jarrett, N. and Ley, T. 2012. *Psychology for Nurses and the Caring Professions*, 4th edn. Maidenhead: Open University Press.

Webb, L. 2020. *Communication Skills in Nursing Practice*, 2nd edn. London: Sage.

While, A.E. and Clark, L.L. 2010. Overcoming ignorance and stigma relating to intellectual disability in healthcare: a potential solution. *Journal of Nursing Management* 18: 166–72.

Wilschut, V., Pianosi, B., van Os-Medendorp, H. et al. 2020. Knowledge and attitude of nursing students regarding older adults' sexuality: A cross-sectional study. *Nurse Education Today*. doi:10.1016/j.nedt.2020.104643.

World Health Organization (WHO). 2017. *Sexual Health, Human Rights and the Law*. Geneva: WHO.

World Health Organization (WHO). 2020. Depression. Available from: https://www.who.int/en/news-room/fact-sheets/detail/depression (Accessed on 8 February 2021).

Wray, A. 2020. *The Dynamics of Dementia Communication*. New York: Oxford University Press.

Zendedel, R. et al. 2015. Informal interpreting in general practice: Comparing the perspectives of general practitioners, migrant patients and family interpreters. Available from: https://pure.uva.nl/ws/files/16232057/Informal_Interpreting_in_General_Practice.pdf (Accessed on 15 April 2021).

Zigmund, A.S. and Snaith, R.P. 1983. The hospital anxiety and depression scale. *Acta Psychiatrica Scandinavica* 67(6): 361–70.

Fundamentals of mental health assessment for non–mental health practitioners

Joanne Sale and Skye Capolucci

The NMC (2018a, p. 3) in their Future Nurse Standards proficiency for Registered Nurses suggest that Registered Nurses play a key role in providing nursing care for people with complex mental, physical, cognitive and behavioural care needs. They must be able to meet the needs of people they encounter in their practice in a person-centered, holistic way. This includes all nurses being able to assess and meet the mental health needs of the people they encounter in the care setting and understanding the proficiencies in Annex A and B in respect of their field of nursing. This is also included in the standards of proficiencies for nursing associates.

(NMC 2018b)

Assessment is the foundation of nursing in all disciplines and is the underlying component of skilled practice. Assessment skills are a key factor in initially identifying a person's healthcare needs. Nevertheless, assessment as a continuous fundamental process not only initiates nursing care, but it is also an ongoing cycle, a process that is implemented throughout all points of nursing practice. Assessment plays an essential role in identifying suitable nursing interventions and planning of care together with identifying functioning baselines and evaluating response to treatments (Carniaux-Moran 2013).

This chapter will focus on assessment in relation to mental health; however, it is likely in practice that you will be assessing both mental health and physical health combined. Someone may attend your service for a physical health complaint but present with a mental health problem and contrariwise. This chapter will also suggest how healthcare workers can increase their understanding of mental health, mental ill health and undertake a mental health assessment. Whilst it is acknowledged that the purpose of assessment is to inform the referral to the mental health specialists who will complete a full assessment, it is also important, that the information communicated is accurate and demonstrates that the person is currently safe and receiving quality care.

DOI: 10.4324/9781003020660-3

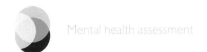

PRACTICE SCENARIOS

Adult

Diane Beck is a 50-year-old woman with multiple sclerosis who lives at home with her husband and two teenaged children. She has difficulty walking. She has tingling and burning pains and spasms in her legs, so she uses walking sticks or a wheelchair. She has a suprapubic catheter for her bladder problems.

Mental Health

Natalie Turney is 21 years old. She has been admitted as a voluntary person to an acute mental health ward with severe depression. After going home for a day, she returns, appearing unsteady on her feet and she has a strong smell of alcohol. Her speech is very slurred, and she is quite uncommunicative. When the staff ask her if she has taken any tablets, she mentions some 'little yellow pills' and paracetamol. However, she will not give details about the quantity or when she took them.

Farah Muhammed, a 45-year-old female who lives alone, has three adult children and has a diagnosis of **bipolar affective disorder** with a history of several hospital admissions to a mental health unit. Farah is currently an inpatient on an acute mental health inpatient ward due to a relapse in mental state; she is experiencing mania. Prior to her admission to hospital, she was undergoing investigation for her physical health. Farah has recently been diagnosed with stage 3 bowel cancer. Farah has made the decision not to accept treatment for her cancer diagnosis, she has also declined for her children to be informed. Professionals are concerned about Farah's decision, suspecting she is lacking capacity and is unable to make an informed decision about her care and treatment. Due to her current mental state, a capacity assessment is completed.

Violet Davies, aged 76, has moderate Alzheimer's disease. She has been admitted to a care home for respite as her husband is physically and emotionally exhausted and needs a break. He has refused help in the past as he has been determined to look after his wife, but he has now agreed to take a holiday visiting friends. Violet is physically well, but she is also known to have osteoarthritis in her right hip. She looks permanently worried and is agitated; she keeps repeating the same phrase over and over. Mr. Davies looks shaky and tearful at the thought of leaving his wife for a week.

Learning Disability

Maria is a 68-year-old woman with a moderate learning disability who has been living in a group home for the past five years. She has long-standing diabetes mellitus (Type 1) treated with insulin and has recently developed painful diabetic neuropathy. She has pain in both legs below the knees, which she finds particularly distressing when she is walking and during the night; her sleep is disturbed. She is in the care of both her general practitioner and the diabetic team at her local hospital. Maria's mother, who is 90 years old and recently widowed, visits weekly and is concerned about Maria's distress. Her community learning disability nurse would like to understand more about how he can support Maria, her mother and the group home staff on how to manage Maria's pain and increase her comfort.

UNDERSTANDING THE DIFFERENCE BETWEEN MENTAL HEALTH AND MENTAL ILL HEALTH

Box 3.1 Learning outcomes

By the end of this section, you will be able to

1 explain what mental health entails and how it differs from mental ill health
2 explain how mental ill health is categorised

Learning outcome 1: explain what mental health entails and how it differs from mental ill health

Defining what constitutes health can be problematical as it is often impacted by personal, cultural and societal norms and expectations. A frequently applied definition is the one given by the World Health Organization (1948 para 1) that health is 'a state of complete physical, mental and social wellbeing, not merely the absence of disease or infirmity'. However, this seems to be quite limiting as it does not take into account aspects that we may feel are important to our overall health such as our emotions, our environment, our cultural expectations and norms or our spiritual well-being. It is also true that this list is not likely to be definitive and may well change over time. So, health can mean many things to us as individuals and can alter from moment to moment.

Box 3.2 Activity: what makes you feel well?

ACTIVITY

Write down what makes you feel well.
And what makes you feel unwell.

You may have said; I sleep well, can relax, enjoy meeting with my family and friends; I have interests and hobbies that I enjoy; I get on well with work and feel I can cope with whatever I face.

When it comes to mental health, defining what this means can be challenging. The World Health Organization (2003, p. 9) says that it is a

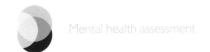

state of well-being in which the individual realises his/her own potential, can cope with normal stresses of life can work productively and fruitfully and is able to make a contribution to his/her community.

What is important to note here is that mental health and well-being are more than just the absence of an illness. However, this definition alone can raise many questions, for example how do we measure potential? Therefore, how do we truly know if and when someone has realised or is realising it? What are the normal stresses of life? How does just having received bad news fit in here; is this a normal stressor? What if a person receiving a diagnosis takes longer to absorb the new facts or perhaps they continue to deny them – are they mentally healthy? Is this an understandable and expected reaction to the news they have just been given? This takes us to other contestable issues as how we measure coping. For the person who copes with their anxieties by spending increasing amounts of time at the gym or drinking wine, at what point is their coping strategy causing them harm and not keeping them healthy?

National Institute of Clinical Excellence [NICE] (2013) states that mental well-being includes areas that are key to optimum functioning and independence such as life satisfaction, optimism, self-esteem, feeling in control, having a purpose in life and a sense of belonging and support. As with the previous definition, this attempt at understanding mental well-being leaves many questions unanswered and does not seem to reflect the dynamic nature of mental well-being. Concepts such as life satisfaction, and a sense of control and optimism can alter in seconds due to changes in the internal or external environment. Therefore, exacting a clear understanding that is widely shared, as to what constitutes mental health and well-being may be too much to expect. A better approach to understanding may be to aim to understand from the individual's perspective – how they are feeling, what is their life like and how is their relationship with others.

If defining mental well-being is so complicated, then it is not surprising that defining mental illness is also fraught with difficulties. In fact, even the Mental Health Act (Great Britain 2007) does not attempt to define mental illness, instead turns to mental disorder. Mental disorder is defined for the purposes of the Act as 'any disorder or disability of the mind'. Good practice suggests that 'relevant professionals should determine whether a person has a disorder or disability of the mind in accordance with good clinical practice and accepted standards of what constitutes such a disorder or disability' (Department of Health 2015a p. 26). One of the reasons that mental illness is so hard to define is that how it is understood and defined changes within and between societies and cultures. Behaviours that were once seen as reflective of a mental illness in the UK such as homosexuality and having a child out of wedlock (see Mental Deficiency Act 1913 – Education England 2021) are no longer viewed in such a manner. However, there are societies around the world that still view homosexuality as an illness and/or a crime [(for example, you can still be stoned to death in Mauritania or be sentenced to death in Nigeria, Iran, Saudi Arabia and Somalia (Human Dignity Trust 2021)]. Equally some

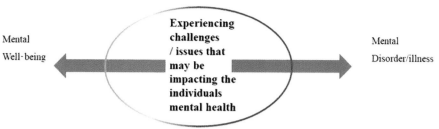

Figure 3.1: Conceptualising mental health and mental illness.

societies still lock up, disown or kill women who dishonour their families by having a child out of a marriage.

We can consider mental health and mental illness to be at opposite ends of a continuum. In between, a person's mental well-being may be challenged by anything that may impact this sense, however temporary; Figure 3.1 conceptualises this relationship. Someone who would generally see themselves as mentally well may be experiencing relationship issues, at the same time as they prepare for an exam. This may start to impact on their sleep due to the constant worry or even anxiety. This in turn may affect their dietary intake; they may stop cooking for themselves; feeling that they do not have time. Thus, they end up eating take-away food and snacking. The person may also start drinking more alcohol, especially at night, in a vain attempt to get to sleep or may avoid going out, stop attending their classes or responding to social media as they feel overwhelmed by what is happening. At this point, they may still be relatively healthy, but if this continues for a longer term, it may be that their mental health is at risk, and if they were to continue like this and their behaviour were to escalate, they may even end up with a diagnosis of a mental illness. On the other hand, the person may seek support (from friends to deal with their relationship issues and from the university to deal with their assessment concerns) and their sense of mental well-being may improve, so that they never have a diagnosis of a mental illness.

Box 3.3 Activity: mental well-being and physical deterioration

ACTIVITY

Consider Diane Beck who has Multiple Sclerosis (MS) and has recently had a suprapubic catheter inserted. Reflecting on what you know of her and MS, how might her mental well-being be affected by her recent deterioration?

You may have considered how Diane's recent health concerns might have worried her; she may feel embarrassed by the catheter, worried that it will smell or leak. She may also be concerned at losing the ability to walk altogether. These worries may affect her ability to sleep; she may well want to avoid others, and to spend more time alone. At this point, her mental well-being may be threatened by her new situation and is uncertain as a result.

Perinatal mental illness affects up to 20% of new and expectant mothers and covers a wide range of conditions.

If left untreated, mental health issues can have significant and long-lasting effects on the woman, the child, and the wider family.

In response to the need to improve PMH care in the long-term plan, Department of Health Northern Ireland (2020) put out a Mental Health Action Plan. Available from: www.health-ni.gov.uk/publications/mental-health-action-plan (Accessed on 9 June 2021).

NHS England (2020) set out the English and Welsh Government's response to the need to improve PMH care in the long-term plan. Available from: www.england.nhs.uk/mental-health/perinatal/ (Accessed on 9 June 2021).

NHS Scotland (2019) sets out the service development guidance. Available from: https://www.pmhn.scot.nhs.uk/professionals-2/guidance-resources/ (Accessed on 9 June 2021).

The general principles are that there should be distinctive service provision and:

- Increased availability of specialist PMH services
- Improved access to evidence-based psychological therapies for women and their partners
- Mental health checks for partners of those accessing specialist PMH community services and signposting to support as required.

Learning outcome 2: explain how mental ill health is categorised

Psychologically, we like the world to be ordered and to make sense. This is important when we are assessing people, helping us to work with the individual whilst making a nursing diagnosis and agreeing on plans to meet the person's needs. We tend to put people's experiences into boxes for our ease; this enables a greater understanding and in healthcare, it leads to a diagnosis.

In mental health, these are called classification systems and there are two that are mainly used. These being the International Classification of Disease (ICD-10) (WHO 2010) and the Diagnostic and Statistical Manual of Mental Disorders (DSM-5) (American Psychiatrist Association 2013). These systems are fraught with controversy and criticisms, but they remain widely used and from a positive point, they enable the person's presenting issues and behaviour to be categorised. This helps with nursing diagnosis, and more importantly, the formulation of the care plan and identification of appropriate interventions to meet the person's needs.

We can all experience some behaviours that may characterise a mental illness, but we will not be diagnosed with one. This is mainly because the impact the symptoms/ experiences may have on us may not be great, or the person may be in control of them or they may not last for long. For example, Maria, who has been experiencing pain, and may not really understand what is happening, perhaps due to her learning difficulty, and this could also cause her anxiety. However, this anxiety may be temporary and reduce quickly as her pain is better managed. Also, with the use of effective and sensitive communication skills, the care team can help her to develop an understanding of what is happening and how she can herself reduce the pain through seeking support when the pain is starting.

To see a more in-depth consideration of these classification systems and how they are applied, please read the chapter on Classification of Mental Illness by Kingdon et al. (2017) in Chambers (2017).

Box 3.5 Activity: listing mental illnesses

ACTIVITY

Write down a list of all the mental disorders that you can think of.

Box 3.6 The most common mental disorders

Dementia – such as Alzheimer's dementia, vascular dementia, Lewy's body dementia

Mood disorders – such as depression, bipolar affective disorder

Anxiety disorders – such as generalised anxiety disorder, panic, phobias, obsessive compulsive disorder, post-traumatic stress disorder

Schizophrenia and other psychotic disorders

Eating disorders – such as anorexia nervosa and bulimia nervosa

Personality disorders – such as emotionally unstable personality disorder

---

There are many mental disorders that you might have considered, too many to fully list here. But in Box 3.6 are some of the main illnesses that you may have considered.

Think back to the scenario's you may have put self-harm and suicide (or suicidal intention) on your list; however, these are not mental disorders, they are behaviours that are not always linked to mental disorders. They may be helpful to the person as a form of coping; however, they can also be very risky, and we will discuss risk later in this chapter.

Suggested further reading:

To find out more about mental disorder, access the Royal College of Psychiatrists; https://www.rcpsych.ac.uk/mental-health/problems-disorders

Summary

- you should have started to develop your understanding of what mental health means
- how mental illness/disorder differs from mental health
- how people's experiences/behaviours can be categorised into mental illness/ disorders
- the importance of you being able to recognise some of the major mental illnesses/disorders that you may encounter.

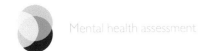

Demonstrate an awareness of the underpinning legal and ethical principles involved in undertaking a holistic comprehensive assessment of needs.

Box 3.7 Learning outcomes

By the end of this section, you will be able to:

1 outline the importance of legislation that is relevant to mental health assessment
2 discuss the importance of engaging and communicating in a holistic and non-judgemental manner
3 discuss the interplay between mental and physical health, particularly in relation to assessment.

Learning outcome 1: outline the importance of legislation as relevant to mental health assessment

Underpinning legislation

Nursing and nurse associate training and practice in all fields is guided by the NMC code (NMC 2018a, 2018b) and the NMC standards of proficiency (NMC 2018a, 2018b), which are devised with a deontological ethical approach, with their primary role and core focus to protect and safeguard the health, rights and well-being of the public (Tee et al. 2012). To meet and maintain the standards of the NMC monitor, the education, training and conduct of midwives, nurses, nursing associates and nursing students who need to ensure that their skills and knowledge are up to date and the standards of their professional code upheld (NMC 2018a, 2018b).

Nurses and nurse associates have a duty to abide by the law and deliver services in accordance with legislation that underpin their practice; in particular, the Human Rights Act (Great Britain 1983), Mental Health Act (Great Britain 2007), Health and Social Care Act (Great Britain 2012), Mental Capacity Act (Great Britain 2005) (see below) and NICE Guidelines (2020). Legislation governs policies and frameworks, determining the provision of service. Nursing staff are compelled to comply with policies, as well as the Code, to deliver care that will fulfil; respect beneficence or non-maleficence, challenge stigma and discrimination, promoting equality, diversity and inclusion (Department of Health 2011) (see Table 3.1).

Table 3.1: Care should *mirror* these concepts

Respect	To act in a manner that reflects an understanding of the person's uniqueness, their wishes, likes and dislikes
Beneficence	Moral duty to act in the best interests of the person
Non-maleficence	Nurses must do no intentional harm to people – no negligence
Stigma/discrimination	Challenge and abstain from discrimination and disgrace associated with diagnosis or any aspect of the person
Equality, diversity and inclusion	Treat people fairly, without bias or prejudice, increase opportunities for all and not judge people

During your assessment, you may identify concerns around an individual's capacity and whether they have the capacity to make decisions, and, therefore, in addition, complete a capacity assessment, and this should be done before any treatment is commenced.

We will now go on to consider a couple of relevant pieces of legislation; the Mental Capacity Act (Great Britain 2005) and the Mental Health Act (Great Britain 2007).

Mental capacity

Mental capacity means having a state of mind that is sound to make your own decisions, although, being able to make decision can often be problematic for anyone, with many day-to-day circumstances hindering decision-making, including tiredness, indecisiveness, environmental factors, physical and emotional factors and in particular mental illness. The purpose of the Mental Capacity Act [MCA] (Great Britain 2005) is to safeguard and empower vulnerable individuals over the age of 16 who may be unable to make decisions on their own due to their capacity being hindered by disability or illness. However, deciding that someone lacks capacity must not be established by his or her age, appearance, condition or behaviour alone (Great Britain 2005).

Assessing capacity

The MCA Code of Practice (2007) states that the person who is responsible for carrying out a capacity assessment, is the carer (or professional) who is caring for (or delivering a professional intervention to) the person who lacks capacity. Therefore, when working with service users, we should all be considering their capacity when agreeing on the care required. Simply put, the person who is asking the question is the one who does the capacity assessment.

It should always be assumed that an individual has capacity to make a decision and endeavour to support and encourage individuals to make their own decisions in relation to their care and treatment (Great Britain 2005). There may be circumstances where an individual makes a decision that you believe is negligent or unconventional; however, this does not fundamentally mean that the individual is lacking the capacity to make that decision. If we have capacity, we have the right to make unwise decisions; think about the time you stayed out for an extra hour and regretted it in the morning as you got ready for an early shift, or the relationship you got involved in despite having a gut instinct that it was not a good idea.

Capacity is decision- and time-specific, and it is possible to have capacity for some decisions and still lack capacity for others. The complexity of the decision is often the deciding factor in this, consenting to having a bandage changed is easier than consenting to surgery and its risks.

If someone lacks capacity to make major decisions such as their choice of treatment or accommodation or finances, this does not mean they are unable to make minor decisions such as what they would like to eat or clothing they would like to wear (CQC 2011). However, it is essential under the MCA (Great Britain 2005) that before carrying out any care or treatment, an assessment of capacity is completed.

If you have a plausible doubt that the individual has capacity, and that they are unable to make a sound decision themselves, then an assessment of capacity needs to be completed, with it being more formal, the more consequential the decision is. Lack of capacity is often not permanent and can change, which is why capacity assessments must be time- and decision-specific – an individual may be unable to make a particular decision at a particular time, due to specific factors. This is particularly relevant in the mental health field as you can see in this next scenario.

Thinking back to Farah Muhammed, who is currently experiencing mania and has had a recent diagnosis with stage 3 bowel cancer: Farah has made the decision not to accept treatment for her cancer diagnosis; she has also declined for her children to be informed. If following an assessment of capacity it is deemed that Farah does not have capacity, it will need to be determined what care and treatment will be in her **best interests**. Should treatments be initiated, and if Farah were to make a significant level of recovery, she should then be re-assessed to see if she has regained capacity. If Farah now has capacity, then she can make decisions about her care and treatment and would also attend a review meeting of her care and treatment.

For a full explanation, read Office of the Public Guardian, (2009). Making decisions… about your health, welfare or finances. Who decides when you can't? Available from: https://assets.publishing.service.gov.uk/government/uploads/system/uploads/attachment_data/file/365631/making_decisions-op601.pdf (Accessed on 9 June 2021).

The MCA (Great Britain 2005) specifies that someone lacks capacity if they are unable to make their own decision and if they are unable do one or more of the following four criteria:

- Understand information given to them
- Retain that information long enough to be able to make the decision
- Weigh up the information available to make the decision
- Communicate their decision – Verbally, using sign language or even muscle movements such as squeezing a hand or blinking (Figure 3.2).

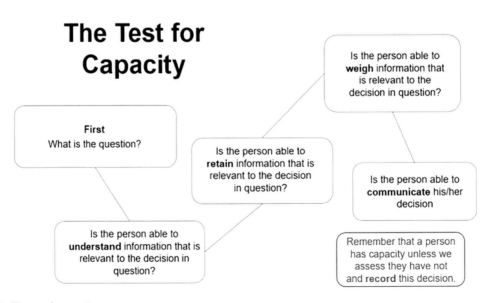

The Test for Capacity

First
What is the question?

Is the person able to **understand** information that is relevant to the decision in question?

Is the person able to **retain** information that is relevant to the decision in question?

Is the person able to **weigh** information that is relevant to the decision in question?

Is the person able to **communicate** his/her decision

Remember that a person has capacity unless we assess they have not and **record** this decision.

Figure 3.2: The test for capacity.

Source: Developed by D. Roberts, learning disability consultant.

For individuals who present with communication barriers, for example, language or physiological barriers such as hearing difficulties, poor eyesight and speech impediments, it is vital that individuals are supported with the facilitation of an interpreter or communication aids. All efforts of communicating with the individual should be made before making the conclusion that they lack capacity to make a decision.

Who can assess capacity?

The Mental Capacity Act applies to all those who work in health and social care and is designed to empower all to complete capacity assessments themselves (MCA 2005) – good professional training is key. However, should you find that cases involve complex or major decisions like Farah's you may need to involve other professionals, including ward doctors/consultants, a general practitioner (GP) or a specialist (consultant psychiatrist or psychologist).

Consent

It should never be assumed an individual would absolutely accept assessment, care and treatment. Therefore, it is essential that at every stage of contact you seek consent. If they agree to accept an assessment, again it should not be assumed that they will also accept treatment. Continually seeking consent and discussing care and treatment plans with the person is pivotal, ensuring you provide as much information as possible. Treatment plan options should be explored, and you must enable the individual to exercise their rights and make informed choices (Baillie 2014). In circumstances when a person withholds their consent, this constitutes a refusal of care. Should a person decline care and treatment and they have the capacity, their decision should be respected; however, it is fundamental that the consequences of their refusal to care and treatment should be clearly explained, specifically the effects on their health and well-being. The nurse must be assured that they are making an informed decision, has understanding of the consequences of that decision and have it recorded.

However, if a person lacks mental capacity as evidenced by a capacity assessment, to consent to treatment or even their information being shared, professionals must make a best-interests decision in accordance with the MCA (Great Britain 2005) and Code of Practice (Department of Constitutional Affairs 2007) to determine that the considered care and treatment would be in the best interests of the person.

Mental Health Act (Great Britain 2007)

The Mental Health Act (MHA) 1983 (as amended, Great Britain [GB], 2007) is the key piece of legislation formulated for the purpose of the care management and treatment of individuals with mental health disorders. It permits health professionals to use legal powers, in the best interests and for the health and safety of individuals and the public. The Mental Health Act [MHA] (GB 2007) allows appropriate professionals to detain, assess and treat people who present with a mental disorder and present with risk of harm to themselves or others. The legislation is equally there to protect and safeguard individuals from unethical and incongruous care and treatment under the provisions of the Act.

The MHA (GB 2007) solely authorises treatment for mental disorder only; therefore, treatment for physical illness cannot be given without consent. However, treatment can be given in only two circumstances: if the presenting physical health problem is the cause of the mental disorder, for example, hypothyroidism in depression. And if the physical health problems are a direct result of the mental health disorder such as the requirement for enteral feeds required for those with an eating disorder. This is usually only contemplated as a last resort and as such is often literally lifesaving. It can be a very distressing situation for all involved, so a very sensitive and professional approach is required. Support and debriefing within the care team are essential.

Powers set out in the 1983 Act (as amended, GB 2007) allow for both 'civil' admissions to hospital and criminal justice admissions from the courts or prison (The Kings Fund 2008). Overall, in adult nursing practice, you are most likely to care and treat individuals that are subject to Section 2 and/or Section 3 of the MHA. In some circumstances you may also treat and care for those under a forensic section if they are transported from prison into hospital. However, in these circumstances, individuals who are detained under the MHA will be accompanied and under constant observation from a chaperoning mental health professional.

The MHA 1983 amended 2007 applies to England and Wales. The Scottish Parliament in 2003 passed its own MHA (the Mental Health (Care and Treatment) (Scotland) Act 2003 amended 2015). However, the two legislations have corresponding, comprehensive purpose, the two Acts differ significantly in material, so comparisons need to be treated with caution (The Kings Fund 2008).

You may not be directly involved in administering the MHA, but you should know what it means for the people under your care and for you and your colleagues.

Further reading:

Mental Health Act: www.nhs.uk/mental-health/social-care-and-your-rights/mental-health-and-the-law/mental-health-act/

MIND: www.mind.org.uk/information-support/legal-rights/sectioning/about-sectioning/

Learning outcome 2: discuss the importance of engaging and communicating in a holistic and non-judgemental manner

Engagement and communication

To achieve a broad and precise assessment, it is imperative to establish a rapport with the person. It may be that for some people the nursing assessment may be the only meaningful engagement they have had, or the only opportunity they may have had, to be open about their mental health. Furthermore, assessing someone's mental health can come with some complexities; it requires the ability to be unprejudiced and free from bias. Implementation of core nursing values and principles is pivotal during all aspects of nursing care upholding conduct in line with Royal College of Nursing (RCN) Principles; see below. People with mental health problems experience stigma and discrimination in almost every aspect of their lives (Turner 2017, cited in Chambers 2017). Many have said the stigma of mental ill health is more disabling than the illness itself; research has shown that people with mental health problems are pre-judged and find it hard to access healthcare for physical health (Mental Health Care 2015).

Nursing principles

- Treat everyone in your care with dignity and humanity.
- Nurses and nursing staff take responsibility for the care they provide and answer for their own judgements and actions.
- Nurses and nursing staff manage risk and are vigilant about risk and safety.
- Nurses and nursing staff provide and promote person-centred care.
- Nurses and nursing staff are at the heart of the communication process, assessing, recording and reporting on treatment and care.
- Nurses and nursing staff have up-to-date knowledge and skills.
- Nurses and nursing staff work closely with their own team and with other professionals
- Nurses and nursing staff lead by example and influence the approach to person-centred care.

(Adapted from RCN 2020)

Engaging with the person when completing the assessment stage will allow the nurse to recognise or identify normal or abnormal psychological presentations in the person, this will also help prioritise interventions and care. It is important to remember there are many types of questions such as closed/open-ended questions, probing questions, leading questions and affective questions (Sale and Neale 2014). It is essential to use the right type of questioning during an assessment to ensure you do not hinder the rapport, do not cause the person to become distressed or for them to feel inadequate, but to also encourage them and give them opportunity to contribute more detail that could help with your assessment. It is also important to use the assessment to identify any risks they may pose to themselves or others. By completing risk assessments from the information you have obtained, for example, if the person tells you they have had suicidal thoughts, it needs to be assessed as to what level of risk this is, this will be discussed further under risk; nevertheless, it is an essential part of the assessment.

Learning outcome 3: discuss the interplay between mental and physical health, particularly in relation to assessment

Understanding the connections between mental health and physical health
Unfortunately, there still remains inequality between mental health and physical healthcare, with many barriers including the individual's presentation. However, stigma and socioeconomic inequalities can be a major contributing factor that hinders access to physical healthcare for individuals with mental illness (The Kings Fund 2016). Often, individuals will present with physical health complaints, which can be exacerbated by mental health conditions such as anxiety, depression

and psychosis. This is where comprehensive holistic assessments will help ensure an individual is in the right care setting for their need presented. It will identify whether indications of either their physical health or mental health are impacting on the other and whether treating one will reduce the intensity of other symptoms or presentations.

Parity of esteem

Mental health frameworks and strategies date back many years, with frameworks such as National Service Framework for Mental Health (National Health Service 1999). This was then followed by the 'No Health without Mental Health' Strategy (Department of Health 2011), and its supporting guidance 'Closing the Gap' (Department of Health 2014).

All of the abovementioned set clear modern standards and service models for the improvement of mental health services, as each standard is based on evidence. In more recent years, there has been greater focus on integration and parity of esteem between care provision, to promote health and greater care for the increasing older population and those with long-term health conditions (The Kings Fund 2019). In comparison, each framework highlights the need for improvement in relation to, parity of esteem, integrated care and the fundamental need for collaboration between all agencies involved in individuals care needs. Parity of esteem illustrates the essential need for mental health to be valued equally to physical health, and there is a great ambition for this across both mental health and physical health (O'Brien et al. 2019). Everyone, whether they experience short-term difficulties with their mental illness or with complex mental health needs have the equal right to access healthcare treatment and support as those devoid of mental health conditions (RCN 2019):

> Patient surveys completed by CQC highlighted that patients with a pre-existing mental health condition who were in hospital for physical health treatment, reported poor experiences of care. These areas included information sharing, respect and dignity, coordination of care, confidence and trust, respect for patient centred needs and values, and perceptions of overall experience of care.
>
> (NICE 2019a, p. 17)

There unfortunately remains an inequality between mental health and physical health, despite many years of strategies to change this. Many health professionals continue to fail to take people with mental illness seriously when they raise concerns about their physical health. Or those concerns are overlooked once they are recognised to have a mental illness, meaning recovery from the physical condition is hindered, increasing the risk of long-term health condition and premature death (The Kings Fund 2016).

Individuals who have mental health conditions are more likely to suffer with at least one physical health problem along with their mental health problems, which is known as comorbidities or multi-morbidities if they have multiple health conditions (The Kings Fund 2016). Individuals with severe mental illness are also at higher risk of premature mortality, an average of 15–20 years earlier than the general population; this is often due to preventable physical illnesses (Public Health England 2018).

The common causes of death in individuals with severe mental illness include chronic physical medical conditions such as cardiovascular disease, respiratory disease, diabetes and hypertension (Public Health England 2018). This is often caused by a poor lifestyle; people with mental illness are more likely to smoke tobacco, but they are less likely to be given support to quit, increasing their risk of cardiovascular and respiratory diseases (The Kings Fund 2016).

Health and social inequalities are avertible; studies on inequalities linked to mental health show that those living in areas of poverty with poor access to employment and income are less likely to engage in healthy activities such as exercise, healthy eating and have poorer access to healthcare (The Kings Fund 2020). As a result of this, many individuals with mental health conditions are not receiving basic annual physical health checks. Monitoring of physical health in individuals with mental illness is vital due to all contributing factors including the effects of psychiatric medications. Psychiatric medications themselves can impact on someone's physical health; for example, they can impact someone's weight; people on average gain around 13lbs in weight during the first two months of taking psychiatric medications and this continues over the first year, which increases the risk of diabetes and heart disease, high blood pressure, problems with cholesterol and hormone levels (NICE 2015).

In extreme cases, the person can come to believe that they are a burden on their family or the hospital and would be better off dead, increasing risk of self-harm and suicide. For example, physical illness in the elderly is a major risk factor for suicide, often due to having complex health complications that requires they receive a lot of support, that they feel guilty for seeking from family members; therefore, it is also important to assess the risk associated with both their mental and physical health (NICE 2004). The next section will consider how to undertake an assessment of someone's mental health and well-being.

Summary

- An overview of the underpinning legislation has been highlighted, particularly those related to capacity, consent and metal ill health/disorders.
- The importance of engagement and communication when undertaking an assessment has been shown.
- The relationship between a person's physical and mental health has been highlighted.
- The importance of taking a holistic approach to a person's care has been recommended.

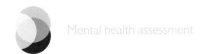

UNDERTAKING A MENTAL HEALTH ASSESSMENT

> **Box 3.8 Learning outcomes**
>
> By the end of this section, you will be able to:
>
> 1 outline the role of assessment within the nursing process
> 2 explain the different forms that assessment of mental health may take
> 3 explain importance of family/social support and of sharing information in the assessment process

Learning outcome 1: outline the role of assessment within the nursing process

There are five components to the nursing process, comprising assessment, diagnosis, planning, implementation and evaluation (Peate 2020). This chapter will focus on assessment.

Nursing process

- Assessment (gather subjective and objective data, family history, medical history, medication history, psychosocial history)
- Diagnosis (formulate a nursing diagnosis by using clinical judgement on what is wrong with the individual)
- Planning (develop a care plan that incorporates goals, potential outcomes and interventions)
- Implementation (perform the task or intervention)
- Evaluation (was the intervention successful or unsuccessful).

(Lappin 2018)

Nursing assessment is the first step of the nursing process. A simple interpretation of the nursing assessment process is, where the nurse or nursing associate takes a history, examines the person, makes a nursing diagnosis and identifies treatment. However, the nursing assessment requires more in-depth understanding, to be able to make adequate assessments that ensure all individuals receive high standards of care and are offered best evidence treatment through the correct care pathway. Assessment starts from the first point of referral to your service. This may be referral documentation or the person attending your area of practice. They may even have seen you regularly or their health may be being reviewed, for example someone with a long-term physical health condition. However, what may be important is that they are now presenting with a change in their mental state. Therefore, you should consider your first point of contact as the first stage to initiate your assessment and the start of your data collection. Assessment is, first of all, identifying the person's needs. You cannot follow the other components of the nursing process without, first of all, an assessment to identify what needs they have.

Assessments should be completed holistically, which involves gathering of information concerning the individual's physiological, psychological, sociological and spiritual needs. Holistic assessments improve the quality of care provided to the individual and also improve the person's outcomes. Individuals with mental illness have a greater susceptibility to poor physical health with high mortality rates than the general population (Tranter and Robertson 2019). Therefore, it is imperative that assessments are completed holistically and with a person-centred approach, to ensure their care needs are addressed to both improve their mental health, physical health and lifestyle, reducing the risk of further health complications.

Box 3.9 Children and young people practice points – assessment of mental well-being

The NHS (2020) suggests that around one in eight children and young people experience behavioural or emotional problems growing up.

Look out for:

- significant changes in behaviour
- ongoing difficulty sleeping
- withdrawing from social situations
- not wanting to do things they usually like
- self-harm or neglecting themselves
- declining performance at school/difficulty with school attendance
- weight loss/changed eating habits
- persistent aggression.

Everyone feels low, angry or anxious at times. But when these changes last for a long time or are significantly affecting them, then the child or young person may need extra support and help.

Sources:

MindEd for Families, Health Education England. 2017. Should I be worried? Available from: https://mindedforfamilies.org.uk/Content/should_i_be_worried_support_available_for_parents/course/assets/d16fba428026e7a81b246ad6035696ce4e9b117d.pdf (Accessed on 9 June 2021).

NHS. 2020. Looking after a child or young person's mental health. Available from: https://www.nhs.uk/oneyou/every-mind-matters/childrens-mental-health/ (Accessed on 9 June 2021).

Learning outcome 2: explain the different forms that assessment of mental health may take

Methods of assessment

The starting point of assessing someone's mental state involves making observations of the individual's presentation and behaviours. Much of this involves looking for visual cues; for example, how do they appear? Are their clothes appropriate, clean and well fitting? Are they agitated or relaxed? Does the person look to be in good physical health or not? Are there any injuries that could identify risk? We will also use our other senses to inform our observations such as smell, hearing and even touch.

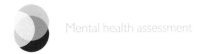
Box 3.10 Activity: Natalie Turney

Read Natalie's scenario below and complete this activity in relation to assessing her appearance and behaviour.

If you are the admitting nurse in the Emergency Department, what would you look out for in relation to Natalie and her behaviour? (Bear in mind that she may have drunk some alcohol so this too may have an impact.)

Natalie Turney is 21 years old. She has been admitted as a voluntary person to an acute mental health ward with severe depression. After going home for a day, she returns, appearing unsteady on her feet and she has a strong smell of alcohol. Her speech is very slurred, and she is quite uncommunicative. When the staff asks her if she has taken any tablets, she mentions some 'little yellow pills' or paracetamol. However, she will not give details about the quantity or when she took them.

You may have considered some of the following: is Natalie calm or is she agitated? Does she make eye contact when you try to communicate with her? To what extent can Natalie follow simple questions and answer them, or does she struggle with this? Is Natalie able to concentrate or is she distracted?

You may have also considered the impact of alcohol on Natalie; is she slurring her words? Falling asleep? Is she unsteady on her feet? Can you smell alcohol on her breath?

Once you know the extent and possible impact of the overdose and any treatment for this has been completed. Then you may need to leave Natalie, in a safe place, to sleep off the effect of the alcohol before a fuller assessment can be undertaken.

The observations above are very subjective and can be biased by a lack of cultural sensitivity and understanding. Therefore, it is important to garner more information from the individual. Interview style assessments are the most common techniques used to collect and gather information from individuals in relation to mental health. There are two main components to interview assessment method, these being the subjective and objective. They each require significant skills such as, being able to think critically, problem-solve, employ communication skills, and most importantly, the skill of listening. The overall aim of the assessment is to gather and scrutinise the information, interpret the information and identify the problem.

The first component is a systematic collection of subjective information; this is information given by the person (Weber 2014), their personal view and description of their experiences and needs. It is important at this stage to implement the skill of listening, avoid asking too many questions, but prompt where needed. You may wish to document in note form, important information or information you wish to expand on during the assessment. However, always inform the person that you will be making notes for your reference and be mindful not to appear as though you are too busy writing and not engaging with them. Allowing the individual to talk about how they are experiencing things will give a broader understanding of their condition, symptoms and what their specific needs are. This also allows the person to take lead in their care;

it is also essential to remember when making decisions related to the formulation of a care plan that the decision is made jointly with the individual. This allows the individual to feel supported and empowered to make informed decisions, it also acknowledges that care and treatment is tailored to the individual's needs (NICE 2020).

The second component is the objective assessment, the nursing assessment. This element of the assessment identifies current and future care needs of the person by allowing the formation of a nursing diagnosis. It is at this stage, that the nurse will ask relevant clinical questions, expand on the subjective information given by the individual, and obtain history if not already given as well as working collaboratively to identify an end goal and care plan.

Assessing someone's mental health and well-being
Mental status examination

Mental status examination (MSE) is the equivalent of a nursing physical examination: it is a structure of significant observations and investigations that focus on revealing normal and abnormal clinical findings in relation to one's mental health (Chambers 2017). The most common method of a mental state assessment occurs in the context of an interview. Each assessment should be individualised, taking a person–centred approach. Therefore, there may be no particular sequence in relation to what information you would need to acquire to develop an understanding of the person's presentation.

Box 3.11 Outline of the mental status examination tool

General observations

Someone's physical appearance may evidently support the assessment by indicating the type of lifestyle they have, their current mental state and their ability to care for themselves.

- Appearance – hygiene: clean, body odour, shaven, grooming
- Dress: clean, dirty, neat, ragged, climate appropriate – anything unusual?
- Jewellery: rings, earrings – anything unusual?
- Makeup: lipstick, nail polish, eye makeup – anything unusual?
- Other: prominent scars, tattoos.

Speech

- General: accent, clarity, stuttering, lisp
- Rate: fast (push of speech) or slow
- Latency (pauses between questions and answers): increased or decreased
- Volume: whispered, soft, normal, loud
- Tones: decreased (monotone), normal
- Content: relevant to topic, appropriate, logical and consistent.

Behaviour

- General: increased activity (restlessness, agitation), decreased activity
- Eye contact: decreased, normal, excessive, intrusive
- Mannerisms: stereotypical, posturing, withdrawn, threatening, relaxed
- Cooperativeness – cooperative, friendly, reluctant, hostile, engaged.

(Continued)

Box 3.11 (Continued)

Thoughts

- Thought process – tight, logical, goal-directed, loosened, circumstantial, tangential, flight of ideas, word salad
- Thought content – future-oriented, suicidal ideation, homicidal ideation, fears, ruminative ideas
- Perceptions: hallucinations (auditory, visual, olfactory), delusions (paranoid, grandiose, bizarre).

Emotions

- Mood: subjective (individual describes in own words and rates on a scale 1–10)
- Affect: objective: depressed/sad, anxious, euphoric, angry
    - Range: full range, labile, restricted, blunted/flattened
    - Appropriateness to content and congruence with stated mood.

Cognition

- Memory: immediate recall, three- and five-minute delayed recall of three unrelated words
- Orientation/attention: day, date, month, year, place
- Insight/judgement: good, limited or poor (based on actions, awareness of illness, plans for the future).

As a non–mental health specialist, having this information would aid any referral you make to the mental health specialist services.

Box 3.12 Explanations of terms used within the MSE

Emotion Mood and affect both relate to emotion, although profoundly different.

Affect (Observed) One's current expressed and observed emotion, the individual's complete conduct during the assessment and how you objectively perceive their emotion.

Mood (What you are told) is the subjective, internal emotion described by the person themselves

Delusions These are beliefs or ideas that the person believes in 100 per cent, without a single doubt, and which nobody else seems to accept. These beliefs or ideas cannot be explained by the person's culture, religion or background. Other people may find these ideas strange, unrealistic or even bizarre.

Hallucinations A hallucination happens when a person can hear, smell, feel, taste or see something, but it is not caused by anything (or anybody) around them. The most common one is hearing voices. These seem very real to the person, so they can be frightening or consoling depending on the content and context.

Word Salad A number of unrelated, unintelligible words that are linked together in someone's speech or writing. This can be a symptom of schizophrenia.

(Continued)

Box 3.12 (Continued)

Flight of ideas A form of thought disorder, where the person is bombarded with copious thoughts/ideas, and these may or may not then be expressed in disconnected garbled speech. This can be experienced by someone in a manic episode.

Tangential thinking The person skips from thought to thought but never seems to get to the point.

The information you gather from using this tool and related questions, will go some way to understanding the person and their presenting issues and needs. This would be essential information to pass on to other colleagues and as part of a mental health referral.

For some people with a learning disability, it may be necessary to use a specific mental health assessment tool. NICE guidance: Involving people with learning disabilities, and their family members, carers or care workers, in mental health assessment and treatment. Available from: www.nice.org.uk/guidance/ng54/chapter/Recommendations#assessment (Accessed on 9 June 2021).

Talking to the individual, their carer/family or learning disability nurse (or any other specialist involved in their care) will help you to decide on the best approach to take.

Learning outcome 3: explain the role of family/social support and the importance of sharing information in the assessment process

Family/social support

An important part of the assessment should include identifying an individual's support network; whether an individual has a support network or lacks a support network can add important information to your assessment (Chambers 2017). If the person attends your service with a friend or family member or gives you the contact details of a member of their support network, with the consent of the individual, it can add value to your assessment if you make contact to obtain further information in relation to the person and their presentation. In some cases, you may also want to identify areas of support that the carer/family/support network may need, are they able to care for the individual, is it impacting on their own health. Support can be identified for them if needed via a referral for a carer's assessment.

Scenario

Violet Davies, aged 76, has moderate Alzheimer's disease. She has been admitted to a care home for respite as her husband is physically and emotionally exhausted and needs a break. He has refused help in the past as he has been determined to look after his wife, but he has now agreed to take a holiday, visiting friends. Violet is physically well, but she is also known to have osteoarthritis in her right hip. She looks permanently worried and is agitated; she keeps repeating the same phrase over and over. Mr. Davies looks shaky and tearful at the thought of leaving his wife for a week.

Box 3.13 Activity: Mr. Davies

What information would you ask Mr. Davies in relation to Violet that may be of value in informing her caretaker during her respite stay?

What information would you ask Mr. Davies in relation to his own health and social needs?

You may have thought about asking: how can you reassure Violet, bearing in mind she is being taken out of her familiar environment and her husband is spending some time away from her. Has he noticed any changes in Violet's behaviour recently; if so, what? Are there any particular things that Violet likes to do or things she dislikes – such as foods?

How is Mr Davies managing? Does he appear well? How do his care responsibilities impact on his mental health? Does he need any longer-term support or help?

Although never fully complete, as information gathering will continue throughout contact and care, once data is collected, it will initiate the next aspect of the process. Or it may be that at this point you will complete your referral to a specialist mental health team for them to undertake a full in-depth mental health assessment.

- Analysis or diagnosis (formulate a nursing diagnosis by using clinical judgement; what is wrong with the person): depression, psychosis, substance abuse? How is their physical health?
- Planning (develop a care plan that incorporates goals, potential outcomes, interventions) – referral to another service, hospital admission treatment/medication/discharge with or without aftercare.
- Implementation (perform the task or intervention).
- Evaluation (was the intervention successful or unsuccessful) – assessing and evaluating.

(Lappin 2018)

Information-sharing

Information-sharing contributes greatly to care continuity. With continuity being fundamental to care quality, discrepancies are likely to cause inefficient and less cost-effective services. Continuity of care matters to everyone, increasingly so, for individuals who develop multiple morbidities, complex problems or become socially or psychologically vulnerable (World Health Organization 2018). Failures in care continuity increase the likeliness of individuals being put at risk of harm whilst adding avoidable costs (National Health Service 2019). Therefore, timely sharing of information is fundamental to succeeding seamless and accurate provisions of care. The increasing obligations to develop sound partnership working between services makes it imperative to have consistent lawful procedures for sharing confidential information (Caldicott 2013).

Information-sharing is classified as a form of communication (Caldicott 2013) whereby sharing information enhances care and health outcomes. However, confidentiality is a long-standing concept of ethical healthcare provision. Therefore, gaining consent is pivotal; as observed in practice, this is done on first contact, with delayed information-sharing being one of the primary contributing factors towards medical errors and harm (Woolf et al. 2004).

An inquiry by the Equality and Human Rights Commission found that deaths and other harmful incidents related to mental health can be prevented if sharing of information was improved in all settings (Equality and Human Rights Commission 2015). A study carried out by the CQC (2009) found concerns on timeliness of sharing information, which hindered the integration of care. They suggested that sharing of information in a timely manner is fundamental to enabling, enhancing care outcomes and decreasing risk of harm, whilst enabling consistency in the care provided. It is important to consider that not every personal detail needs to be shared with professionals; whether family or carers, sharing of information should be specific and relevant, appropriate and justifiable (HM Government 2018).

Summary

- You will understand the role of assessment within mental health
- You will have some guidance as to how a mental health assessment is conducted and some of the areas to be considered
- You will understand the importance of involving significant others in the assessment process
- Also, the importance of information-sharing.

Undertaking Assessment of risk

Box 3.14 Learning outcomes

By the end of this section, you will be able to:

1 describe what risk and risk assessment mean in relation to mental health
2 discuss what crisis means in a mental health risk situation
3 explain what to consider when undertaking an assessment of risk
4 discuss recommendations with regard to level of risk, especially in regard to self-harm and suicide.

Learning outcome 1: describe what risk and risk assessment mean in relation to mental health

Definition of risk and risk assessment

Individuals encounter risk on a day-to-day basis; throughout life, we are exposed to risk. However, some risk factors can have greater impacts on people than others such as attachment issues, childhood abuse, poverty, racism and poor education (Elliott 2016). Throughout life, the more we are exposed to multiple risk, particularly in childhood and adolescence, the ability to overcome the impact weakens and causes vulnerability to the individual's health and well-being, whilst also increasing the risk of them engaging in further risk behaviours that continue through adulthood (Newman 2002). The impact and vulnerability developed by risk exposure to individuals can be detected by the observation of the risk behaviours they engage in and the outcome of those risks. Jessor (2017) defines risk factors as circumstances that lead to undesirable and negative outcomes, including on health, well-being and social status; however, protective factors have the opposite effect and can reduce negative consequences and enhance positive outcomes. Fischhoff et al. (2001 p. 56) state that 'the consequences of a given level of vulnerability in either short or long term cannot be predicted without knowing the protective process that operate to reduce the impact of risk/vulnerability'.

Studies have shown that individuals who have less exposure to risk during childhood and adolescence, such as the experiences of a positive upbringing, good education and positive support, are more likely to develop protective factors (Elder et al. 2011). This helps develop resilience and resistance of fear, through a level of awareness that allows us to cope with circumstances that would otherwise have an impact on mental health, well-being and social status, as opposed to leading to further risk. However, a change in level of vulnerability caused by stress, life-changing events or bereavement along with contributing influences such as environmental, biological or psychological factors can diminish resilience. 'Risk is a natural occurrence, but with implied possibility of loss or hazard' (Hart 2014 p. 9).

Risk associated with mental health is defined as behaviours, negative characteristics or situations that have the probability to cause harm to oneself or others (Callaghan and Gamble 2015). Risk can also be beneficial in the sense of positive risk-taking, which means enabling individuals to do things others may take for granted (Department of Health 2015b). Risk assessment involves scrutinising likely outcomes associated with characteristics, behaviours and situations. Then, risk management comprises formulating a plan to decrease the likelihood of harm occurring and to optimise beneficial behaviour (Callaghan and Gamble 2015). Increase in risk is associated with a change in mental state, which is often caused by an individual being in a state of severe mental distress and crisis. It is important to remember, 'Risk cannot be eliminated, but it can be rigorously assessed and managed or mitigated' (Royal College of Psychiatrists 2016, p. 3).

Box 3.15 Children and young people practice points: suicide and self-harm in children and young people

Suicide rates in children are low compared with other demographic groups but the rate in the under 20s has been rising in England and Wales since around 2010.

Young people in their late teens also have the highest rate of non-fatal self-harm, a key suicide risk factor, and this rate appears to have risen in recent years.

Children and young people are therefore seen as a high priority for suicide prevention in the UK and many other countries.

Multiple factors contribute to an individual's risk of suicide. Additional stressors during the pandemic may include fears that a family member or oneself will develop COVID-19, the impact of bereavement, isolation, loneliness and loss of social supports, disruptions to care and support and fears about accessing it, school closure and exam disruption, and exposure to domestic violence and family tensions.

National Child Mortality Database (2020). Child suicide rates during the COVID-19 pandemic in England: real-time surveillance. Available from:

www.ncmd.info/wp-content/uploads/2020/07/REF253-2020-NCMD-Summary-Report-on-Child-Suicide-July-2020.pdf (Accessed on 9 June 2021).

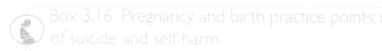

Box 3.16 Pregnancy and birth practice points: risk of suicide and self-harm

Maternal suicide remains the leading direct cause of maternal death between six weeks and a year after the end of pregnancy (MBRRACE 2020). NICE guidance suggests that the healthcare professional should carry out a risk assessment in conjunction with the woman and, if she agrees, her partner, family or carer. Focusing on areas that are likely to present possible risk such as self-neglect, self-harm, suicidal thoughts and intent, risks to others (including the baby), smoking, drug or alcohol misuse and domestic violence and abuse.

If there is a risk of, or there are concerns about, suspected child maltreatment, follow local safeguarding protocols.

If there is a risk of self-harm or suicide:

- assess whether the woman has adequate social support and is aware of sources of help
- arrange help appropriate to the level of risk
- inform all relevant care professionals (including the GP and those identified in the care plan)
- advise the woman, and her partner, family or carer, to seek further help if the situation deteriorates.

Sources:

National Institute for Health and Care Excellence [NICE] 2020. Identifying and assessing mental health problems in pregnancy and the postnatal period. Available from: https://pathways.nice.org.uk/pathways/antenatal-and-postnatal-mental-health/identifying-and-assessing-mental-health-problems-in-pregnancy-and-the-postnatal-period#content=view-node%3Anodes-assessment (Accessed on 9 June 2021).

MBRRACE. 2020. Mothers and Babies: Reducing Risk through Audits and Confidential Enquiries across the UK. Available from: https://www.npeu.ox.ac.uk/mbrrace-uk (Accessed on 9 June 2021).

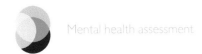

Learning outcome 2: discuss what crisis means in a mental health risk situation

Definition of crisis

ACTIVITY

Box 3.17 Activity: Maria

Thinking about Maria's situation:

- How may the following scenario lead to a mental health crisis?
- Can you define crisis from the perspective of the service user?

You may have thought about Maria's situation: she is in constant pain; her sleep is poor; she has an elderly mother that she is concerned about; her father also recently died; so she is grieving. Maria may feel, at present, that she is unable to cope with everything; she may feel overwhelmed by all that is happening – out of control. She may not understand elements of what is happening, and this would increase its impact.

An important concept is that the event itself is not the concern but the service user's perception of the event. That is – it is perceived as hazardous, threatening or extremely upsetting. Crisis situations are unique to each individual, and crisis can be defined as 'A perception or experience of a situation as an intolerable difficulty that exceeds current resources and coping mechanisms' (James and Gilliland 2016, p. 9). When an individual finds their current circumstances irresolvable, it may result in an increase in stress and anxiety, emotional distress and inability to function at their normal level of functioning for prolonged periods.

During the recent pandemic, the Office for National Statistics (2020) found that the number of adults experiencing depression had doubled and stood at 1:5 of the population. This was particularly the case for younger adults, females, those with a disability and those who were financially affected. The pandemic had been the trigger for them to develop mental ill health – it had threatened their resilience and the cause would be multi-faceted; for some, it would be the enforced isolation as a result of the lockdown, the lack of physical proximity, loss of employment or massive changes to working practices, financial concerns or even concerns related to Covid-19. This was an international event, but individuals can be similarly impacted by events that they find threatening. Someone with a mild learning difficulty would need person-centred approaches identifying their needs as anyone else in society would do. They would have some coping mechanisms and some areas where support would be needed.

Signs of crisis
How to recognise the signs of crisis

Individuals who are experiencing a time of crisis may present with some of the following signs:

Sudden changes in mood including, extreme depressive mood, persistent agitation or even mania (found in **bipolar affective disorder**).

Someone in crisis may express or experience suicidal thoughts or behaviour such as engaging in reckless activities posing a risk to self or others, including increased drug and alcohol use, impulsive spending, they may be organising finances so that family members are not left to deal with it should they have suicidal plans and intent.

They may experience changes in their mental well-being and experience an increase in intensity of symptoms including an increase in psychotic symptoms.

Physically, they may present with dramatic changes in sleeping patterns, changes in weight and even start to present with neglect of personal care and hygiene, not changing clothing, showering or even simple tasks such as brushing their teeth and combing their hair.

Social changes may include withdrawal from normal activities, decreased performance at work or school. Each individual will present with different responses when in crisis, so it is important to take a holistic view and identify what changes they are presenting with and what is considered 'normal' for them.

Box 3.18 Activity: factors leading to mental health crisis

ACTIVITY

It is fundamental when assessing crisis and risk that you assess the person taking a holistic approach, as this will help you to understand the triggers and contributing factors for their distress.

Consider the impact that Diane's physical health has on the social and psychological aspects of her life, why this might lead to mental health crisis and what risks might she present with?

You may have considered the impact of increasing pain on Diane, she may as a result lose sleep and withdraw from activities and people. Her mobility is already limited so she may find it easier to stay at home and very quickly become isolated, and this could impact her mood. Due to her isolation, she may ruminate a lot, and, as a result, she may find it hard to see positive aspects of her life; so, she may develop depression, and as her worries increase about her future, she may also become anxious.

Learning outcome 3: explain what to consider when undertaking an assessment of risk

Risk assessment

You should first consider the ABCs of risk assessment (Callaghan 2012, p. 14)

a. Antecedents – What has provoked behaviours/presentation?
b. Behaviour – What are the presenting reactive behaviours?
c. Consequences – What are the consequences of those behavioural reactions?

Box 3.19 Applying ABC

ACTIVITY

Consider Natalie, from the scenario and apply ABC to what you know or might think about her situation. How might this inform the starting point of your risk assessment?

You might have thought about what provoked her to drink when at home: was she alone or with others? Can she explain why she has taken the overdose? Has she done this before or after drinking alcohol? What was she feeling/thinking at the time of taking them?

How much alcohol did she consume? Where did she get it from? Was it at home already or did she have to go out to buy it? In relation to the overdose, what has she taken? How many? Where did she get these from? Does she understand the possible consequences of taking these? How is she feeling now about the overdose?

Box 3.20 Risk and contributory factors

Actuarial/static risk factor – These are unchanging factors:

- Age
- Gender
- Ethnicity
- Genetic predisposition – family history of mental illness/suicide/self-harm
- Demographic/locations
- History of abuse/trauma
- Historical static risk – drug/alcohol/history of exposure to suicide (also family factors)
- Historical criminal activity
- Historical violence or aggression.

Dynamic/clinical risk factors: (related to mental health/physical health) changing factors – when present can increase risk:

- Mental state – low mood, psychotic symptoms, increased anxiety, manic depression
- Risk history – suicide attempts/self-harm
- Current presentation (level of distress/capacity/lack of insight)
- Suicidal/self-harm ideation
- Diagnosis
- Physical illness/smoking/obesity/high cholesterol
- Capacity to self-care
- Engagement levels – engaging well/disengaged
- Impulsivity
- Unresponsive to treatment.

Other contributing factors to current presentation and level of risk – including biopsychosocial events, factors or dynamics occurring in the broader environment

- Bereavement
- Family dynamics/relationship difficulties/lack of support
- Time of year (seasonal affective disorder, Christmas, birthdays, anniversaries, loss of loved ones)
- Poor sleep hygiene and nutritional intake
- Debt/financial difficulties/financial abuse

(Continued)

Box 3.20 (Continued)

- Domestic abuse/sexual abuse, bullying (children and adolescents)
- Homelessness/accommodation adequacy
- Drug use
  - Exposure to suicidal behaviours
  - Lack of support
  - Bullying (children and adolescents)
  - Poor sleep hygiene
  - Poor nutritional intake.

The factors in Box 3.20 could contribute to the level of risk, but this list is not exhaustive. These are the factors that may contribute to the person's risk vulnerability, which should be considered during your assessment, as should the risk categories below. In reality, many of these will be considered simultaneously during the assessment, and this will be easier the more confident and proficient the practitioner becomes.

Risk categories should assist healthcare professionals in their assessment and management of the presenting risk. These are aspects that should be considered with the person during risk assessment:

- self-harm
- suicide
- violence and aggression
- abuse
- self-neglect
- risk associated with disability
- physical health complications.

NICE guidelines (2009a) state that during commencement or increasing anti-depressant pharmacological treatment, there is an increased risk period of mood changes and suicidal ideations. In accordance with the NMC (2018c) Code of Conduct, it is the nurse's and nurse associate's responsibility to act immediately if there is a risk to the person's safety and therefore their responsibility to acknowledge and act on concerns.

Formulation of risk

When formulating your risk, if the responses are not disclosed with specific information, ask more open-ended questions to identify specific details. For example, if an individual states, 'I want to die', ask if they have plans or intentions to end their life? It is important to clarify the information they are giving you by asking for more details. This will also aid your clinical judgement and decision-making. A good example of how to ask relevant questions, depending on responses is given below.

Formulation of Risk (Royal College of Psychiatrists 2016) with examples:

- How serious is the risk? Can the risk be minimised or contained?
- Is the risk specific or general? I want to die (general)? I am going to end my life by taking an overdose (specific)?

- How immediate is the risk? I do not know when I will do it (not planned/ not immediate). I am going this afternoon when my husband leaves for work (planned/immediate)
- How volatile is the risk? Suicide, suicide including children, harm to others, involving potential death.
- Are circumstances likely to arise to increase risk? Non-compliance with treatment, being sent home alone, stressful situations, change in physical health, use of alcohol/drugs.
- What treatment or management plan can best reduce risk? Psychiatric assessment, hospital admission, crisis support, family support, community referral.

NICE guidance (2009b) suggests that when supporting a person with a physical health problem, you should be alert to the possibility of the person becoming depressed and even suicidal. They suggest that you should ask a couple of important questions:

- Be alert to possible depression (particularly with individuals with a past history of depression or a chronic physical health problem with associated functional impairment) and consider asking the person who may have depression two questions, specifically:

  - During the last month, have you often been bothered by feeling down, depressed or hopeless?
  - During the last month, have you often been bothered by having little interest or pleasure in doing things?

They then go on to suggest:

If a person with chronic physical health problems answers 'yes' to either of the depression identification questions (above), a practitioner who is competent to perform a mental health assessment should:

- ask three further questions to improve the accuracy of the assessment of depression, specifically:

  - during the last month, have you often been bothered by feelings of worthlessness?
  - during the last month, have you often been bothered by poor concentration?
  - during the last month, have you often been bothered by thoughts of death?

You may feel that you are not 'competent' to ask these questions and you would rather wait for a mental health specialist; however, not having this level of awareness means that the decisions you make about the person's care may be compromised. You may decide to leave the person alone in a cubicle or side room whilst you wait for the specialist team to attend. This may put the person at greater risk as the environment is not safe for a person who may have suicidal ideation. You may also feel uncomfortable asking these questions, but what they show is that having a full understanding of the level of risk is essential. If you consider there to be a risk, then, a timely referral to specialist services is essential (see Box 3.21).

Box 3.21 NICE (2021) guidance

If the person presents considerable immediate risk to themselves or others, refer them urgently to specialist mental health services.

Advise the person and their family or carer of the following, and ensure they know how to seek help promptly, if required:

- the potential for increased agitation, anxiety and suicidal ideation early in treatment; actively seek out these symptoms and review treatment if they develop marked and/or prolonged agitation
- the need to be vigilant for mood changes, negativity, hopelessness and suicidal ideation, particularly when starting or changing treatment and at times of increased stress

Available from: www.pathways.nice.org.uk/pathways/common-mental-health-disorders-in-primary-care

If the person you are assessing has any form of cognitive impairment such as a learning disability or dementia, then taking your time with the assessment is important, using clear English and giving the person time to think about what you have asked (see Box 3.22).

Box 3.22 NICE (2021) guidance

If the person has a learning disability or acquired cognitive impairment:

- consider consulting a relevant specialist when developing treatment plans
- where possible, provide the same interventions as for other people with depression; adjust the method of delivery or duration if necessary.

Clinical judgement, intuition, reflection and critical thinking along with systems, policies and procedure that are then combined with the information you have obtained through assessment all contribute to decision-making and outcomes (Standing 2017). One of the biggest challenges as a professional is making decisions that may have either positive or negative impacts on the individual's life. In particular, when making decisions around risk, the presentation of risk can be complex and the information you have may be incomplete. This may be due either to conflicting information or lack of information divulged by the individual you are assessing, decision-making becomes a complex task. It often feels like you are trying to predict the unpredictable. As health professionals, we make decisions continuously; therefore, it is valuable to know how we make decisions and how this can change as you gain experience and knowledge.

Critical decision-making with risk

Decision-making is a fundamental aspect of the health professional's role, whether these are ethical, political, practice-related or clinical and non-clinical decisions; they will have an influence on the care, safety and outcomes (Simmons et al. 2003; Tanner 2006). Decision-making can be a complex yet imperative process (Coulter et al. 2011) and is an essential and intricate part of the nurse's role to provide appropriate and harmless care. To protect the person and act in their best interests, in particular, when caring for an individual who is presenting with risk, it is important to know how we make decisions.

Decision-making in nursing can be not only complex but accompanied by uncertainty, which also requires the enforcement of policies and evidence-based practice, knowledge, and safe judgement, to preserve a person's rights and safety (Walker et al. 2013). For instance, the implementation and application of standards were set by the NMC Code (2018c), whereby nurses must maintain knowledge and skills to practice safely and effectively, which would include making decisions in the best interests of the person and being accountable for the decisions made.

The process of decision-making may sound simple; everyone makes decisions continuously throughout the day; it is claimed to be an unconscious cognitive process (Newell and Shanks 2014). However, despite this, it could be argued that decisions are not made unconsciously, often we need to actively think about them. Nevertheless, there are foundations that determine how we make decisions relating to the type of decision-maker we are. Therefore, within the individual's approach to decision-making, it is pivotal to take a look at the evidence in that moment to ensure any decision made will reduce risk and preserve the safety of the person.

It is important to consider people's views and engage them in the decision-making process, according to evidence, people who are actively involved and participate in the management of their healthcare have better quality outcomes than those who have decisions made for them (Coulter, Collins and Kings Fund 2011). The primary role of a nurse is to work towards restoring an optimum degree of autonomy for the person who has been affected as a result of illness or risk (Thompson et al. 2006). Equally, a lack of capacity may hinder an individual's ability to make decisions; therefore, during this process, capacity must be taken into consideration.

Learning outcome 4: discuss recommendations with regard to level of risk, especially with regard to self-harm and suicide

There is a growing concentration on addressing the needs of individuals who self-harm and/or are suicidal. As can be seen by the statistics in Box 3.23, this is an area of national and international concern. As a healthcare professional, you may come into contact with individuals who are experiencing suicidal ideation and/or self-harm, and this may be on many occasions; therefore, you have a vital role to play in the prevention of suicide and self-harm. The National Collaborating Centre for Mental Health and Health Education England (2018) have commissioned a framework designed to educate all individuals in a broad range of professions that have a significant part to play in self-harm and suicide prevention, to be able to support individuals that present with self-harm and suicide risks, in particular in relation to signposting and providing support. In the first instance, the priority is for individuals to be kept safe from harm, minimising immediate risk to self and or others. In any situation, you can work with the individual to create an 'immediate safety plan', which is a co-produced plan with the individual with pragmatic methods to help keep the individual safe whilst you identify the plan of care (Health Education England 2018). The contents of the safety plan will depend of the situation, location and presentation. For example it may mean reducing access to means of harming oneself, or it may require contacting of a family member or friend to offer support. It may require that the person's normal coping strategies are compromised, in the short term, for example, going out for a walk may not be a good idea as it can increase the risk of absconding.

Completing this with the individual will give them the opportunity to raise any questions they have about the plan.

Suicide and self-harm prevention

In the UK, suicide is defined as deaths given an underlying cause of intentional self-harm or injury/poisoning of undetermined intent.

Self-harm is when somebody intentionally damages or injures their body.

As we have seen previously from the statistics, suicide and self-harm present significant issues in the UK. Therefore, anyone who is in your care, who you think may be a risk, should have a management plan related to their safety.

Throughout your assessment, but in particular when identifying a safety plan, using empathy and compassion is vital and will ensure that the individual feels understood, supported and not judged. There are many misconceptions about suicide, not everyone who experiences suicidal ideation, actually wants to die; they just do not see any other alternative to their current experience or situation (Kakar and Nandy 2017). Hence the important need for a biopsychosocial approach in assessments, to identify the trigger and contributing factor of these thoughts and support them to identify safe and effective ways to manage them. You should always take into consideration the individual's capacity.

Box 3.23 Statistics

- In 2019, there were 5,691 suicides registered in England and Wales, an age-standardised rate of 11.0 deaths per 100,000 population and consistent with the rate in 2018.
- The England and Wales male suicide rate of 16.9 deaths per 100,000 is the highest since 2000 and remains in line with the rate in 2018; for females, the rate was 5.3 deaths per 100,000, consistent with 2018 and the highest since 2004.
- Males aged 45–49 years had the highest age-specific suicide rate (25.5 deaths per 100,000 males); for females, the age group with the highest rate was 50–54 years at 7.4 deaths per 100,000.
- Despite having a low number of deaths overall, rates among the under 25s have generally increased in recent years, particularly 10–24-year-old females where the rate has increased significantly since 2012 to its highest level with 3.1 deaths per 100,000 females in 2019.
- As seen in previous years, the most common method of suicide in England and Wales was hanging, accounting for 61.7% of all suicides among males and 46.7% of all suicides among females.
- Among the general population, 20.6% of people have had suicidal thoughts at some time, 6.7% have attempted suicide and 7.3% have self-harmed.

(Continued)

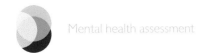

Box 3.23 (Continued)

- Mental Health Foundation statistics show that only 27% of people who died by suicide between 2005 and 2015 had been in contact with mental health services in the year before they died.
- People under the influence of drugs and alcohol are more likely to act on suicidal thoughts.

(Office of National Statistics 2019)

An essential aspect to include in a safety plan is any identified protective factors. We discussed how individuals develop protective factors at the beginning of this chapter, but what role do protective factors have? Protective factors are aspects or attributes in an individual's life that help them deal more effectively with stressful situations and can aid the mitigation of risk (Newman 2002). Protective factors act by reducing exposure to risk, as well as, decreasing the impact of risk should it manifest, and examples of some can be seen in Box 3.24. When completing a risk assessment, it is important to identify protective factors to identify the likelihood of risk, which may even include previous means and strategies of coping during difficult times (Simpson and Brenner 2019). For example, if an individual presents with suicidal ideation, you may ask them 'Can you identify a reason for living', and they may identify their family and support network as a protective factor. If the family and support network are actively involved and support the individual, the risk is likely to reduce, although not remove the risk altogether. Of course, with consent, involving family members, carers and friends in an assessment can add valuable information to keep them safe, and they can also aid and assist in supporting and keeping a person who has suicidal thoughts or plans safe (NICE 2019a). However, it is important to consider that should someone report their children as protective factors that you explore the risk to the children, in case they are included in any suicide plans or in particular if an act of self-harm has already taken place (Royal College of Psychiatry 2020).

It is also important to assess the likelihood of whether risk would change if their protective factor was taken away; for example, if the family/support network withdrew support, or were unable to support the individual, would this cause an increase in risk?

Box 3.24 Types of limitless protective factors

- Optimism, coping and problem-solving skills
- Social support – family and friends, community support
- Economic security
- Sense of self-worth
- Children and partner
- Pets
- Access to services – availability of physical and mental healthcare
- Cultural and religious beliefs that discourage suicide
- Supportive relationships with care providers
- Limited access to lethal means

Should an individual in your care present with a deterioration in their mental state and or present with a risk, following your assessment and implementing an immediate safety plan to ensure immediate safety, a referral to psychiatric services will be required, as previously stated (see Boxes 3.21 and 3.22).

Should you find yourself in the community or public space, then support should be sought from the police to support the individual to a place of safety (136 Suite/A&E) if you cannot do this yourself.

SECTION 136

Section 136 of the Mental Health Act 1983 (2007)

'Gives the police lawful powers to detain someone in a public place, who they believe may have a mental disorder and who may cause harm to themselves or another person and take them to a safe place where a mental health assessment can be carried out'.

A 'place of safety' is defined as:

A residential accommodation provided by a local social services authority under part III of the National Assistance Act 1948 (the Mental Health Act, 1983); A police station; An independent hospital or care home for mentally disordered persons (CQC 2014).

Urgent referrals should not be delayed, the timelier you intervene, the more chances of suicide prevention you have (NICE 2019b). Handover of clinical responsibilities should involve an effective, comprehensive sharing of all relevant information; it must also include the sharing of the management plan. The handover of responsibility of the individuals care to another clinician or service, must be successfully and explicitly accepted (Royal College of Psychiatrist 2020).

Summary
- You will understand what risk is, within a mental health situation
- You will also understand how a crisis can increase the level of risk
- You will understand what aspects to consider when assessing risk
- You will also understand aspects that may impact on the level of risk, especially in relation to self-harm and suicide.

CHAPTER SUMMARY

All nurses, whatever their primary care focus, must be able to keep people safe and provide an excellent quality of care. Within this chapter, you will have seen the importance of considering someone's mental health state and the care that they need. Undertaking an informed mental health assessment is essential if the person's care and risk are to be managed successfully.

Whilst it is excellent that current practice is for more collaborative work across specialities, mental health liaison staff are frequently found in acute mental health trusts. It is still important that all healthcare staff have mental health knowledge so that they can ensure that the person remains safe whilst in their care. Mental health and risk can change very quickly, so this is a very dynamic area and the nurse and nurse associate have to be aware of this potential. This chapter addresses many of the pertinent issues that you will need to consider and also identifies areas for further reading and learning.

REFERENCES

American Psychiatric Association. 2013. Diagnostic and Statistical Manual of Mental Disorders (DSM-5) Available from: https://www.psychiatry.org/psychiatrists/practice/dsm (Accessed on 15 January 2021).

Baillie, L. 2014. *Developing Practical Nursing Skills*, 4th edn. Boca Raton, FL: Taylor and Francis.

Caldicott, F. 2013. *Caldicott Committee Information: To Share or Not To Share? The Information Governance Review.* London: Department of Health.

Callaghan, P. 2012. *Emergencies in Mental Health Nursing.* Oxford: Oxford University Press.

Callaghan, P. and Gamble, C. 2015. *Oxford Handbook of Mental Health Nursing*, 2nd edn. Oxford: Oxford University Press.

Care Quality Commission (CQC). 2009. National study: The right information, in the right place, at the right time. Available from: http://systems.hscic.gov.uk/infogov/links/cqcigstudy.pdf Accessed (Accessed on 29 November 2020).

Care Quality Commission (CQC). 2011. *The Mental Capacity Act 2005: Guidance for Providers: A New system of registration.* Available from: https://www.cqc.org.uk/sites/default/files/documents/rp_poc1b2b_100563_20111223_v4_00_guidance_for_providers_mca_for_external_publication.pdf (Accessed on 29 November 2020).

Care Quality Commission (CQC). 2014. A safer place to be, findings from our survey of health-based places of safety for people detained under section 136 of the MHA [Online] Available from: https://www.cqc.org.uk/sites/default/files/20141021%20CQC_SaferPlace_2014_07_FINAL%20for%20WEB.pdf (Accessed on 9 March 2021).

Carniaux-Moran, C. 2013. *The Psychiatric Nursing Assessment.* Burlington: Jones and Bartlett Learning.

Chambers, M. 2017. *Psychiatric and Mental Health Nursing; The Craft of Caring*, 3rd edn. Oxon: Taylor and Francis.

Coulter, A., Collins, A. and Kings Fund. 2011. Making shared decision-making a reality, no decision about me, without me. Available from: http://www.kingsfund.org.uk/sites/files/kf/Making-shared-decision-making-a-reality-paper-Angela-Coulter-Alf-Collins-July-2011_0.pdf (Accessed on 21 January 2021).

Department of Constitutional Affairs. 2007. Mental Capacity Act: Code of practice. Available from: https://assets.publishing.service.gov.uk/government/uploads/system/uploads/attachment_data/file/921428/Mental-capacity-act-code-of-practice.pdf (Accessed on 1 March 2021).

Department of Health. 2011. No health without mental health: A cross- government mental health outcomes strategy for people of all ages, Analysis of the Impact on Equality (AIE). Available from: https://assets.publishing.service.gov.uk/government/uploads/system/uploads/attachment_data/file/138253/dh_124058.pdf (Accessed on 9 June 2021).

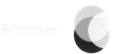

Department of Health. 2014. Closing the gap; priorities for essential change in mental health [Online] Available from: https://assets.publishing.service.gov.uk/government/uploads/system/uploads/attachment_data/file/281250/Closing_the_gap_V2_-_17_Feb_2014.pdf (Accessed on 18 December 2020)

Department of Health. 2015a. MHA 1983: Code of practice. Available from: https://assets.publishing.service.gov.uk/government/uploads/system/uploads/attachment_data/file/435512/MHA_Code_of_Practice.PDF (Accessed on 29 November 2020).

Department of Health. 2015b. 'Nothing ventured, nothing gained': Risk guidance for people with dementia [online] Available from: https://assets.publishing.service.gov.uk/government/uploads/system/uploads/attachment_data/file/215960/dh_121493.pdf (Accessed on 18 December 2020).

Education England. 2021. Mental Deficiency Act 1913. Available from: http://www.educationengland.org.uk/documents/acts/1913-mental-deficiency-act.html#:~:text=Mental%20Deficiency%20Act%201913%20%2D%20full%20text&text=This%20Act%20sets%20out%20arrangements,%20of%20appropriate%20accommodation%20for%20them (Accessed on 12 April 2021).

Elder, R., Evans, K. and Nizette, D. 2011. *Psychiatric & Mental Health Nursing – E-Book*. Australia-New Zealand: Elsevier Health Science.

Elliott, I. 2016. *Poverty and Mental Health: A Review to Inform the Joseph Rowntree Foundation's Anti-Poverty Strategy*. London: Mental Health Foundation.

Equality and Human Rights Commission. 2015. *Preventing Deaths in Detention of Adults with Mental Health Conditions*, An Inquiry by the Equality and Human Rights Commission [Online] Available from: http://www.equalityhumanrights.com/sites/default/files/publication_pdf/Adult%20Deaths%20in%20Detention%20Inquiry%20Report.pdf (Accessed on 1 November 2020).

Fischhoff, B., Nightingale, E. and Iannotta, J. 2001. *Adolescent Risk and Vulnerability, Concepts and Measurement*. Washington D.C: National Academies Press, p. 56.

Great Britain. 1998. Human Rights Act. Available from: https://www.legislation.gov.uk/ukpa/1998/42/contents (Accessed on 1 March 2021).

Great Britain. 2005. Mental Capacity Act 2005. Available from: https://www.legislation.gov.uk/ukpa/2005/9/pdfs/ukpa_20050009_en.pdf (Accessed on 1 March 2021).

Great Britain. 2007. Mental Health Act (MHA) 2007(amended the MHA 1983). Available from: https://www.legislation.gov.uk/ukpa/2007/12/contents (Accessed on 1 March 2021).

Great Britain. 2012. Health and Social Care Act 2012. Available from: https://www.legislation.gov.uk/ukpa/2012/7/contents/enacted (Accessed on 1 March 2021).

Hart, C. 2014. *A Pocket Guide to Risk Assessment and Management in Mental Health*. Oxon: Taylor and Francis, p. 9.

Health Education England. 2018. Self-harm and suicide prevention competence frameworks; Community and Public health. Available from: https://www.rcpsych.ac.uk/docs/default-source/improving-care/nccmh/self-harm-and-suicide-prevention-competence-framework/nccmh-self-harm-and-suicide-prevention-competence-framework-public-health.pdf?sfvrsn=341fb3cd_6 (Accessed on 18 December 2020).

HM Government. 2018. Information sharing; Advice for practitioners providing safeguarding services to children, young people, parents and careers. Available from: https://assets.publishing.service.gov.uk/government/uploads/system/uploads/attachment_data/file/721581/Information_sharing_advice_practitioners_safeguarding_services.pdf (Accessed on 18 December 2020).

Human Dignity Trust. 2021. Map of countries that criminalise LGBT people. Available from: https://www.humandignitytrust.org/lgbt-the-law/map-of-criminalisation/ (Accessed on 5 February 2021).

James, R.K. and Gilliland, B.E. 2016. *Crisis Intervention Strategies*, 8th edn. Boston, MA: Cengage Learning, p. 9.

Jessor, R. 2017. *Problem Behaviour Theory and Adolescent Health; The Collected Works of Richard Jessor*, Volume 2. Switzerland: Springer International Publishing.

Kakar, A. and Nandy, S. 2017. *Understanding Mental Illness*. India: Elsevier Health Sciences.

Kingdon, D., Rathod, S. and Asher, C. 2017. Classification of mental illness. In Chambers M. (ed.) *Psychiatric and Mental Health Nursing. The Craft of Caring*, 3rd edn. Oxon: Routledge, pp. 127–134.

The Kings Fund. 2008. Mental Health Act 2007. Available from: https://www.kingsfund.org.uk/sites/default/files/briefing-mental-health-act-2007-simon-lawton-smith-kings-fund-december-2008.pdf (Accessed on 9 March 2021).

The Kings Fund. 2016. Bringing together physical and mental health; a new frontier for integrated care. Available from: https://www.kingsfund.org.uk/publications/physical-and-mental-health (Accessed on 18 December 2020).

The Kings Fund. 2019. Leading for integrated care. Available from: https://www.kingsfund.org.uk/sites/default/files/2019-11/leading-for-integrated-care.pdf (Accessed on 18 December 2020).

The Kings Fund. 2020. What are health inequalities? Available from: https://www.kingsfund.org.uk/publications/what-are-health-inequalities (Accessed on 9 January 2021).

Lappin, M. 2018. The nursing process. In: Peate, I. and Wild, K. (eds.) *Nursing Practice: Knowledge and Care*, 2nd edn. Oxford: Wiley, pp. 111–128.

Mental Health (Care and Treatment) (Scotland) Act. 2015. Available from: https://www.gov.scot/policies/mental-health/legislation-and-guidance/ (Accessed on 9 March 2021).

Mental Health Care. 2015. Stigma and discrimination. Available from: http://www.mentalhealthcare.org.uk/discrimination_and_stigma (Accessed on 20 November 2020).

The National Collaborating Centre for Mental Health and Health Education England. 2018. Self-harm and suicide prevention competence framework, Community and Public Health. Available from: https://www.ucl.ac.uk/pals/sites/pals/files/self-harm_and_suicide_prevention_competence_framework_-_public_health_8th_oct_18.pdf (Accessed on 9 January 2021).

National Health Service. 1999. A national service framework for mental health. Available from: https://assets.publishing.service.gov.uk/government/uploads/system/uploads/attachment_data/file/198051/National_Service_Framework_for_Mental_Health.pdf (Accessed 20 November 2020).

National Health Service. 2019. The NHS long term plan. Available from: https://www.longtermplan.nhs.uk/ (Accessed on 15 January 2021).

National Institute for Clinical Excellence (NICE) 2004 Self harm: Clinical Guidance CG16. Available from: https://www.nice.org.uk/guidance/cg16/chapter/1-Guidance#special-issues-for-older-people-older-than-65-years. (Accessed on 18 December 2020).

National Institute for Clinical Excellence (NICE). 2009a. Depression in adults: Recognition and management. Available from: https://www.nice.org.uk/guidance/CG90/chapter/1-Guidance (Accessed on 18 December 2020).

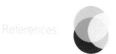

National Institute for Clinical Excellence (NICE). 2009b. Depression in adults with a chronic physical health problem; recognition and management. NICE guideline CG91. Available from: https://www.nice.org.uk/guidance/cg91/chapter/Recommendations (Accessed on 15 February 2021).

National Institute for Clinical Excellence (NICE). 2013. Mental well-being of older people in care homes QS50. Available from: https://www.nice.org.uk/guidance/qs50/resources/mental-wellbeing-of-older-people-in-care-homes-pdf-2098720457413 (Accessed on 10 December 2020).

National institute for Clinical Excellence (NICE). 2015. BiPolar, Psychosis and Schizophrenia in children and young people; Quality Statement 6 Monitoring for side effects of anti-psychotic medication. Available from https://www.nice.org.uk/guidance/qs102/chapter/quality-statement-6-monitoring-for-side-effects-of-antipsychotic-medication. (Accessed on 27 October 2021)

National Institute for Clinical Excellence (NICE). 2019a. NICE impact mental health. Available from: https://www.nice.org.uk/Media/Default/About/what-we-do/Into-practice/measuring-uptake/NICEimpact-mental-health.pdf (Accessed on 10 December 2020).

National Institute for Clinical Excellence (NICE). 2019b. Suicide prevention 1.3.1. Available from: https://www.nice.org.uk/guidance/qs189 (Accessed on 10 December 2020).

National Institute for Clinical Excellence (NICE). 2020. Mental health and wellbeing. Available from: https://www.nice.org.uk/guidance/lifestyle-and-wellbeing/mental-health-and-wellbeing (Accessed on 16 November 2020).

National Institute for Clinical Excellence (NICE). 2021. Step 1 Recognition, assessment and initial management of depression in adults/ Available from https://pathways.nice.org.uk/pathways/depression. (Accessed on 18 December 2020).

Newell, B. and Shanks, D. 2014. Unconscious influences on decision making: A critical review. Available from: http://www.ncbi.nlm.nih.gov/pubmed/24461214 (Accessed on 18 December 2020).

Newman, T. 2002. *Promoting Resilience: A Review of Effective Strategies for Child Care Services.* Centre for Evidence Based Social Services: University of Exeter.

Nursing Midwifery Council (NMC). 2018a. Standards for pre registration nursing programmes. Available from: https://www.nmc.org.uk/globalassets/sitedocuments/standards-of-proficiency/standards-for-pre-registration-nursing-programmes/programme-standards-nursing.pdf (Accessed on 16 November 2020).

Nursing Midwifery Council (NMC). 2018b. The Code: Professional standards of practice and behaviour for Nurses, Midwives and Nursing Associates. Available from: https://www.nmc.org.uk/globalassets/sitedocuments/nmc-publications/nmc-code.pdf (Accessed on 16 November 2020).

Nursing Midwifery Council (NMC). 2018c. The Code: Professional standards of practice and behaviour for nurses and midwives. Available from: http://www.nmc.org.uk/standards/code/ (Accessed on 18 December 2020).

O'Brien, A., Johnson, C., Nizette, D and Evans, K. 2019. *Psychiatric and Mental Health Nursing in the UK*, 4th edn. Australia: Elsevier Health Sciences.

Office of National Statistics. 2019. Suicides in England and Wales: 2019 registrations, Registered deaths in England and Wales from suicide analysed by sex, age, area of usual residence of the deceased and suicide method. Available from: https://www.ons.gov.

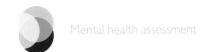

uk/peoplepopulationandcommunity/birthsdeathsandmarriages/deaths/bulletins/suicid esintheunitedkingdom/2019registrations (Accessed on 9 January 2021).

Office of National Statistics. 2020. Coronavirus and depression in adults, Great Britain: June 2020. Available from: https://www.ons.gov.uk/peoplepopulationandcommunity/ wellbeing/articles/coronavirusanddepressioninadultsgreatbritain/june2020. (Accessed on 18 March 2021).

Peate, I. 2020. *Fundamentals of Assessment and Care Planning for Nurses.* Oxford: John Wiley and sons.

Public Health England. 2018. Severe mental illness (SMI) and physical health inequalities: Briefing. Available from: https://www.gov.uk/government/publications/severe-mental-illness-smi-physical-health-inequalities/severe-mental-illness-and-physical-health-inequalities-briefing#main-findings\ (Accessed on 16 November 2020).

Royal College of Nursing. 2019. *Parity of esteem, delivering physical health equality for those with serious mental health needs.* London: Royal College of Nursing.

Royal College of Nursing. 2020. Principles of nursing practice. Available from: https:// www.rcn.org.uk/professional-development/principles-of-nursing-practice (Accessed on 18 December 2020).

Royal College of Psychiatrists. 2016. Assessment and management of risk to others; good practice guide, p. 3. Available from: https://www.rcpsych.ac.uk/docs/default-source/ members/supporting-you/managing-and-assessing-risk/assessmentandmanage-mentrisktoothers.pdf?sfvrsn=a614e4f9_4 (Accessed on 18 December 2020).

Royal College of Psychiatrists. 2020. Self-harm and suicide in adults; Final report of the Patient Safety Group 2020. Available from: https://www.rcpsych.ac.uk/docs/default-source/improving-care/better-mh-policy/college-reports/college-report-cr229-self-harm-and-suicide.pdf?sfvrsn=b6fdf395_10 (Accessed on 9 January 2021).

Sale, J. and Neale, N.M. 2014. The nurse's approach and communication: Foundations for compassionate care. In: Baillie, L. (ed.) *Developing Practical Nursing Skills*, 4th edn. Boca Raton, FL: Taylor and Francis.

Simmons, B., Lanuza, D. and Fonteyn, M. et al. 2003. Clinical reasoning in experienced nurses. *Western Journal of Nursing Research* 25(6): 701–19. Available from: http://www. ncbi.nlm.nih.gov/pubmed/14528618 (Accessed on 18 December 2020).

Simpson, K. and Brenner, L. 2019. *Suicide Prevention after Neurodisability; An Evidence-Informed Approach.* Oxford: Oxford University Press.

Standing, M. 2017. *Clinical Judgement and Decision Making in Nursing*, 3rd edn. London: SAGE Publications.

Tanner, C.A. 2006. Thinking like a nurse: A research-based model of clinical judgement in nursing. *Journal of Nursing Education* 45(6): 204–11. Available from: http://www. mccc.edu/nursing/documents/Thinking_Like_A_Nurse_Tanner.pdf (Accessed on 18 December 2020).

Tee, S., Brown, J. and Carpenter, D. 2012. *Handbook of Mental Health Nursing.* Boca Raton, FL: CRC Press.

Thompson, I., Melia, K., Boyd, K. and Horsburgh, D. 2006. *Nursing Ethics*, 5th edn. London: Elsevier.

Tranter, S. and Robertson, M. 2019. Improving the physical health of people with a mental illness: holistic nursing assessments. *Mental Health Practice* 22(4): 34–41.

Walker, S., Carpenter, D. and Middlewick, Y. 2013. *Assessment and Decision making in Mental Health Nursing.* London: Sage Publications.

Weber, J. 2014. *Nurse's Handbook of Health Assessment*, 8th edn. China: Wolters Kluwer Lippincott Williams and Wilkins.

Woolf, S., Kuzel, A., Dovey, S., Phillips, R. 2004. A string of mistakes: The importance of cascade analysis in describing, counting, and preventing medical errors. *Journal of Department of Family Medicine Virginia Commonwealth University, Richmond* 2(4): 317–26. Available from: http://www.annfammed.org/content/2/4/317.full.pdf+html (Accessed on 16 November 2020).

World Health Organization (WHO). 1948. Basic documents- constitution of the World Health Organization. Available from: https://apps.who.int/gb/bd/pdf_files/BD_49th-en.pdf. (Accessed on 1 March 2021).

World Health Organization (WHO). 2003 Investing in mental health. Available from: https://www.who.int/mental_health/media/investing_mnh.pdf. (Accessed on 1 March 2021).

World Health Organization (WHO). 2010. International Classification of Disease (ICD-10) Available from: https://icd.who.int/browse10/2010/en#/V (Accessed on 18 December 2020).

World Health Organization (WHO). 2018. Continuity and coordination of care; a practice brief to support implementation of the WHO Framework on integrated people-centred health services. Available from: https://apps.who.int/iris/bitstream/handle/10665/274628/9789241514033-eng.pdf?ua=1 (Accessed on 18 December 2020).

RECOMMENDED FURTHER READING

https://www.rcpsych.ac.uk/docs/default-source/improving-care/better-mh-policy/college-reports/college-report-cr229-self-harm-and-suicide.pdf?sfvrsn=b6fdf395_10

https://assets.publishing.service.gov.uk/government/uploads/system/uploads/attachment_data/file/939479/PHE_LA_Guidance_25_Nov.pdf

https://fingertips.phe.org.uk/profile-group/mental-health/profile/suicide/da

For specific ante and post natal concerns go to;

Knight, M., Bunch, K., Tuffnell, D., Jayakody, H., Shakespeare, J., Kotnis, R., Kenyon, S. and Kurinczuk, J.J. (eds.) on behalf of MBRRACE-UK. 2018. *Saving Lives, Improving Mothers' Care – Lessons Learned to Inform Maternity Care from the UK and Ireland Confidential Enquiries into Maternal Deaths and Morbidity 2014–16*. Oxford: National Perinatal Epidemiology Unit, University of Oxford.

Or

NPEU, University of Oxford. 2013. Maternal health and wellbeing in the perinatal period. Available from: https://www.npeu.ox.ac.uk/research/projects/103-maternal-health-and-wellbeing-in-the-perinatal-period?highlight=WyJwZXJpbmF0YWwiLCIncGVyaW5hdGFsJyIsIidwZXJpbmF0YWwiLCJtZW50YWwiLCJoZWFsdGgiLCJoZWFsdGgnLiIsIidoZWFsdGgiLCJwZXJpbmF0YWwgbWVudGFsIiwicGVyaW5hdGFsIGllbnRhbCBoZWFsdGgiLCJtZW50YWwgaGVhbHRoIl0=

4

Measuring and monitoring vital signs

Sue Maddex

Measuring and monitoring the six vital signs of respiratory rate (RR), oxygen saturation SpO$_2$ blood pressure (BP), pulse (HR), ACVPU scale (alert, new confusion, voice, pain, and unresponsive) and temperature (T) are essential to health care professionals each day. Collectively they are referred to as vital signs and make up the components of the National Early-Warning Score 2 (NEWS2). All student nurses and nursing associates should learn to measure and record vital signs accurately (Nursing and Midwifery Council [NMC] 2018a, 2018b). Acting upon vital sign measurements in a timely and appropriate manner can contribute to the recognition of deterioration of the individual's condition and help to gain an understanding of their well-being.

This chapter includes the following topics:

Box 4.1 Recommended biology reading

Recommended biology reading

To gain an understanding of vital signs measurement and monitoring, reviewing the following questions will help you focus on biology, underpinning the skills outlined in this chapter. Use your university course recommended anatomy and physiology textbook to find answers to the following questions:

What is homeostasis and why is it important?

Respiratory system

- What are the components of the respiratory system (e.g. airways, respiratory muscles, control mechanisms) and what are their functions?
- How do these functions contribute to maintaining homeostasis?
- What is the main function of the respiratory system?
- How is ventilation controlled?
- How is oxygen transported in the body?
- Where does gaseous exchange occur? Which gases are being exchanged?
- Why does this exchange occur? What may affect this exchange?
- How does inspiration occur? What is the stimulus for us to breathe?
- What are the proportions of gases in atmospheric, alveolar and expired air?
- What factors are required for adequate tissue oxygenation to occur? Consider the role blood plays in this oxygenation

(Continued)

DOI: 10.4324/9781003020660-4

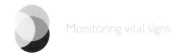

Box 4.1 (Continued)

Cardiovascular system

- What are the components of the cardiovascular system?
- Which vessels usually carry oxygenated blood?
- Why does blood travel in one direction?
- Name the four chambers of the heart, the great vessels and valves. Draw a diagram of the heart and label these structures. Indicate the direction in which oxygenated and deoxygenated blood flows through the heart.
- What are the layers of the heart wall and what types of tissue are they composed of?
- How does the heart contract in such a coordinated way? Explore the route taken by impulses through the myocardium.
- Myocardial tissue needs its own blood supply. Where are the coronary vessels located? What would result from their blockage?
- Compare the structures of arteries, capillaries and veins. Which vessels permit gaseous exchange and why? Which vessels contain valves?
- When tissues are damaged, an inflammatory process is initiated to repair the damage. What are the clinical signs of inflammation? What role does histamine play in inflammation? Why is inflammation of brain tissue potentially life-threatening?
- What role does blood play in maintaining cellular homeostasis?
- What are the components of blood and what specific roles do they play?
- Where are blood cells produced?
- What is haemostasis? Why is it important?
- What is BP and how is it maintained?

Temperature control

- Which body systems are involved in thermoregulation?
- How is heat generated within the body?
- How is heat lost from the body?
- What effect does temperature have on cellular function?
- What happens if the body starts to get too hot or too cold?
- Why do we appear flushed when too warm?

Nervous system

- What are the different areas of the brain?
- What are the components of the nervous system?
- What is the role of the autonomic nervous system?
- What are the functions of the parasympathetic and sympathetic nervous systems?

PRACTICE SCENARIOS

Observation and recording of a person's vital signs are carried out for many reasons. NMC (2018a) in their nursing procedures recommendations state that registered nurses should be able to demonstrate proficiency in vital signs measurement and interpretation. The following scenarios are used to assist you with putting these skills you learnt to practical use with people you might encounter in practice settings.

Adult

Mrs Anne Parkinson is a 56-year-old woman who has been taken to the Emergency Department by ambulance after a head injury as a result of her falling from her bicycle. She cannot remember the accident but was apparently unresponsive for 2–3 min afterwards. She is alert but appears disorientated. Her husband is present.

Learning disability

Ken O'Reilly is a 49-year-old man with Down's syndrome and a moderate learning disability. He has some verbal communication difficulties. He lives in a small group home with a live-in staff team. Ken is known to the community learning disability nurse (CLDN) as he is prone to chronic chest infections. He has oxygen therapy and a nebuliser at home, which the staff team have been trained to support him with. The nurse, while carrying out routine **health facilitator's** training with the staff team, is informed that Ken is unwell and is asked for advice. The nurse records Ken's vital signs and advises the staff to arrange for the general practitioner (GP) to visit to carry out further health assessment.

Mental health

Natalie Turney is 21 years old. She has been admitted as a voluntary inpatient to an acute mental health ward with severe depression. After going home for a day, she returns to the ward, appearing unsteady on her feet and she has a strong smell of alcohol. Her speech is very slurred and she is quite uncommunicative. When the staff ask her if she has taken any tablets, she mentions some little yellow pills and paracetamol. However, she will not give details about the quantity or when she took them.

EQUIPMENT REQUIRED FOR THIS CHAPTER

Before working through this chapter, find out what vital signs recording equipment is available within the skills laboratory or your practice area. Look for:

- thermometers: may be tympanic, electronic probes, chemical disposable.
- sphygmomanometers: electronic and/or manual equipment.
- pulse oximeter for recording oxygen saturations.
- technological monitoring devices that record temperature, pulse, BP, oxygen saturation – check your local trust to identify which devices are regularly used and check that you are aware of how these should be operated.

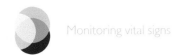

- NEWS2 chart or technological devices for vital signs recording, e.g. e-observations.
- Glasgow coma scale (GCS) chart or technological device with GCS programme.

You may wish to work through the sections with a colleague so that you can practise skills mentioned in this chapter.

Recent advancements in vital signs monitoring

Numerous changes have been seen in clinical areas regarding measuring, monitoring and escalating vital signs. Many major clinical NHS trusts are now implementing the use of bedside handheld and mobile devices to monitor vital signs (NHS England 2019). They highlight how their use has the potential to improve individual care and assist staff experience in handover situations. The increase in the use of handheld devices and the move away from paper charts have changed the face of vital signs monitoring. The handheld devices, technology and Wi-Fi devices (e-observations) have significantly improved healthcare workers' understanding of vital signs and assist in the recognition of possible deterioration. For example, e-observation systems enable vital signs to be measured, recorded and escalated throughout a person's care. Hence early deterioration can be tracked and acted upon immediately.

The digital systems used for vital signs in hospital settings enable data to be shared with prehospital situations, e.g. ambulance trust and community settings. Individual vital signs from the community setting can also be used to inform their care within a hospital stay. This enables vital signs monitoring to follow from home, hospital setting and back to a community setting. For example, while in hospital, a person can be tracked for sepsis, acute kidney injury and other signs of deterioration. Communication can be improved between fellow healthcare professionals for the benefit of both individual and healthcare professionals.

Purpose of vital signs monitoring

The purpose of vital signs measurement is part of the overall primary assessment of the person. It establishes a baseline for their physical health and offers future comparison to help identify abnormalities of well-being. The Royal College of Physicians, [RCP] (2017) identify that physiological observations should be recorded and interpreted accurately for all adults admitted to acute hospitals so that deterioration is recognised and responded to early. They report how vital signs are primary indicators of physiological status and demonstrate signs of deterioration. However, there is a potential that vital signs can be misinterpreted, mismanaged and often omitted (Bucknall et al. 2017). The move towards handheld devices used in the prehospital situation and at the bedside has attempted to address this issue in many clinical areas. When recorded accurately and responded to quickly, vital signs can provide person-centred healthcare assessments. Their recording and reporting enable the best interests of the person to be considered, promoting health and preventing ill health. They can provide information in accessible ways to help people understand and make decisions about their health requirements. For example, a person who has a high BP can be monitored to see if they require medication to reduce their risk factors of **stroke** or coronary heart disease. A person with a high temperature and of a non-healing wound can be reviewed to consider for potential signs of infection.

How vital signs change in times of injury or disease is important to understand. The NMC (2018a: 3.2) proficiency indicates that registered nurses should be able to "demonstrate and apply knowledge of body systems and homeostasis, human anatomy and physiology, biology genomics, pharmacology and social and behavioural sciences" when undertaking full and accurate assessments and developing appropriate care plans, and from nursing associates, a similar proficiency is expected when delivering care (2018b: 3.2). Gaining an understanding of relevant physiology will assist practitioners in understanding the significance of monitoring the six parameters of vital signs and the necessity of measuring and recording and escalating a NEWS2 score (RCP 2017). Brekke et al. (2019) highlight how vital signs monitoring show changes in a person's condition and thus detect preventable outcomes. Sepsis and acute kidney injury alerts within such systems can potentially offer life-changing alerts to improve care.

The use of technological devices to monitor a person's vital signs is a healthcare procedure that is carried out many times in a shift in a clinical setting. The frequency of their measurement is dependent upon the person's health condition. Over recent years, since 2012, a national early-warning scoring system (NEWS) has been adopted by many clinical areas. Firstly, the systems are available in paper chart form (RCP 2012) and secondly, those available from 2017 NEWS2 are also included in technological devices to measure vital signs, e.g. e-observation systems. The development and refinement of this tool continues with updates being offered frequently to reflect current and contemporary practices.

The recording of a national early-warning score (NEWS2) for all those hospitalised has now been implemented in many clinical areas and is approved and endorsed by NHS England and NHS Improvement. Prehospital practitioners, GPs, 999 call handlers and community-based clinicians are using this tool to measure, monitor and escalate concerns about a person's deterioration (RCP 2017). This system has been endorsed for electronic notification and documentation of data about a person's vital signs and is an evidence-based digital charting system for vital signs observations and facilitates calculation of the NEWS score. This subject along with individual deterioration is addressed further in Chapter 14.

Before proceeding with this chapter's activities, please familiarise yourself with the NEWS2 chart (RCP 2017). Available from: https://www.rcplondon.ac.uk/projects/outputs/national-early-warning-score-news-2 (Accessed 9 June 2021).

KEY PRINCIPLES IN VITAL SIGNS MEASUREMENT

When measuring, monitoring and recording vital signs, there are some key principles that you should always apply. These principles are explored in this section.

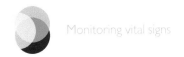

Learning outcome 1: explain key principles that apply to the measurement of vital signs

As explained in the introduction to this chapter, vital signs measurement is a key aspect of a person's assessment. The results contribute to decisions about further investigations and treatment, including future goals that might include medication prescriptions. Accurate measurement is therefore crucial. Effective communication with the person who is having their vital signs recorded is imperative and it is important to recognise that vital sign parameters can change in times of anxiety and stress. Fernandez–Ayuso et al. (2018) reported that nursing students undergoing cardiopulmonary resuscitation (CPR) training experienced both physiological and psychological effects on their vital signs. With this in mind, try to alleviate anxiety for a person when recording their vital signs. This can be achieved by explaining what you are doing and why, and the results of your findings and explaining how these act as a baseline for their care.

Box 4.3 Activity: accuracy of vital signs measurement

ACTIVITY

Now consider what might affect the accuracy of vital signs measurement?

You might have considered the following:

The equipment used. The National Institute for Health and Clinical Excellence (NICE 2016) highlights that electronic devices and manual equipment used for vital signs measurement should be properly validated. Equipment should be maintained and regularly recalibrated according to manufacturer's instructions. When new devices are introduced into clinical settings, staff must be trained to use them correctly, in accordance with manufacturers' instructions.

The competence of the person recording vital signs. The NMC (2018a, 2018b) state that a registered nurse and nursing associate should be able to take, record and interpret vital signs manually and via technological devices. To attain these skills, consider how competence can be developed. This can include how to carry out the practical skill, including documentation, the approach of the healthcare worker (discussed further in learning outcome 3). The underpinning knowledge and understanding of how to interpret the results and plan appropriate actions are also important considerations. Documenting the skills and reporting the measurements are crucial to ensure that abnormalities or potential problems are identified and addressed promptly. In any practice setting, ensure that you become familiar with the documentation in use, including national early-warning score/track and trigger systems (NEWS2) (also see Chapter 14). After recording vital signs via technological devices, discuss the results with a qualified nurse, so that appropriate actions can be taken if the recordings fall outside the normal parameters.

It is essential that you learn and then rehearse vital signs measurement frequently to develop competence and confidence. Practising vital signs skills within simulated environments can help you to contextualise these skills and support the acquisition of your clinical skills. Take every opportunity to practice vital signs measurement in different situations, for example, emergencies, and with people across the life span. Consider practising your skills in using a variety of equipment including manual and electronic devices to maintain your clinical proficiency. If you are using technological devices, ensure that you understand the system fully, including how to enter data and how this will be monitored and escalated and by whom. Ensure that the vital signs monitored are viewed in the context of the person's overall physical and mental health. The value of using vital signs trends for predicting and monitoring clinical deterioration should not be underestimated. They play an important role in the nursing assessment.

Vital signs measurement across the life span. The Royal College of Nursing [RCN] (2017) highlighted that practitioners who assess, measure and monitor vital signs in infants, children and young people should be competent in observing their physiological status and be aware of vital signs parameters for different age ranges. This is further supported by NMC (2018a and b) standards to ensure all nurses, and nursing associates in all fields of nursing understand how to measure and monitor vital signs. This book focuses on adults, but in each section, you will be advised about the normal parameters across the age range and guided to further resources. How vital signs may alter during pregnancy and key factors in interpreting vital signs in pregnancy are also highlighted, as a nurse may care for pregnant mothers when they have other health issues.

Learning outcome 2: reflect on how the healthcare provider's approach will affect vital signs measurement

Box 4.4 Activity: reflecting on the importance of accurate vital signs measurement

Reflect on how the healthcare worker's approach to a person might affect both the accuracy of vital signs measurement and the person's care experience.

When carrying out clinical observations, effective non-verbal and verbal communication skills are essential (covered in Chapter 2). You may be aware that HR, RR and BP are affected by emotions, for example, fear, anxiety or anger. Therefore,

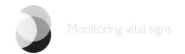
for accurate measurements, individuals need to feel comfortable with you and well informed. Ensure that you introduce yourself, are friendly and kind, gain consent (e.g. 'Is it ok if I check your blood pressure?') and explain what you are doing. Taking this approach will promote accurate measurements and dignity in care. You must also foster confidence in your ability to perform these skills accurately, hence the need to develop your competence. Displaying uncertainty in your skills may produce fear and anxiety in people, thus altering their vital signs measurements.

Learning outcome 3: consider how technological developments are influencing vital signs measurement

The future of vital signs monitoring lies in the development and production of electronic devices that further record, interpret and analyse vital signs to enhance care.

Box 4.5 Activity: technological developments relating to vital signs measurement

Are you aware of any technological developments relating to vital signs measurement?
Consider: What might be the associated advantages and safety issues?

ACTIVITY

The increasing world of technology, smartphones and tablet applications and Wi-Fi availability is undoubtedly assisting healthcare professionals in their care delivery. This wireless technology for healthcare workers enables practitioners to offer immediate advice regarding vital signs readings to the individual or other healthcare professionals. For example, those being monitored for hypertension (high BP) can send their BP readings to GP surgeries for monitoring and interpretation. Paramedic crews can liaise with emergency departments regarding vital signs when caring for those who are critically ill. Recording and reporting and escalating on NEWS2 scores and using these as a common language between healthcare professionals from prehospital situations to discharge inevitably can improve the person's care. In a community setting, the individual's vital signs results can be sent to the doctor's or senior nurse's smartphone or tablet device to ensure that the critically ill are assessed and treated in a timely manner. Safety issues include the validity of devices and applications; only those tools that are validated and accepted within your practice area should be used. Security of individual data and confidentiality must be maintained when using technology. While it is acknowledged that older client's health can be monitored through a variety of wireless devices, the act of monitoring the movements and activities of an individual should be considered and discussed with the individual prior to such devices being fitted. You are advised to seek guidance regarding the local use of technological devices in practice and ensure you are fully compliant with protocols and data protection (Data Protection Act 2018).

Learning outcome 4: how to record and interpret the NEWS2 score

NEWS2, (RCP 2017), indicates the individual physiological parameters and enables early recognition of acute deterioration in a person's condition, whether in hospital or in a community setting. The six parameters that are measured including: RR, SpO_2, HR, BP, ACVPU and temperature, become an aggregate score, known as the NEWS2 score.

Each vital sign component of RR, SpO_2, pulse, BP, ACVPU and temperature has a scoring system score of 0–3 for each parameter with an additional two added to the score if the person is requiring oxygen therapy. The total NEWS2 score ranges from 0 to 20. The higher the score, the higher the clinical deterioration of the person. The score also includes a section that encourages the practitioner to escalate this to their seniors to ensure immediate intervention. The score is subsequently used to ensure that practitioners are aware of individual care needs and enables the practitioner to know if more advanced care is required, i.e. community rapid response, hospitalisation or intensive care nursing.

The overall goal of NEWS2 in healthcare is to ensure that there will be a single standardised system across the NHS. This enables the recording, aggregate scoring and response to physiological changes to be in routinely measured and acted upon. This is particularly pertinent for the acutely ill (RCP 2017).

The structure of the NEWS2 system follows the Resuscitation Council Airway, Breathing, Circulation, Disability and Exposure approach, ensuring that life-threatening issues are recognised and managed effectively. It offers a practitioner an opportunity to escalate and to identify a LOW, MEDIUM and HIGH risk of deterioration and by using the score system, practitioners can alert other staff to the severity of deterioration. Recommendations by the RCP (2017) include using NEWS2 for everyone, excluding children, young people and pregnant mothers as their vital signs are measured and recorded using an early-warning score system pertinent to their own user group. The elements of NEWS2 are used in electronic observation recording on handheld devices. Whether using paper charts or handheld technological devices, using the same assessment tool for vital signs monitoring can improve the response and escalation thus improving response times to those who are unwell.

Components of the NEWS2

The sections of the NEWS2 chart will now be discussed to offer you an outline. Each vital sign will then be discussed.

Respiratory rate

This section requires you to measure the person's RR for 1 min to identify the rate. You should note that this may be raised or significantly low in signs of deterioration.

Oxygen saturation: SPO_2 use of scale 1 or 2

This section requires you to follow directions from a senior member of the clinical team on using scale 1 or scale 2 to record SpO_2.

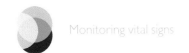
Decisions to use scale 1 or 2 SpO_2 is derived from a senior healthcare professional's review of the person and a scale adopted and used consistently. For example, scale 2 should be used primarily for those presenting with hypercapnia (excessive carbon dioxide in bloodstream), usually due to chronic obstructive pulmonary disease (COPD).

Supplementary oxygen use or air

When recording people's vital signs and using NEWS2, it is important to consider if they are receiving oxygen therapy or breathing air. If receiving oxygen therapy, this would indicate that the person is unwell. Oxygen is given to support the individual's SpO_2 in accordance with British Thoracic Society [BTS] guidelines (BTS 2017). The NEWS2 requires the practitioner to document the rate by L/min and record this in the NEWS2 chart or e-observation system. This would mean that a person would have an additional two points added to their NEWS2 score to identify that they are dependent upon oxygen therapy.

Pulse

This section requires you to measure the pulse for 1 min and note regularity and strength. You will note on the chart that a low or high pulse can signify signs of deterioration.

Blood pressure

You will next move to record the person's BP using the device that is recommended in your clinical area. The BP is recorded as systolic and diastolic, with the systolic measurement being used to calculate the NEWS2 score.

ACVPU scale

ACVPU scale – asks that you assess the person's level of consciousness. Using the ACVPU scale, as shown below, can be an effective and fast tool to use in this assessment.

- Alert (A)
- Confusion (C) (new to the person)
- Verbal response (V)
- Pain – responds to pain (P)
- Unresponsive (U).

Remember that individual neurological compromise may be subtle, so ask the person an open-ended question. An open-ended question requires the person to formulate an answer in a sentence and cannot be answered with "Yes" or "No".

Temperature

This final vital sign on the NEWS2, requires you to record the person's temperature using a valid tool recommended by the clinical area.

Calculating the NEWS2 score

The chart or electronic system used includes a colour coding of red, amber and white to initiate a response to the severity of deterioration. The vital signs measured on the NEWS2 chart or technological device are now added up. The sections give an aggregate score to indicate individual physiological status.

Continued use of NEWS2

The initial purpose of NEWS2 is to assess the severity of the acutely ill person, detect clinical deterioration and initiate timely and a competent clinical response (RCP 2017). However, vital signs monitoring, forms part of the national early-warning track and trigger systems that alert staff to potential deterioration. This system continues to be used in a clinical area to identify further signs or improvement of a person's condition. Deteriorating health is discussed in more detail in Chapter 14. A NEWS2 score of five or more is a key threshold for an urgent alert and clinical response. NEWS2 is an aid to clinical decision-making and judgement and enables practitioners to escalate and discuss concerns using a standardised process. While vital signs are important to identify physiological status, pain can be an indicator of ill health, and therefore, it is also important to assess this when recording vital signs and its assessment and management are crucial in enabling the individual to enjoy health and well-being.

Summary

- Accuracy of vital signs measurement is crucial; equipment used must be well maintained and used correctly and competently.
- The nurse's approach to people when recording vital signs should promote their comfort, confidence and dignity.
- Technological advances are affecting how vital signs are recorded, monitored and communicated; any devices should be validated and used safely.
- Healthcare workers should maintain competency in using NEWS2 scoring systems and subsequent escalation handovers.

MEASURING AND RECORDING RESPIRATIONS (AIRWAY AND BREATHING)

The major function of the respiratory system is to supply the body with oxygen and remove carbon dioxide. When the RR is measured, it is the act of ventilation that is observed. One respiration consists of one inspiration (breathing in) and one expiration (breathing out). Respiratory rate measurement is an important aspect of the person's assessment. Churpek et al. (2016) state that this is the most accurate predictor of deterioration in a person. Deterioration of respiratory effort leads to low levels of oxygen in the blood and raised levels of carbon dioxide. Chapter 14 provides further detail about respiratory assessment.

Box 4.6 Learning outcomes

By the end of this section, you will be able to:

1. explain when and why observation of respiration is performed and state the range of normal RRs for adults;
2. discuss other aspects of breathing to observe when measuring RRs;
3. accurately measure and record the RR.

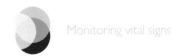

Learning outcome 1: explain when and why observation of respiration is performed and state the range of normal respiratory rates for adults

Box 4.7 Activity: observing respiration

ACTIVITY

Why would a person's respiration be observed? The practice scenarios will give you some clues. List the possible reasons.

You may have thought of the following situations:

- To provide a baseline for future comparison, for example, when a person is admitted to hospital or has a preoperative assessment
- To monitor a person in hospital or in the community following injury or during an illness, for example, loss of consciousness, chest injury, difficulty with breathing, chest pain (so Anne, Ken and Natalie should all have their respiration rates measured)
- To monitor the individual's condition – for example, after surgery, or during treatment, such as a morphine infusion
- To monitor the person's response to treatments or medication that affect the respiratory system

When assessing RR, you should know the expected normal rate; if a baseline reading is available, you can make a comparison with this rate. The RR varies according to age, size and gender and can fluctuate in healthy people, for example, if metabolic demands change. The normal adult RR is about 12–20 breaths per minute (RCP 2017). Exercise, stress and fear all increase the RR and this increase is a normal bodily response. If you count RRs when an individual has just arrived at the hospital, anxiety may lead to a raised RR, which would not be an accurate baseline. In deep sleep (see Chapter 8), the RR drops to its lowest normal level. Knowledge of normal biological functioning will help you to recognise abnormalities and causes for concern.

An increased RR is termed tachypnoea. On a NEWS2 scale, the rate may be 21–24, indicating a score of 2. A RR of above 25 would gain a score of 3. This would indicate the severity of the deterioration and the RR is often the first vital sign to alter when the person's condition is deteriorating, so it is imperative that this vital sign is monitored and recorded. Ken's RR may increase due to his chest infection. Having a baseline for Ken's observations is important as he will not have his usual carers with him. A decreased RR is termed bradypnoea. On a NEWS2, a RR of 9–11 would be scored as a 1, while a RR of less than 8 would be scored as a 3. In the case of Natalie's RR, this may decrease owing to the drugs she has taken. A serious side effect of opioid drugs, such as morphine, is a depressed RR.

In healthy people, the relationship between pulse and respiration is relatively constant, being a ratio of one respiration to every four or five heartbeats. Very rapid respirations, such as over 40 per minute in an adult (in the absence of exercise), or very slow respirations, such as 8 per minute, are cause for alarm and should be reported promptly.

Learning outcome 2: discuss other aspects of breathing to observe when measuring RR

ACTIVITY

Box 4.8 Activity: counting RRs of people

When you are counting the RRs of the people in the scenarios, what else about their respiration should you observe?

You should observe the difficulty, sound, depth and pattern of breathing, as discussed next.

Difficulty in breathing

Respirations are normally effortless, and you should therefore observe whether breathing is difficult (termed dyspnoea). People with dyspnoea may use accessory muscles of respiration such as their neck and abdominal muscles. If Ken has a chest infection, he is likely to experience dyspnoea and this should be noted in his health action plan for future reference. People with dyspnoea often mouth breathe because there is less resistance to airflow through the mouth than the nose. Mouth breathing can lead to drying of the oral mucus membrane and so oral hygiene (discussed in Chapter 7) is essential.

People with dyspnoea need to sit up, either in an armchair or on a bed well supported by pillows, to optimise ventilation. 'Orthopnoea' is the term used when people cannot breathe unless they are upright. Dyspnoea is frightening and psychological support is essential.

Sound of breathing

Asthma

Asthma is a respiratory disorder characterised by recurrent episodes of difficulty in breathing, wheezing on expiration, coughing and viscous mucoid bronchial secretions.

You should also observe the sound of breathing, which is normally quiet. You may hear a variety of abnormal breath sounds. A wheeze, often heard in people with **asthma,** is a high-pitched sound occurring when air is forced through narrowed respiratory passages. A wheeze may also occur with chest infections. A stridor is a harsh, high-pitched sound that is heard during respiration when the larynx is obstructed.

Depth of breathing

The person's depth of breathing should be observed, which relates to the volume of air moving in and out of the respiratory tract with each breath – the tidal volume. An adult male's tidal volume should be approximately 500 mL and a female's, approximately 400 mL (Hallett et al. 2020). However, this can be altered to fit physiological needs, for example during exercise. The term hyperventilation refers to prolonged, rapid and deep ventilations that can occur during an anxiety attack, causing dizziness and fainting as the resulting low carbon dioxide level causes cerebral vasoconstriction.

Hypoventilation is the term used for slow and shallow breathing, which could lead to inadequate gaseous exchange. You should also observe whether the chest expands equally on both sides, particularly if there is a history of chest injury.

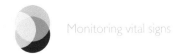

Pattern of breathing

The pattern of breathing should be observed. Terms are given to certain abnormalities.

Apnoea: is a period without breathing. It could occur during hypoventilation, with another breath only occurring when arterial carbon dioxide levels rise and breathing is stimulated.

Cheyne–Stokes respirations: are when there is a gradual increase in the depth of respirations, leading to an episode of hyperventilation, followed by a gradual decrease in the depth of respirations, and then a period of apnoea lasting about 15–20 seconds.

Kussmaul's respiration: is very deep and laboured breathing, sometimes associated with people in a diabetic coma. The deep breathing is due to metabolic acidosis.

The person's RR should be equal between each breath, with a short pause at the end of inspiration and expiration. Irregularities of breathing rate may indicate respiratory disease.

Learning outcome 3: accurately measure and record the RR

For the following activities, you need a willing volunteer. If a colleague is not available, another friend or family member may oblige!

ACTIVITY

> ### Box 4.9 Activity: measuring respiratory rate
>
> Measure your volunteer's RR, using the instructions in Box 4.11.

Respiratory rates, particularly on admission, may be recorded simply as a number (the number of respirations per minute). If the person's RR is recorded regularly over a period of time, a NEWS chart/e-observation is used according to local policy.

ACTIVITY

> ### Box 4.10 Activity: respiratory rate post exercise
>
> Ask your volunteer to spend a couple of minutes exercising (e.g. jogging on the spot) and then count the RR again.

> ### Box 4.11 Measuring respiratory rate
>
> Note the placement of the second hand of your watch or zero your timing device
>
> - Count each rise and fall of the chest for 1 min (remember one respiration is the breath in and the breath out). Note the depth and regularity of their breathing. In practice you should do this count when people are unaware that they are being observed, otherwise they may alter their breathing pattern. It is often useful to count the RR immediately after counting the pulse for this reason.
>
> For an unresponsive person, this precaution is not relevant.
>
> - Review the NEWS2 chart or handheld device and identify how this will score on the NEWS2.

Box 4.12 Children and young people: practice points – respiration

It is important to observe the child's breathing when they are not aware that you are doing, so which will allow for a more accurate assessment. Thorough assessment of the child's respiratory function is vital as their condition can deteriorate very quickly if left unmanaged. The range of RRs varies with the age of the child so understanding the normal parameters is vital:

- <1 year 30–40
- 1–2 years 25–35
- 2–5 years 25–30
- 5–12 years 20–25
- Over 12 years 15–20

For further guidance on respiratory assessment of infants and children and young people, see:

Crawford D, Davies K (2020) Biological basis of child health 5: Development of the respiratory system and elements of respiratory assessment. *Nursing Children and Young People*. doi: 10.7748/ncyp.2020.e1246

Royal College of Nursing. 2017. Standards for assessing, measuring and monitoring vital signs in infants, children and young people. Available from: https://www.rcn.org.uk/professional-development/publications/pub-005942 (Accessed on May 13 2021).

Box 4.13 Pregnancy and birth: practice points – respiration

During pregnancy, mothers are encouraged to adopt the left lateral position when lying down, to prevent pressure on major blood vessels. If the mother lies on her back, then her blood flow may be affected and in turn affect her general well-being, the well-being of her unborn baby and will impact on her vital signs. That is why mothers are recommended to sleep on their side in later pregnancy (Heazell et al. 2017). During pregnancy, some mothers experience fluid retention that can seriously affect, amongst other things, respiratory function. Fluid retention may affect gaseous exchange, and changes to oxygen saturation and RR may be seen. Seek midwifery advice regarding positioning of a pregnant woman once she is in your care.

In later pregnancy, breathing becomes largely diaphragmatic due to the enlarging uterus. However, RR remains unchanged. Therefore, breathlessness (RR > 20) is one of several significant symptoms in pregnancy or the postnatal period indicating deteriorating health or signs of puerperal sepsis that will require accurate regular monitoring. It is easy to monitor RR even if other

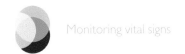
monitoring equipment is not available. (MBRRACE 2020) The use of Modified Early-Obstetric Warning Scores (MEOWS) is strongly recommended and are different to NEWS2 (see Chapter 14).

Heazell, A.E.P., Li, M., Budd, J. et al. 2017. Association between maternal sleep practice and late stillbirth findings from a stillbirth case-control study. BJOG, *International Journal of Obstetrics and Gynaecology*. Doi:10.1111/1471–0528 14967.

MBRRACE. 2020. Saving lives improving mothers' care. Available from: https://www.npeu.ox.ac.uk/assets/downloads/mbrrace-uk/reports/maternal-report-2020/MBRRACE-UK_Maternal_Report_Dec_2020_v10_ONLINE_VERSION_1404.pdf

(Accessed on 3 June 2021).

Summary

- Respirations are measured as part of an acutely ill person's assessment, as a baseline for future comparison, and to monitor and evaluate a person's condition and response to treatment.
- It is important to be aware of normal RRs and of possible abnormalities that can occur.

MEASURING OXYGEN SATURATION BY PULSE OXIMETRY (SPO_2) SCALE 1 AND SCALE 2 (NEWS2: AIRWAY AND BREATHING)

Pulse oximetry enables continuous non-invasive monitoring of the oxygen saturation of haemoglobin (Hb) (SpO_2) in arterial blood, updated with each pulse wave, via a microprocessor with a probe attached to the individual. Haemoglobin is a molecule present in erythrocytes (red blood cells) that transports gases – especially oxygen – around the body. About 98% of the oxygen in the blood is transported and attached to these Hb molecules, to form what is called oxyhaemoglobin (HbO_2), and about 2% of the oxygen is carried and dissolved in the plasma. Pulse oximetry measures how saturated with oxygen are the Hb molecules. RCP (2017) NEWS2 charts and e-observation systems include two scales SpO_2 scale 1 oxygen saturations show a range of maintaining SpO_2 between 96% and 100%. Scores of 94–95% indicate a score of 1, 92–93% indicate a score of 2, below 91% indicate a score of 3.

Scale 2 to be used if target SpO_2 is 88–92% in hypercapnia respiratory failure, less than 97% on O_2 scores 3 95–96 on O_2 scores 2, 93–94 on O_2 scores 1. 86–87% scores 1, 84–85% scores 2, less than 83% scores 3. The scale should only be used when directed by a senior clinician, while scale 2 of the SpO_2 scale should only be used under the direction of a qualified clinician. This scale is used for those who present with hypercapnia respiratory failure 88–92% on air. The use of bedside mobile devices for measuring oxygen saturation enables the practitioner to decide if oxygen therapy should be commenced. BTS (2017) indicate that oxygen can be administered in an emergency when SpO_2 levels fall below 94–98% or 88–92% in a person who has hypercapnia.

Box 4.14 Learning outcomes

By the end of this section, you will be able to:

1 explain how pulse oximetry works and how it is used;
2 identify when pulse oximetry is used and discuss its advantages and limitations.

You may be able to access a pulse oximeter in the skills laboratory or your practice setting.

Learning outcome 1: Explain how pulse oximetry works and how it is used

---

Box 4.15 Activity: pulse oximetry

ACTIVITY

Have you seen pulse oximetry used in practice? If so, can you remember what the equipment looked like, and do you know how it works? What is a normal reading?

Pulse oximeters range from small handheld devices, displaying the percentage of oxygen saturation and the pulse rate, to more substantial devices that also show the pulsatile waveform (Figure 4.1). The box has a wire leading to the sensor or probe clip or sleeve that is placed on a finger, toe or earlobe. It should be noted that a probe designed for each anatomical area should be used only in its designated area and is not interchangeable, i.e. a finger probe should only be used on a finger and an ear probe used only on the ear lobe. This is to ensure the accuracy of the reading. Mc Dermott et al. (2018) warn of the potential inaccuracies of some commercially available devices; therefore, caution is needed when using these devices to commence treatment. For example, when relying on these devices to commence oxygen therapy or medications. Probes can be disposable or reusable and are available in different sizes. Ambulatory devices allow monitoring while still maintaining some independence and mobility. Mobile devices can monitor SpO2, RR and HR. Radius tetherless pulse oximetry devices enable a person to be fully mobile and not restricted in personal activities but can still be monitored by their care provider. The diagram in Figure 4.2 shows how the sensor works.

Pulse oximeters monitor only light absorption from tissue with a pulsatile flow, thereby preventing false readings from fat, bone, connective tissue and venous blood. It is essential that the person has sufficient arterial blood flow to the extremities to produce a reliable reading.

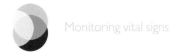

Box 4.16 Activity: measuring oxygen saturation

If you have access to a pulse oximeter or vital signs monitoring device with SpO_2 probe attachment, measure your oxygen saturation using the instructions in Box 4.17.

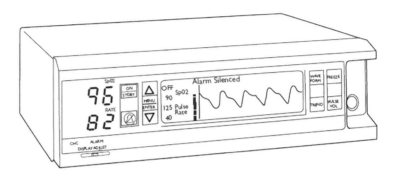

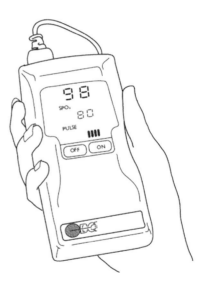

Figure 4.1: Examples of pulse oximeters showing SpO_2 reading and heart rate.

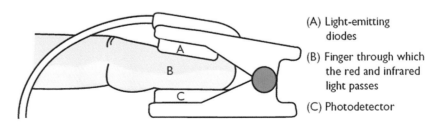

(A) Light-emitting diodes

(B) Finger through which the red and infrared light passes

(C) Photodetector

Figure 4.2: Diagram showing how a pulse oximeter works.

Hypercapnic respiratory failure

Inadequate gas exchange by the respiratory system occurs where there is a buildup of carbon dioxide.

The normal value of oxygen saturation is 96–100%, so hopefully your reading was within that range. This figure refers to the percentage of Hb molecules that are fully saturated with oxygen. RCP (2017) suggests that the recommended target saturation range for those acutely ill and not at risk of **hypercapnic respiratory failure** is 96–98%. However, some people, especially if aged 70 years, may have oxygen saturation measurements below 96% and do not require oxygen therapy when clinically stable. Repositioning the person to a more upright position, if not contraindicated, may provide significant improvement. Pulse oximeters have alarm systems that sound if the measurement falls below a normal level.

Box 4.17 Use of pulse oximeter

Turn the pulse oximeter on and allow the device to go through its checking and calibration procedure.

- Select the appropriate probe; ensure correct fitting and positioning on the digit. Avoid placing probe on false nails, or nail-polished fingernails.
- Allow several seconds for the oximeter to detect your pulse and calculate your reading.
- Look at the waveform displayed.
- Read percentage (%) displayed and record this number on the observation chart.
- In practice you should record whether the person is receiving oxygen (and if so, the percentage) or breathing air.

Source: Adapted from Hill, Stoneham and Fearnley 2008 Practical applications of pulse oximetry

http://e-safe-anaesthesia.org/e_library/04/Pulse_oximetry_-_practical_applications_Update_2008.pdf

---

Most manufacturers claim that their devices are accurate to ±2% at oxygen saturations of 70–99%. The ability of pulse oximeters to detect hypoxaemia (insufficient oxygenation of blood) was confirmed by Louie et al (2018). However, as hypoxaemia rises, pulse oximetry becomes less accurate. An SpO_2 of less than 80% can lead to inaccurate readings, so at 80–85%, a more detailed assessment is necessary. If there is any doubt about the accuracy of pulse oximetry, blood gas analysis (analysis of a sample of arterial blood) should be performed (see Chapter 14). If the person is peripherally shut down or has a weak pulse, pulse oximetry readings will not be precise. Cardiac arrhythmias such as atrial fibrillation can interfere with capture of the pulsatile signal and thus reduce accuracy.

Hypoxia

A condition in which inadequate oxygen is available to the tissues to allow normal function.

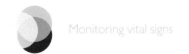

Fingertips, toes, earlobes and the bridge of the nose can be used to measure oxygen saturation. However, the appropriate probe for the anatomical area should be used. Movement of the fingers or toes can cause artefact leading to inaccurate readings, so, if possible, the sensor should be attached to a part of the body that is most likely to keep still. Louie et al. (2018) explained that pulse oximetry does not necessarily provide information on Hb concentration, oxygen delivery to the tissues or ventilatory function, so the person may have normal oxygen saturations yet still be hypoxic. In the clinical setting, you are advised to ensure that you observe, monitor and report any changes in the individual's appearance along with measuring their oxygen saturation.

Learning outcome 2: identify when pulse oximetry is used and discuss its advantages and limitations

Oxygen saturation should be checked by pulse oximetry for everyone as part of their vital signs monitoring and is an inexpensive and non-invasive method of assessing this. Pulse oximetry should be available wherever emergency oxygen is used. Hypoxaemia can rapidly lead to tissue damage however assessing through observation is notoriously inaccurate and unreliable. The brain is very sensitive to oxygen depletion, and visual and cognitive changes can occur when oxygen saturation falls to 80–85%. Other signs of hypoxaemia include restlessness, agitation, hypotension and tachycardia. However, all these signs can be missed or wrongly interpreted.

Cyanosis

Cyanosis is a bluish, greyish or purplish discoloration of the skin due to the presence of abnormal amounts of reduced haemoglobin in the blood.

Cyanosis is the visible sign of hypoxaemia, but it is only detected at a saturation of about 75% in normally perfused people. Pulse oximetry should therefore be a more accurate and objective measure of hypoxaemia, alerting health professionals at an early stage.

Box 4.18 Activity: practice placement experiences

ACTIVITY

Think about your practice placement experiences. In what situations have you seen pulse oximetry being used?

You may have considered the following:

- **Acute illness.** Pulse oximetry is part of the assessment of anyone who is acutely ill, particularly during initial assessment and management.
- **Investigations and surgery.** Pulse oximetry is used during and after procedures and investigations involving general anaesthesia, or sedation.
- **Chronic obstructive pulmonary disease**

    A chronic disease that includes conditions such as emphysema, chronic bronchitis and chronic asthma. It causes debilitating breathlessness, which affects day-to-day living.

- **Respiratory and circulatory problems.** People with respiratory disease, particularly if receiving oxygen therapy, will have SpO_2 monitoring. The amount of oxygen administered may be adjusted according to the SpO_2. Oxygen should be prescribed to achieve 94–98% oxygen saturations for most acutely ill people, or 88–92% for those at risk of **hypercapnic respiratory failure** – and the target saturation should be written on the NEWS2 chart and e-observation system. Anyone who is at risk of hypoxaemia – such as those with pneumonia, congestive heart failure, **COPD** exacerbation or acute lung injury – may have continuous SpO_2 monitoring via a pulse oximeter. People whose cardiorespiratory status is unstable, and who are undergoing transfer, often have pulse oximetry *in situ*.

- **Cystic fibrosis**

    Cystic fibrosis is a genetic disease causing oversecretion of viscous mucous, thus predisposing to respiratory infections.

    Pulse oximetry can be used in the community with chronically ill people who are at risk of hypoxaemia, for example, those with **cystic fibrosis**.

Limitations of pulse oximetry

Although pulse oximetry has allowed for non-invasive measurements of arterial oxygen saturation, monitoring of pulse oximetry should be viewed with caution. Pulse oximetry complements measurement of other vital signs, but it does not replace them; oxygen saturations are only a single physiological variable and should not be over relied upon. Pulse oximeters cannot differentiate between different forms of saturated Hb and therefore cannot identify hypoxaemia. When carbon monoxide is inhaled, carboxyhaemoglobin (COHb) is formed and is absorbed and registered as oxyhaemoglobin, leading to the overestimation of oxygen saturation. Thus, for people who have been involved in accidents involving smoke, or who are affected by carbon monoxide poisoning, pulse oximetry is not recommended. COHb readings are also high in tobacco smokers.

Holmes and Peffers (2013) highlight various conditions that can influence pulse oximetry, such as **asthma**, peripheral vascular disease in older people, some antiretroviral medication (HIV drugs), anaemia and sickle cell anaemia (a genetic condition causing red blood cells to have a sickle shape affecting oxygen transport). They also identify that nail polish, dirt or artificial nails on the fingertip, movement leading to artefacts and dark or pigmented skin can alter readings. Barnett et al. (2012) and McDermott et al. (2018) describe the choice of sites in pulse oximetry readings and note that ear and finger sites may offer different readings. Therefore, it is important that you identify which site is used routinely in your clinical area, to aim to eliminate errors of reading. If you consider the factors mentioned above, you can try to increase accuracy in measurement of pulse oximetry, and you must report any abnormal findings immediately to a registered nurse or doctor.

Note that it is the quality of oxygen delivery to the tissues that is of most importance – which depends on cardiac output, tissue perfusion and Hb concentration – not just oxygen saturation of arterial blood. Oxyhaemoglobin saturation could be 99%, but this saturation is of no value if the heart cannot deliver it to the tissues.

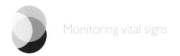

Box 4.19 Activity: symptoms of hypoxia

What signs and symptoms might indicate a lack of oxygen to the tissues (hypoxia)?

Signs that you could observe for include the warmth of peripheral areas of the body, colour of skin and tongue, urine output and mental state.

Box 4.20 Children and young people: practice points – measuring oxygen saturation

For infants, children and young people, smaller probes are used. Different sizes are available, and for infants, the device used is usually wrapped around the foot. The normal values are the same across the life span. For further guidance on measuring oxygen saturations, see:

Gormley-Fleming, E. 2018. Pulse oximetry. In Gormley-Fleming, E. and Martin, D. (eds.) *Children and Young People's Nursing Skills at a Glance*. Chichester: Wiley, 40–41.

Royal College of Nursing. 2017. Standards for assessing, measuring and monitoring vital signs in infants, children and young people. Available at. https://www.rcn.org.uk/professional-development/publications/pub-005942

Summary

- Pulse oximetry is widely used and has many applications.
- Pulse oximetry is non-invasive and easy to apply and provides a continuous measurement.
- It is important to understand the limitations of pulse oximetry and to be aware of its role as complementary to the overall clinical picture.

Air or oxygen?

In this section of the NEWS2, you are required to note if the person is receiving oxygen therapy or breathing air. If they are not requiring oxygen and breathing air, then a 0 is given to this score. However, if a person is on oxygen therapy, this would indicate that they are unwell and requiring oxygen to support their oxygen saturation and possibly their respiration. An additional two points are added to the aggregate NEWS2 score in this case. It is important to record the litres of oxygen and device that it is delivered via too.

MEASURING AND RECORDING BLOOD PRESSURE (CIRCULATION)

Once the above parameters have been measured and recorded, BP is then taken. Blood pressure is the pressure that the blood exerts on the walls of the blood vessels (Waugh and Grant 2018). Arterial pressure is determined by the volume ejected by the heart into the arteries, the elasticity of the walls of the arteries, and the rate at which the blood flows out of the arteries (Magder 2018). Blood pressure is different in different blood vessels, but in everyday clinical practice, the term BP is used to mean systemic arterial BP. Blood pressure is regulated by complex neural and hormonal systems (Tortora and Derrikson 2017). Blood pressure is a key vital sign to assist in monitoring general health and recognising signs of clinical deterioration (Brekke et al 2019). An accurate recording is imperative if treatment is to be based upon this. Blood pressure measuring and recording to ensure escalation of a person's deterioration is part of the NEWS2 scoring system and is included in e-observation software. The NEWS2 uses systolic BP as a measurement and a low or falling systolic BP (hypotension) enables a practitioner to note deterioration, for example, loss of fluid volume in shock or acute kidney injury. An elevated BP (hypertension) is a risk factor of coronary heart disease, **stroke** or diabetes. In the NEWS2 score, severe hypertension, i.e. above 220 mmHg, could indicate pain or distress. The diastolic BP recording should be routinely recorded as it may indicate signs of accelerated hypertension. NICE CG 136 (2019a) explains this as a significant increase over baseline BP that is associated with organ damage. A BP of greater than 220 mmHg would lead to a practitioner initiating an escalation process for the person to receive immediate treatment for hypertension.

Box 4.21 Learning outcomes

By the end of this section, you will be able to:

1. explain what makes up BP and when BP should be measured;
2. discuss the equipment used for BP measurements and the meaning of the reading obtained;
3. identify the normal values for BP and factors affecting BP recordings;
4. accurately measure a person's BP using manual and electronic equipment.

Learning outcome 1: explain what makes up BP and when blood pressure should be measured

Understanding BP and its effects on the body is complex. Marieb and Hoehn (2018) explain that BP results from cardiac output (CO), multiplied by systemic vascular resistance (SVR), which is in opposition to blood flow from friction between blood and blood vessel walls. CO is the production of HR and stroke volume (SV), which is the amount of blood ejected with each beat. SV is determined by preload (volume of blood in the ventricle waiting to be ejected), afterload (resistance of moving the preload) and contractility (strength of heart muscle). If a person's BP is high or low, then some of these factors are out of balance.

Currently, BP is measured in millimetres of mercury (mmHg) using a sphygmomanometer or electronic device (British Heart Foundation 2020).

A BP reading has two values, systolic and diastolic. Systolic BP is primarily determined by CO and diastolic, by SVR.

- The systolic pressure occurs during ventricular contraction and is the maximum pressure of the blood against the wall of the artery. This pressure is recorded as the top figure when documenting the BP. In recognising and responding to a person's

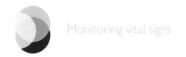

deterioration, the systolic pressure is usually the reading that is monitored. NEWS2 and e-observation systems include this measurement.

- The diastolic pressure is the minimum pressure of the blood against the wall of the artery, which occurs following closure of the aortic valve. This measurement assesses the pressure when the ventricles are at rest and is recorded as the bottom figure.

Thus, a BP recorded as 120/70 means that the systolic pressure is 120 mmHg and the diastolic pressure is 70 mmHg. The measurements of systolic and diastolic pressure should be judged as one reading.

Blood pressure measurement and monitoring are now increasingly performed to detect a person's physiological health status. Ambulatory recording of BP, where the person takes a device home to record their BP over a period, can be beneficial and has also become more popular; see later discussion (Learning outcome 3). Ken's **Health Action Plan** should include his BP measurement, and an ambulatory BP device may well be used for him.

Learning outcome 2: discuss the equipment used for blood pressure measurements and the meaning of the reading obtained

Box 4.22 Activity: using a sphygmomanometer

What equipment have you seen used to measure BP? If you are not familiar with the sphygmomanometer ('sphygmo'), try to access one in the skills laboratory or the practice setting. If possible, look at electronic equipment too, as many devices are now used in the clinical setting.

There are two main ways of measuring BP:

- **Indirect method**: Pressure can be measured indirectly, using electronic/digital equipment – for example, an oscillometer. An oscillometer is a machine that is attached to the arm by means of a cuff. The cuff is inflated by the machine, which then reads the pressure within the artery. The result is displayed as two readings – the systolic and the diastolic pressure. In clinical practice, BP recording is most frequently performed using an electronic device; however, it is important that you learn to use both manual and electronic devices.
- **Non-invasive auscultation method**: The pressure is taken manually by using a sphygmomanometer and stethoscope.

Blood pressure was traditionally recorded manually but is now increasingly recorded electronically. Mercury sphygmomanometer use is discouraged, due to the risks of mercury spillage (Medicines and Healthcare Regulatory Agency [MHRA] 2019) and a drive to reduce mercury use in healthcare. Mercury sphygmomanometers have been largely replaced with aneroid sphygmomanometers (Figure 4.3), but there is debate about their accuracy; these devices must be calibrated and serviced as per manufacturer's guidelines. Oscillometric devices are increasingly used for

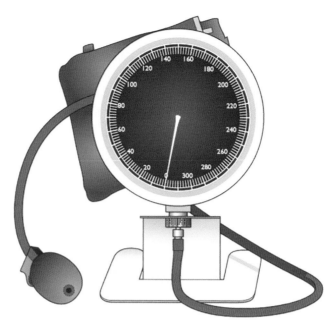

Figure 4.3: An aneroid sphygmomanometer.

measurement, although their accuracy continues to be critically debated. Healthcare workers should learn how to record a BP manually, as electronic devices are not always available, particularly in community and non-acute settings.

On oscillometers and monitoring devices you will notice the term MAP, which refers to mean arterial pressure, or the average BP during the cardiac cycle. MAP can indicate when the person's condition is deteriorating (for more information, see Chapter 14).

Learning outcome 3: identify the normal values for BP and factors affecting BP recordings

When measuring BP, as with any other vital signs, you should be aware of expected normal ranges. Variability in BP from person to person exists. Normal adult BP is generally considered to range from 100/60 to 140/90. However, the NICE guidelines CG 127 (2011a) for hypertension, written in conjunction with the British Hypertension Society (BHS), offer more detailed classification of BP levels to indicate acceptable/unacceptable parameters. The term used for high BP is hypertension, and the term used for low BP is hypotension. According to RCP recommendations, NEWS2, uses the systolic BP only to indicate a score. A BP above 220 indicates a score of 3. Low BP (hypotension), systolic BP of 101–110 scores a 1, systolic BP 91–100 scores a 2 and systolic BP 81–50 indicates a score of 3.

Box 4.23 Activity: factors affecting BP measurements

ACTIVITY

What factors do you know of that might affect BP measurements?

Would any of these apply to the people in this chapter's scenarios?

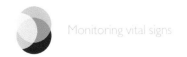

Age, disease, injury, and medicines all influence BP (Peate 2019) and could be factors relevant to all three scenarios. There are many other factors too.

- Blood volume: Regulatory mechanisms can cope with minor fluctuations in circulating blood volume, but losses of 10% or more – due to trauma, haemorrhage or severe dehydration – result in a fall in BP (Tortora and Derrikson 2017).
- Age: Blood pressure increases from birth and throughout life (Marieb and Hoehn 2018). Anne and Ken may have a higher BP than Natalie, who is a younger adult.
- Disease: Atherosclerosis can affect the elasticity of the arteries. Many other diseases can raise BP, including heart disease, kidney disease, endocrine disorders and neurological conditions (Marieb and Hoehn 2018; Odya and Du Pree 2018). In these instances, high BP is termed secondary hypertension.
- Posture and gravity: A decrease in BP may occur from lying to sitting or standing position, but Kallioinen et al. (2017) asserted that this positioning is unlikely to lead to a significant error in recording, provided the arm is supported at the level of the heart. Some people's BP falls more significantly on standing (termed orthostatic hypotension). This effect is more common in older people (Marieb 2018) and is a complication of immobility (see Chapter 11).
- Drug use: Prescription and recreational drug can influence the BP. Some with dramatic affects and consequences. Prescribed drugs affect BP; examples are diuretics and tranquillisers (Tortora and Derrikson 2017). If Natalie has taken an overdose of a tranquilliser, depending on the quantity, this drug intake could lower her BP. It may be beneficial when the person is taking medication to note the time of drug ingestion in association with the BP being monitored.
- Emotional factors: Stress, fear and anxiety all increase BP. Staff who fail to explain the procedure or rush the procedure and people who are anxious about the outcome are factors that can affect the reading (Kallioinen et al. 2017). In people with dementia, remember to explain the procedure, show the person the equipment and allow them time to comprehend what you are doing.
- Weight: An obese person's heart must work harder, so the BP may be higher (Marieb and Hoehn 2018; Odya and Du Pree 2018).
- Diet: High-salt and low-calcium dietary intakes may lead to a rise in BP (Marieb and Hoehn 2018).
- Exercise: People who take regular exercise may have a lower BP (British Heart Foundation [BHF] 2020).
- Arm support and position: Diastolic BP may increase by 10% if the arm is left unsupported (Kallioinen et al. 2017). An overestimation of BP can result if the arm is placed below the heart level.
- Arm used: During the initial assessment, bilateral BP measurements should be recorded to identify any differences in the readings (BHS 2012a, 2012b; Reinberg 2020). It is normal to have a small difference in BP readings between arms, but a big difference is a cause for concern. Differences could indicate abnormalities or disease of the aorta, such as aortic coarctation or an aneurysm. Surgical and cardiac procedures, for example, cardiac catheterisation, may also result in differences. If people are found to

Aortic coarctation

A congenital narrowing of the aorta.

Aneurysm

A weakness in the arterial wall leading to a bulge, with the risk of rupture.

have big differences in systolic pressure between arms, they are more likely to require further vascular assessment to exclude heart disease (Reinberg 2020).

- White coat hypertension: White coat hypertension is a term used when a person's BP is consistently higher when recorded in a medical situation, such as a hospital, clinic or GP's surgery, than at home (Kallioinen et al. 2017). It is a common phenomenon, affecting some people when becoming assessed in the community or hospitalised. NICE (2011a) highlighted that treatment regimens could be based upon false readings and therefore recommended that those with long-term hypertension should have their BP measured at home, using ambulatory devices, over a period of time before treatment is commenced.
- Observer bias: When recording routine observations, healthcare professionals may be at risk of expecting the measurement to be normal, for example, when recording BP for a person who they know well or when recording several BP measurements in a shift.

Learning outcome 4: accurately measure a person's BP using manual and electronic equipment

Attaining accurate results for BP recordings, both manual and electronic, is very important. Many treatment schedules and clinical decisions are made based upon BP-monitoring. It is therefore imperative that readings are accurate.

Although many clinical settings predominantly use electronic devices, it is imperative to learn the technique of manual BP recording and ensure you are competent in this skill. This will also allow you to be able to gain a better understanding of Korotkoff sounds and what we refer to as systolic and diastolic BP readings. Although BP can be measured at several sites, in most clinical situations, the brachial artery is used as it is convenient and easily accessible, so it is the artery you are most likely to have seen used in practice. Some electronic devices measure BP at the radial artery. It is advisable to avoid recording the BP on an arm that is affected by disability (e.g. weakness due to a stroke, lymph node removal), or where an intravenous infusion is in place. When a person has suffered trauma or surgery affecting both arms, the thigh can be used for which a larger cuff is needed. Skinner et al. (2013) explain that BP is a key vital sign that should be recorded in trauma. Measuring BPs in both arms is sometimes practised when a person presents with chest pain or unexplained back pain (Skerrett 2012). This practice can help establish blood flow issues around the person's body.

Recording Korotkoff sounds in manual blood pressure measurement
The Korotkoff sounds are heard through the stethoscope when you manually record a BP value (Table 4.1). These sounds are not audible using electronic/ digital devices. The sounds are named after Nikolai Korotkoff, who first identified the audible sounds of BP in 1905 (Korotkoff 1905, cited in O'Brien et al. 2003). There may be a period between phases 2 and 3 where no sounds are audible, but they become audible again at a lower pressure. This phenomenon is known as an auscultatory gap (Campbell et al. 2020). This phenomenon is seen in approximately 20% of elderly people with hypertension (McGee 2018). This is the reason that the correct procedure involves palpation to find the systolic BP before using the sphygmomanometer. This technique is explained later.

Table 4.1: Korotkoff sounds

Phase	Sound	When they are normally heard (mmHg)
1	Clear tapping	Usually above 120
2	Blowing or whistling	Around 110
3	Soft thud	Around 100
4	Low-pitched, muffled sound	Around 90
5	Disappearance of all sounds	Around 80

BP British and Irish Hypertension Society (BIHSOC 2020).

There is debate about whether the diastolic pressure should be recorded at phase 4 or 5. Generally, guidelines recommend phase 5 as the point of diastolic pressure (BHS 2012a).

Steps in recording blood pressure

Blood pressure recording is frequently carried out by healthcare workers and is a common experience for most people, but remember that for some people, it will be their first time. Always give adequate explanation and warning about the tightness of the cuff, which some people find quite uncomfortable. Box 4.24 provides the steps in measuring BP using both manual and electronic equipment. Selection of correct cuff size is essential for an accurate reading. There are a variety of sizes of cuffs available: small adult, standard and large adult as well as a thigh cuff. Ensure that you note the size of the person's arm and use an appropriate cuff (Table 4.2).

Accurate BP readings obtained manually via cuff and stethoscope are still a vital aspect of clinical decision-making about a person's condition.

Box 4.24 Steps in recording blood pressure manually and electronically

Blood pressure can be monitored using manual or electronic BP monitors:

- The person should be seated for at least 5 min, relaxed and not moving or speaking.
- The arm must be supported at the level of the heart. Ensure no tight clothing constricts the arm.
- Place the cuff on neatly with the centre of the bladder over the brachial artery. The bladder should encircle at least 80% of the arm (but not more than 100%).
- Estimate the systolic value beforehand:

  (a) Palpate the brachial artery.
  (b) Inflate cuff until pulsation disappears.
  (c) Deflate cuff.
  (d) Estimate systolic pressure.

- Then, inflate to 30 mmHg above the estimated systolic level needed to occlude the pulse.
- Place the stethoscope diaphragm over the brachial artery and deflate at a rate of 2–3 mm/s until you hear regular tapping sounds.
- Measure systolic (first sound) and diastolic (disappearance) to nearest 2 mmHg.

- Some monitors allow manual BP setting selection where you choose the appropriate setting. Other monitors will automatically inflate and reinflate to the next setting if required.
- Repeat three times and record measurement as displayed. Initially, test blood pressure in both arms and use arm with highest reading for subsequent measurement.

(Continued)

Box 4.24 (Continued)

Source: Reproduced with kind permission from British Hypertension Society. 2012a. Blood pressure measurement with manual blood pressure *monitors*. Available from: http://www.bhsoc.org/files/9013/4390/7747/BP_Measurement_Poster_-_Manual.pdf; British Hypertension Society. 2012b. Blood pressure measurement with electronic blood pressure monitors. Available from: http://www.bhsoc.org/files/8413/4390/7770/BP_MeasurementPoster__Electronic.pdf

Measuring blood pressure

NICE CG 136 guidelines (2019a)

The guidelines recommend that practitioners adhere to the following when measuring BP:

1.1.1 Ensure that healthcare professionals taking BP measurements have adequate initial training and periodic review of their performance. [2004]

1.1.2 Because automated devices may not measure BP accurately if there is pulse irregularity (for example, due to atrial fibrillation), palpate the radial or brachial pulse before measuring BP. If pulse irregularity is present, measure BP manually using direct auscultation over the brachial artery. [2011]

1.1.3 Healthcare providers must ensure that devices for measuring BP are properly validated,[1] maintained and regularly recalibrated according to manufacturers' instructions. [2004]

1.1.4 When measuring BP in the clinic or in the home, standardise the environment and provide a relaxed, temperate setting, with the person quiet and seated, and their arm outstretched and supported. Use an appropriate cuff size for the person's arm. [2011, amended 2019]

1.1.5 In people with symptoms of postural hypotension (falls or postural dizziness):
- measure BP with the person either supine or seated
- measure BP again with the person standing for at least 1 min before measurement. [2004, amended 2011]

1.1.6 If the systolic BP falls by 20 mmHg or more, when the person is standing:
- review medication
- measure subsequent BPs with the person standing
- consider referral to specialist care if symptoms of postural hypotension persist. [2004, amended 2011]

Table 4.2: Selection of blood pressure cuff size

	Indication	Width (cm)[a,b]	Length (cm)[a,b]	BHS Guidelines Bladder width and length (cm)[a]	Arm circumference (cm)[a]
	Small adult/child	10–12	18–24	12 × 18	<23
Cuff size	Standard adult	12–13	23–35	12 × 26	<33
	Large adult	12–16	35–40	22 × 40	<50
	Adult thigh cuff[c]	20	42		<53

[a] The range for columns 2 and 3 are derived from recommendations from the BHS, European Hypertension Society (ESH) and the American Heart Association. Columns 4 and 5 are derived from only the BHS guidelines.

[b] Bladders of varying sizes are available, so a range is provided for each indication (applies to columns 2 and 3).

[c] Large bladders for arm circumferences >42 cm may be required.

Source: Reproduced from British Hypertension Society. 2012a. Blood pressure measurement with manual BP monitors. Available from: http://www.bhsoc.org/files/9013/4390/7747/BP_Measurement_Poster_-_Manual.pdf; British Hypertension Society. 2012b. Blood pressure measurement with electronic BP monitors. Available from: http://www.bhsoc.org/files/8413/4390/7770/BP_Measurement_Poster_-_Electronic.pdf. With permission.

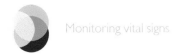

Box 4.25 Activity: a sphygmomanometer and stethoscope

If you can access manual BP recording equipment – a sphygmomanometer and a stethoscope – practise measuring and recording BP with a colleague, using the guidance in Box 4.24. Ensure you choose a correct size cuff (see Table 4.2).

Table 4.3: Common problems with manual BP measurement and suggested solutions

Problem	Solution
Incorrect BP reading	Ensure that the measurement is made to the nearest 2 mmHg
Incorrect size and position of cuff	Use the appropriate size of cuff for the individual: the cuff bladder should cover 80% of the arm's circumference
Confusion about diastolic BP reading	A too large or too small cuff will give a false reading
	Diastolic measurement taken at cessation of sounds
Poorly maintained equipment causing errors in measurement	Ensure that the manometer starts at zero and that the machine is calibrated according to the manufacturer's instructions
	The tubing and all connections should be carefully checked before use
	(O'Brien et al. 2019)

Errors in blood pressure measurement

Errors in BP measurement, including equipment failure and operator error, can significantly affect a person's investigations and treatment. Healthcare workers should be aware of the potential pitfalls in recording and overcome the risk of errors. Table 4.3 lists possible problems you may encounter and how to resolve them.

Recording blood pressure in people with postural hypotension or requiring sitting and standing blood pressure recordings

Some people experience a drop in BP when they suddenly stand up. For example, older people often experience postural drops in BP that may lead to falls or injury, and some mothers experience postural drops while pregnant. Identifying postural drop in BP and managing these drops appropriately is essential, thus recordings of laying and standing BPs are needed. To record lying and standing BP values, first lay the person down for 5 min, ensuring they are as relaxed as possible and not eating, drinking or talking. Measure the BP using an appropriate device. Stand the person up for a minute taking care of your own and their safety. Measure the BP again. Seat the person or lay them down again before documenting your findings. Remember that they may feel dizzy, faint or sick at this time, so have someone to assist you. If you are concerned about your own or their safety, abandon the procedure ensuring safety. Repeat the procedure with colleagues to assist you.

Ambulatory blood pressure monitoring and monitoring blood pressure away from the hospital environment and the use of the individual's own devices

The ambulatory device is an electronic device that is worn on the person's arm for 24 h while they continue their normal daily routine. Ambulatory BP devices are now used frequently to establish a person's BP average reading over a period of 24 h. NICE (2019a) guidelines and MHRA (2019) recommended that ambulatory devices are used to identify, measure and monitor BP in the home setting before treatment regimens are commenced. The use of ambulatory vital signs monitoring and BP devices has increased to track individual medication response and potential future management requirements. Such monitoring allows the healthcare team to review the person's BP over a longer period than their hospital visit, providing a more accurate view of their BP measurement. Ambulatory devices are used for people with an unusual variability of readings, possible white coat hypertension, to decide treatment, to review drug therapy effectiveness, to review hypertension treatment in potential heart disease or pregnancy and evaluate symptomatic hypotension in all groups.

MHRA (2020) highlighted that it is important to measure and monitor people with high BP to ensure correct management of their hypertension is achieved. This is due to the potential increased risk of, for example, **stroke** and **acute coronary syndrome**. The introduction of safe and well clinics has seen the ability to monitor people's risk factors of **acute coronary syndrome**, **stroke** and potential deterioration. MHRA (2021) recommends the use of an action plan if a person's BP is high with the intention of recognising those at risk of further insult or injury.

Accessibility to BP-monitoring devices has grown within the community setting. Many people now have greater access to BP-monitoring devices in pharmacies, GP surgeries and gyms. This can assist in people having a greater awareness of their own health and well-being. Availability of devices and purchasing of such devices for the home can assist with frequent BP-monitoring and review the effectiveness of treatments and medications. The reliability of purchased devices should however be considered. Seongil et al. (2018) highlight that several types of BP-monitoring devices can lead to errors in recording and suggest caution when using home BP devices. It is therefore important to ensure that a person uses the device correctly and that it is maintained and serviced at manufacturers' recommended intervals. Ringrose et al. (2017) note that some home devices are less accurate in monitoring BP and suggest that home devices may differ at a rate within 5 mmHg, and, therefore, users will initially need support.

Considerations with self-monitoring of blood pressure

McManus et al. (2012), The British Hypertension Society (2020) and British Heart Foundation (2020) report that this growing trend allows people to be more aware of their own BP. Self-monitoring results can often be lower than those taken by medical personnel. However, there are some inaccuracies in measuring devices and/or techniques used by people who monitor their own BP. The British Hypertension Society (2020) and British Heart Foundation (2020) offer guidance on which ambulatory devices should be used for these purposes. It is important to be aware that some individuals will be well informed about their own BP and obtaining their views and understanding of this procedure will be beneficial. Normal parameters of the person's BP will be obtained, and potential home-monitoring problems with BP recording can be reduced or avoided.

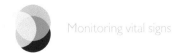

 Box 4.26 Children and young people: practice points – BP

When measuring BP for an infant or child, the correct size cuff must be used to obtain an accurate reading. For children, BP readings vary with age; see ranges below.

Systolic blood pressure (mmHg)

- <1 year 70–90
- 1–2 years 80–95
- 2–5 years 80–100
- 5–12 years 90–110
- >12 years 100–120

For further guidance on BP in infants and children, see the following:

Gormley-Fleming, E. Measuring blood pressure. In Gormley-Fleming, E. and Martin, D.(eds.) 2018 *Children and Young People's Nursing Skills at a Glance*. Chichester: Wiley, 26–27.

Royal College of Nursing. 2017. Standards for assessing, measuring and monitoring vital signs in infants, children and young people. Available from: https://www.rcn.org.uk/professional-development/publications/pub-005942 (Accessed on 4 June 2021).

Box 4.27 Pregnancy and birth: practice points – BP

Blood pressure is measured regularly throughout pregnancy as an indication of maternal health. Pregnancy itself is not normally associated with significant changes in arterial BP because any potential rise due to increased blood volume as pregnancy progresses is counterbalanced by the hormone progesterone, which reduces resistance in blood vessel walls. This effect results in a lowering of systolic pressure of 5–10 mmHg and diastolic pressure of 10–15 mmHg up to 24 weeks of pregnancy. However, serious conditions can occur. Blood pressure is monitored at every antenatal appointment and very frequently during labour. Some mothers at risk of hypertension in pregnancy need additional monitoring and care planning and the thresholds for managing hypertension in pregnancy may be different from other people.

Some mothers develop high BP alone during pregnancy with no other symptoms; however, some develop serious complications. Pre-eclampsia can occur, where the mother's BP may be raised along with protein detected in the urine, after 20 weeks gestation and over. If symptoms are not recognised, this condition can lead to reduced oxygen through the placenta to the fetus (hypoxia) and, in its severest form, lead to eclampsia and eclamptic seizures, potentially life-threatening for mother and fetus. Following the guidelines (NICE 2011b) 'Hypertension in pregnancy: diagnosis and management' ensures that these conditions are recognised, monitored and treated. (Available from: https://www.nice.org.uk/guidance/NG133 Accessed on 4 June 2021)

Summary

● Blood pressure is an important indicator of health and well-being.
● Readings can be affected by psychological, physical and environmental factors; however, technique and equipment are also important aspects.
● Electronic devices are increasingly used for recording pulse, BP and oxygen saturation. However, an understanding of how to use manual equipment accurately remains important for healthcare workers.
● There is increasing use of ambulatory devices and self-monitoring of BP, which can lead to greater accuracy as BP is measured over time, rather than as a one-off, and the person may be more relaxed.

MEASURING AND RECORDING THE PULSE (CIRCULATION)

When the left ventricle of the heart pumps blood into the already full aorta and out into the arterial system, this causes a wave of expansion throughout the arteries. Where arteries are near the surface of the body, this expansion – the pulse – can be felt when lightly pressing (palpating) the artery against bone. The pulse thus represents each ventricular contraction of the heart, and in the healthy heart, one heartbeat corresponds to one pulse beat.

Disease can affect the cardiac cycle, leading to a difference between the HR and the pulse rate. The pulse rate is the number of heart beats in a 60-s period. Pulse measurement provides very useful information about health status.

Box 4.28 Learning outcomes

By the end of this section, you will be able to:

1 explain the rationale for monitoring pulse rate and the normal values of the pulse;
2 locate pulses in different areas of the body and identify which area might be palpated in specific situations;
3 accurately measure a person's pulse rate.

Learning outcome 1: explain the rationale for monitoring pulse rate and the normal values of the pulse

Box 4.29 Activity: what can a pulse tell us?

ACTIVITY

Look again at the definition of a pulse, and then identify what a person's pulse might tell you about their health.

The pulse is measured to identify the rate and strength of the ventricular contraction and to gain information regarding a person's health. For example, in the case of

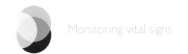
trauma and severe bleeding, the pulse rate might be weak and fast. When measuring a pulse, the following should be observed:

- **The frequency of the pulse.** The frequency of the pulse indicates the rate of contraction of the left ventricle. It is affected by numerous factors, including age, exercise, stress, injury and disease. The normal adult HR ranges from 51 to 90 beats per minute (bpm) (RCP 2020). The HR is influenced by the autonomic nervous system during sleep, producing sinus bradycardia (a slow HR); the HR can diminish during sleep by about 10–20 bpm (Waugh and Grant 2018). An abnormally slow pulse is termed bradycardia, and in an adult, would usually be a pulse rate below 51 bpm. An underactive thyroid gland, hypothermia and some drugs slow the pulse. An abnormally fast pulse is termed tachycardia – usually a pulse rate above 90 bpm in an adult. There are many reasons for a fast pulse – for example, a fever, an overactive thyroid gland and certain drugs. The thickness and tension of a person's arteriole walls influence the pulse. Atherosclerosis develops in many people over the age of 40 years and can lead to structural changes in the arteries, thus altering the pulse rate.
- **The volume.** Volume indicates the strength of the ventricular contraction. A weak contraction produces a pulse that feels weak, or it may not be strong enough to produce a pulse at the periphery – such as the wrist – at all. A lack of blood volume also leads to a weak pulse. For example, loss of blood due to trauma could lead to hypovolaemia (low blood volume) and thus eventually affect the volume of the pulse.

Atrial fibrillation

Atrial fibrillation comprises fibrillation (quivering) of the atria leading to irregular and often fast ventricular contraction and thus a highly irregular pulse rate. This is known as an arrhythmia.

- **The rhythm.** Rhythm helps to establish whether the heart is beating regularly. An irregular pulse indicates a possible abnormality in the heart's conduction system. NICE (2019b) recommends that manual pulse palpation should be performed to identify an irregular pulse, which can indicate **atrial fibrillation**. Electronic devices may not be able to record irregular pulse rates, so learn how to record a pulse manually.

Learning outcome 2: locate pulses in different areas of the body and identify which might be palpated in specific situations

It is important to know the sites where a pulse can be found.

Box 4.30 Activity: list of pulses that can be palpated

ACTIVITY

Here is a list of pulses that can be palpated (Figure 4.4). How many can you find on yourself?

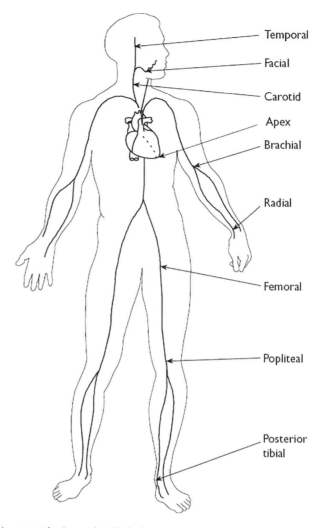

Location of pulses within the body.

- Temporal artery – on the side of the forehead
- Facial artery – on the side of the face
- Carotid artery – at the neck
- Brachial artery – in the antecubital fossa of the arm
- Radial artery – at the wrist
- Femoral artery – in the groin
- Popliteal artery – behind the knee
- Posterior tibial artery – at the inner side of each ankle.

The choice of site for pulse measurement depends on the individual and the situation. For adults in a non-emergency situation, the radial pulse is usually recorded because this site is non-invasive and easily accessible. Anne, Ken and Natalie could all have their radial pulses taken. It may be difficult to palpate some pulse sites in people with contractures. Pulses in the lower legs are usually only palpated when assessing the presence of circulation to the limbs, which might be after trauma or surgery.

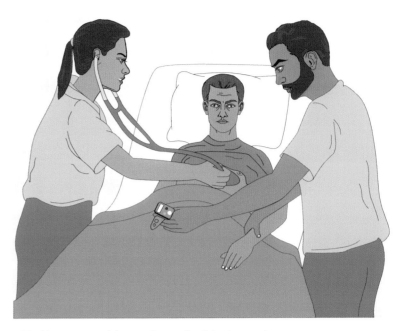

Figure 4.5: Measurement of the apex beat and radial pulse together.

Some pulses are easier to palpate and more accessible than others. In an emergency when a person has collapsed, it is often difficult to locate peripheral pulses (including the radial pulse), so the carotid or femoral pulse may be checked. You may see these pulses being checked during prolonged resuscitation attempts and monitoring of those who have deteriorated in a clinical area. However, the Resuscitation Council UK (2021) guidelines specify that only staff who are trained and experienced in clinical assessment should check the carotid and femoral pulse when assessing signs of life in a collapsed person. Checking a person's pulse as part of basic life-support guidelines is not advised as this check is time-consuming and slows down the response time for resuscitation attempts.

Note that the apex beat (site shown in Figure 4.5) can be listened to with a stethoscope, and it is located to the left side of the sternum over the heart. The apex beat may be measured when the person has a cardiac condition and is usually measured along with the radial beat. Two healthcare workers are required to perform this skill. With the person either sitting or lying still, they use the same watch over 1 min. Healthcare worker 1 counts the radial pulse and healthcare worker 2 counts the apex beat of the heart, listening with a stethoscope (Figure 4.5). The measurement is usually recorded as apex (A) and radial (R), for example, A72, R72. The numbers should be the same but in some instances, the pulse will differ, for example, A80, R72. This situation is known as a pulse deficit. People who have atrial fibrillation sometimes show these observation variations.

Learning outcome 3: accurately measure a person's pulse rate

With all individuals, psychological state needs to be considered, and consent and cooperation sought, before measuring the pulse. This cooperation involves explaining why the pulse needs to be measured.

Box 4.31 Activity: measuring and recording radial pulse

You need a willing volunteer, a watch with a second hand or a digital watch and an observation chart from your skills laboratory. Now, follow the steps in Box 4.33 to measure and record the radial pulse.

When measuring the pulse rate, healthcare workers often count the pulse for 30s and multiply by two. With a regular pulse, this count gives a reasonably accurate measurement, but an irregular pulse should always be counted for a full minute – and the word 'irregular' should be written by the recorded rate.

Box 4.32 Activity: pulse rate after exercise

Now ask your volunteer to jog on the spot for 1 min and then record the pulse rate again. You will probably find that their pulse rate has risen, due to the extra oxygen demands caused by exercise. Can you remember any other reasons why the pulse may be faster in a healthy person?

Anxiety or stress raise the pulse rate. Thus, Anne's pulse rate could be raised due to the anxiety about her situation. As discussed earlier, you need to put people at ease when recording vital signs, thereby relieving anxiety and gaining an accurate measurement.

Box 4.33 Locating and measuring a radial pulse

- Identify the radial artery. This artery is found with the palm of the hand facing upward and gently pressing at the wrist region at the thumb side (see the diagram).
- Press the artery gently against the bone with your fingers (not your thumb, which itself has a pulse) and feel the pulse bounding.
- For example, 70 beats indicate the person's pulse rate is 70.

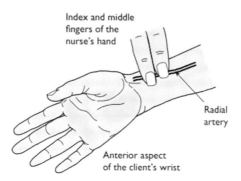

Index and middle fingers of the nurse's hand

Radial artery

Anterior aspect of the client's wrist

Figure 4.6: Measuring radial pulse.

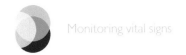
Electronic measurement of the pulse rate

The following devices can electronically record the pulse rate:

- **Oscillometer.** An oscillometer can be used for BP measurement (discussed earlier in this chapter) and the pulse rate is usually displayed too.
- **Pulse oximeter.** A pulse oximeter (discussed earlier in this chapter) measures oxygen saturation, and the pulse rate is usually displayed too.
- **Cardiac monitor.** A cardiac monitor displays the HR as well as the rhythm of the person's heart. Chapter 14 discusses cardiac monitoring.

Although these devices provide a pulse rate, they will not all indicate either the volume of the pulse or its regularity. With the pulse oximeter and cardiac monitor, movement may cause an artefact, leading to an inaccurate figure being displayed. Ensure that the pulse rate accurately represents the person's physical appearance and your own assessment. If during measuring vital signs, an electronic device shows a low reading or that the pulse is unrecordable, always attempt to record a pulse manually. If you doubt the accuracy of any observation, rerecord it manually and inform a qualified member of the healthcare team.

 Box 4.34 Children and young people: practice points – pulse measurement

In children under two years of age, the HR is measured by listening to the apical beat with a stethoscope. For children over two years, HR can be measured by palpating the radial or carotid artery. The range of pulse rates varies with the age of the child. Having an understanding of the normal parameters is vital.

- <1 year 110–160
- 1–2 years 100–150
- 2–5 years 95–140
- 5–12 years 80–120
- Over 12 years 60–100

For further guidance on pulse measurement for infants and children, see:

Akers, E. 2018. Circulatory assessment. In Gormley- Fleming, E. and Martin, D. (eds.) *Children and Young People's Nursing Skills at a Glance*. Chichester: Wiley, 24–25.

Royal College of Nursing. 2017. Standards for assessing, measuring and monitoring vital signs in infants, children and young people. Available from: https://www.rcn.org.uk/professional-development/publications/pub-005942 (Accessed on 4 June 2021).

Box 4.35 Pregnancy and birth: practice points – pulse measurement

You should ascertain what the woman's normal pulse rate is and use this rate as a guide. The technique for assessing and recording the pulse is the same as for any other adult. It is easy to take a pulse rate even if other monitoring equipment is not available. Until 32 weeks of pregnancy, maternal HR increases by 10–20 bpm (healthy non-pregnant female value = 65–85 bpm) as CO must cope with the increased blood volume that occurs. This can adversely affect women with associated pre-existing cardiac disease due to the additional stress on the cardiovascular system (CMACE 2011). In the sudden onset of severe shock, the presence of a pulse may be an unreliable indicator of an adequate cardiac output (MBRRACE 2020)

Centre for Maternal and Child Enquiries (CMACE) 2011. Saving mothers' lives. *BJOG: International Journal of Obstetrics and Gynaecology* 118(1): 1–203.

MBRRACE. 2020. Saving lives improving mothers' care. Available from: https://www.npeu.ox.ac.uk/assets/downloads/mbrrace-uk/reports/maternal-report-2020/MBRRACE-UK_Maternal_Report_Dec_2020_v10_ONLINE_VERSION_1404.pdf

(Accessed on 3 June 2021).

Summary

- Measuring a person's pulse is minimally invasive and uses little equipment but is a useful vital sign giving insight into health status.
- Nurses must be able to palpate a range of pulses and be aware of which pulse is appropriate to measure in different situations.
- It is important to be aware of the normal pulse range and to assess the volume and regularity of the pulse as well as the rate.

ACVPU (NEWS2) AND NEUROLOGICAL ASSESSMENT (GCS) (DISABILITY CONSCIOUSNESS)

ACVPU scale

A = Alert
C = Confusion (new onset)
V = (responds to) voice
P = (responds to) pain
U = Unresponsive

Neurological assessment is performed to assess a person's neurological status and is appropriate whenever there is impaired consciousness, a history of loss of consciousness or a risk that the level of consciousness might deteriorate. Neurological assessment consists of either a quick review of the person's neurological state using the ACVPU scale, or an evaluation of the level of consciousness using the GCS, pupil size and reaction, motor and sensory function and vital signs. The ACVPU scale is used to rapidly ascertain the alertness of a person and is part of a track and trigger system seen on e-observations and NEWS2. Cooksley and Rose (2018) highlight that NEWS2 is a time-sensitive assessment tool that enables a practitioner to review ACVPU along with other vital signs. If the person is ALERT, a score of 0 is recorded in the consciousness section. If, however, they are newly CONFUSED, are able to talk to you VERBALLY, respond to PAIN or are UNRESPONSIVE, a score of 3 is recorded.

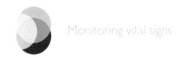

Following the initial assessment, the GCS will be used to assess and monitor a person's neurological status in more detail. This will enable the practitioner to note and respond to any change or deterioration in the person's clinical condition. See Chapter 14 for more information regarding the management of a person who is deteriorating.

Learning outcome 1: appreciate why a neurological assessment would be needed and what instruments are used

ACTIVITY

Neurological assessment would be particularly important for Anne and Natalie because they have histories of impaired consciousness. Anne has a head injury and was unconscious briefly. Natalie is not fully alert, and she has ingested an unknown quantity and variety of drugs that may affect her neurological function.

A head injury (as in Anne's case) is a particularly important reason for performing neurological assessment. Neurological observations should be conducted only by professionals competent in the assessment of head injury. The GCS, which forms part of this assessment, directly affects subsequent investigations and management.

Extradural haematoma

Extradural haematoma is an accumulation of blood between the dura and the skull. The meningeal artery passes through the extradural space and can become torn after a head injury, resulting in an arterial bleed into the extradural space. The brain then becomes compressed and displaced. This condition is life-threatening and requires urgent treatment.

Subdural haematoma

Blood accumulates in the subdural space and gradually builds up to produce a haematoma. This haematoma can lead to compression of the brain, which in turn can result in loss of brain function.

Accurate neurological assessment is particularly important where there is a concern about the development of raised intracranial pressure (Box 4.38). Being a rigid vault, the skull (cranium) cannot accommodate any swelling without the function of the brain being impaired. In disease or injury, the brain tissue, blood, or cerebral spinal fluid (CSF) can increase in volume or size, causing a rise in intracranial pressure and thereby affecting cerebral blood flow (Pinto et al. 2019). In some situations, particularly with a head injury where an extradural or subdural haematoma can develop, detection of deteriorating consciousness level is paramount because life-saving treatment could be needed. Neurological observations should be carried out under supervision of a registered nurse, and any concerns should be reported immediately.

Instruments used to assess neurological status

The GCS was developed by Jennett and Teasdale (1974) and is widely used and recognised as a scale to review a person's conscious level. The scale enables practitioners to review decision-making and monitoring trends to review conscious levels.

Box 4.39 Activity: neurological observation scale

Access a neurological observation scale from your local practice setting – either a paper chart or an e-observation technological device. Look at the sections and how they are laid out. They should include the GCS, pupil reactions and limb movements and a section for recording vital signs.

The GCS is used to assist healthcare professionals in providing a consistent and standard measurement of people's neurological status. Scoring using the GCS is done in three sections: eye-opening, motor response and verbal response (Figure 4.7). Each section is given a score, and these scores are totalled to give a score ranging from 15 (best) to 3 (worst). As a person's neurological condition improves, their GCS score should improve.

The severity of a head injury can be indicated by the score attained (Jennett and Teasdale 1974 and Jennett 2005). A score of 8 or less indicates a severe head injury, and the person will be in a coma. The rhyme 'If the Glasgow score is 8, then it is time to intubate' may help you to remember that a GCS score of 8 or below is a serious clinical situation where the person is unconscious. Maintenance of the airway by intubation of the trachea or nasopharyngeal airway using an advanced airway is a specialised clinical skill, performed by advanced practitioners who have undergone training for this procedure. You may, however, be required to observe or assist with this skill in an emergency (for more information, see Chapter 14).

A GCS score of more than 8 indicates that the person is conscious. People with a minor head injury might have a score between 13 and 15. Use of the GCS for people with head injuries is well documented, but it can be used for anyone who requires a neurological assessment, regardless of the underlying cause – so it may be relevant for Natalie and Ken, as well as for Anne.

For further information regarding how to use the scale and record and report your findings watch the videos on www.glasgowcomascale.org

	Score
Eye opening	
Spontaneous	4
To speech	3
To pain	2
None	1
Motor response	
Obeys commands	6
Localises to pain	5
Withdraws to pain	4
Abnormal flexion to pain	3
Extensor response to pain	2
No movement	1
Verbal response	
Oriented	5
Confused	4
Inappropriate words	3
Incomprehensible speech	2
None	1

Figure 4.7: Glasgow coma scale. (Adapted from Jennett, B. 2005. Development of Glasgow coma and outcome scales. *Nepal Journal of Neuroscience* 2(1): 24–8.) Also available at Glasgow coma scale – www. glasgowcomascale.org

Learning outcome 2: accurately perform and record an assessment of an adult's neurological status

When assessing any person in your care, the first priorities are to check responsiveness, ensure an open airway, check breathing and maintain adequate circulation after the basic life-support algorithms (Resuscitation Council UK 2021). Systematic assessment of acutely ill people is discussed further in Chapter 14. It should be quickly established whether the person lost consciousness at any stage and appears to be deteriorating, particularly after an accident. Thus, the person and any bystanders should be asked about the incident. Witnesses to a cardiac or respiratory event can be a valuable source of information regarding a person's condition (Resuscitation Council UK 2021) so it will be essential to gain a detailed history from Anne's husband about exactly what he observed. The onset and duration of signs and symptoms, previous medical history and any recent illnesses are all useful to note. After taking the history, a person's neurological status can be assessed using the GCS. This assessment provides a quantitative score for assessing eye-opening, verbal response and motor response.

Box 4.40 Activity: GCS score

Find a willing adult volunteer to help you to work through the GCS. Look at the scale in Figure 4.7 and consider how you might assess whether your volunteer's GCS score was 15 – the best response.

A person with a GCS score of 15 will have airway, breathing and circulation that is present and normal and will speak to you and answer questions appropriately. In brief, a talking, breathing, alert, coherent and orientated person will have a score of 15. It is to be hoped that your volunteer attained this score.

The website at www.glasgowcomascale.org recommends that the scores for each of the three sections – eye-opening (E), motor response (M) and verbal response (V) – should be documented separately to explain exactly what score has been awarded in each category.

The approach to assessing a person is outlined by RCPs and Surgeons of Glasgow – The GCS (www.glasgowcomascale.org) recommend practitioners should:

- **CHECK:** to identify any factors that might interfere with your assessment
- **OBSERVE**: for spontaneous behaviours in any three aspects of EMV
- **STIMULATE:** verbal and physical stimuli will be required in people without spontaneous behaviours
- **RATE**: judge observed response against presence or absence of defined criteria.

Each section of the scale is now explained in more detail and linking to how Anne, who has sustained a head injury might be assessed.

Eye-opening (E)

Assessment of Anne's eye-opening response indicates the arousal mechanisms found within her brainstem. When observing her eye-opening response, gently touch her arm when you ask a question. Touch is an important way of communicating non–verbally and is particularly important for people with hearing and visual deficits. Anne's husband could inform you if these deficits apply to Anne. Some people with a head injury might have difficulty opening their eyes due to eyelid swelling, particularly if there is an accompanying facial injury.

- **Spontaneous** (score 4). Anne will score 4 if she opens her eyes or already has her eyes open when you approach her.
- **To speech** (score 3). It is important to differentiate between a person sleeping and being unresponsive. This distinction can be done by asking a simple question, such as 'Can you open your eyes?'
- **To pain** (score 2). If Anne does not open her eyes to speech, you should assess whether she responds to pain. How pain should be inflicted remains controversial. You may only use appropriate touch and must take care not to cause damage such as bruising. Cook and Woodward (2011) suggest that squeezing the trapezius muscle is the most suitable method, achieved through grasping approximately 3 cm

of muscle between the thumb and forefinger, where the neck meets the shoulder, and gently twisting for 30 s. Alternatively, you can apply supraorbital pressure by pressing the skin just below the eyebrow or apply the sternal rub by using the knuckles of a clenched fist to apply pressure to Anne's sternum. Underlying injuries must be considered when applying these techniques to avoid causing more pain or injury to people. For example, do not press over the sternum if you know the person has fractured ribs, and do not apply supraorbital pressure if there is an injury in this area. Only the minimum stimulus to elicit a response should be used. You should discuss the accepted practice within your area with your supervising practitioner.

- **None** (score 1). This score is recorded where applying pain causes no eye-opening response.

Box 4.41 Activity: techniques for applying painful stimuli

ACTIVITY

If your volunteer agrees, you could try out the different techniques for applying painful stimuli, or even try them on yourself!

Motor response (M)

When assessing motor response, you should consider pre-existing disabilities and any new injuries, which in Anne's case could have been sustained in her fall. Motor response assessment is performed in relation to upper limbs because lower limb responses can reflect spinal function. *Note:* Assessment of limb movement (discussed later) is carried out on both upper and lower limbs.

- **Obeys commands** (score 6). When you are carrying out Anne's other observations, you can assess whether she coordinates her actions in response to your requests. For example, you might ask Anne to roll up her sleeve for BP measurement. Alternatives would be to ask her to close/open her eyes or stick out her tongue. If Anne were unable to obey commands, you would next apply painful stimuli (as discussed previously) and note her motor response to pain.
- **Localises** (score 5). Anne would move her hand towards the pain. For example, if you apply supraorbital pressure, she would try to push your hand away.
- **Withdraws** (score 4). If Anne's limb flexes normally to pain, this response scores a 4.
- **Abnormal flexion** (score 3). Anne's flexion to pain would be slow and abnormal.
- **Extensor response** (score 2). Anne would straighten her arm as a response to painful stimuli.
- **No movement** (score 1). Here, no motor response to any painful stimulus is made.

Verbal responses (V)

The verbal response should be assessed in relation to a person's usual communication, so you need to be aware of how they would communicate normally. Anne's neurological status is being assessed by staff who do not know her and how she communicates, so her husband's input would be particularly helpful.

- **Orientated** (score 5). If Anne is fully orientated, she should be able to answer your questions appropriately. She will tell you her name, where she is and the date.
- **Confused** (score 4). In this case, Anne can discuss something with you but may not give accurate information. For example, when asked 'Where are you?' she may respond: 'I'm in the town'.
- **Inappropriate words** (score 3). Here, Anne will use words that do not make sense. She may appear agitated and at times aggressive when you ask questions.
- **Incomprehensible speech** (score 2). Anne will not use any understandable words but will make verbal noises such as mumbling, moaning or groaning.
- **None** (score 1). Anne will not respond verbally at all. If a person is intubated, they will be unable to talk and should be recorded as 'I'.
- **Hearing loss**. If the person has impaired hearing, it may be difficult to communicate verbally, which could affect the accuracy of the result in all three categories. Sign language could be used or a communication board, if this is appropriate to the person's level of consciousness and their vision is not impaired. The person may lip-read and therefore be able to communicate effectively with you. Written responses are also valuable in this situation.
- **Language barrier**. If a person cannot understand or speak English, it could lead to difficulties with obtaining an accurate response, for example, assessing orientation or whether commands are obeyed. A communication board may help, or assistance from a professional interpreter.
- **Speech difficulties or physical impairment**. A person with learning disabilities, for example, may communicate by a signing system, in which case information from family or carers would be important.
- **Face coverings, visors and noisy environments** can lead to a person mis-understanding what you are saying. Try to consider eliminating what factors you can around the person's bedside when possible but always maintain your own personal protection and that of others.
- **Alcohol use**. If a person has ingested alcohol and has a suspected head injury, it is difficult to assess accurately. However, healthcare workers should always err on the side of caution. A person's neurological assessment should never be assumed to be due to alcohol until other causes, for example, a head injury, have been ruled out.

Box 4.42 Activity: factors affecting the accuracy of a GCS score

ACTIVITY

When assessing a person's GCS score, what factors could affect the accuracy of the assessment and how could you overcome these?

A healthcare worker carrying out neurological assessment of any of the people in the scenarios would need to be aware of all the above-mentioned factors. For example, any of them could have impaired hearing. Involvement by family or significant others who know the person's usual level of response is invaluable.

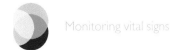

Pupil reaction

Assessment of pupil reaction usually forms part of neurological observation, as alteration in pupil sizes and reaction could indicate a rise in intracranial pressure. Look at the pupil sizes shown in Figure 4.8. You will see that they are shown in varying sizes from 1 to 8 mm. The person should be examined in dim light because bright light affects pupil reactions to the torchlight.

> ### Box 4.43 Activity: assessing pupil dilation
>
> ACTIVITY
>
> Ask your willing volunteer to walk into a brightly lit room and observe what happens to their pupils. Now observe the pupils in a dimly lit room. When did the pupil size appear the greatest?

When recording pupil reactions, the size and reaction of each eye are checked and recorded individually, for example, L5 for left eye and R5 for right eye. A light beam (usually from a pen torch) is directed into the eye to assess the reaction to the light and the size of the pupil against the chart.

- **Pupil sizes and equality.** Before shining the light in the eyes consider the following: Are the pupils equal? Do they look between 2 and 5 mm? Do they look round?
- **Reaction.** What happens when a light is shone into the eyes? Are the reactions brisk? (If yes, record **B**.) Are they sluggish? (If yes, record **SL**.) Is there no reaction? (If so, record **None**.)

Always note whether a person is wearing contact lenses or has a false eye because these conditions will affect the results. In Figure 4.8, both the left and right pupils have been recorded as 4B, meaning that the pupils are approximately 4 mm in size and react to light briskly (Figure 4.8).

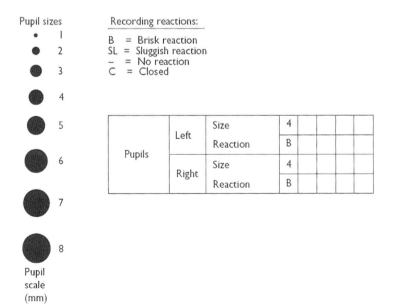

Figure 4.8: Pupil sizes and recording reactions.

Box 4.44 Activity: assessing pupil size

Now assess the size and reaction of your volunteer's pupils.

Glaucoma

An increase in the intraocular pressure of the eye causing reduced vision in the affected eye. People with visual impairment or people who have had ocular surgery or disease may have altered pupil reactions, so you should establish what is normal for this person. For example, a person who has **glaucoma** may use eyedrops that constrict the pupil.

Limb movements

A neurological chart contains a section for recording limb movements. There are different versions used in practice, and Table 4.4 gives one example. Verbal commands are used to examine these movements. For example, the healthcare worker may ask the person to push and pull against them with each limb. The responses are recorded for arms and legs separately. If there is a difference between the limbs, they are recorded separately.

In Table 4.4 the assessment indicates normal power in both legs, a mild weakness in the left arm and normal power in the right arm.

- **Normal power** is recorded when the person responds appropriately to commands and shows normal function and strength of the limb.
- **Mild weakness** implies that the limb can be moved but with reduced power. The arm weakness recorded on the chart shown may be due to a stroke or other pre-existing conditions such as cerebral palsy.
- **Severe weakness** implies movement is possible but with no real strength. Flexion is recorded when the knee or elbow is bent, and extension is recorded when the arm or leg straightens, when a painful stimulus is applied.
- **No response** is recorded when no stimulus (as used in best motor response) obtains any motor response from the person.

Table 4.4: Recording limb movements

Limb	Movements	Arms	Normal power	R
			Mild weakness	L
			Severe weakness	
			Flexion	
			Extension	
			No response	
		Legs	Normal power	R/L
			Mild weakness	
			Severe weakness	
			Flexion	
			Extension	
			No response	

Box 4.45 Activity: recording a full set of neurological observations

Practise all the skills included in this chapter by recording a full set of neurological observations with your willing volunteer. This full set should include vital signs as well as level of consciousness, pupil reactions and limb movements.

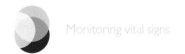

Consistency and frequency of neurological recordings

Neurological assessment is complex and requires practice in the clinical setting (www.glasgowcomascale.org). You should first observe a registered nurse recording a neurological assessment and then take part under supervision, according to local policy. The first set of neurological observations forms the baseline for future assessment. To improve reliability, handover between two healthcare professionals should be completed before a new healthcare worker takes over the care of the person. The previous healthcare worker should demonstrate the neurological assessment during this handover to gauge the person responses.

Neurological assessment should be conducted at a frequency recommended by the clinician who is caring for the person. Changes of eyes, motor and verbal responses should be monitored and tracked, and these changes should be escalated immediately.

 Box 4.46 Children and young people: practice points – neurological assessment

Neurological assessment of children is a complex procedure that must be conducted by a skilled, experienced practitioner. Eye movement, motor responses and vocal responses are measured using a scale of 15/15 with a modified GCS chart (Kirkham et al. 2008). If you have the opportunity, compare the different charts used for different age groups in practice. NICE (2014) guidelines for head injury include ones for infants and children as well as adults.

For further guidance on neurological assessment of infants and children, see:

Crawford, D. (2020) Biological basis of Child Health 4: an overview of the central nervous system and principles of neurological assessment. *Nursing Children and Young People*. doi: 10.7748/ncyp.2020.e1249

 Box 4.47 Pregnancy and birth: practice points – neurological assessment

In pregnancy, neurological assessment remains the same as in the adult and validated tools such as FAST (Face Arms Speech Test) are supported; however, consideration must be given to the parameters of vital signs where possible use a Modified Early Obstetric Warning Score (MEOWS). Remember to seek advice about the positioning of the pregnant mother who has become unwell. The unborn child and the life of the mother will be of urgent concern if a neurological condition develops as a change in vital signs can be harmful to both.

Summary
- An initial ACVPU scale should be used on all people. Thereafter, neurological observations using the GCS should be carried out if a neurological deficit is observed. Neurological assessments are frequently performed by healthcare professionals and are very important when monitoring the condition of a person with actual or potential neurological impairment.
- The GCS has been developed to promote consistency in assessment. Nevertheless, slight variations of terminology in the categories of eye-opening, motor responses and vocal responses can be found, and there may be variation in how the scale is used in practice. To promote reliability between readings, one healthcare worker should carry out the observations and demonstrate how they were carried out to any other healthcare worker who is taking over the care.
- The GCS score can be highly influential in terms of treatment, further investigation and predicting the individual's eventual outcome. Therefore, students carrying out these observations should be working under supervision and report immediately any concerns.
- Most head injuries are mild, but some people suffer serious injuries to their brain, resulting in severe disability or death. Healthcare workers who observe, measure and record neurological observations must be aware that people who have experienced neurological trauma can deteriorate very quickly. Noticing any changes in neurological function and notifying senior nursing and medical colleagues of these changes are imperative so that life-saving procedures can be carried out.

MEASURING AND RECORDING TEMPERATURE (EXPOSURE)

Healthcare workers frequently measure temperature to assess whether body temperature is within the normal range. A person's body temperature is measured by a thermometer in degree Celsius (°C). Body temperature results from a balance between heat production within the body and heat loss from the body (Marieb and Hoehn 2018). In a healthy individual, the normal core body temperature – the temperature of the organs within the cranial, thoracic and abdominal cavities – is maintained within a range of 36.1–38°C (RCP 2017) the process is called thermoregulation and is controlled by the hypothalamus, which acts as a thermostat (Tortora and Derrikson 2017). There may be times when this process is ineffective for various reasons. Body temperature higher than 37.5°C is termed pyrexia, and a body temperature lower than 35°C is termed hypothermia (Robertson and Hill 2019). Raises in temperature can be seen in hot weather but can also indicate signs of infection and a potential for underlying diseases. While low temperature can be due

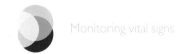

to cold weather, more worryingly, it can indicate severe infection and possible sepsis. Alcohol, medication and disease can affect temperature and it is therefore important to consider all aspects which may affect the individual's temperature during your assessment.

Box 4.48 Learning outcomes

By the end of this section, you will be able to:

1 explain the rationale for monitoring temperature;
2 identify the sites and equipment used for measuring temperature;
3 accurately measure a person's temperature.

Learning outcome 1: explain the rationale for monitoring temperature

---

Box 4.49 Activity: factors that might influence a person's body temperature

ACTIVITY

What factors might influence a person's body temperature?

You may have identified the following factors:

- **Age**. Older people often have a lower body temperature as metabolic rate falls after the age of 50 years (Childs 2019). Newborn infants' ability to regulate temperature is not fully developed. Young children grow rapidly, producing heat as a by-product of metabolism, so they have a slightly higher temperature.
- **Environment**. Heat loss is influenced by environmental temperature and humidity. The body's ability to thermoregulate cannot accommodate extremes of heat and cold for long periods. Hence, hypothermia may result from prolonged exposure to cold, and heat exhaustion can arise in a very hot environment. If thermoregulation is impaired, people become susceptible to overheating or cooling. Older people are less able to respond metabolically to falling body temperature and may have decreased perception of cold thus increasing risk for hypothermia (Tortora and Derrikson 2017). People with impaired cognitive function, confusion or perceptual disturbance may be unable to recognise and respond appropriately to environmental temperature changes; for example, they may go out inadequately dressed in cold weather.
- **Level of physical activity**. Muscular activity produces heat energy that contributes to maintaining body temperature; changes to muscle activity are an important part of thermoregulation (Marieb and Hoehn 2018). Muscle movement brings about heat production in the body (Norris and Siegfried 2017). In the adult, the body's natural response to cold brings about shivering leading to a large amount of heat being produced. This shivering is a physiological response to cold and is the body's

attempt to raise its temperature. In the young child, however, the underdeveloped hypothalamus inhibits this action. Strenuous exercise may lead to a higher core body temperature for several hours afterwards due to heat production by muscles. People with diminished mobility, due to conditions such as cerebral palsy or arthritis, may be susceptible to cold and unable to respond behaviourally by, for example, adding extra clothing, without assistance.

- **Metabolic rate**. The body's metabolic processes are a source of heat production. People with an excessive metabolic rate, for example, people with an overactive thyroid gland, may have a higher than normal body temperature. Underactivity of the thyroid gland results in a condition termed myxoedema and a low metabolic rate. Low metabolic rates may cause low body temperatures.

- **Time of day**. A roughly 24 h cycle in a physiological process in living human beings, such as body temperature, is referred to as a circadian rhythm. Body temperature normally falls during sleep and so tends to be lowest at night and rises during the day, peaking in the early evening.

- **Drugs**. Alcohol diminishes perception of cold, impairs shivering and causes vasodilation, thus predisposing an individual to a lowered body temperature. Sedative and narcotic drugs may reduce perception of cold and thus the likelihood of appropriate behavioural responses (Marieb and Hoehn 2018).

- **Infection**. One of the body's responses to infection is to raise body temperature; the thermostat of the hypothalamus is reset, causing increased heat production and inhibition of heat loss (Marieb and Hoehn 2018).

- **Menstrual cycle**. Many women have higher body temperature around ovulation (Childs 2019).

- **Eating**. Digesting and metabolising food can produce enough heat to raise body temperature slightly (Childs 2019).

Practitioners must take all these factors into account when interpreting temperature measurements.

Box 4.50 Activity: reasons for recording a person's temperature

ACTIVITY

For each of this chapter's scenarios, explain reasons why you might record the person's temperature.

You would measure Anne's temperature during her initial assessment and as a baseline for future recordings. Also, she may have become hypothermic if she was lying on the ground outside in very cold weather. Ken's temperature would be recorded as part of his general assessment, particularly if he feels hot or cold to touch and he may have had an annual check to provide a good baseline. He may have an infection, causing him to feel unwell. Natalie's temperature would have been recorded during her admission assessment; this temperature acts as a baseline against which future measurements can be compared. Her body temperature may be lower due to alcohol consumption.

Body temperature is routinely recorded when a person is in a community setting, admitted to hospital, pre- and postoperatively, after invasive procedures and during various treatments. For people with learning disabilities, recording body temperature can help identify whether behavioural changes are due to a physical health problem. Also, recording temperature regularly for people with learning disabilities, perhaps during routine health checkups, promotes familiarity with the equipment and procedure so that temperature measurement should not cause undue distress during ill health. Frequency of measurements may range from just one recording on admission to hourly in a person with high temperature.

Learning outcome 2: identify the sites and equipment used for measuring temperature

Ideally, the same site and method should be used for a person's temperature measurement each time to promote greater consistency. However, different sites and methods are appropriate in different circumstances.

Box 4.51 Activity: equipment and sites used to record body temperature

ACTIVITY

From your experience in practice, as well as personal experience of having your temperature taken, list the equipment and sites that can be used to record body temperature. What might be their advantages and disadvantages?

Sites for temperature recording

You are likely to have seen the following sites used:

- Mouth
- Axilla (armpit)
- Tympanic membrane (in the ear)
- Forehead
- Rectal
- Bladder (via urinary catheter)

Considering the choice of site and their associated accuracy

Geijer et al. (2016), in their systematic review of temporal scanners to measure temperature, highlight that temperature is one of the most used parameters in healthcare. There is no universal agreement on how accurate a thermometer must be. They explain how temperature has historically been measured using invasive methods. However, a non-invasive method may be suitable on some occasions. Temporal artery temperature measurement offers such a solution. Their findings indicate that temporal measurement is not accurate enough to replace monitoring via rectal or bladder. Interestingly, they did, however, conclude that temporal temperature may be as inaccurate as the tympanic route (Geijer et al. 2016).

The rectum can also be used to measure temperature, but this site is rarely used, except in a few special circumstances. Taking temperatures rectally is invasive and can cause embarrassment. Temporal artery temperature measurement is sometimes used. The device is held over the forehead and senses infrared omissions to note the temperature. Oral measurements are unsuitable for people who are confused, unconscious or breathless. A breathless person tends to mouth breathe so oral temperature measurement would then be both distressing and inaccurate. Axillary temperature measurement requires good contact between the two skin surfaces, so this site will probably be inaccurate with very thin people. The person must be able to keep the arm still by the side of the chest. The axillary temperature is not an accurate indicator of core body temperature if the person is vasoconstricted or chilled, as Anne may be if she has been outside for a prolonged period. The tympanic membrane is a convenient site for temperature recording and can be used with most people if the equipment is available.

Box 4.52 Activity: routes for temperature measurement and rationale for their use

ACTIVITY

When you are next in the practice setting, observe which routes are used for temperature measurement for different people and identify the rationale for their choice.

Equipment

You may have seen chemical disposable, electronic and infrared light reflectance thermometers and forehead bands or stickers. In the past, mercury thermometers were used, but they are no longer used due to concerns about the potential risks of mercury spillage from broken glass thermometers.

Noncontact infrared thermometers have developed over recent years offering a quicker less invasive way to monitor a person's temperature. Many are available to be purchased for children in the form of head stickers or monitor bands. These bands or stickers monitor the temperature at the temporal artery. Kiekkas et al. (2016) in their systematic review noted some issues related to using such devices, such as inaccuracy due to poor placement. They suggest that such devices are low in sensitivity. NICE (2019b) recommends that temporal devices to monitor temperature are not used.

Chemical disposable thermometers

In some clinical situations, the oral route is recommended. For example, Gates et al. (2018) highlight that accurate temperature measurements for individuals with cancer are critical. They recommend the oral route is used to ensure this.

Chemical disposable thermometers can be used in the mouth to record oral temperature. These are thin plastic strips with small dots of thermosensitive chemicals that change colour with increasing temperature and may be used in the mouth or axilla (Figure 4.10). They are disposed of after use, so there is no cross-infection risk. Accuracy depends on correct technique in relation to timing and positioning. Also, they must be stored at under 30°C. When using these

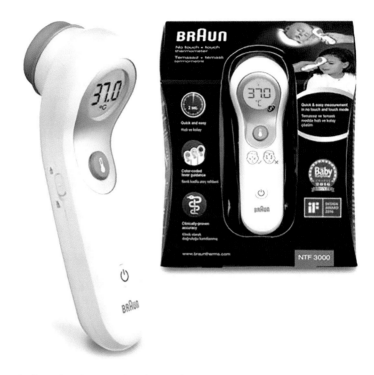

Figure 4.9: Examples of non-touch and touch thermometers.

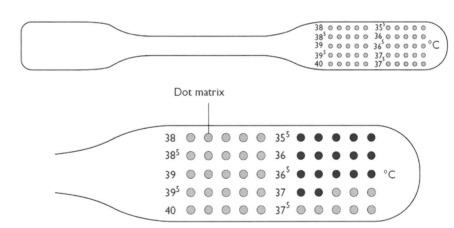

Figure 4.10: A chemical dot matrix thermometer showing 37.1°C.

thermometers, ensure the mouth is closed for 60 s and leave them *in situ* no longer than 2 min. In the axilla, the thermometer should be placed against the torso and completely covered by body surfaces for 3 min (3M™ 2020). It should be read after 10 s. Read the thermometer by looking at the last dot. If the thermometer is left in the mouth for longer than 2 min or in the axilla longer than 5 min, it must be rerecorded with a new thermometer as it could be inaccurate otherwise (www.medicalindicators.com 2020) (Figure 4.10).

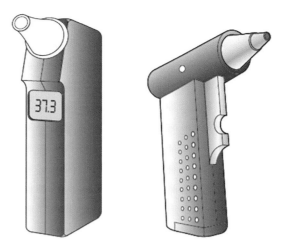

Figure 4.11: An infrared tympanic thermometer.

Electronic thermometers

Electronic thermometers consist of a probe that is placed in the mouth, the axilla or the rectum, usually connected to a power supply and display unit. The purchase cost is significant, as are the ongoing costs of probe covers needed for each use. Most of these thermometers produce an auditory signal after a preset time or when maximum temperature is reached, so the user does not determine the timing.

Infrared thermometers

Infrared thermometers detect heat radiated as infrared energy from the tympanic membrane (Figure 4.11). Temperature is recorded within a few seconds, causing little inconvenience or discomfort. The thermometers are designed to detect heat from the tympanic membrane, but they also detect heat from the ear canal (which may be 2°C lower) if not correctly placed to provide a snug fit (MHRA 2019 and NICE 2013); therefore, correct placement of the probe is essential. Bridges and Thomas (2009) and Arslan and Khorsid (2011) warned against taking the temperature immediately after the person has been lying on the ear that you use to record temperature as this can affect the reading. If the individual is lying on their ear, use the upward facing ear if possible, but if this is not possible, due to surgery or trauma for example, wait 3 min before recording the temperature in the ear that they have been lying on.

Rectal and invasive measurement devices

Rectal thermometry is seen to be accurate, the procedure is however poorly tolerated and invasive, so alternatives have been developed to assist practitioners to monitor temperature. However, in some critically ill people, temperature monitoring may be performed via the rectal route (Figure 4.12).

Bladder temperature using urinary catheters

In critically unwell people, recording temperature is significant and requires more invasive equipment for temperature measurement than can be seen in the prehospital

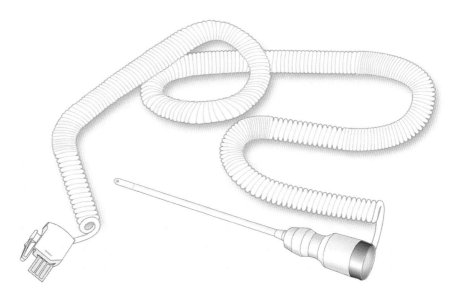

Figure 4.12: Rectal thermometer and probe.

or ward situation. Temperature sensing urinary catheters can be used to continuously monitor core body temperature. This is a urinary Foley catheter with an inbuilt temperature sensor that is inserted into the bladder and therefore urine output can be measured along with temperature in the bladder. Thus, two measurements and functions can be obtained via one device (Figure 4.13).

Box 4.53 Activity: methods and sites appropriate to individuals

ACTIVITY

Which method and site are most appropriate for each of the people in this chapter's scenarios, and why?

Compare your answers with the points below:

- **Adult** – For Anne, a tympanic thermometer would probably be used. The oral route is not appropriate as she is disorientated, and she may be in pain, anxious and receiving oxygen via a mask. A tympanic thermometer would record her temperature without affecting her other treatments and observations.
- **Learning disability** – Ken's temperature could be measured in the axilla using either a disposable or an electronic thermometer. A tympanic thermometer could be used if the equipment is available. Ken may have preferences about the type of equipment used and method, and these preferences should be respected if possible. The nurse should explain carefully first, especially if the equipment used is unfamiliar to him – showing him the equipment first will help lessen any anxiety he may have.
- **Mental health** – Natalie's temperature could be recorded using a tympanic thermometer. The oral route is not suitable as she is not fully conscious. The axilla

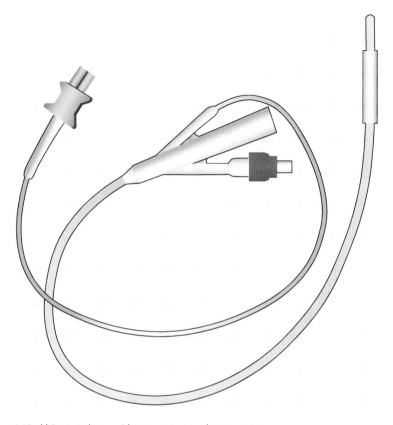

Figure 4.13: Urinary catheter with temperature probe connector.

route could be used, using a disposable thermometer or electronic thermometer. The nurse would need to help her keep her arm by her side for the required length of time.

Learning outcome 3: accurately measure a person's oral temperature measurements

Box 4.54 Activity: chemical disposable thermometer use

ACTIVITY

Find a willing volunteer with whom to practise this activity. You will need a chemical disposable thermometer. Follow the steps in Box 4.55.

Remember that this route is not frequently used; however, it is important to gain clinical competency in recording temperature via the oral route. Please refer to local clinical trust protocols to identify which anatomical areas are recommended.

Factors that might affect the oral temperature measurement include:

* eating or drinking hot or cold substances shortly before the procedure;
* smoking;
* talking;

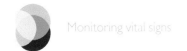
- breathing through the mouth;
- incorrect positioning of the thermometer;
- thermometer in the mouth for too short a time.

Oral temperature should not be recorded within 15 min of the person eating, drinking or smoking.

Box 4.55 Measuring oral temperature

Diagram of oral cavity and placement of thermometer (Figure 4.14).

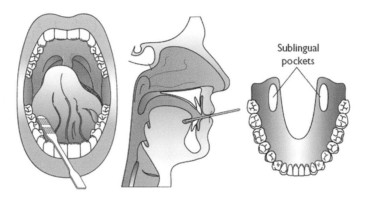

Sublingual pockets

Figure 4.14: Measuring an oral temperature.

- Explain the procedure to the person, including the need to keep the lips closed while the thermometer is in position.
- Position the plastic strip in the person's mouth under the tongue to the side; see the diagram for correct positioning. The face with the dots on (dot matrix) can be placed either way up and must be left in for 1 min.
- Remove the thermometer. Wait 10 s and read the last blue dot, ignoring any dots in between that have not changed colour (3M™ 2020). Dispose of the thermometer.
- Record the measurement on a NEWS2 observation chart or e-observation systems, for example, a temperature of 38.5°C. Report abnormal temperatures.

Axilla measurements

Box 4.56 Activity: measuring axillary temperature

ACTIVITY

Now try using a chemical disposable thermometer to measure axillary temperature using the instructions in Box 4.58. Compare this reading with the previous oral measurement.

Electronic devices

Box 4.59 lays out instructions for using electronic thermometers. You may be able to practise using these devices if the equipment is available. Note that the tympanic temperature should not be taken with a hearing aid in place, in an ear that is infected or after ear surgery. If the person has experienced any trauma in and around the ear, then seek medical advice as to whether the tympanic thermometer is suitable. Consideration of ottorhoea (discharge from the ear) also needs to be made. Several manufacturers of tympanic thermometers advise not using a tympanic thermometer in an ear that has been operated on for a week postoperatively, so check the manufacturer's instructions regarding this issue.

ACTIVITY

Box 4.57 Activity: other observations to assess body temperature

Using a thermometer will give you an accurate measurement of temperature, but what other observations could help you to assess body temperature?

You can feel whether the person has cold extremities or is hot to touch, whether the person is shivering or sweating and ask them how they feel. It is particularly important to use these observations if people are unable to communicate verbally about whether they feel cold or hot. Your observations may prompt you to record their temperature.

Box 4.58 Measurement of a temperature in the axilla, using a chemical, disposable thermometer

- Explain the procedure to the person, including the need to remain still while the thermometer is in position (Figure 4.15).

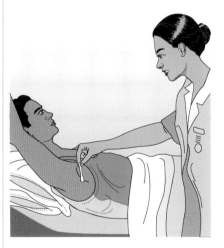
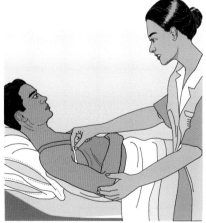

Figure 4.15: Measurement of a temperature in the axilla.

- Raise the person's arm. Place the thermometer in the centre of the person's axilla (see the diagram), positioning it with the dot matrix against the torso.

(Continued)

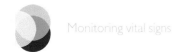

Box 4.58 (Continued)

- Check to ensure there is good contact with the skin when the arm is lowered.
- Rest the person's arm across the chest and maintain the thermometer in position for a minimum of 3 min.
- Remove the thermometer, read and record the result described as in Box 4.7.
- Dispose of the chemical thermometer.
- Report abnormal temperatures.

Box 4.59 Temperature measurement using electronic devices

Using an electronic thermometer to record oral or axilla temperature

- The positioning of electronic probes in the mouth or the axilla is the same as for chemical disposable thermometers (see Boxes 4.55 and 4.58).
- A new probe cover should be used for each person.
- Devices have either an auditory (e.g. bleeping sound) or visual (e.g. flashing) indicator when maximum temperature is reached; the probe should remain in place until this indicator is noted.

Using an infrared tympanic membrane thermometer

- The speculum is covered with a disposable cover.
- The ear is pulled gently but firmly to straighten the ear canal, pulling the ear up and back.
- The speculum is inserted gently into the ear canal, ensuring a snug fit.
- The start button is pressed.
- The reading is obtained within 1 or 2 s, indicated by a bleeping sound.

 Box 4.60 Children and young people: practice points – temperature measurement

All children and young people who attend a healthcare setting should have their temperature taken as part of their assessment. They can present with mottled skin, feel hot or cold to touch or may have a rash, so it is appropriate to take a temperature within the assessment using a measurement device suitable for the child or young person's age.

Infants under four weeks: Axilla route using an electronic thermometer

Four weeks to five years: Axilla route using an electronic or chemical dot thermometer, or tympanic, using an infrared tympanic thermometer

Five years and over: oral or axilla (with electronic or chemical dot thermometer) or tympanic, using an infrared tympanic thermometer

See:

Gormley-Fleming, E. 2018. Measuring temperature. In Gormley-Fleming, E. and Martin, D. (eds.) *Children and Young People's Nursing Skills at a Glance.* Chichester: Wiley, 32–33.

Royal College of Nursing. 2017. Standards for assessing, measuring and monitoring vital signs in infants, children and young people. Available from: https://www.rcn.org.uk/professional-development/publications/pub-005942 (Accessed on 13 May 2021).

Box 4.61 Pregnancy and birth: practice points – body temperature

- The hormone progesterone, as well as a raised metabolic rate during pregnancy, increases the amount of heat generated by the body by 30–35%. Even though the body compensates for this increase by losing heat, maternal temperature can be increased by 0.5°C.
- A high maternal temperature raises the fetal temperature and HR, which can lead to serious complications for the fetus (Advanced Life Support in Obstetrics, [ALSO] 2017), such as preterm labour and hypoxia (Centre for Maternal and Child Enquiries, [CMACE] 2011).
- A newborn baby's inability to thermoregulate effectively, due to having a large surface area and little subcutaneous fat to insulate them, makes them vulnerable to cold air and draughts.
- In addition, care must be taken with overheating, which is one of the risk factors for sudden unexpected death in infancy cot death. See: The Lullaby Trust. Available from: https://www.lullabytrust.org.uk/ (Accessed 9 June 2021).

Centre for Maternal and Child Enquiries (CMACE) 2011. Saving Mothers Lives. *British Journal of Obstetrics and Gynaecology.* 118(1). Available from: https://obgyn.onlinelibrary. wiley.com/doi/abs/10.1111/j.1471-0528.2010.02847.x (Accessed on 10 June 2021).

Advanced Life Support in Obstetrics (ALSO) 2017. American Academy of Family Physicians. Available from:

https://www.cascadetraining.com/offered_classes/advanced_life_support_in_ obstetrics_also.cfm (Accessed on 10 June 2021).

Summary

- Choice of route and equipment for measuring temperature should consider individual factors such as physical and mental conditions as well as the devices available.
- For each route and device used, the measurement should be conducted and recorded carefully and accurately.
- Abnormal measurements should be reported and appropriate action taken.
- As temperature can vary between body sites, the measurement site should be recorded and the same site used for subsequent recordings whenever possible.

CHAPTER SUMMARY

Following the recording of all vital signs, the NEWS2 will be calculated and the appropriate actions taken as per the clinical guidelines of your practice area. This chapter aimed to help you develop your skills in assessing vital signs and recording NEWS2 scores within the practice setting. These vital signs should not be considered in isolation but as part of a person's holistic assessment, which will include a range of other observations and information from various sources. It is imperative that you observe, question, discuss and practise recording vital signs first in a simulated environment and then in a clinical area. It is necessary to become familiar with clinical equipment used for vital signs monitoring to ensure that this equipment is used correctly. Overreliance of electronic equipment should be avoided because there is a potential to become deskilled in monitoring vital signs. Observation, rehearsal and supervised practice will initially develop your confidence in performing this set of skills.

Vital signs must be measured, assessed and recorded accurately, using the appropriate equipment in the recommended manner, as per trust protocols and manufacturers' instructions. They must also be reported, and guidance sought in their interpretation. Ensure you use technology devices that include the NEWS2 score and note a person's potential for deterioration. Bedside technology can ensure changes to the individual's condition are noted in real time and help ensure early recognition and quick action. Indeed, Lang et al. (2019) in their safety literature, reported the importance of early recognition of deterioration. E-observation systems deployment has seen approximately 50% reduction in NEWS policy-related person safety incidents (Lang et al. 2019). This is attributed to ease of calculation, prompt treatment and timely escalation, for example, recognition of sepsis or acute kidney injury. Some vital signs can change quickly along with the person's level of consciousness, so their observation must be carried out at the required frequency. Chapter 14 offers further guidance regarding the assessment of people whose condition is deteriorating. It can take considerable practice with a range of people in a variety of settings to become confident and competent in these skills. See it, record it and report it should be your motto in vital signs monitoring.

REFERENCES

3M™. 2020. 3M *Tempa DOT™ Single-use Clinical Thermometers: How to Read 3M Tempa DOT™ Thermometers*. US: 3M™ Medical Division. Available from: www.medicalindicators.com (Accessed on 25 February 2020).

Arslan, G. and Khorsid, L. 2011. Analysis of the effects of lying on the ear on body temperature measurement using a tympanic thermometer. *Journal Pak Medical Association* 61(11): 1065–8.

Barnett, E., Duck, A. and Barraclough, R. 2012. Effect of recording site on pulse oximetry readings. *Nursing Times* 108(1–2): 22–3.

Brekke, I.J., Puntervoll Pederson, P., Kellett, L. and Brabrand, M. 2019. The value of vital sign trends in predicting and monitoring clinical deterioration: A systematic review. doi: 10.1371/journal.pone.0210875

Bridges, E., and Thomas, K. 2009. Noninvasive measurement of body temperature in critically ill patients Literature review. *Critical Care Nurse* 29(3): 94–7.

British Heart Foundation (BHF). 2020. Heart matters How to choose a blood pressure monitor and measure your blood pressure at home available at www.bhf.org.uk (Accessed on 27 February 2020).

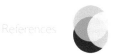

British Hypertension Society. 2012a. Blood pressure measurement with manual blood pressure monitors. Available from: http://www.bhsoc.org/files/9013/4390/7747/BP_Measurement_Poster_-_Manual.pdf

British Hypertension Society. 2012b. Blood pressure measurement with electronic blood pressure monitors. Available from: http://www.bhsoc.org/files/8413/4390/7770/BP_Measurement_Poster_-_Electronic.pdf

British and Irish Hypertension Society (BIHSOC). 2020. How to measure blood pressure www.bihsoc.org (Accessed 26 February 2020).

British Thoracic Society Guidelines. 2017. For oxygen use in healthcare and emergency settings www.brit-thoracic.org.uk (Accessed on 19 February 2020).

Bucknall, T., Harvey, G., Considine, J. et al. 2007. Prioritising responses of nurses to deteriorating patient observations (PRONTO): testing the effectiveness of a facilitation intervention in a pragmatic, cluster randomised trial with an embedded process evaluation and cost analysis *Implementation Science* 12. 85.

Campbell, M., Sultan, A. and Pillarisetty, L. 2020. Physiology, Korotkoff sound. Available from: https://pubmed.ncbi.nlm.nih.gov/30969600/ (Accessed on 9 June 2021).

Centres for Disease Control and Prevention. 2020. Measure your blood pressure available at www.cdc. gov (Accessed on 27 February 2020).

Childs, C. 2019. Maintaining body temperature. In: Brooker, C. and Nicol, M. (eds.) *Alexander's Nursing Practice: Hospital and Home*, 5th edn. Edinburgh: Churchill Livingstone.

Choi, S., Yu, C., Mi, K., Jinho, S. et al. 2018. Comparison of the accuracy and errors of BP measured by 2 types of non-mercury sphygmomanometers in an epidemiological survey. *Medicine* June, 97(25): e10851. doi: 10.1097/MD.0000000000010851.

Churpek, M., Adhikari, R. and Edelson, D.P. 2016. The value of vital sign trends for detecting clinical deterioration on the wards. *Resuscitation*. doi:10.1016/j.resuscitation.2016.02.005

Clark, C.E., Taylor, R.S., Shore, A.C. et al. 2012. Association of a difference in systolic blood pressure between arms with vascular disease and mortality: A systematic review and meta-analysis. *The Lancet* 379(9819): 905–14.

Cook, N. and Woodward, S. 2011. Assessment, interpretation and management of altered consciousness. In: Woodward, S. and Mestecky, A. (eds.) *Neuroscience: Evidence-Based Practice*. Chichester: Blackwell Science, 107–22.

Cooksley, T. and Rose, S. 2018. A systematic approach to the unconscious patient. *Clinical Medicine* 18(1): 88–92.

Data Protection Act. 2018. General Data Protection Regulation (GDPR). Available from: www legislation.gov.uk (Accessed on 27 February 2020).

Department of Health (DH). 2009. *Health Action Planning and Health Facilitation for People with Learning Disabilities: Good Practice Guidance*. London: DH.

European Parliament and Council of European Union. 2016. GDRP Regulation. Available from: https://eur-lex.europa.eu/legal-content/EN/TXT/HTML/?uri=CELEX:32016 R0679&from=EN (Accessed on 25 February 2020).

Fernandez–Ayuso, D., Fernandez Ayusho, R. and Calvo Lobo, C. 2018. The modification of vital signs according to nursing student's experiences undergoing cardiopulmonary resuscitation training via high fidelity simulation Quasi experimental study. *JMIR Serious Games* 6(3): e11061.

Gates, D., Horner, V., Bradley, L. et al. 2018. Temperature measurements comparison of different thermometer types for patient with cancer. *Clinical Journal of Oncology Nursing* December 1, 22(6): 611–17. doi 10.1188/18 CJoN 611–617 PMID 22 (6).

Geijer, H., Udumyan, R. and Lohse Nilsagard, Y. 2016. Temperature measurements with a temporal scanner: Systematic review and meta-analysis. *BMJ Open* 6: e009509. doi 10.1136/bmjopen 2015–009509.

Glasgow Coma Scale. Available from: www.glasgowcomascale.org (Accessed on 26 February 2020).

Hallett, S. Toro, F. and Ashurst, J. 2020. Physiology, Tidal Volume Jun 1 In StatPearls (Internet) Treasure Island (FL) Stat Pearls publishing. Available from: www.ncbi.nlm. nih.gov (PMID 29494108 (Accessed on 8 March 2021).

Hill, E., Stoneham, M. and Fearnley, S.J. 2008. Practical applications of pulse oximetry. Available from: http://www.nda.ox.ac.uk (Accessed on 25 February 2020).

Holmes, S. and Peffers, S. 2013. PCRS-UK opinion sheet No 28. Pulse oximetry in primary care. Available from: http://www.pcrs-uk.org (Accessed on 25 February 2020).

Jennett, B. 2005. Development of Glasgow coma and outcome scales. *Nepal Journal of Neuroscience* 2(1): 24–8.

Jennett, B. and Teasdale, G. 1974. Assessment of the coma and impaired consciousness. *The Lancet* 2: 81–4.

Kallioinen, N., Hill, A., Horswill, M. et al. 2017. Sources of inaccuracy in the measurement of adult patients resting blood pressure in clinical settings a systematic review. *Journal of Hypertension* 35(3): 421–41.

Kiekkas, P., Stefanopoulos, N., Bakalis, N. et al. 2016. Agreement of infrared temporal artery thermometery with other thermometry methods in adults: Systematic review. *Journal of Clinical Nursing* 25(7–8): 894–905.

Kirkham, F., Newton, C. and Whitehouse, W. 2008. Paediatric coma scales. *Developmental Medicine & Child Neurology* 50(4): 267–74.

Lang, A., Simmonds, M. and Swinscoe, C. 2019. The impact of an electronic patient bedside observation and handover system on clinical practice: Mixed methods evaluation. *JMIR Medical Information* Jan–Mar 7(1): e11678.

Louie, A., Feiner, M., Bickler, P. et al. 2018. Four types of pulse oximeters accurately detect hypoxia during low perfusion and motion. *Anesthesiology* 3(28): 520–30.

Magder, S. 2018. The meaning of blood pressure. *Critical Care* 22(257). https://doi. org/10.1186/s13054-018-2171-1.

Marieb, E.N. and Hoehn, K. 2018. *Human Anatomy and Physiology*, 11th edn. London: Pearson Education.

McDermott, R., Liddicoat, H., Moore, A.J. et al. 2018. Evaluating the accuracy of commercially available finger pulse oximeters in a hospital setting. *European Respiratory Journal* 52(Suppl 62): PA4452.

McGee, S. 2018. *Part 17 Blood Pressure in Evidence-Based Physical Diagnosis*, 4th edn. London: Elsevier.

McManus, J., Glasziou, P., Haye, A. et al. 2012. Self-monitoring: Question and answers from a national conference. *British Medical Journal* 337(10): 2732.

Medicines and Healthcare Products Regulatory Agency (MHRA). 2009. Kid's stuff – paediatric special. *One-liners* (73). Available from: http://www.mhra.gov.uk (Accessed on 10 February 2013).

Medicines and Healthcare Products Regulatory Agency (MHRA). 2020. *Device Bulletin: Blood Pressure Measurement Devices* October. Available from: http://www.mhra.gov.uk (Accessed on 18 March 2021).

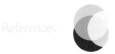

Mestecky, A. 2013. Assessment and management of raised intracranial pressure. In: Woodward, S. and Mestecky, A. (eds.) *Neuroscience Nursing Evidence Based Practice*, Ist edn. Oxford: Wiley Blackwell, Kindle Edition.

National Institute for Health and Clinical Excellence (NICE). 2007a. *Quick Reference Guide. Acutely Ill Patients in Hospital: Recognition of and Response to Acute Illness in Adults in Hospital.* Clinical Guidelines 50. London: NICE.

National Institute for Health and Clinical Excellence (NICE). 2007b. *Head Injury: Triage, Assessment, Investigation and Early Management of Head Injury in Infants, Children and Adults.* Clinical Guidelines 56. London: NICE.

National Institute for Health and Clinical Excellence (NICE). 2011a. *Hypertension: Clinical Management of Primary Hypotension in Adults.* Clinical Guidelines 127. London: NICE.

National Institute for Health and Clinical Excellence (NICE). 2011b. *Hypertension in Pregnancy: The Management of Hypertensive Disorders during Pregnancy.* Clinical Guidelines 107. London: NICE.

National Institute for Health and Clinical Excellence (NICE). 2013. Full guideline Feverish illness in children assessment and initial management in children younger than 5 years. Clinical Guideline 160. Available from: www.nice.org.uk (Accessed on 25 February 2020).

National Institute for Health and Clinical Excellence (NICE). 2017. Sepsis recognition, diagnosis and early management. Clinical Guideline 51.Available from: www.nice.org.uk (Accessed on 25 February 2020).

National Institute for Health and Clinical Excellence (NICE). 2019a. Hypertension in adults: Diagnosis and management. Available from: www.nice.org.uk (Accessed on 3 March 2020).

National Institute for Health and Clinical Excellence (NICE). 2019b. Atrial Fibrillation. The Management of Atrial Fibrillation. Clinical Guidelines 36. London: NICE. Available from: www.cks.nice.org.uk (Accessed on 3 March 2020).

NHS England. 2019. The atlas of shared learning introducing bedside vital signs devices at Imperial College Healthcare NHS Trust. Available from: https://www.england.nhs.uk/atlas_case_study/introducing-bedside-vital-signs-devices-at-imperial-college-healthcare-nhs-trust/ (Accessed on 26 February 2020).

Nicholas, A. 2012. Oscillometric sphygmomanometers: A critical appraisal of current technology. *Blood Pressure Monitoring Journal* 17(2): 80–8.

Odya, E. and Norris, M. 2017. *Anatomy and Physiology for Dummies*, 3rd edn. Indianapolis: Wiley and Sons.

Nursing and Midwifery Council. (NMC). 2018a. *Standards of Proficiency for Registered Nurses.* London: NMC.

Nursing and Midwifery Council. (NMC). 2018b. *Standards of Proficiency for Nursing Associates.* London: NMC.

O'Brien, E. et al. 2013. European society of hypertension position paper on ambulatory blood pressure monitoring. *Journal of Hypertension* Sep 31(9): 1731–68.

O'Brien, E., Petrie, J., Littler, W. et al 2019. *Blood Pressure Measurement Recommendations of the British Hypertension Society.* London: BMJ Publications.

Odya, E. and Du Pree, P. 2018. *Anatomy and Physiology Workbook for Dummies with Online Practice*, 3rd edn. London: Wiley and Sons.

Peate, I. 2019. Nursing patients with cardiovascular disorders. *Alexander's Nursing Practice Hospital and Home*, 5th edn. Edinburgh: Churchill Livingstone.

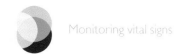

Pedersen, T., Hovhannisyan, K. and Møller, A.M. 2009. Pulse oximetry for perioperative monitoring. *Cochrane Database of Systematic Reviews Issue* (4): Art. No.: CD002013. DOI: 10.1002/14651858.CD002013.pub2.

Pinto, V., Prasanna, T. and Adeyinka, A. 2019. Increased intracranial pressure. Available from: https://pubmed.ncbi.nlm.nih.gov/29489250/ (Accessed on 9 May 2020).

Reinberg, S. 2020. Blood pressure differences between arms could signal heart risk. Available from: https://www.medicinenet.com/script/main/art.asp?articlekey=154135 (Accessed on 20 May 2020).

Resuscitation Council (UK). 2021. Resuscitation guidelines. Available from: http://www.resus.org.uk (Accessed on 8 March 2021).

Ringrose, J., Polle, G., McLean, D. et al. 2019. An assessment of the accuracy of home blood pressure monitors when used in device owners. *American Journal of Hypertension* 30(7): 683–9.

Robertson, M. and Hill, B. 2019. Monitoring temperature. *British Journal of Nursing* 28(6). https://doi.org/10.12968/bjon.2019.28.6.344

Royal College of Nursing. 2017. *Standards for Assessing, Measuring and Monitoring Vital Signs in Infants, Children and Young People.* London: RCN.

Royal College of Physicians (RCP). 2012. National early-warning score (NEWS) standardising the assessment of acute illness severity in the NHS. Available from: www.rcplondon.ac.uk

Royal College of Physician (RCP). 2017. *National Early Warning Score (NEWS2) Standardising the Assessment of Acute – Illness Severity in the NHS.* London: RCP.

Skerrett, P.J. 2012. *Different Blood Pressure in Right and Left Arms Could Signal Trouble.* Available from: http://www.health.harvard.edu/blog/different-blood-pressure-in-rightand-left-arms-could-signal-trouble-201202014174 (Accessed on 19 May 2021).

Skinner, D. and Driscoll, P. 2013. *ABC of Major Trauma, ABC Series,* 4th edn. London: Wiley Blackwell BMJ.

Tortora, G. and Derrikson, B. 2017. *Principles of Anatomy and Physiology,* Global edn. New York: John Wiley.

Waugh, A. and Grant, A. 2018 *Ross and Wilson's Anatomy and Physiology in Health and Illness,* 13th edn. London: Churchill Livingstone.

USEFUL WEBSITES

British Heart foundation: www.bhf.org
British Hypertension Society: www.bhsoc.org
Glasgow Coma Scale: www.glasgowcomascale.org/
Stroke Association: www.stroke.org.uk

Meeting personal needs: hydration and nutrition

Sue Maddex

Nutrition and hydration are essential to maintain health. Meeting human basic needs of air, water, food, shelter, sanitation, touch, sleep and personal space are all fundamental to support well-being. In healthcare, people strive to meet nutritional and hydration needs of their client groups to promote recovery from illness. Recognising people who need nutritional support and preventing malnutrition are key skills required of nurses and healthcare workers. NICE (2017) guidelines CG 32 aim to assist practitioners identify and care for adults who are malnourished or at risk of malnutrition in hospital or in their own home. NICE (2017) offers a flow chart to assist practitioners make decisions regarding nutritional interventions. They express the importance of this role in healthcare. While adequate nutrition and hydration are essential for people's recovery, it is reported that it is often difficult to achieve optimum nutrition during times of illness or injury. Across the world, malnutrition continues to compromise people's quality of life, health and well-being, delays the speed of recovery from disease and increases mortality rates. Often in a world of plenty, appropriate nutrition and hydration are lacking in many social situations. Malnutrition is frequently undetected and untreated, causing a wide range of adverse consequences (Carers UK 2020), with one in four adults being seen to be malnourished upon hospitalisation (The British Association of Parenteral and Enteral Nutrition [BAPEN] 2020). Concern has been expressed for what happens to a person's nutritional state when they are in crisis, become unwell or are hospitalised or isolated (BAPEN 2020). Malnutrition is associated with negative outcomes for the individual. Limited nutrition and hydration inhibit cellular function and affect the function and recovery of every organ system. The consequences of malnutrition include vulnerability to infection, delayed wound healing, impaired function of the heart and lungs, decreased muscle strength and depression (NHS Improvements 2020). It is therefore a fundamental part of a healthcare worker's role to ensure that individuals have adequate nutrition and hydration when receiving care. This role is sometimes overlooked while other care and treatments are prioritised. Local and national organisations, such as Age UK, work tirelessly to make older people and their carers and significant others aware of the dangers of poor diet and hydration. End-of-life care support services exist to ensure people at the end of life receive appropriate and relevant nutritional and

DOI: 10.4324/9781003020660-5

hydration support. However, the Supreme Court in 2018 confirmed that judicial approval for withdrawing life-prolonging treatments for individuals was not always required. Following this legislation, the British Medical Association (2020) and Royal College of Physicians have developed guidance regarding withdrawal of fluid and nutrition in end-of-life care situations. Recommended Summary Plan for Emergency Care and Treatment (ReSPECT) is a process where people are encouraged to have an individual plan regarding their emergency and clinical care. This system allows people to express their choices in emergency and end-of-life situations or when a person is no longer able to make their own choices. The process facilitates open conversations with families and significant others and healthcare workers. The document produced sets out people's preferences and clinical judgements. This can include dietary requirements and hydration choices. It is, however, important to remember that this document is not legally binding, so a practitioner's clinical judgement in given situations is required. The British Association of Parenteral and Enteral Nutrition (2020) offers a decision tree for considering ethics and clinically assisted nutrition or hydration approaching the end of life. Please review these resources, available at www.bapen.org.uk to find out more.

Many procedures to supplement a person's fluid and nutritional status are seen to pose risks to the person and practitioner. This is potentially due to misplacement of lines and tubes and inducing coughing or swallowing issues. Recent COVID 19 disease has led to a review of what constitutes an aerosol-generated procedure (AGP). The safeguarding of the person and their carers is paramount at this time. In view of this, an independent high-risk AGP panel has been set up in 2020 (Public Health England 2021). Their role is to review the available evidence to advise and support practitioners in their ever changing role in the COVID-19 pandemic. They conclude that coughing is a major factor in individuals diagnosed with COVID-19. The use of droplet precautions equipment and appropriate levels of personal protective equipment (PPE) should be adopted in all such procedures that have the potential to induce coughing. Please review current government guidance at www.gov.uk on AGP before providing and supporting anyone with additional fluid and nutritional needs.

This chapter includes and now addresses the following topics:

- Nutrition in healthcare: Concerns and initiatives
- Recognising the contribution of nutrition to health
- Assessing and maintaining hydration
- Promoting healthy eating and addressing people's choices
- Nutritional screening – Malnutrition Universal Screening Tool (MUST) tool
- Assisting people with eating and drinking
- Additional nutritional support strategies
- Enteral and parenteral feeding

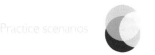

Box 5.1 Recommended biology reading

The following questions will help you to focus on the biology underpinning the skills in this chapter. Use your recommended textbook to find out:

- What are nutrients?
- Where do nutrients come from?
- What is a balanced diet?
- What advice would you give to people regarding their '5-a-day' intake?
- How is food digested in the body?
- What process does the body adopt to use water in the body?
- Briefly explain these processes: mastication, consumption, absorption, defecation.
- How does fluid shift in the body?
- In a cell, what is the process of fluid shift across a membrane known as?
- What percent of your body weight is water?
- What should be the average fluid intake of a person each day?
- What is a calorie?
- How many calories should be ingested by a man each day?
- How many calories should be ingested by a woman each day?
- What is the difference between a macronutrient and a micronutrient?
- Why do we need these nutrients? What are their roles?
- How are macronutrients digested?
- Once digested, where do they go?
- What factors may affect the absorption of digested nutrients?
- How does nutrition affect health?
- What are the consequences of under-nutrition and over-nutrition?
- How do nutritional requirements alter across lifespan?
- What features of different age groups (e.g. teenagers, young adults and older people) may impinge upon nutritional status?
- How does a 'health need' alter our nutritional demands (or supply)?

PRACTICE SCENARIOS

Nutrition is relevant for everybody. The following practice scenarios highlight situations where nutritional issues would be particularly important, and they will be referred to throughout this chapter.

Adult

Miss Alice West is 84 years old and has been transferred from a medical ward to a rehabilitation unit following a **stroke** that has caused right-sided weakness. The medical ward staff who transferred her said that, although she initially had swallowing problems, she has since been assessed as being able to swallow. However, her appetite is very poor, and she often eats only a few small mouthfuls, refusing any more. The staff have been keeping a food chart and a fluid chart, which confirm her poor intake. She has dentures but they appear loose. Her niece is concerned that she is 'looking thin' and seems depressed. Miss West is often uncommunicative but on occasions expresses herself clearly. She is also registered partially sighted. Her weight on admission was 58 kg and is now 53 kg. Her height is 1.64 m.

Learning disability

Phillip Picton is a 31-year-old man with a learning disability who lives in a supported living scheme with three other people. Recently, he has become increasingly overweight. His obesity is beginning to interfere with his day-to-day activities. He has expressed concern about two issues: bending over to put his socks on and getting out of breath walking to the local shops. His carers took him to see his GP who referred him to the community team for people with learning disabilities. The community nurse for learning disabilities and the occupational therapist, who is Phillip's **health facilitator**, are going to visit him to carry out an assessment. Phillip does his own food shopping with support. His weight 3 years ago was 58 kg and is now 92 kg.

Mental health

Charles Cooper is an 88-year-old widower (his wife died 15 years ago). He lives alone in a bungalow in a small village. The village has very poor public transport services. The local shop has recently closed. Mr Cooper has a diagnosis or **dementia** for which he is prescribed medication. He is prompted to take this by a home carer who calls twice a day. Recently, community mental health nurse noticed that Mr Cooper had lost weight. When questioned about his dietary intake, Mr Cooper stated that he has a 'good appetite' and manages to prepare his own meals. On checking the kitchen, the nurse observed little evidence of recent food preparation or cooking. The refrigerator contained some dairy products, and these had all expired and were beginning to smell.

Your role in nutrition and hydration

Nurses have historically been involved in assisting people with their nutrition and hydration needs. In 1859, Florence Nightingale, recognised that starvation existed in the midst of plenty. She was influential in seeing that during the Civil War, people received adequate nutrition. To date, nutrition and hydration remains on the agenda for many healthcare workers. Many identify how they can improve people's lives through providing and supporting eating and drinking requirements of people in their care.

The Nursing and Midwifery Council (NMC) (2018a) in their Future Nurse Standards proficiency for Registered Nurses Platform 2 – Promoting health and preventing ill health, identifies how Registered Nurses play a key role in improving and maintaining the mental, physical and behavioural health and well-being of people, families, communities and populations. Registered nurses support and enable people at all stages of life and in all care settings to make informed choices about how to manage health challenges to maximise their quality of life and improve health outcomes. The standards promote nurses to take an active role in the prevention of and protection against disease and ill health and to engage in public health, community development and global health agendas, and in the reduction of health inequalities. Thus, providing nutritional and hydration support is seen as a key role of healthcare workers.

The next sections of this chapter will discuss how healthcare workers can understand about nutrients, what happens if we have a lack of them and how healthcare workers can assist in supporting nutrition.

NUTRITION IN HEALTHCARE: CONCERNS AND INITIATIVES

Poor nutrition and hydration

Malnutrition

Malnutrition is a condition in which a deficiency, excess or imbalance of food intake, protein and other nutrients causes measurable adverse effects on tissue, body form (shape, size or composition), function, clinical outcome and quality of life. The term malnutrition is associated with both under- and over-nutrition (Malhi 2018). The term can be associated with disease-related malnutrition as a result of or a cause of an illness.

BAPEN (2020) report that while malnutrition includes both over-nutrition (overweight and obesity) and under-nutrition, there has been a concentration on the problem of obesity, while the problem of under-nutrition has been largely neglected. In 70% of individuals, **malnutrition** remains undiagnosed (RCN 2020).

Stratton et al. (2018) explain how malnutrition is a public health problem. They explore the costs of malnutrition and identify a cost of at least £ 23.5 billion in the UK. Older adults (over 65 years) account for 52% of the total costs with the remainder from younger people and children.

Box 5.2 Learning outcomes

By the end of this section, you will be able to:

1 review reports that have highlighted concerns about malnutrition, particularly in hospital
2 discuss recommendations and initiatives to improve nutrition in healthcare.

Learning outcome 1: review reports that have highlighted concerns about malnutrition, particularly in hospital

This chapter's introduction highlighted the continuing problem of malnutrition in community and in hospitals.

Box 5.3 Activity: malnutrition

ACTIVITY

Drawing on your practice experiences, reflect on why people could be at risk of malnutrition, particularly in hospital?

Compare your thoughts with those from some of the reports:
Concerns about hospital nutrition include

- Appropriateness of the food on offer
- Availability of help with eating the food
- Monitoring of people for signs of malnutrition

- Involvement of the person, their relatives and carers
- Knowing how and who to raise concerns with

Age UK (2020) identified that some of the problems associated with poor nutrition and hydration are closely linked to relationships between staff and the individual and between different groups of staff, such as healthcare workers and catering staff. Historically much has been discussed and published regarding malnutrition and dehydration in the care sector. Age Concern's (2006) original *Hungry to Be Heard: The Scandal of Malnourished Older People in Hospital* included harrowing case studies of nutritional needs being neglected. In 2010, a further report *Still Hungry to Be Heard* suggests that this issue is still something for consideration in many care environments. For example, access to snacks and additional fluid and nutritional support outside of mealtimes in a hospital is sometimes problematic. This problem is not just isolated to hospital settings and is seen in care facilities in the non-acute setting. Carers UK (2020) revealed that the vital role of carers providing nutrition for their significant others is often overlooked; 60% reported worrying about the nutrition of the person they care for. In addition, 16% cared for someone underweight and with a small appetite. All these are indicators of malnutrition risk and carers need to be equipped with knowledge and understanding as to why nutrition and hydration is particularly important for people who require care. Age UK (2020) added how some carers were worried about nutrition and identified how they felt they received little support regarding nutrition in the community setting. Referrals to healthcare professionals, including dieticians, were sadly found to be suboptimal. In light of these reports, highlighting how malnutrition and dehydration are commonplace, various recommendations and improvements continue to be initiated. These are set to address human costs by reviewing people's vulnerability to malnutrition. Considering how to address malnutrition is key as this has a huge financial cost of approximately £90 billion annually on the NHS (Malnutrition Pathway 2017, www.malnutritionpathway.co.uk). Increasing public awareness of the hazards of poor diet and fluid intake is required. Royal College of Nursing (RCN 2021) identify factors that could develop greater understanding in health and social care services about people's nutritional needs and how these can be addressed in the clinical situation would potentially reduce malnutrition.

Some recommendations and initiatives are now discussed in view of these findings. It is anticipated that you will develop your knowledge and skills in nutrition and thus help reduce malnutrition and dehydration in a care setting.

Learning outcome 2: discuss recommendations and initiatives to improve nutrition in healthcare

Box 5.4 Activity: initiatives to improve nutrition

ACTIVITY

What initiatives have you seen in practice to try to improve nutrition in healthcare settings?

You may have seen the following:

Malnutrition screening tool (MUST): an assessment tool to enable recognition, identification and treatment of malnutrition. This has been revolutionary in changing how malnutrition and dehydration are addressed in the clinical setting. This tool is explored in more detail later in this chapter.

Protected mealtimes: These are periods on hospital wards/care homes when all non-urgent clinical activity stops so that the person can eat their meals uninterrupted, assisted by staff. Generally, visiting is stopped during protected mealtimes, but a family or significant other coming to assist a person with eating should be welcomed.

Red trays/red jugs: The 'red tray' system is a simple way of alerting healthcare staff that a person needs help with eating. A red dot sticker on the person's menu sheet (or similar agreed system) signals to the catering department that the meal must be served on a red tray. Clinical staff can then easily identify people who require help by looking out for a red tray and providing assistance quickly so that there is no compromise to the dignity of the person or the quality of the meal (Royal College of Nursing [RCN] 2012). Red jugs may be used in a similar way, to alert staff to people who need help drinking.

NHS stickers for glasses or mugs: this initiative consists of a sticker that is affixed to a person's glass or mug to alert staff to top up a drink when passing an individual. Clearly, this is done is coordination with the persons consent and clinical teams' advice with consideration to their health and well-being. These act as a prompt to consider fluid intake on a regular basis for the individual.

24-hour catering: Previously hot food was not always available outside mealtimes. The tradition of setting times for breakfast, lunch and supper needs to be challenged to meet the ever-changing clinical needs of the individual. Offering a 24-hour catering services can ensure that hot food, snacks and drinks are available to people at any time of day, to meet their needs, thus eliminating the situation of missed meals or snacks due to individuals attending investigations and seeing medical and significant others.

Familiar foods and snacks: Some wards and clinical areas with people with dementia have implemented tables with a variety of familiar snacks that people can help themselves to. Some clinical areas have implemented 'afternoon tea', where cakes are served mid-afternoon. These simple initiatives can improve calorific intake for the individual. Other initiatives include themed events where food is served to include family members and significant others. For example, Italian evenings and sing along sessions where samples of food are tried and tasted.

Sustainability and seasonality: This includes sourcing local food, which is likely to be fresher, using organic or fairly traded goods and reducing food waste.

Flexi-menu systems: These offer a fixed menu for lunch and evening meals, so that people can choose food they like more than once.

Mealtime volunteers: Volunteers registered with the care setting who attend to people assisting them to eat.

Nutrition champions: Staff members who have up-to-date knowledge about nutrition and strive to promote this to other staff.

Easy handling or assisted drinking devices: Devices such as the 'Hydrant bottle' to promote independence in drinking (see later discussion).

Take-aways and food from home: These can offer individuals familiar choices in their diet. Caution must be noted here to ensure that products meet health and safety requirements regarding content, temperature and allowed substances. It is advisable to check your local trust or care home policy before embarking upon this option.

Shops in hospital foyers and reception area cafes in care homes: café areas and social spaces in hospital foyers and care home reception areas have facilitated the ability for relatives, significant others and individuals to meet and share food and drink experiences together outside of the busy clinical setting.

Missed meals and replacements: Individualising mealtimes for people and offering replacement meals if a meal is missed.

Other innovations to address poor nutrition and hydration could include action prior to admission, the ambulance crew or significant other could give staff an overview of their nutritional needs on admission, if a person is unable to do this for themselves. The Alzheimer's Society (2020) promotes the use of 'This is me', which is a simple tool to offer a snapshot view of people with dementia and their likes and dislikes, which includes preferences for food and drink.

In the UK, government policies and action groups continue to ensure that nutrition stays at the forefront in the healthcare setting. Various UK organisations have made recommendations for improving nutrition in healthcare settings; some of the initiatives outlined earlier relate to these recommendations. Age UK (2017) in their study "*Still Hungry to Be Heard*" highlighted how there are an unacceptable number of people who become malnourished when in hospital with malnutrition costing the NHS £7.3 billion every year.

Age UK (2017) recommends the following: seven steps to address issues, which include that staff:

1. should listen to individuals, relatives, significant others and carers about the person's diet;
2. should be food aware;
3. should follow their professional codes and be directed by their professional or regulatory bodies;
4. should assess the person for signs of risks for malnutrition on admission and at regular intervals during their stay;
5. should follow guidance for protected mealtimes;
6. should implement systems for red tray meals;
7. should involve volunteers to help at mealtimes.

Addressing malnutrition in the community setting

In the community, initiatives can be seen for clients '*A guide to managing adult malnutrition in the community*' offers comprehensive advice regarding supporting clients with their nutritional needs (www.malnutritionpathway.co.uk 2017). They offer guidance on how to recognise, optimise and manage malnutrition in the community setting. NICE guidance CG 32 (2017) recommends includes optimising nutritional intake for people in a community setting or care home. They suggest considering oral nutritional support to improve nutritional intake for people who can swallow safely and are malnourished. NICE (2017) further explains that practitioners should attempt to overcome barriers to optimise oral intake, offering small frequent meals and snacks, a dentition review, a swallow assessment and changes in taste should be investigated. They also warn of taking care with food fortifications to ensure that requirements for all nutrients are met. The Association of UK Dieticians (2018) produces a food fact sheet to spot the signs of malnutrition, and how to stop and treat malnutrition. It suggests how malnutrition can affect anyone, while it is common in the older person and socially isolated. They describe how a balanced diet is crucial for health and well-being. They suggest ways in which carers can consider ways to improve people's diet by following simple recommendations in their diet. NHS England (2015) in their Guidance; Commissioning Excellent Nutrition and Hydration (2015–18) recommend factors that care providers should address including developing nutrition and hydration care pathways to meet the populations' needs. The World Health Organization (WHO) (2019) also recommends how we should adopt a life approach to nutrition and hydration, they identify how tackling malnutrition requires intervention at all stages throughout the entire life course.

The Care Quality Commission (CQC) plays an important role in ensuring people in care facilities receive adequate nutrition. The CQC inspects all health and social care providers who provide care for individuals. With specific reference to nutrition, the CQC's regulation 14 (2020), www.cqc.org.uk, asks all providers of healthcare to meet nutritional and hydration needs. This means that a service user should be in receipt of suitable and nutritious food and hydration that is adequate to sustain life and good health (CQC, 2020). Its role amongst others is to inspect care provider facilities of nutrition in care settings. The CQC identified some problem areas in meeting the nutritional needs of the person and residents. In a minority of hospitals and care settings, some people were not helped to eat and drink, some meals and snacks remained untouched by the individual due to lack of dexterity on behalf of the person / resident. They also highlighted how some individuals were not given food choices, or appropriate food that they could eat, nor were they helped to wash their hands before eating. However, it was highlighted how most care settings were meeting the nutritional needs of people in residence (CQC 2020). Many were found to now provide flexible catering facilities. Hospital canteens were seen to be offering choices in meals, including portion size and adjusting times when meals and snacks could be ordered. In hospitals with good nutritional systems in place, staff completed nutritional risk assessments, including MUST assessments, recorded food and fluid intake accurately and recorded and monitored peoples' weights as needed. The CQC continues to offer each care facility it assesses recommendations on how they may improve meeting the nutritional and hydration needs of their client group. Many initiatives have been suggested and taken up, thus improving the nutritional intake of clients.

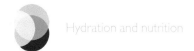

Fluid and nutritional support in worldwide disease

As a person recovers from a disease, injury and illness, their fluid and nutritional demand may need to be increased to promote recovery. For example, during the recent COVID-19 pandemic, the need to consider fluid and nutritional support for those recovering from the disease is paramount to support the individual's recovery. People who are receiving ventilator support require additional nutritional support to promote recovery, and in COVID-19, it is seen to be important to their recovery (British Dieticians Association 2020). Community people who have recovered from COVID still require additional fluid and nutritional support to enable their recovery. During this time, Age UK (2020) recommends people have a balanced diet of three protein items, three dairy items and five fruits and vegetables each day to support their recovery post COVID.

Supportive measures of enteral and parenteral nutritional supplements have a place in supporting such individuals; however, all additional routes that are used can potentially lead to an AGP being used. Public Health England (2021) highlights the risk factors of many procedures associated with supporting people with fluid and nutrition. To address these, for all AEG, practitioners are required to wear the appropriate PPE level.

Summary

- Peoples' nutritional needs should be given high priority, but a number of reports have highlighted that individuals' nutritional needs are not always met effectively, particularly in hospitals and care homes.
- Many initiatives are being implemented to address these concerns, and recommendations have been made.
- Healthcare workers are well-placed to implement improvements, working with families and the multidisciplinary team, and other departments, for example, catering units.
- Consider nutrition and hydration needs as part of your daily routine when you are involved in the care of individuals.

RECOGNISING THE CONTRIBUTION OF NUTRITION TO HEALTH

An adequate supply of essential nutrients is required in the diet to maintain health. The term 'diet' usually refers to the total food eaten, while nutrients refer to components of foodstuffs that have a role in body functioning. For example, bread is composed of carbohydrate, protein, fat and some vitamins. It is important to understand the key components of a nutritious diet and to be able to identify factors that might prevent adequate nutrition.

Box 5.5 Learning outcomes

By the end of this section, you will be able to:

1 explain the major nutrients in the body;
2 discuss factors that might influence healthy people's nutritional needs;
3 reflect on situations in which an individual's nutritional status might be impaired.

Learning outcome 1: explain the major nutrients in the body

Nutrients are derived from foods that we eat to promote normal growth, maintenance and repair. Most foods contain a variety of nutrients.

Box 5.6 Activity: major nutrients

ACTIVITY

The major nutrients are listed below. For each of these, consider what are their main uses in the body? Refer to your biology book for details about:

- Carbohydrates and glucose
- Protein
- Fats (lipids)
- Vitamins
- Minerals
- Water

Some brief notes on each are given below:

Carbohydrates and glucose: These are used for body cells. Your brain and red blood cells rely on glucose to supply their energy: think of these as brain foods.

Protein: Essential to the body for growth, repair and maintenance.

Fats (lipids): Phospholipids are used to make up cell membranes; triglycerides are fuel for the body. Fats act as insulation for your body and help the body absorb vitamins.

Vitamins: A, B group, C, D, E and K are crucial in helping the body use other nutrients.

Minerals: Calcium, phosphorus, potassium, sulphur, sodium, chloride and magnesium are required for living organisms.

Water: An essential nutrient for hydration.

In the body, these nutrients become involved in a variety of biomechanical processes. Refer to your biology book to find out more about the important groups of nutrients and their role in maintaining health.

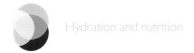

Box 5.7 Activity: analysis of the nutrients in your most recent meal

Consider your last meal and think about the nutrients in it:

- What nutrient(s) did you eat in large quantities?
- Were any nutrients missing?
- Now consider: On an average day, what quantity of water do you consume?
- Before moving on, think about what, if anything, you could change about your water and food intake.

We are all perhaps guilty of a missed meal, a reluctance to drink or not having time to drink enough. However, looking after ourselves is essential for us, as carers, to care for others. Sprake et al. (2018) reviewed factors that may affect university students' eating habits, they highlight how university represents a key transition in adulthood. They found that students may consume poor quality diets. This they reported has a potential implication for body weight and long-term health. They also found that students had a greater potential to snack while studying and commented that economic factors affected diet choices when shopping for food. They concluded that university students were at risk of having a poor diet and needed to eat healthy foods to prepare them for their future and avoid chronic diseases.

While the media may bombard you with messages about what to eat, remember people in your care may often look to you for advice about their diet, particularly if they are newly diagnosed with a disease or have experienced an illness or accident recently. Try to educate yourself about the components of a healthy diet and why this is essential and gain an understanding of the role of nutrients in the body so that you may share your knowledge.

Learning outcome 2: discuss factors that might influence healthy people's nutritional needs

The amounts of various nutrients required for health vary from individual to individual and throughout life.

Box 5.8 Activity: factors influencing a person's nutritional needs

What factors might influence a healthy person's nutritional needs?

You may have thought of the following:

- **Age**. In adulthood, the energy requirement decreases with age because older people have a lower metabolic rate than younger adults.
- **Gender**. Men require more energy because their relatively greater muscle mass results in a higher metabolic rate than that in women.
- **Height and build**. The bigger the body, the greater the amount of nutrients required to maintain cells.

- **Amount of physical activity**. As energy is used as fuel, the greater the physical activity, the higher the energy utilisation.
- **Pregnancy**. During the second and third trimesters of pregnancy, rapid growth of the fetus alters the woman's nutritional needs – see the 'Pregnancy and birth practice points' box at the end of this section.
- **Lactation**. A breast-feeding mother requires increased energy (as much as 500 calories/day or more), increased intake of calcium and vitamins A, C and D. She should drink enough fluids to satisfy her thirst.

Being aware of factors affecting nutritional demands in healthy people is important prior to considering factors that compromise nutritional status.

Learning outcome 3: reflect on situations in which an individual's nutritional status might be impaired

There are many situations where people may be unable to meet their nutritional needs, leading to malnutrition, this may be as a result of inadequate intake, inappropriate intake, increased nutritional demands or any combination of these factors.

> **Box 5.9 Activity: predisposition to inadequate nutritional intake**
>
> What might predispose to an inadequate nutritional intake? The scenarios will give you some clues but also reflect on your experience in practice. Remember to think about psychological and socio-economic factors as well as physical factors.

There are many factors you could have identified and many of these interlink. Here are examples:

Loss of appetite. As you read, Miss West currently has a poor appetite. Appetite loss may be seen in older people and can be caused by pain, stress, anxiety, reduced physical activity and fatigue, which often accompany illnesses.

Stress. Digestion slows when adrenaline is produced; thus, people who are stressed may feel less urge to eat.

Lack of knowledge and skills. People may not understand the importance of eating and may be unable to buy suitable food and prepare it. For example, although Phillip can eat independently and can shop with help, he might be unaware of the different nutrients he needs to stay healthy. Therefore, he may not be eating enough of the right food while eating too much of the food that might lead to obesity, such as a high-fat diet or excess sugar.

Dementia. Mr Cooper has dementia, which could affect his appetite and his ability to shop and prepare food, leading to an inadequate and inappropriate intake. People with dementia may not be able to eat independently, and in very severe cognitive impairment they may no longer recognise food (www.alzheimers.org.uk)

Paranoia. Some people may not eat because of fear of being poisoned; for example, people who have psychological problems may see food as poisonous.

Nausea and vomiting. Various diseases and illnesses and some medication can reduce people's appetite or prevent them from eating.

Nil by mouth. Some people may be unable to eat for prolonged periods due to their condition (e.g. if they are unconscious) or treatment (e.g. following some types of surgery).

End of life. People nearing the end of their life may wish to withdraw from eating or drinking either due to physical lack of strength or loss of interest in food.

Physical factors. One example is dysphagia (difficulty in swallowing), which results from delayed or absent swallow reflex, for example, following a stroke (see www.rcslt.org). Initially, Miss West had this problem. Difficulty in chewing and pain caused by decayed teeth or ill-fitting dentures or mouth ulcers are other physical causes of inadequate intake. Limited dexterity causing difficulty in manipulating cutlery may make eating slow and difficult (e.g. people with cerebral palsy, stroke or rheumatoid arthritis). For example, Miss West's weak right arm will cause difficulty manipulating eating utensils. The physical effort of eating may be too great for some people with chronic diseases such as heart failure or emphysema. Loss of taste (**dysgeusia)** may occur due to illness, for example, after a stroke (Stroke Association 2012). A loss of taste can make a big difference to the quality of life, and people find it to be a distressing and unexpected after-effect of a stroke. This has been evident during COVID 19 where people have reported a loss of sense of smell and appetite.

Medication. Some medications hinder the taste of food, for example, ferrous sulphate or steroids, often giving people a metallic taste in their mouth. Some medicines suppress the appetite or bring on nausea making eating less desirable.

Basal metabolic rate. It is the amount of energy needed by the body for essential processes when at complete rest but awake.

Increased nutritional demands: The body's reaction to injury, infection and surgery raises the **basal metabolic rate** and hence increases nutritional demands. Healing of wounds and fractures requires additional nutrients (see Chapter 13 for discussion of nutrition and wound healing). Some neurological conditions such as some types of cerebral palsy, can cause excessive body movements, using up energy and thus increasing nutritional demands.

Dependency. People who are dependent on others and unable to express their needs are at risk of inadequate intake. Examples would be people unable to communicate as a result of intellectual or neurological impairment, or dementia.

Lack of finance. People who are living on a low income often have many demands on their limited funds, so nutrition may not be the top priority.

Food is sometimes found to be a source of comfort in periods of stress or anxiety. With Phillip, it would be important to consider whether these social and psychological factors are relevant. For example, are there sufficient activities for him to be involved

Emphysema

It is a lung disease characterised by over-inflation and destructive changes leading to lack of elasticity in the alveolar walls.

in? Fad diets and erroneous health beliefs may lead people to follow diets that are too restricted to meet their needs. It is important that dietetic advice is sought.

Making mealtimes matter

As a member of the care team, it is important to think of the importance of your own personal requirements of food and drink. Try to consider how a person may feel when unable to eat and drink at any given time. Try to take actions to ensure that clients' needs are met before, during and after mealtimes; before mealtimes people are prepared to eat and during mealtimes protect the time that people eat, avoiding interruptions for investigations, visitors and visits to other clinical test areas. However, it should be remembered that visitors can on many occasions play a vital role in supporting their significant other to eat. It should be also remembered that eating and drinking is a social event and not always done in isolation. Practitioners should be mindful to what assists their client to eat and drink. After meals people should be able to have time to digest food and attend to their personal hygiene needs. Staff should complete food charts, clean work surfaces around the bed space or eating area and tidy used dishes and crockery away. Drinks should be left in place to encourage constant hydration for your client.

Activity coordinators, volunteers and catering staff play a vital role in encouraging people to be involved in their own dietary intake. Initiatives like care home facilities encouraging tasting sessions, clients preparing their own food with safety in mind may help. Offer tasting sessions to encourage people to be familiar with trying different food and textures. Remember to consider ethnic preferences and ensure these are addressed on specific dates in the calendar. Also, religious festivities could be marked, for example during festive celebrations, try different foods which the person may have enjoyed at home, also enable others to share the food. Encourage visitors to be involved in their significant others' mealtimes. Invite relatives and significant others to share mealtimes with their friend or relative when appropriate. Offer choice at all times and facilitate snack and drinks when able to in the clinical area.

Altered food intake due to mental health issues

Anorexia nervosa

Anorexia nervosa is an eating disorder in which people feel they need to have an unnatural control of what they are eating to avoid putting on weight. It is associated with irrational thoughts about becoming overweight. Extensive weight loss is often seen as an individual's attempt to keep their weight under control.

Bulimia

Bulimia is an eating disorder that begins as a psychological issue, which in turn affects the person's ability to consume a balanced and nutritional diet. Bulimia is associated with eating too much in a short space of time, often referred to as a binge.

Eating disorders, for example, **anorexia nervosa** or **bulimia** as well as mental health issues such as obsessive-compulsive disorder, addiction to drugs and alcohol, personality disorders, depression, bipolar disorder and schizophrenia could all affect a person's nutritional intake. Some people who experience mental health issues need to take medication as part of their treatment. Certain sedative medication may alter the person's desire for food either increasing or decreasing their appetite.

There is a lot of relevant information on which to draw, to help you to understand how to support someone who has an eating disorder, for example; MIND (www.mind.org.uk) and BEAT (https://www.beateatingdisorders.org.uk/) for information about eating disorders. The Royal College of Psychiatrists (2012) also provides guidance for healthcare professionals and the public, aiming to ensure that those caring for people with eating disorders address such issues as diet and exercise and electrolyte imbalance.

Box 5.10 Children and young people practice points: nutrition

The WHO recommends exclusive breast feeding for 6 months for optimum health.

World Health Organization (undated) The World Health Organization's infant-feeding recommendation. Available from:

https://www.who.int/nutrition/topics/infantfeeding_recommendation/en/

The UNICEF website provides useful information on infant feeding:

Formula feeding: http://www.unicef.org.uk/BabyFriendly/Resources/Resources-for-parents/A-guide-to-infant-formula-for-parents-who-are-bottle-feeding/

Breast-feeding: http://www.unicef.org.uk/UNICEFs-Work/What-we-do/Our-UK-work/Breastfeeding/

Bottle feeds must be prepared with scrupulous attention to hygiene.

In Weaning: Starting Solid Food, the DH (2008) recommends that solid foods are introduced from about 6 months and never before 4 months old. For further reading, see:

UNICEF guidance, Available from: https://www.unicef.org.uk/babyfriendly/wp-content/uploads/sites/2/2008/02/start4life_guide_to_bottle_-feeding.pdf

All NHS trusts will have infant-feeding protocols or guidelines, so make a point of reading these, also if interested in how to support breast feeding read:

RCN (2019) Promoting Optimal Breastfeeding in Children's Wards and Departments Guidance for good practice available from:

https://www.rcn.org.uk/-/media/royal-college-of-nursing/documents/publications/2021/january/009-470.pdf?la=en

Box 5.11 Pregnancy and birth practice points: nutrition

A healthy, balanced diet is important for both the mother and her baby throughout pregnancy and after birth. Pregnant mothers have a number of additional dietary requirements. These include folic acid supplementation to prevent fetal neural tube defects/spina bifida and vitamin D supplementation to increase the mother's own stores and reduce the risk of her baby developing rickets in childhood. While most foods and drinks are safe, there are some that are best avoided, these include alcohol, caffeinated foods and drinks, some cheeses, meats, fish, eggs and dairy. This is to reduce the risk of harm to the woman and her baby during pregnancy and afterwards.

Obesity in women can significantly increase the risk of additional complications occurring in pregnancy and childbirth (these include raised blood pressure; preeclampsia; gestational diabetes; venous thromboembolism; and difficulty with intubation during general anaesthetic). This means that all healthcare staff have a public health obligation in supporting pregnant mothers to eat healthily and exercise appropriately, to achieve the best possible birth outcome.

When caring for breast-feeding mothers, staff must ensure that they have access to adequate hydration and a balanced diet with sufficient calories to maintain a good breast milk supply.

Further reading:

NHS. 2020. Have a Healthy Diet in Pregnancy Available from: www.nhs.uk/pregnancy/keeping-well/have-a-healthy-diet/

Royal College of Obstetricians and Gynaecologists. 2018. Care of Women With Obesity in Pregnancy Available from: https://www.rcog.org.uk/en/guidelines-research-services/guidelines/gtg72/

UNICEF. 2018. Breastfeeding: A mother's gift, for every child Available from: https://data.unicef.org/resources/breastfeeding-a-mothers-gift-for-every-child/

Summary

- An adequate intake of the correct balance of nutrients is essential to maintain health and prevent malnutrition.
- The nutritional needs of healthy people are affected by various factors, including their stage in the lifespan.
- Healthcare workers care for many people who are unable to meet their nutritional needs due to a wide range of issues, and some will also have increased nutritional demands.
- Various mental and physical health conditions affect nutritional intake, with a potential adverse effect on health.

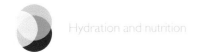

ASSESSING AND MAINTAINING HYDRATION

While obtaining the necessary nutrients from food is important, water is also essential to life. The NMC (2018a) states that healthcare workers must be able to assess fluid status of the person and act to ensure there is adequate intake, in partnership with the individual. The body's fluid intake is mainly regulated by thirst. Dehydration refers to a fluid loss of 1% or greater of the total body mass (Campbell 2014). Medical conditions may inhibit or promote fluid intake; for example, when a person has dementia, the person may think they have just had a drink; at the onset of diabetes, the person cannot quench their thirst. Causes of inadequate fluid intake include dependency on healthcare workers, prolonged preoperative fasting, weakness, illness, reduced taste, loss of sensation due to ageing and restricted access to drinks. While thirst and the need to have oral fluids is a situation where individuals require oral supplements of fluids, dehydration can become very serious. Acute dehydration is a medical emergency and requires immediate intervention by administering fluids to a person via the intravenous route. Poor fluid intake can lead to reduction of bodily functions with acute kidney injury seen when fluid intake reaches extreme low levels (Scanlon and Sanders 2018).

Box 5.12 Learning outcomes

By the end of this section, you will be able to:

1. identify the percentage of water in the body and the recommended fluid intake;
2. explain how to assess and monitor a person's fluid status;
3. discuss ways of promoting adequate oral fluid intake for people and initiatives in practice;
4. explain how supplementary fluids can be administered when the oral route is not available or sufficient.

Learning outcome 1: identify the percentage of water in the body and the recommended fluid intake

Approximately 60% of the body is made up of water; for example, a 70 kg man is made up of about 42 L of total water. Two-thirds of body fluid is found within body cells and is termed intracellular fluid (ICF). The other third is extracellular fluid (ECF), which is found in plasma, lymph, tissue fluid and specialised body fluids such as cerebrospinal fluid, ocular, pleural, peritoneal and synovial fluids.

The proportion of water in the body varies according to age. A new-born baby is composed of approximately 75% water while an older person is composed of approximately 50% water (Roland 2019). The more muscular a person's body is, the more water it contains while, conversely, the greater the fat content in the human body, the lesser the water content.

Box 5.13 Activity: recommended fluid intake

ACTIVITY

What do you think the recommended fluid intake is? Reflect on your own fluid intake yesterday: do you think you drank sufficient fluids?

There is currently no agreed recommended daily intake level for water in the UK, but estimates suggest the average is approximately 1.9 litres per day (Antwi-Ahima 2020). Effective hydration in older peoples care facilities ranges from 1500 to 2000 mL (Antwi-Ahima 2020). She suggests an 8 × 8 rule, i.e. eight 8 oz. glasses a day. How do these figures compare with your own fluid intake? Healthcare professionals are best placed to ensure that individuals receive sufficient fluid whether it is oral or via other routes (see learning outcome 4). Simply administering fluids orally, when the person's condition allows, can be lifesaving and life preserving. Occasionally, people have medically restricted fluid intake, for example, in renal failure, but for all others, the recommended fluid intake should be the target.

Learning outcome 2: explain how to assess and monitor a person's fluid status

Healthcare workers must be able to assess and monitor fluid balance (NMC 2018a, 2018b). Fluid balance refers to the amount of fluid that is taken into the body (input) and the amount that is excreted (output). A negative fluid balance is where the output is greater than fluid ingested, and a positive fluid balance is where intake is greater than output.

ACTIVITY

Box 5.14 Activity: fluid balance chart

Review a fluid balance chart in your practice area.

- What do you note about the person's input and output?
- Are they in a negative or positive fluid balance?
- Why do you think this might be?

Now, review the possible causes of positive or negative fluid balance below and compare them with your answer:

Negative fluid balance: Could be due to dehydration resulting from excessive fluid loss from the body, through sweating, urination, vomiting, diarrhoea or haemorrhage, or may result from insufficient fluid intake.

Positive fluid balance: It is caused by fluid overload and electrolyte imbalance, in particular sodium. Could also be due to conditions that reduce the body's ability to eliminate fluid, for example, heart or renal failure.

A fluid balance chart to record input and output is readily available in many clinical care settings, and regular reviews of fluid balance charts is part of many clinical areas' routine. This tool assists you in identifying over a period of 24 hours if a person is in a negative or positive fluid balance. CQC (2020) recommends that carers should use a fluid balance chart if a person is at risk of dehydration. They stress the importance of this as dehydration can increase the risk of hospitalisation and mortality. Dehydration is often seen as a result of underlying health issues, which leads to further ill health. People should be monitored via blood tests with biochemistry results acting to

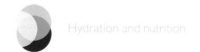
inform clinicians about underlying disease processes, for example, acute kidney injury. Consider employing the following to assist in your assessment; MUST tool scoring, vital signs and NEWS2 scoring, capillary refill time, elasticity of skin, body weight (BMI) and urine output.

Box 5.15 Activity: clinical signs of dehydration

ACTIVITY

What clinical signs would alert you that an adult is dehydrated?

Box 5.16 gives a summary of the signs of dehydration in adults, which you should be aware of.

Learning outcome 3: discuss ways of promoting adequate oral fluid intake for people and initiatives in practice

Fluid intake should be a consideration for all individuals. Remember, if a person is embarrassed about asking for the toilet or is worried about how they might manage in the hospital bathroom, even the most mobile of persons may refrain from drinking; thus, fluid intake should be considered for all people in care settings.

Box 5.16 Clinical signs of dehydration in adults

Mild to moderate dehydration:

- Thirst
- *Dizziness* or light-headedness
- Headache
- Tiredness
- Dry mouth, lips and eyes
- Concentrated urine (dark yellow)
- Passing only small amounts of urine infrequently (less than 3 or 4 times a day)

If mild or moderate dehydration is untreated, the person may become severely dehydrated.

Severe dehydration:

- Dry, wrinkled skin that sags slowly into position when pinched up
- An inability to urinate, or not passing urine for 8 hours
- Irritability
- Sunken eyes
- Hypotension
- A rapid, weak pulse
- Cool hands and feet
- Seizures
- Reduced consciousness, lethargy or confusion
- Blood in the stools or vomit

Source: NHS Choices. 2020. Signs of dehydration. www.nhs.uk and www.nhsinform.scot

Box 5.17 Activity: ability to take on fluids

In your practice area, observe several mobile people who are able to take oral fluids independently and reflect on whether they readily help themselves to drinks on a regular basis. If not, try to find a way to discuss this with them. Remember to offer them drinks when other less mobile individuals are offered drinks too.

Do not assume that people know they need to drink more while they are unwell nor assume that they know they are 'allowed' to drink outside mealtimes. Consider ways in which you can portray this message to individuals in your practice area. Observe whether signage to drinks machines and water fountains are easily visible. If not, what could you do to rectify this? Is it ward or department policy that individuals and their visitors can help themselves to drinks?

Remember that drinking is a social event too. Events of happiness and sadness are often accompanied by drinking (alcoholic or non-alcoholic). If it is not policy for individuals and family to drink together, then explore how to address this issue, which is especially important where people are in hospital for long periods. In long-stay settings, check if there are canteen facilities where individuals and visitors can socialise and get beverages together and, if so, direct them to these facilities. Be proactive and see how you might bring about changes in your area.

In the community setting, consider ways in which you can assist people to increase their fluid intake. Look at the placing of taps, kettles, cups, tea and coffee facilities when you visit their home. Consider ways in which you might assist them to easily make a cup of tea. Does the person have a flask made up for them or is there someone who could assist them with drinks when you are not there? With the person's permission, are there items that can be placed nearer so that they can maintain their independence for accessing a drink? Again, be proactive, consider ways in which you may promote peoples' hydration at home and with their permission set up their environment to promote their independence. Ask the person to keep a log of when they take a drink and monitor this when you visit them. Offer information about why fluid intake is important and why omitting fluids for a long period of time is potentially harmful to them.

Box 5.18 Activity: promoting hydration

Have you observed any initiatives to promote hydration for people?

There have been many initiatives within the NHS recently to try to ensure that people receive enough hydration. Examples include the provision of a red jug to individuals who require assistance to drink or need to drink more (Campbell 2014; Hollis 2011). The 'Hydrant' bottle is a water bottle devised for easy handling to assist people with limited mobility with their fluid intake (see http://www.hydrateforhealth. co.uk/the-hydrant.html). Ensuring people receive adequate hydration has economic benefits and long-term health benefits for the person. In their extensive toolkit, they identify factors associated with poor hydration and offer tips on how to increase water intake each day. Carers play a vital role in ensuring people receive adequate hydration.

McIntyre et al. (2012) proposed an 'intelligent fluid management bundle', aimed at getting the basics of hydration right. They recommended that all people are assessed in terms of hydration needs, a plan is devised to ensure optimum hydration and fluid intake is continuously monitored. The aim is that dehydration is detected early and staff are educated regarding hydration (McIntyre et al. 2012). The use of this approach continues to date.

Learning outcome 4: explain how supplementary fluids can be administered when the oral route is not available or sufficient

Healthcare workers must be able to safely administer fluids when individuals cannot take them independently (NMC 2018a, 2018b). In some instances, fluid intake by the oral route is not possible or insufficient to maintain hydration.

Box 5.19 Activity: alternative ways to administer fluids

ACTIVITY

Reflect on experiences in practice and write down a list of routes for administering fluids, if the oral route is not suitable or sufficient.

You may have thought of the following:

- Intravenously (IV): into the vein.
- Subcutaneous (SC) (hypodermoclysis): into subcutaneous tissue. This route is a valuable alternative method of fluid delivery to the traditional intravenous route, particularly used for older people. It has many advantages over parenteral fluid administration, including ease of administration and fewer systemic side effects.
- Intra-osseous (IO): directly into the bone marrow of the antero-medial aspect of the tibia (most popular), femur, iliac crest or humerus.

In an emergency, the IV and IO routes are more likely to be used. The SC route is used for fluid administration when the intravenous route is not available, for hydration of an older person or at the end stages of life for rehydration.

Box 5.20 Children and young people practice points: dehydration

Dehydration can develop very quickly in infants and young children as such a large proportion of body weight is water. There is a risk of dehydration if diarrhoea and vomiting occur or with other conditions, for example, acute respiratory conditions where the infant may not be feeding adequately. Dehydration can escalate quickly and lead to shock and death but is challenging to assess. Healthcare workers working with infants and young children should be alert and able to recognise signs of dehydration, which may be the following:

> Mild: loss of body weight (<5%), slightly dry mucous membranes, slightly decreased urine output, increased thirst, irritability.
>
> Moderate: loss of body weight (5–10%), raised heart rate, poor tear production, decreased skin turgor, sunken eyes and fontanelles, decreased urine output, restless to lethargic.
>
> Severe: loss of body weight (10–15%), low blood pressure, absent urine output, lethargic to comatose.
>
> For mild to moderate dehydration, oral rehydration therapy is used as a supplement to continue infant/formula feeding.
>
> For moderate to severe dehydration, IV fluids are required.
>
> For further reading, see:
>
> Veal, Z. and Veal, C. 2018. Care of children and young people with fluid and electrolyte imbalance. In: McAlinden, O. and Pryce, J. (eds.) *Essentials of Nursing Children and Young People*. London: Sage, 426–437.

Summary

- Maintaining hydration is a fundamental part of care, along with other important care principles such as hand hygiene.
- Healthcare workers must be proactive in ensuring that people in their care have an adequate fluid intake, whether in the hospital or community setting, to maintain hydration. Ease of access to fluids must be in place, 24 hours a day.
- Fluid intake must be assessed on admission to hospital and then monitored to ensure that adequate hydration is maintained during each person's care.
- Healthcare workers must be alert to any signs of dehydration so that hydration status can be promptly addressed.
- When people cannot take sufficient oral fluids to maintain hydration, other methods must be used that are suitable for the individual.

PROMOTING HEALTHY EATING AND ADDRESSING PEOPLE'S CHOICES

Age UK (2020) identifies how food and fluid are a significant part of services provided to older people in residential care and are key to satisfaction with services. A balanced diet consists of a particular selection of foods, in the correct proportions to meet the body cells' requirements and is essential for maintaining a healthy body that functions efficiently. We have already considered the nutrients necessary for a healthy diet and factors that affect nutritional status, but in care settings, achieving a healthy diet poses particular challenges. Considering people's food preferences is an important aspect of promoting healthy eating.

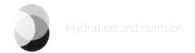

Box 5.21 Learning outcomes

By the end of this section, you will be able to:

1. discuss factors that should be considered to enable individuals to make healthy food choices that are acceptable to them;
2. assist people to select a healthy diet from a menu in a care setting.

Learning outcome 1: discuss factors that should be considered to enable individuals to make healthy food choices that are acceptable to them

The NMC (2018a, 2018b) expects that healthcare workers should assist individuals to choose a diet that provides an adequate nutritional and fluid intake.

Box 5.22 Activity: helping people to make healthy food choices

Thinking about the scenarios at the start of this chapter, reflect on factors that you would consider when helping people to make healthy food choices.

Recognising and responding to a persons' food preferences is paramount if people are to consume a balanced nutritional diet while in your care. Therefore, spending time with Miss West, Philip and Mr Cooper to find out what they like to eat and drink is key to promoting healthy eating for them. Family can also be involved, for example, Miss West's niece should be able to help with information about her usual diet. There is no replacement for asking the person or significant other about personal preferences and making sure that you recognise the individual's choices. As mentioned earlier in this chapter, there should be written documentation of food preferences. For example, the Alzheimer's Society (2020) have developed 'This is me', which is a leaflet that, when completed, helps people with dementia to communicate their needs, preferences, likes and dislikes (see http://www.alzheimers.org.uk/thisisme).

Healthcare workers must ensure that persons' cultural and religious beliefs are respected during food selection. Cultural differences in food preparation, serving and eating routines need to be considered to enable people to have choices in their diet. People's beliefs and values may lead them to require a vegetarian or vegan diet, for example. You should consider the person's religion as food preferences of some people are related to religious beliefs. It is important not to make assumptions about what people might eat according to their culture/religion, instead it is to be found out from the individual or the family concerned. For example, a person who follows Sikhism may refrain from eating beef, eggs or fish or may be a vegetarian. A person following Judaism is required to eat kosher food (food fit to be eaten in accordance with Jewish law), but there are many diverse practices concerning this.

You should become familiar with any dietary restrictions that are advised for chronic diseases as some people in your care may receive prescribed diets as part of their medical treatment, for example, low fat for a person who has heart disease or high protein for an individual who has had extensive surgery. Dietary supplements may also be prescribed, and it is important that you work with the dietician to ensure that the person receives these in a timely manner.

ACTIVITY

Box 5.23 Diet in your care environment

Arrange to meet with the dietician in your care environment and discuss with them what types of diet are recommended for people in your care setting.

Learning outcome 2: assist people to select a healthy diet from a menu in a care setting

ACTIVITY

Box 5.24 Activity: choosing a healthy diet from a menu

How might you assist a person to choose a healthy diet from a menu?

When looking at the menu with an individual, you need to be prepared to explain the foods, as some items may be unfamiliar to people. You may need to read out menus and complete them for people; this would be necessary for Miss West, who is partially sighted. You can guide the person towards appropriate foods on the menu, ensuring there is a balance of the important food groups discussed earlier in this chapter, while taking preferences into account. Miss West requires food that is not only nourishing but also weight inducing, so you might encourage her to eat more carbohydrates and dairy products. Murphy et al. (2017) highlight how showing a person a picture of food on offer, picture menus, may support people in making informed choices. It can also assist them to try new foods that they have perhaps not considered. For some people, seeing pictures may help prompt them to make choices of their favourite foods.

Summary

- When promoting healthy eating, healthcare workers should find out persons' food preferences, from the individual, their family or written information.
- People may need help with understanding and completing menus; pictures of food available will be helpful in some situations.
- Healthcare workers should guide people regarding appropriate food choices, with respect for individual preferences, culture, religion, values and beliefs.
- Healthcare workers should take account of any specific nutritional requirements, relating to the persons' health conditions, liaising with the dietician accordingly.

NUTRITIONAL SCREENING

Healthcare workers must be actively involved in the assessment and monitoring of a person's nutrition. It is imperative that practitioners can establish a person's nutritional status and formulate a plan of care in partnership with the individual, their carers and other healthcare professionals. To achieve this, it is important to gain an understanding of how to use nutritional screening tools. Healthcare workers are in a unique position to identify people at risk of malnourishment and then take appropriate action. As recognised already in this chapter, there are many factors that can affect nutritional status. If healthcare providers do not carry out nutritional screening carefully, people can be put at unnecessary risk from the effects of malnourishment. A range of nutritional screening tools are available, but the MUST is recommended by BAPEN (2020).

BAPEN, also, offers an online web-based nutritional tool kit (see www. bapen.org. uk). The tool helps to monitor the individual's status. The MUST calculator is a useful tool to access and begin to use in a practice situation and then in a clinical situation to gain a good understanding. People can also use the tool in a community setting to review their body mass index (BMI) and monitor their weight. This self-screening can enable objective assessment of a person's BMI.

In critical care situations, it is sometimes difficult to be aware of a person's height or weight due to the person having reduced mobility and potentially being bed bound. BAPEN (2020) offer a part of the tool that will enable you to carry out an estimation of a person's height using ulnar length, i.e. measuring the ulna (lower arm) with the arm bent, using the left arm if possible. This is done by placing the palm across the persons chest, fingers pointing to the opposite shoulder, use a tape to measure the length from the elbow (olecranon) and to the wrist – styloid bone. This enables a calculation to be made to estimate a person height as the measurement is converted in a table thus eliminating the requirement of knowing the person's height (see www.bapen.org.uk/screening-and-must/must-calculator).

Box 5.25 Learning outcomes

By the end of this section, you will be able to:

1. discuss how observations can contribute to nutritional assessment;
2. explain the purpose and use of nutritional screening tools;
3. carry out nutritional screening and recognise if people are at risk of malnutrition.

Learning outcome 1: discuss how observations can contribute to nutritional assessment

Assessment should include a range of observations to gain insight into nutritional status and contribute to screening.

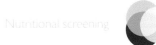

Box 5.26 Activity: observations to assist nutritional assessment

With reference to the scenarios, what observations could be carried out to assist nutritional assessment?

You may have identified many of the aspects listed below – most would be useful in assessing the people in the scenarios.

- Observe whether clothing, rings and dentures are fitting comfortably. If not, this could suggest an alteration in weight. These could be useful indicators as to whether Mr. Cooper is losing weight. You will remember that Miss West's dentures are loose, and her niece might know whether her aunt's loose dentures are a new problem. Remember that the person may be deliberately trying to lose weight and so do not make assumptions.
- Look at the skin and check for excessive dryness, scaling and temperature.
- Check the eyes for brightness and whether they are sunken into their sockets, which could indicate dehydration. These would be important observations with both Mr. Cooper (who may not be drinking enough) and Miss West, whose fluid intake we know is poor.
- Note the smell of the breath. Halitosis can indicate poor dental health or dehydration. This could lead you to review the state of the mouth, and to identify a problem, if any, with the teeth or gums. A sore mouth can indicate a poor diet. Chapter 7 considers oral hygiene in detail.
- Observe the level of mobility, for example, whether the person can move their arms adequately to eat independently, or can walk or manoeuvre to get access to food. This is particularly relevant to Miss West, but the community mental health nurse should also consider Mr. Cooper's mobility in relation to obtaining and preparing food.
- Observe for drooling, which could be a sign of poor swallowing, as well as poor lip seal. Although Miss West has been assessed as being able to swallow now, these are signs that healthcare workers should be aware of owing to her previous history.
- While the person is eating and drinking, observe their sequence of breathing and swallowing.
- Observe for non-verbal signals, gestures or signs that the person may use to communicate their wishes, such as pushing the dish away. It is important to respect people's wishes.
- In people's own homes, community healthcare workers can observe what food is around and whether it is within the sell-by date. Out-of-date food could indicate that food is being bought but not actually eaten. These were important observations for Mr. Cooper's community mental health nurse to make. Regarding Phillip, the community nurse for learning disability and occupational therapist could observe what food he is buying and storing.
- Observe food intake, which will indicate the amount of food that is actually being consumed. Such details recorded over several days allow for any day-to-day

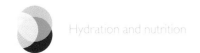

fluctuations. It was good practice that the staff on the medical ward from which Miss West was transferred were recording her food and fluid intake on a food chart. The healthcare workers on the rehabilitation unit should check back over charts from previous days. Three days should be sufficient to assess a person's eating habits, and then a decision can be made as to what additional support is needed. This may involve a nurse or a dietician.

Learning outcome 2: explain the purpose and use of nutritional screening tools

The purpose of nutritional screening is a process of identifying people at risk of malnourishment. The Malnutrition Advisory Group (MAG), part of BAPEN, developed MUST for use with adults at risk of malnutrition (Todorovic et al. 2003). The MUST tool is downloadable from www.bapen.org.uk and is available as an online calculator to assess a person's nutritional status and provides detailed screening guidelines to use in the clinical setting. MUST is advocated as the tool that all healthcare settings should be using. NICE (2017) has stated that a validated assessment tool be used for all nutritional assessments, recommending the use of MUST for all adults in your care. MUST use is further supported by the British Dietetic Association, Royal College of Nursing and Royal College of Physicians. Additional information for use of MUST is also available, in *The MUST Explanatory Booklet* (Todorovic et al. 2003 and www.bapen.org.uk).

The components of the tool and their usage are presented next, but do refer to the website documents for further explanation and these documents may also be updated periodically (www.bapen.org.uk 2020) originally Todorovic et al. (2003). Nutritional screening is the first step in identifying people who may be at nutritional risk or potentially at risk, and who may benefit from appropriate nutritional intervention. It is a rapid, simple and general procedure used by nursing, medical or other staff on first contact with the person so that clear guidelines for action can be implemented and appropriate nutritional advice provided. Todorovic et al. (2003) point out that repeated screening may be necessary when a person's condition and nutritional risk change, and that it is always better to prevent or detect problems early by screening than discover serious problems later. Box 5.27 presents the five steps in screening using MUST. These steps are explained next.

Step 1: Body mass index (BMI)

The BMI provides a 'rapid interpretation of chronic protein-energy status based on an individual's height and weight' (Todorovic et al. 2003 www.bapen.org.uk). Box 5.28 explains how to measure height and weight accurately.

The formula to calculate BMI is:

$$\frac{\text{Weight in kilogrammes}}{\left(\text{Height in metres}\right)^2}$$

The chart in Figure 5.2 displays BMI scores based on weight and height and the corresponding MUST score. In some care settings, entering the weight and height into an electronic record will automatically generate the BMI measurement. MAG (2017) suggests a variety of other indicators if weight and height measurements are not available.

Box 5.27 The five MUST steps (use the following steps or access the MUST calculator via www.bapen.org.uk)

Step 1

Measure height and weight to get a BMI score using the chart provided. If unable to obtain height and weight, use alternative procedures, detailed in MUST (MAG 2017).

Step 2

Note percentage of unplanned weight loss and score using tables provided in MUST (MAG 2017).

Step 3

Establish acute disease effect and score.

Step 4

Add scores from Steps 1–3 together to obtain overall risk of malnutrition.

Step 5

Use management guidelines and/or local policy to develop care plan.

Source: Reproduced with the kind permission of BAPEN. Available from: http://www.bapen.org.uk/pdfs/must/must-full.pdf

---

Box 5.28 Measuring height and weight

Height

- Use a height stick (stadiometer), if available. Ensure it is correctly positioned against the wall.
- Ask the person to remove their shoes and to stand upright, feet flat, heels against the height stick or wall (if height stick not used).
- Ask the person to look straight ahead. Lower the head plate until it gently touches the top of the head.
- Read and document height.
- Some people's height may need to be measured while lying in bed.

Weight

- Use clinical scales wherever possible and make sure they have been regularly checked for accuracy.
- Ensure that the scales read zero without the person standing on them.
- Weigh the person in light clothing and without shoes.
- Bed scales are available to weigh someone restricted to bed. Hoist scales are also available.

Source: www.bapen.org.uk

Alternative method for estimating height using the measurement of the persons ulnar length.

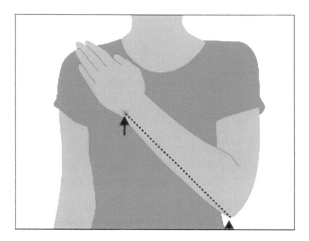

Figure 5.1: Height estimation.
Source: www.bapen.org.uk › pdfs › nsw › nsw11 › ulna-measurement-nsw11.

Measure between the point of the elbow (olecranon process) and the midpoint of the prominent bone of the wrist (styloid process) (left side if possible).

If possible, using the left arm – it should be bent at the elbow at a 90-degree angle with the upper arm held parallel to the body (see Figure 5.1). The distance should be measured between the acromion process (bony protrusion of shoulder) and the olecranon process (elbow). Mark the midpoint here.

Ask the person to let their arm hang loose and measure around the marked area with the tape measure. Note the result in centimetres.

If mid-upper arm circumference (MUAC) is less than 23.5 cm, BMI is likely to be less than 20 kg/m².

If MUAC is greater than 32.0 cm, BMI is likely to be greater than 30 kg/m².

A score cannot be attributed to this calculation, but an estimation of BMI can be obtained by this method.

Box 5.29 Activity: BMI calculation

ACTIVITY

Calculate:

- Phillip's BMI, if his weight is 92 kg and his height is 1.68 m;
- Mr. Cooper's BMI, if his height is 1.9 m and his weight is 64 kg.
- Looking at Figure 5.2, what would their BMI scores be for the MUST screening?

Phillip's BMI is 33. The chart classifies this as 'obese', and his score for Step 1 of the MUST is 0. Mr. Cooper's BMI is 18, giving his score for Step 1 of the MUST as 2.

Step 2

Todorovic et al. (2003) (available at www.bapen.org.uk) identify that unplanned weight loss over 3–6 months is 'a more acute risk factor for malnutrition than BMI' (p. 6). You can ask the person whether they have lost weight in the last 3–6 months

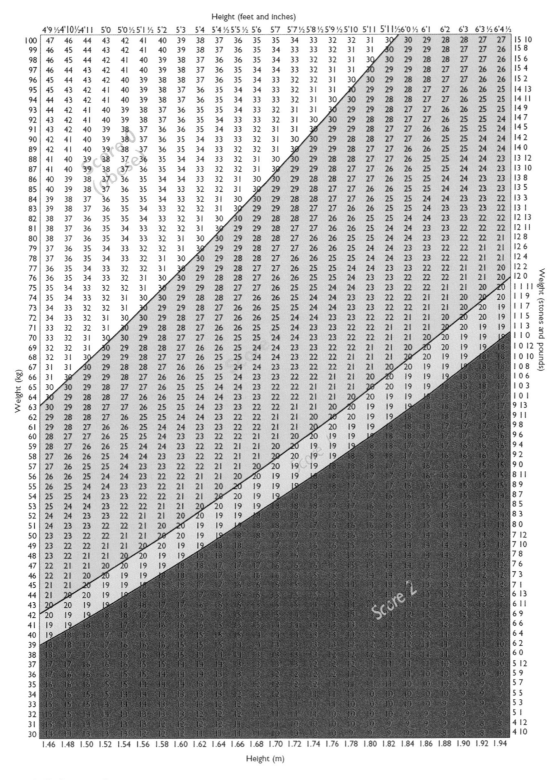

Figure 5.2: Body mass index score.

(Reproduced with kind permission of BAPEN. Available from: http://www.bapen.org.uk/pdfs/must/bmi-weight-loss-charts/must-table-up-to-100kg.pdf.)

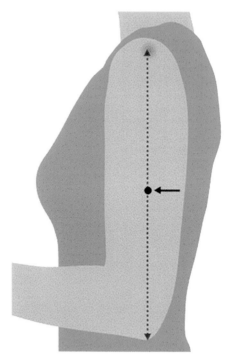

Figure 5.3: Estimating BMI category from MUAC.

and, if so, how much. You can also check their records. Then calculate how much weight has been lost using weight-loss tables (see MAG 2003) and identify the weight-loss score:

<5% = 0
5–10% =1
>10% = 2

Note: Take care when interpreting a persons' BMI or percentage weight loss in some circumstances, for example, fluid disturbances, pregnancy, lactation, critical illness and presence of plaster casts. Adjustments of body weight can be made for amputations (for details, see Todorovic et al. 2003, www.bapen.org.uk).

Step 3
If the person has an acute illness and there has been no nutritional intake, or it is likely that there will be none for more than 5 days, they score 2.

Step 4: overall risk of malnutrition
The scores from Steps 1–3 are added to provide the overall risk of malnutrition:

Score 0 = low risk; Score 1 = medium risk; Score 2 or more = high risk.

Note: If neither BMI nor weight loss could be calculated, the score is assessed taking other criteria into account (see Table 5.1). The observations discussed earlier (in learning outcome 1) will contribute to this estimation.

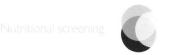

Table 5.1: Other criteria (adapted from MUST, www.BAPEN.org.uk)

If height, weight or BMI cannot be obtained, use the below criteria to help form a clinical impression of a patient's overall nutritional risk.

Note: Use of this criteria will not result in an accurate indication of nutritional risk. It can, however, be used as an indication of *an increased risk* of malnutrition.

BMI	Weight loss	Acute disease
Clinical impression Does the individual appear thin/acceptable weight? Does the individual appear overweight? Note: Obvious wasting very thin) and obesity (very overweight) can be noted.	Are clothes or jewellery notably loose? Over the last 3–6 months, is there a history of decreased food intake, reduced appetite, or dysphagia (issues with swallowing)? Presence of any psychosocial or physical disabilities likely to cause weight loss?	Has there been no (or likelihood of no) nutritional intake for more than 5 days?

Table 5.2: Management guidelines based on MUST score

0 Low risk Routine care	1 Medium risk Observe	2 or more High risk Treat*
Repeat screening: · Hospital – weekly · Care Home – monthly · Community – annually for special groups, for example, those >75 years	Document dietary intake for 3 days If adequate – little concern and repeat screening: · Hospital – weekly · Care Home – at least monthly · Community – at least every 2–3 months If inadequate – clinical concern – follow local policy, set goals, improve and increase overall nutritional intake, monitor and review care plan regularly	Refer to dietitian, nutritional support team or implement local policy Set goals, improve and increase overall nutritional intake Monitor and review care plan: · Hospital – weekly · Care Home – monthly · Community – monthly * Unless detrimental or no benefit is expected from nutritional support, for example, imminent death.

All risk categories:

· Treat underlying condition and provide help and advice on food choices, eating and drinking, when necessary.
· Record malnutrition risk category.
· Record need for special diets and follow local policy.

Source: Malnutrition Universal Screening Tool. Available from: http://www.bapen.org.uk. Reproduced with kind permission of BAPEN.

Step 5: management guidelines

Table 5.2 presents action required according to the MUST score. The MUST management guidelines advise that if the screening identifies a person is obese, this should be noted and that for those with underlying conditions, these are generally controlled before treating obesity.

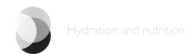

Learning outcome 3: carry out nutritional screening and recognise if people are at risk of malnutrition

Nutritional screening tools have been designed to enable healthcare workers to make an accurate and quick assessment of individuals.

ACTIVITY

Box 5.30 Activity: risk of malnutrition

Using the information provided about Miss West in the scenario and MUST, work out her risk of malnutrition. Remember to use Figure 5.2 to calculate her BMI score. As discussed previously, you can use weight-loss tables to calculate her percentage weight loss – available from BAPEN (http://www. bapen.org.uk/pdfs/must/must-full.pdf).

Your assessment should have clearly identified Miss West as being at high risk. Compare your scoring with that given below:

- Step 1 – BMI. Figure 5.2 shows that Miss West's BMI is 20, so she scores 1.
- Step 2 – weight loss. Miss West has lost 5 kg since admission. The weight-loss table calculates that she has lost 5–10% of her body weight, thus scoring 1. Miss West's loose dentures also suggest some weight loss.
- Step 3 – acute disease can affect risk of malnutrition. Miss West is eating small amounts, but this needs to be monitored, and she has had a stroke, so she scores 2 on this step.
- Step 4 – overall risk of malnutrition. Miss West scores 4, so she is at high risk; therefore, a plan of care needs to be initiated.
- Step 5 – management guidelines. According to MAG (2017); www.bapen.org.uk, Miss West should be referred to the dietician. Goals to improve her nutritional intake must be set, and her weight should be monitored weekly. The next sections in this chapter detail likely interventions to improve her nutrition.

ACTIVITY

Box 5.31 Activity: using MUST

Practise using MUST with some other people:

- Find a willing colleague and assess their nutritional status by working through the screening tool; hopefully, their result falls into the low-risk category.
- Think back to a person you have been caring for recently and work through the tool. Are you surprised at the score you obtained?

You have now practised using the screening tool with several individuals. Once you have established that a person is at risk of malnutrition, you need to develop a plan of action. If the person is at high risk (like Miss West), she will need referral to a dietician for an in-depth nutritional assessment, and additional nutritional support may be needed. However, there are many ways in which healthcare workers can help people to meet their nutritional needs, based on their individual assessment.

> Box 5.32 Children and young people
> practice points: nutritional assessment
>
> Assessment on admission will include the method of feeding for infants (mother's milk, formula or combination) and likes and dislikes for children. Weight is an important measurement; infants should be weighed without clothes or nappy on. Weights must be recorded with total accuracy; medication doses are calculated on weight. Infant growth is recorded on standard percentile charts.
>
> For further reading, see:
>
> Howe, R., Forbes, D. and Baker, C. 2010. Providing optimum nutrition and hydration. In: Glasper, A., Aylott, M. and Battrick, C. (eds.) *Developing Practical Skills for Nursing Children and Young People*. London: Hodder Arnold, 203–9.
>
> Chapman, S. 2012. Assessment. In: Macqueen, S., Bruce, E.A. and Gibson, F. (eds.) *The Great Ormond Street Hospital Manual of Children's Nursing Practices*. Chichester: Wiley-Blackwell, 16–17.

Summary

- Observations can usefully contribute to assessment of nutritional status.
- Nutritional screening allows rapid identification of people at risk of malnutrition, and MUST is recommended for adults in all settings.
- After screening is completed, an appropriate action plan must be developed and implemented.

ASSISTING PEOPLE WITH EATING AND DRINKING

Most people eat independently. However, physical or mental impairment, debilitating illness or generalised weakness may make people physically unable to eat and drink without assistance. NICE (2017) guidelines specify that individuals should be provided with an adequate quality and quantity of food and fluid in an environment conducive to eating, with encouragement and help given as needed. Some people will be able to eat independently, as long as they are well prepared and supported (e.g. by positioning and the use of appropriate equipment). These aspects are discussed in detail in this section. Other people will need complete assistance with eating, and then healthcare workers must do everything possible to make this a pleasant experience and to ensure that their nutritional intake is adequate. When handling food in care settings, good food hygiene is essential, and this is also discussed.

To gain the most from this section, you need the opportunity to assist someone with eating, so you might like to work through the section with a colleague, or another willing volunteer. You will also need a variety of foods: hot, cold, chewy and soft.

By the end of this section, you will be able to:

1 identify how food hygiene can be promoted;
2 assist people with eating and drinking.

Learning outcome 1: identify how food hygiene can be promoted

The NMC (2018a, 2018b) requires that healthcare workers should assist in creating an environment that is conducive to eating and drinking. One aspect of this is food hygiene. Chapter 12 focused on preventing cross-infection, and when involved with food, healthcare workers must adhere to the principles discussed. This is important for people of all age groups but particularly people who are vulnerable to cross-infection, such as people who are immune-compromised and older people, such as Miss West and Mr. Cooper. Hand hygiene is a key skill in relation to food hygiene.

Box 5.34 Activity: precautions taken when handling food

ACTIVITY

When next in the practice setting, actively observe what precautions healthcare workers and other staff take when handling food. Also, find out if there is a local policy on food hygiene and, if so, access this to read.

You should have observed staff performing hand hygiene before serving meals donning appropriate PPE for the procedure when necessary, wearing a clean apron (perhaps a different colour to that worn for other care activities), and keeping food covered and utensils clean, with one serving utensil per menu item.

Good food hygiene must be practised in all areas; this is a government requirement under the Food Safety Act (DH, 1990) and Food Safety and Hygiene (England) Regulations (2013). All aspects are covered in the legislation and regulations, including how food is stored and handled. Food poisoning outbreaks in healthcare settings are not uncommon; stringent steps to prevent occurrences are essential. See the Food Standards Agency for further information (www.food.gov.uk/).

Learning outcome 2: assist people with eating and drinking

With one in four adults on hospital admission appearing malnourished (BAPEN 2020), encouraging people to eat and drink is essential to maintain a person's health and well-being. It is important that factors like the ward environment or community setting are considered to assist people to eat. Consider your own mealtimes and think about what helps you to eat and drink. Remember that what works for one person may not be right for another, so ensure that you discuss food and drink with the individual frequently to find out their likes and dislikes with food and drink.

Box 5.35 Activity: an environment conducive to good nutrition

What do you think healthcare workers can do to make the environment in a care setting conducive for eating in?

You might have considered removing any unpleasant odours and sights and making sure that the table is cleaned. Some care settings have a separate dining area, so if possible, assist people in leaving the bedside to sit at a dining table to eat. The table should be set properly. Ward cleaning and bed-making must never be carried out during mealtimes, and people should not be disturbed by other healthcare professionals carrying out ward rounds. As discussed in an earlier section, 'protected mealtimes' are recommended so that people can eat undisturbed and with sufficient staff available to assist.

Box 5.36 Activity: helping people to eat and drink

How might healthcare workers help people eat and drink? Consider how Miss West can be helped to eat independently, and what is the correct technique for assisting her.

The following aspects are all important points to consider.

Oral hygiene
Ensure that the person's mouth is clean and that dentures have been washed. Many people leave dentures to soak overnight, so prior to serving breakfast ensure that they have been cleaned, rinsed and reinserted.

Comfort and hygiene
Offer use of the toilet before eating and offer a handwash prior to meals.

Menu choices
Avoid choosing the person's food without consulting them. Try to involve them in decision-making regarding their dietary needs and encourage them to try a balanced diet.

Environment
Try to create a pleasant and calm environment at mealtimes. Remove obstructions from the individual's eating area (e.g. Zimmer frames, commodes, urine bottles). If appropriate, help Miss West to move to the area she wishes to eat in – people should have the freedom to choose where, and with whom, they sit.

Positioning
Miss West should be helped into a safe and comfortable position for eating. People should always eat and drink in an upright position, as close to 90 degrees as possible and in the midline. This lessens the risk of food passing into the respiratory tract, causing choking. Sitting out of bed in a comfortable chair is preferable to sitting up

in bed. Ideally, the person should sit upright with their feet on the ground, their body well supported and their head tipped slightly forward. There may be circumstances when it is not possible for people to be positioned upright, and then a side-lying position can be substituted. For useful information about how to support people who have had a stroke with eating and drinking, including positioning (see Stroke4Carers at http://www.stroke4carers.org/).

Clothing protection

Offer the person a serviette or protection for their clothing if they would like it. Avoid using plastic bibs or paper towels because this will reduce self-esteem and dignity.

Giving food choices

Tell the person what the choices of food are. Ideally, show the person the food, as the smell can induce appetite and its appearance also influences food choice. Help them choose their meal – ensure you understand what is on the menu, particularly when describing casseroles, for example, whether it is lamb or beef, and so on. Explain clearly anything they do not understand. Encourage them to eat food that is appropriate for their needs, such as soft diet, low in sugar and low in fat.

Individual dietary needs

Ensure that the person has expressed their individual dietary requirements to the staff. Do not presume about ethnic meal requirements.

Food presentation

Try to ensure that food is well presented, at the right consistency and temperature to encourage the person. Food should be prepared on a tray that is clean with an appropriate drink, a napkin and cutlery. Try to set the meal out so that it is appetising and enticing to eat.

Condiments

Provide a range of condiments – individual sachets of salt, pepper, mustard, vinegar, mint sauce, horseradish – and allow the person time to choose.

Portion size

Serve food in sensible portions to suit the person's needs. For an individual with a poor appetite (like Miss West), presentation and portion size might influence whether the food will be eaten. A large meal could be overwhelming, so a small portion is better. Second helpings can then be offered, if wished.

Correct consistency

Ensure specific advice from the multidisciplinary team (MDT) is followed regarding diet as appropriate; for example, puree diet/thickened fluids as recommended by the speech and language therapist (SLT). Many people with eating difficulties (like Miss West) need texture-modified food and fluids, for example, pureed/liquidised or thickened. Where food needs to be liquidised, each item should be liquidised separately to preserve distinctive flavours. The SLT may recommend thickened fluids to help to prevent the choking that can occur with liquid.

Positioning of food

Ensure that the food is within Miss West's reach and inform her that the food is in front of her. This is particularly important as she is partially sighted.

The clock method

As Miss West has a visual impairment, make her aware of the position of the food on the plate using the clock method to explain (see Figure 5.4). Ensure that the plate is not the same colour as the table, as this helps people who have a visual impairment to identify the plate.

Providing the correct equipment

Ensure the person has access to specialist equipment, if required, for eating and drinking (e.g. adaptive cutlery, plate guard, wide-spouted beaker). You may need to liaise with the occupational therapist on this. Non-slip mats prevent the plate from moving around and are useful for people (like Miss West) who can use only one hand. Lipped plates are high-rimmed plates and bowls that prevent the food from being pushed off or over the side. This allows people with erratic hand and arm movements to manage with a degree of independence. Plate guards work in a similar way. Two handle cups and sports bottles may be used to assist a person with drinking. Insulated beakers can be useful for people who are slow to eat or drink as this keeps the liquid hot for longer.

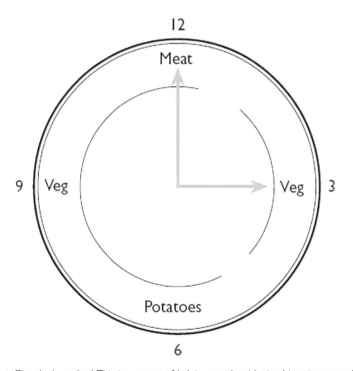

Figure 5.4: The clock method. This is a means of helping people with visual impairment to find their food. Place the food on the plate roughly at the quarter hours. Explain to the person that the meat is at the 12 o'clock position on the plate and that the vegetables are at quarter past and quarter to the hour, and the potatoes are at the half-past position. Ensure that you keep the foods separate.

Knowing people's likes and dislikes

Find out about people's dietary likes and dislikes; if they are unable to communicate these, or to recall what meals or fluids they prefer, then talk to their family or look for other information, for example, accompanying notes from a care home, an Age UK Nutrition card, an Alzheimer's Society (2012) 'This is me' leaflet (discussed earlier).

Cultural and dietary needs

Know what may offend the individual; a vegetarian receiving meat or a Muslim who is fasting receiving food will indicate a lack of understanding of the person. Be aware of allergies and foods that are restricted in the person's diet and avoid offering them these.

Assisting people with eating

You need to assess exactly how much help Miss West needs. This might range from cutting up food and giving verbal encouragement and reinforcement, to total assistance if she is unable to feed herself at all. The technique for this is discussed in detail next. With some people, it is a matter of giving time and not hurrying. If requested, open cartons, remove lids, cut up food and spread butter on bread, because for some people this is all they need to eat independently. Someone who has cerebral palsy might take up to 3 times as long to eat. They would also need some assistance to ensure that they can safely regulate the flow of liquid. You should observe for signs of fatigue and offer to help when necessary.

Assisting people who cannot eat unaided

When assisting with eating, healthcare workers must demonstrate a caring attitude, appreciating that people who cannot eat independently may experience feelings of helplessness and loss of self-esteem and dignity. Try to encourage social contact at mealtimes.

- Review AGP guidance and don appropriate PPE for the procedure when necessary.
- Sit on a chair or stool and sit at eye level with the person to convey a relaxed approach, indicating that you are going to spend time and value them.
- Ask the person in what order they would like the food and drink. They may communicate this through non-verbal rather than verbal communication, and it is important to observe reactions closely. Food should be cut into bite-sized proportions. If a soft diet is being given, adjust the portion according to the size of the mouth.
- Use normal cutlery/crockery appropriate to the food, as in a fork for the main course, a spoon for the pudding.
- Help the person to eat in a socially acceptable manner. If necessary, help the person to wipe away excess food from the mouth, clothes or hands after eating.
- Offer drinks that the individual may enjoy during and after mealtime. Establish when they want it (during or after) and what they would like.
- Allow people to eat at their own pace. Allow time for the person to chew and swallow the food and drink, before offering the next mouthful. Do not hurry the person.

- Observe for any signs of choking, for example, coughing or poor colour, and stop if you suspect this. Be especially vigilant if you know that the person has a history of swallowing problems, which may accompany neurological impairment.
- Ensure specific safe swallowing strategies as recommended by the MDT are followed as appropriate (e.g. encourage clearing swallows, use of teaspoons).
- Offer second helpings, if possible.
- When the person indicates that they have finished, remove the equipment and offer further drink and the opportunity to clean their mouth and teeth. Particles of food left in the mouth may cause dental decay, or sores can develop around the gums.
- Complete documentation (discussed later), evaluate the care provided with the individual, and check whether they have any other care needs.

ACTIVITY

Box 5.37 Activity: positions for eating

With a willing colleague, practise giving each other a variety of food and drink – cold, hot, soft and chewy. Then try some of the following positions for eating:

- review AGP guidance and don appropriate PPE for the procedure when necessary;
- sitting in a scrunched-up position;
- sitting on your hands with a blindfold covering your eyes;
- lying fairly flat on your side and pretending that you cannot move.

(As discussed above, this is not a recommended position for eating and should be used only for a person who, for medical reasons, has to lie flat.) Now ask your colleague about your technique: What did they feel you did well? What do they feel you could do better in? Then reflect on the experience:

- How did this activity feel?
- What would have made the experience better?

What have you learned from this activity?

Reporting/evaluating/documenting

After assisting a person with eating and drinking, you should complete any relevant documentation, such as filling in the food chart and/or fluid balance chart. Remember to report any unusual occurrence to the nurse in charge. Review the plan of care and evaluate. Is it still appropriate? Does it need to be changed?

Other approaches

For people who are in non-acute hospital settings, other approaches may be employed. For example, in some mental health units, healthcare workers eat with clients so that they can encourage and prompt them to eat, while also engaging with them. For people with paranoia, it may dispel fear of poisoning if the nurse is eating the same meal from the same source. In some settings, facilities to make snacks, for example, sandwiches, are available, and for a person with paranoia, it may be less frightening to make their own food from raw materials than to eat pre-cooked food, which they may fear has been poisoned. Alternatively, they may accept food brought in by their own family.

Alzheimer's Society (2020) identified that healthcare workers and carers reported concerns related to eating and drinking for people with dementia. In response, Alzheimer's Society developed some 'Top tips'. Box 5.38 includes some of these additional points. Other members of the healthcare team will be a valuable resource (see next section).

Box 5.38 Eating and drinking for people with dementia: top tips for healthcare workers

- Offer regular prompts and encouragement to eat and drink. Place the cutlery in the person's hands and guide their movements to start with. Similarly, place a cup in the person's hands and guide it to their mouth.
- If using cutlery is difficult, offer finger foods to maintain independence at mealtimes.
- Allow sufficient time for eating as coordination difficulties can make eating slow; prevent the person from feeling pressurised.
- Mealtimes should be relaxed and unhurried; a noisy busy ward can be distracting for people with dementia at mealtimes, resulting in food left uneaten.
- Be flexible as to when food is offered; a person with dementia may develop patterns of eating that fall outside of fixed mealtimes. Ensure there are nutritious snacks available throughout the day and night.
- A person with dementia may struggle to make a menu choice from words alone; pictures of food may help.

Source: Summarised from Alzheimer's Society – Top tips for healthcare workers: Eating and drinking.

Adapted with permission from original information produced by Alzheimer's Society alzheimers.org.uk

---

Murphy et al. (2017) highlight how there is a growing volume of research to offer improvements in nutritional care for people with dementia living in nursing homes. Support with food and drink intake. Training and education tools and the availability of food and drink at frequent intervals can all assist in boosting a person's oral intake of food and drink.

Summary

- Review AGP guidance and don appropriate PPE for this procedure when necessary for assisting with fluid and nutritional support.
- Good food hygiene is essential in care settings.
- When assisting with oral intake of food and drink, the nurse should prepare the person, the environment and the food carefully, and try to promote mealtimes as enjoyable and relaxed events.

- The nurse's approach should ensure that the person feels valued and does not feel rushed.
- Good hygiene should be maintained, including handwashing and oral care for the individual.
- Monitoring and recording food intake is important, especially when a person has been assessed to be at high risk of malnutrition.
- Reviewing the plan of care is vital after every meal.

ADDITIONAL NUTRITIONAL SUPPORT STRATEGIES

Healthcare workers have a responsibility to assist and support people in meeting nutritional needs. This section considers how members of the healthcare team can be involved to support nutrition and how the nutritional value of a person's oral intake can be improved.

Box 5.39 Learning outcomes

At the end of this section, you will be able to:

1. identify other healthcare professionals who may be involved in nutritional care and explain their roles;
2. discuss how the nutritional value of a person's oral intake can be enhanced.

Learning outcome 1: identify other healthcare professionals who may be involved in nutritional care and explain their roles

---

Box 5.40 Activity: meeting nutritional needs

List healthcare professionals who might be able to help people with meeting their nutritional needs; some have already been mentioned in this chapter. Think back to the scenarios and identify healthcare professionals who might support nutrition.

You might have identified that there are a wide range of professionals who contribute to nutritional care. Their roles are explained next.

Dieticians

Dieticians are experts in nutrition, capable of performing comprehensive assessments of people's nutritional status and needs. They are capable of offering general healthy eating advice, guidance for the use of dietary supplements and specific advice for dietary management in relation to medical disorders. Some dieticians specialise in certain age groups, for example, older people. As Miss West's screening identified she was at high risk of malnutrition, she must be referred to the dietician. If Mr. Cooper is found to be at high risk when nutritional screening is carried out, referral to a dietician would be appropriate for him too. A dietician can educate Phillip about eating healthily and his carers too, so that they can support Phillip in making healthy food choices, and also educate Phillip and his carers about the implications of not making dietary changes.

Speech and language therapists

Speech and language therapists are capable of assisting people of all ages and abilities with chewing and swallowing problems; these can occur in people with dementia or people like Miss West, who had dysphagia following a stroke. It could be worthwhile asking an SLT to reassess Miss West's swallowing as she is still having problems eating. Speech and language therapists will advise on whether it is possible for people to take food orally and, if so, whether special precautions are necessary such as using thickening agents.

Physicians

Dietary supplements may need to be prescribed by a doctor. For some people, there may be an underlying medical problem affecting their nutrition, which needs to be treated. In some instances, weight gain, as experienced by Phillip, can be caused by an underlying medical condition, for example, an underactive thyroid gland (hypothyroidism).

Pharmacists

Pharmacists may advise other health professionals in medication-related issues and may be involved in aspects of enteral and parenteral nutrition.

Dentists

Dentists may assist people with dental or denture problems. If Miss West's dentures fitted properly, it could help considerably with her eating. The community mental health nurse should check whether referral to a dentist would be appropriate for Mr. Cooper too.

Community support

Some health centres have health advisers for older people, and this could be relevant to Miss West when she is discharged and for providing additional support for Mr. Cooper.

Psychologists

A referral to a psychologist would be appropriate if a person has an eating disorder but could also be relevant to Miss West in relation to her possible depression.

Physiotherapists

Physiotherapists can assist people with motor problems, for example, following a stroke, and help with their positioning. This is likely to be helpful for Miss West.

Occupational therapists

An occupational therapist may be able to identify suitable aids to assist with eating and drinking and positioning, thus promoting independence. Miss West would be likely to benefit from this help. They may also be able to suggest equipment to assist people with dementia. The occupational therapist could assist Phillip in improving his skills in food preparation.

Social workers

A social worker would be involved in arranging home care packages, including home-carers to serve meals and shop. This may well be essential to enable Miss West to maintain her nutrition after discharge from hospital. The community mental health nurse visiting Mr. Cooper will be part of a multidisciplinary team that will include social workers. The different members of the team will appear on his Care Programme Approach (CPA) plan, with their input identified. His plan may well need reviewing and additional support planned.

Another source of help for Phillip could be attending a 'Healthy lifestyles' course, aimed at his age group, covering a range of issues such as nutrition and exercise, which will be run by a group of professionals, including the dietician, occupational therapist and community nurse for learning disabilities.

Learning outcome 2: discuss how the nutritional value of a person's oral intake can be enhanced

Sometimes, if appetite is poor or a person is very unwell, food intake may be insufficient to meet nutritional needs. Oral supplements may need to be prescribed by the dietician to assist in supplementing oral intake.

> ### Box 5.41 activity: use of supplements
>
> What supplements have you seen in practice to increase the nutritional value of a person's oral intake?

ACTIVITY

A wide range of dietary supplements are available, some of which are designed to be added to the normal diet (e.g. powdered glucose polymers such as Maxijul and Polycal), or to be taken as a drink between normal meals (e.g. Fresubin, Fortisip and Enlive). The purpose of these is to increase the nutritional value of oral intake; some provide just calories, while others provide proteins, vitamins and minerals in addition. A dietician can advise what is most appropriate for an individual person following a comprehensive nutritional assessment. There are a wide variety of flavours available, some probably acceptable to both Miss West and Mr. Cooper. These supplements can be a very good way of increasing nutritional intake. However, it should be remembered that these supplements should be prescribed, monitored and their usefulness assessed on a regular basis. These substances fall into the British National Formulary, Borderline substances category, and as such need close monitoring (Aneurin Bevan Health Board 2013).

Even with the use of supplements, it may not be possible for some people to fully meet their nutritional needs with oral intake. Other people may not be able to take food and drink orally at all owing to an inability to swallow. This may be for a temporary period (e.g. if a person is unconscious for a few days), but for some people, it can be permanent. In these situations, you might have seen people fed by tube (enteral feeding) or through an intravenous infusion (parenteral feeding). The next sections explore these methods.

Summary

- A multidisciplinary approach to promoting nutrition will optimise specialist skills and knowledge, giving people the best chance of having their individual nutritional needs met in full.
- If nutritional needs cannot be met through a person's usual oral diet, other alternatives must be found. These could be oral supplements, enteral feeding or parenteral feeding. The dietician's input and advice are essential in these situations.

ARTIFICIAL FEEDING – ENTERAL AND PARENTERAL FEEDING

The NMC (2018a, 2018b) requires that healthcare workers must ensure that people who cannot take food by mouth receive adequate fluid and nutrition and can safely administer fluids when they cannot be taken independently. Enteral feeding may be achieved via a nasogastric tube (NGT) (a tube passed via the nose down the oesophagus and into the stomach), or via a percutaneous endoscopic gastrostomy tube (PEG) or a percutaneous radiological gastrostomy (PRG), which are an opening in the abdominal wall through which a tube is passed to allow feeds to enter the stomach directly. These procedures are invasive, and informed consent must be gained from the person as per the Mental Capacity Act (Great Britain 2005). As a gastrostomy is a surgical procedure, written consent must be obtained. A PEG tube provides more secure nutritional provision than NGT feeding.

Enteral feeding may be used to supplement or completely replace oral intake. It can be administered by bolus, intermittently or continuously. Enteral feeding might be done to maintain adequate nutrition for a person with severe neurological impairment as a result of cerebral palsy or stroke where swallowing is extremely difficult or hazardous, or for people whose nutritional needs exceed their oral intake, owing to a health problem. All enteral feeding methods have benefits and hazards associated with them. These are discussed later in this section. It is therefore imperative that this procedure is done under the supervision of a qualified practitioner. Medicines may be prescribed via the enteral tube route, and this procedure is also included in this section. In some circumstances, the enteral route cannot be used, and this section also identifies the role of parenteral nutrition and intravenous fluid administration. The use of enteral feeding has gained popularity over recent years, and many people now receive home parenteral and enteral nutrition. Wanten (2011) explains how home parenteral nutrition is the treatment of choice for people with long-term intestinal failure. NICE (2020) provides detailed, evidence-based guidelines relating to enteral and parenteral feeding; these are recommended further reading.

> **Box 5.42 Learning outcomes**
>
> By the end of this section, you will be able to:
>
> 1 discuss nasogastric tube insertion and the associated care;
> 2 explain the specific care needed following gastrostomy;
> 3 identify key principles for administering enteral feeds;
> 4 discuss the process of administering medicines by the enteral route;
> 5 identify the role of parenteral nutrition and intravenous fluid administration in maintaining nutrition.

Learning outcome 1: discuss nasogastric tube insertion and the associated care

Review AGP guidance and don appropriate PPE when necessary before attempting any of the following procedures.

Note: This section focuses mainly on nasogastric tubes for feeding, but the insertion of NGTs for gastric drainage will also be discussed in a subsection.

It is essential that you follow your organisation's policy about who can pass an NGT for feeding and the preparation and competency assessment required.

Prior to NGT insertion, key issues to consider are:

- whether the need for the tube is clinically indicated, appropriate and documented;
- whether the use of an NGT is for drainage or feeding;
- how to ensure the position of the tube is checked after insertion;
- what the ongoing management of the tube will entail.

Inserting a nasogastric tube for feeding

The decision to pass an NGT for feeding must be made by two competent health professionals, to include the person's senior doctor, and the decision must be balanced carefully against the risks with the rationale documented in the person's notes (BAPEN 2020). BAPEN (2020) provides guidance and decision-making trees to support practitioners in their decision-making. They recommend that NGTs must only be inserted by healthcare professionals who have been assessed as competent to do so and should not be inserted out of hours except in emergency situations as there should be radiology staff available to check tube placement, if required. This is due to the limitations that exist with their insertion. In a person who is unconscious and or critically ill and unable to swallow, Sanaie et al. (2020), compare two methods of NGT insertion SORT method (sniffing position, NGT orientation, contralateral rotation and twisting movement) versus neck flexion lateral pressure (NFLP). Sanaie et al. (2020) support the use of the SORT method but highlight how further consideration should be taken with regard to clinical factors, operator experience and preference before NGT insertion.

The recent COVID 19 pandemic has however required practitioners to further review the procedure for the insertion and management of the NGT, to reduce the risk factors for both the individual and staff. Martindale et al. (2020) explain how

NGT insertion is an AGP and as such carries risks to practitioners who insert these devices. They recommend practitioners wear the appropriate level of PPE, follow local organisational guidance and adopt risk-limiting practices in their clinical environment. Najafi (2021) while still recommending the SORT manoeuvre is performed to insert a NGT, advises caution should be adopted. He too expresses how such procedures carry a risk of COVID-19 infection spread. All practitioners are therefore advised to wear the appropriate level of PPE before conducting the insertion of a NG tube.

ACTIVITY

Box 5.43 Activity: nasogastric tubes

Find out what NGTs are used in your care setting. You may also be able to look at these tubes in the skills laboratory. What are their key features?

NGTs used for feeding people vary according to care setting but should be fine-bore feeding tubes. A decision must be made whether or not to insert a tube within 24 h of identifying the need and appropriateness of enteral feeding. Informed consent, as per Mental Capacity Act (Great Britain 2005) must be gained from the person, and any potential contraindications to passing the NGT should be identified, such as:

- previous surgery/trauma to head or neck
- oesophageal varices or other upper gastrointestinal pathology
- complex head and neck problems (e.g. tumour, altered anatomy)
- trauma from poisoning (e.g. oral consumption of bleach)
- nasal fracture or trauma
- reduced level of consciousness when using the ACVPU scale or GCS score
- gastric stasis
- gastro-oesophageal stricture
- base of skull fracture
- caution with anticoagulant therapy due to potential bleeding.

Any of the above should be discussed with the clinical team as the doctor or gastroenterology team may be required to insert the NGT under radiological guidance.

Table 5.3 presents the procedure for passing a nasogastric feeding tube, with the rationale explained; be sure to follow local guidelines. Figure 5.5 shows how to measure the length of tube required, and Figure 5.6 illustrates some of the steps in NGT insertion. Checking of the NGT position is an essential element that is discussed in more detail in the next section.

Don appropriate PPE and then prepare equipment:

Clinically clean tray/trolley, fine-bore NGT with guide wire, sterile receiver, cotton buds and tissues, sterile water, 50 mL syringe, 20 mL syringe, hypoallergenic tape, adhesive patch from NGT packet, glass of water and pH paper/indicator strips.

Table 5.3: Insertion of a nasogastric feeding tube

Action	Rationale
Prepare the person. Arrange a signal by which the individual can communicate, if they want the nurse to stop the procedure (e.g. by raising their hand)	Reduces fear by giving the person some control over the procedure
Assist the person into an upright position in the bed or chair with head supported by pillows; or if unconscious, on their side, supported by pillows	Ensures the person is comfortable and this allows for easy passage of the tube
The head should not be tilted backwards or forwards	Enables easy swallowing and ensures that the epiglottis is not obstructing the oesophagus
Ask the person to blow their nose, if possible	Ensures nostrils are clear, aiding insertion
Clean the mucus/encrustations around the nostrils with cotton buds, moistened with warm water	Helps with ease of insertion and ensures persons' comfort
Perform hand hygiene and put on non-sterile gloves and apron	Minimises the risk of cross-infection. Standard principles must be observed when dealing with body fluids
Estimate the length of the tube to be passed by selecting the appropriate distance mark on the tube by measuring the distance on the tube from the tip of the nose to the earlobe and then to the xiphisternum (see Figure 5.5)	Gives the estimated length of tube required to enable the tip of the tube to rest in the stomach
Assess if the individual has a gag/swallow reflex by consulting medical notes	Absence of a gag/swallow reflex highlights the increased risk of misplacement of the tube, which may lead to aspiration
Lubricate the tube, as per manufacturer's instructions/local policy	Lubrication reduces friction between mucous membranes and tube during insertion
At all times during the procedure, talk to and reassure the individual	Instils confidence in the individual and allays fears
Insert the proximal end of the tube (with the guide wire introducer in position) into the clearest nostril, passing along the floor of the nasopharynx to the oropharynx (see Figure 5.6a). If any obstruction is felt, withdraw the tube and try again in a slightly different direction or try the other nostril	Facilitates the passage of the tube into the oesophagus
As the tube passes down into the oropharynx, ask the person to swallow. To assist the passage of the tube, ask them to take sips of water (if not contraindicated). If the individual is unconscious, then stroking the throat can stimulate the swallow reflex	Swallowing closes the epiglottis and reduces the risk of inadvertent endotracheal placement, enabling the tube to pass into the oesophagus
Advance the tube through the oropharynx, down the oesophagus into the stomach until the estimate mark on the tube reaches the external nares	Sufficient length of tube has been passed for it to enter the stomach
If at any time the individual shows signs of distress, for example, coughing, gasping, cyanosis, remove the tube immediately	The tube may have entered the trachea, not the oesophagus
Confirm the position of the tube by attaching the 50 mL syringe to the guide wire introducer (Figure 5.6b).	A pH reading of 1–5.5, can reliably exclude pulmonary placement of the NGT (NPSA 2011a)
Gently aspirate a small amount of fluid (0.5–1 mL) to test with pH indicator strips (Figure 5.6c). The pH should be 1–5.5. National Patient Safety Agency (NPSA 2011a) recommends that a second competent person checks any readings that fall within the pH range of 5–6, as it may be difficult to differentiate readings in this range	Note: a pH of 1–5.5 does not necessarily confirm gastric placement of the NGT; there is a small possibility that the tube is in the oesophagus, which carries a higher risk of aspiration (NPSA 2011a). See the text for further discussion
If there is any doubt about the position of the tube, and if repeated attempts to obtain aspirate are unsuccessful, a chest X-ray will be required to verify the position of the tube (NPSA 2011a)	To ensure the tube is in the correct position prior to administering anything down it

(Continued)

Table 5.3: (Continued)

Action	Rationale
Remove the guide wire only after the correct position of the tube has been confirmed	While present, it makes the tube more radio-opaque, enabling repositioning of the tube, if necessary
To remove the guide wire, attach a 20 mL syringe and inject 5 mL of fresh tap water down the tube (or as per manufacturers' instructions)	Injecting water activates the lubricant on the guide wire, enabling easy removal
Hold the tube end firmly at the tip of the nose and gently and carefully withdraw the guide wire, disposing of it appropriately	Ensures that the tube stays in position as the guide wire is removed
Secure the tube in place by taping around it and across the nose (a fixing device should be in the pack) (see Figure 5.6d)	Secures the tube easily and comfortably: less likely to cause nasal pressure ulcers
Using an indelible marker, mark the tube at the point where it leaves the nose	To have a visual reference point and allow easy detection of dislodgement of the tube
Document in the person's records, including the method of testing position (NPSA 2011a)	To ensure that there is documented evidence of insertion and confirmation of position of the tube

Note: Ensure that you follow local guidelines for this procedure or visit www.nng, org.uk for further guidance. Below is an overview of the procedure.

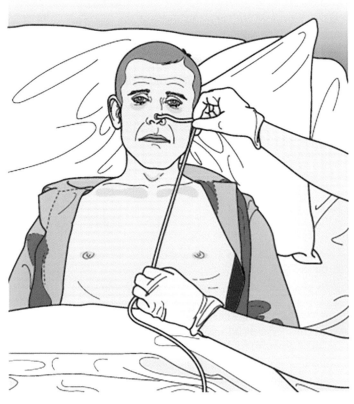

Figure 5.5: Measuring nasogastric tube length.

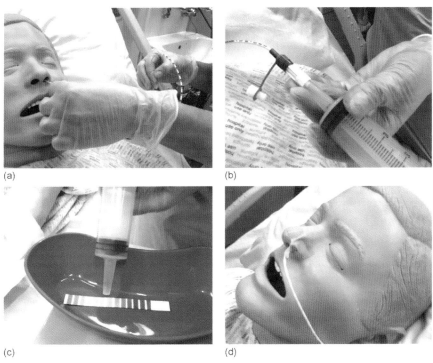

Figure 5.6: Insertion of a nasogastric tube. (a) Inserting the nasogastric tube; (b) Attaching the syringe for aspiration; (c) Testing the aspirate with the pH strip; (d) Securing of the nasogastric tube to the nostril.

Checking nasogastric tube position

Potential position complications include:

- consideration of safety as this is potentially AGP where droplet transmission can occur
- passage of the tube into the trachea
- coiling of the tube into the posterior pharynx
- trauma/haemorrhage or perforation of any of the surrounding tissues.

There have been a number of incidents where incorrect positioning of NGTs for feeding has led to people's deaths or illnesses (NPSA 2016, BAPEN 2020). NPSA (2011b) provides detailed guidelines, and also a 'decision tree', regarding how to confirm the correct position of nasogastric feeding tubes; do access these documents for further information and detailed guidance including the evidence base. NGTs must not be flushed, nor any liquid or feed introduced through the tube following initial placement, until the tube tip is confirmed by pH testing or X-ray, to be in the stomach (NPSA 2016, BAPEN 2020).

If there are problems obtaining aspirate for pH testing, NPSA (2011a) recommends trying each of the following techniques:

- if possible, turn the person, onto their left side;
- inject 10–20 mL air into the tube using a 50 mL syringe;

- wait for 15–30 min before aspirating again;
- advance or withdraw the tube by 1–20 cm;
- give mouth care to people who are nil by mouth as this stimulates gastric secretion of acid.

If aspirate is obtained it can then be tested but otherwise, an X-ray must be performed to check the position of the NGT.

It should be noted that there is potential for harm due to misplaced NG tubes. National Health Service improvements (2016) report how over a period of 5 years, from 2011 to 2016, 95 incidents were reported of fluid or drug therapy being identified within the respiratory tract or pleura of a person, of these 32 people died. Smith et al. (2018), in a study of people in ITU, identified how several individuals showed complications from NG tube insertion including aspiration and death. They advise that the process of NG tube insertion should be carefully planned and constant checks made with regard to feeding and aspiration of the tube carried out. To avoid potential incorrect placement and mortality, BAPEN (2020) advises that further placement checks should be made daily regarding feeding or medication insertion (see BAPEN guidance at www.bapen.org.uk/res_drugs.html). Always check the placement of the tube before administering each feed and before giving medicines. It is also advisable to check the tube's position following vomiting, retching or coughing (as this could dislodge the tube) or if the tube appears to be displaced (e.g. tape undone, tube appears to have moved).

Documentation

It is the responsibility of the professional who inserted or reinserted the NGT to document:

- date and time inserted and by who;
- type, size and batch number of tube;
- length to which the tube was inserted (e.g. '60 cm at right nostril') at the time of its initial placement, the tube must be marked with an indelible pen at the point where it enters the nostril;
- patency of the tube and details of pH testing (NPSA 2011a);
- whether aspirate was obtained;
- what the aspirate pH was;
- who checked the aspirate pH;
- when it was confirmed to be safe to administer feed and/or medication (i.e. gastric pH between 1 and 5.5) (NPSA 2011a);
- any additional comments (difficulties in insertion, etc.);
- expected date for review or removal.

The NGT packaging may include a sticky label with space for these details, for insertion in the person's notes.

After initial insertion, a record of subsequent tube position checks should be maintained, along with the tube length, and any tube-related issues, until it is removed

(BAPEN 2020). If there is any indication that the tube length has changed, appropriate action should be taken to assess tube tip position prior to using the NGT.

ACTIVITY

> **Box 5.44 Activity: insertion of nasogastric tube**
>
> Observe the insertion of NGT and take the opportunity to practise NGT insertion on a manikin, if available. When in practice, if a person has to have a NGT inserted, ask if you can observe the procedure, with the person's consent.

Management of nasogastric tubes and feed administration

When the oral route cannot be used for nutrition support, it is important to still maintain adequate nutrition for the individual. Following the insertion and checking the position of the NGT, feeding can commence via the enteral route.

Nasogastric feeding can be done as a bolus using gravity to assist the feed to the stomach. However, this practice has some limitations and caution must be taken when using this method to avoid further gastrointestinal (GI) symptoms (www.patient.info/doctor/nasogastric-ryles-tubes).

Feeds may also be given intermittently by pump or using gravity. This offers the person a time without feeding and allows the GI tract to rest and digest the feeds given.

For many people, continuous feeding is recommended in the initial stages of maintaining nutrition. This feed is given via a pump system. This is the preferred method of feeding a person as it reduces the risk to the GI tract.

Prior to commencement of any feed, verbal consent must be gained from the individual. Do not carry out this procedure until you are deemed competent by your clinical area. You should adhere to the clinical area procedure and report any abnormalities you find before attempting to adjust any feeds being administered to a person. Please see your clinical area practice guidelines to review the administration of bolus, intermittent and continuous feeding. The tape used to secure the tube in place should be checked daily to highlight any inflammation, irritation or signs of the beginnings of a nasal pressure ulcer on the nose. The tape used to hold the tube should be changed if it is not secure or irritation has occurred. During feeding, the person should be lying at a 45-degree angle (semi-upright position) at all times. The type of feed prescribed and administered should be as recommended by the dietician. Always ensure that the feed has not expired and is in a sealed, sterile bottle. The length of time the tube is *in situ* prior to removal or reinsertion must comply with manufacturer's guidelines. Box 5.45 provides guidelines for removal of NGTs.

If the person's oral route remains unavailable due to injury or disease, the NGT can be used in a community setting to maintain nutrition. This is usually used intermittently to feed the person thus allowing some time away from feeding and also enabling some degree of mobility.

NGT insertion for drainage

The NGT can be used for drainage to empty GI contents prior to surgery and following a trauma. These types of NGT are larger than feeding tubes and produced in various sizes. The clinical need will determine the size of tube that is appropriate, but the smallest (i.e. narrowest) tube appropriate for the individual's management should be used. Prior to inserting an NGT for drainage, first identify whether the tube is being inserted for free drainage, aspiration or intermittent drainage. For free drainage, you will require a bile bag for attachment. Also, identify the purpose of the NGT, for example, is the tube for conservative measures, that is, bowel obstruction or following surgery to prevent aspiration or to relieve vomiting due to gut stasis/ileus?

Box 5.45 Removal of nasogastric tube

Ensure that the tube is clinically no longer required or there is a clear documented reason for removal. Then,

- Don appropriate PPE.
- Prepare equipment – waste bag, tissues and spigot (optional).
- Prepare the person for the removal of the tube. Explain and discuss each step.
- Ensure that the individual is seated upright, if they are able to.
- Ensure the feed has been stopped and detached from the feeding line, and the tube contents have been drained.
- Remove tape from nose that is securing the tube.
- The person may find taking a deep breath during the removal helpful.
- Remove the tube in one swift action and dispose of in the waste bag.
- Wipe the person's nose.
- Remove PPE, wash hands and dispose of waste appropriately.
- Document removal in the individual's medical and nursing notes.

As with any procedure, you should explain and obtain verbal consent from the person according to the Mental Capacity Act (Great Britain 2005). Check for potential contraindications: previous head, face or gut surgery or trauma including basal skull fracture, a reduced level of consciousness, oesophageal varices, cancer/tumour or complex head and neck problems, upper gastrointestinal pathology (i.e. strictures) or coagulation problems should all be taken into account. If contraindications are present, the individual may need a surgeon or gastroenterology team to insert the tube under radiological guidance.

The key principles of passing an NGT for drainage are the same as for insertion of NGTs for feeding (see Table 5.3, and Figures 5.5 and 5.6), including measuring the length of the tube to be passed, checking of tube position and record-keeping. However, the tube should preferably have been stored in a fridge for at least half an hour before the procedure is to begin, to ensure a rigid tube that can be passed easily. Also, have a vomit bowl available or – if there is likely to be a large gastric residual volume – ensure that appropriate suction equipment is available. Prior to passing the tube, check the person's nostrils are patent by asking them to sniff with one nostril closed and repeat with the other nostril. The tube can be passed by oral route if necessary. About 15–20 cm of the tube should be lubricated with a thin coat of lubricating jelly placed on a swab, thus reducing friction between the mucous membrane and the tube.

Learning outcome 2: explain the specific care needed following percutaneous endoscopic gastrostomy tube or percutaneous radiological gastrostomy

Percutaneous endoscopic gastrostomy is indicated in individuals where dysphagia (unable to swallow) has been present or where the nasogastric route cannot be used. If feeding is likely to occur for 28 days or more, PEG feeding should be considered as an alternative to nasogastric feeding. Usually, it is not required in people who have oesophageal obstruction since other methods of treatment are available. Neurological causes of dysphagia (stroke and other chronic diseases such as motor neuron disease) are the most common reasons for referral.

There are two methods of placing gastrostomy; **PEG** is the most frequently used. **Percutaneous radiological gastrostomy** is the other method, and it is particularly indicated for people with a high risk of pulmonary aspiration following gastro-oesophageal reflux. Both techniques can be complicated by abdominal wall sepsis (including necrotising fasciitis) and peritonitis. The type of tube placed and the date of placement are recorded in the medical notes.

In general, gastrostomy is contraindicated where death is likely in a very short time. Even if feeding were started, survival of the individual after gastrostomy is determined mainly by selection criteria. The majority of people who receive gastrostomy feeding have had a stroke. The immediate procedure-related mortality for PEG should be considered when decisions are taken to insert such devices. Onder et al. (2012) explain how risks can be reduced by considering risk factors like hospital bound infections and monitoring of people's blood serum albumin levels. Gastrostomy placement is not a trivial decision, and complications of gastrostomy can increase mortality rates. NPSA (2018) reported how mortality increases with NGT placement.

Necrotising fasciitis

Rare bacterial infection of the deeper layers of skin and subcutaneous tissue.

Peritonitis

Inflammation of the peritoneum, which lines the inside of the abdomen and covers the internal organs, usually due to bacterial infection.

ACTIVITY

Box 5.46 Activity: caring for someone with a gastrostomy

If you are caring for anyone with a gastrostomy currently, discuss the rationale for its insertion with your mentor. Also, find out about local guidelines for immediate and long-term care following insertion.

Learning outcome 3: identify key principles for administering enteral feeds

Most enteral feeds come prepared from the manufacturers. This is a sterile feed specifically designed nutritional liquid with a licence (BAPEN 2020). The feeds vary in volume and content, so need to be prescribed for individuals. Types of feed include whole protein feed (polymeric), pre-digested (peptide/semi elemental/

elemental), which contain proteins in smaller molecules to improve absorption. Disease-specific or immune-enhancing foods formulated for people with organ failure can offer nutrients that can modify the immune system (BAPEN 2020). Feeds may be given continuously, overnight or by bolus at regular intervals, and dieticians will decide on the most appropriate feed regimen. The feeds are administered by an enteral feed pump, so that the rate can be set accurately. It is increasingly common for people to administer their own enteral feeds at home, with training and support from community healthcare workers; BAPEN (2016) offer an explanation as to how this may be achieved in their home enteral nutrition guidance. However, appropriate training should be given to people who wish to support significant others with enteral nutrition and effective levels of PPE must be made available to the individual carrying out these procedures.

Box 5.47 Activity: someone who is being fed enterally

If a person is unable to take food or fluids orally and is being fed enterally, what special care do you think they would need?

You might have included the following:

- Observe fluid intake and output.
- Ensure that the prescribed feeding regimen is adhered to. Store feeds according to manufacturer's instructions.
- Observe for and report any untoward effects (like vomiting, diarrhoea or constipation).
- Maintain mouth care (see Chapter 7).
- Ensure that the position of the tube is maintained (e.g. that a nasogastric tube is secured adequately) (see the earlier section regarding placement checks).
- Take measures to prevent cross-infection (e.g. hand hygiene, aseptic technique when connecting the feed administration set and the feeding tube).
- Ensure that the tube remains patent. Flush with water before and after feeds and medicine are administered.
- Be aware of, and try to minimise, the psychosocial effects of enteral feeding; for example, effects on body image (see Chapter 2) and the loss associated with the inability to enjoy eating and join in with the associated social aspects.

People with enteral tubes may be administered medication via this route, which is discussed next.

Learning outcome 4: discuss the process of administering medicines by the enteral route

Individuals who are unable to take medicines orally and have a NGT or a gastrostomy tube may have some medication administered via a syringe attached to the tube's connector. All medications should be prescribed and administered according to manufacturer instructions and in line with your role and competency. Medicine routes, dosages and prescriptions should be administered as per British National Formula guidance. Other routes (e.g. topical) for drug administration should be used where possible. Self-administration of medications via enteral routes should be addressed and a training programme developed to enable this to take place for individuals who are deemed competent to administer their own medications. For further information regarding drug administration, please see Chapter 10.

Box 5.48 Activity: enteral tube route

What difficulties or risks might there be of administering medicine via the enteral tube route? Consider how these might be addressed.

You could have thought of these points:

- The NGT route can be hazardous as the tube could dislodge from its position in the stomach. Therefore, the tube's position must be checked prior to medicine administration, as discussed earlier.
- Absorption and preparation of medicines for the enteral tube route may differ from oral medication. Therefore, healthcare workers must work with the pharmacist who can advise about medicines being prescribed and dispensed in a suitable format, with consideration of any drug interactions. Some liquid preparations are suspensions of small granules and are therefore not suitable and others contain sorbitol, which is a laxative (BAPEN 2020). The medicines will usually be prescribed as liquids or soluble tablets.

Note: Tablets must not be crushed nor capsules opened as this could alter the medicine's therapeutic action, making it ineffective and thus invalidating the product's licence. Covert administration of medication should be avoided (www.rpharms.com). Medicines should only be administered via a NG tube in accordance with agreed management plans and trust protocols. All medication should be administered as per prescription.

- Enteral tubes can become blocked. Common causes are inadequate flushing and using the wrong formulation of medicine (BAPEN 2020). They suggest that if blockage occurs, aspiration to remove particles can be tried followed by a warm water flush, but excessive pressure must not be applied due to risk of tube fracture. These practices should, however, be carried out under current guidance with regard to COVID 19 and appropriate PPE be donned to conduct such testing.

Box 5.49 Activity: enteral medication syringe

Look at an enteral medication syringe – in practice or in the skills laboratory. Note how it differs from other syringes.

- A syringe is used to prepare the medicine, and there have been reports of enteral medicines being given intravenously by accident with serious consequences (NPSA

2018); this is identified as a Never Event (www.improvment.nhs.uk 2018). Therefore, syringes used to draw up and administer medication via enteral tubes must comply with NPSA (2016) guidance, to prevent administration errors. The syringes used must not be able to be connected to intravenous (IV) cannula, should be labelled and may be of a different colour to distinguish them from IV syringes (NPSA 2016).

All safety aspects of medicine administration (see Chapter 10) must be adhered to when administering medicines by enteral tubes. You must maintain infection control precautions: wash hands and put on non-sterile gloves. You should prepare the correct dose as prescribed in an enteral syringe. The pharmacist's specific instructions regarding the medicine and its preparation and administration must be followed. Liquids should be shaken well and thick liquids diluted with an equal amount of water; soluble tablets should be dissolved in 10–15 mL of water (BAPEN 2018).

> ### Box 5.50 Activity: administering a medicine via the enteral tube route
>
> What specific aspects will be necessary when administering a medicine via the enteral tube route? *Consider:* the individuals who may have a feed in progress, or the tube may be closed off with a spigot.

Remember, as discussed previously, for NGTs, if there is no feed in progress, you must first check if the tube's position is in the stomach (see earlier discussion). BAPEN (2018) advises the following method for administration:

- If the person has a feed in progress, switch this off. Sometimes, there will need to be a break from feeding before and/or after medicine administration – the pharmacist will advise.
- Use a non-touch technique to attach the syringe to the tube's connector. Flush the tube with at least 30 mL of water (or as directed).
- Administer the medicine, flushing with 10 mL of water in between each medicine given.
- Give a final flush of at least 30 mL of water and restart the feed (unless a break is advised).

Learning outcome 5: identify the role of parenteral nutrition and intravenous fluid administration in maintaining nutrition

In some instances, it may not be possible to provide nutrition enterally. Parenteral feeding (often referred to as total parenteral nutrition – TPN) may be used when a person is unable to use the gastrointestinal tract for nutrition, either temporarily or in the long term. An example would be a person who has had major surgery to the gastrointestinal tract. In parenteral nutrition, nutrients and micronutrients are administered directly into the circulation intravenously via a device in the vein and therefore only qualified healthcare workers can administer TPN.

The aim of IV therapy is to maintain or restore normal fluid and electrolyte balance. IV therapy should always be approached with caution if fluid overload, fluid deficit, fluid shifts and unwanted alterations in electrolyte concentrations are to be avoided. It is essential that all fluid replacement regimes are tailored to the individual's requirements.

Assessment of the need for IV fluids and electrolytes should include:

- vital signs monitoring as per NEWS2 score;
- fluid intake and output measurements;
- daily weight;
- skin turgor – this can be assessed by pinching a fold of skin. In a well-hydrated person, the skin will immediately fall back to its normal position when released. It is best practice to pinch the skin over the sternum or the inner thigh;
- capillary refill time (see Chapter 14);
- central venous pressure (CVP) measurements (see Chapter 14);
- serum electrolyte levels in blood sample;
- arterial blood gas results (see Chapter 14);
- routine ward testing of urine to review specific gravity.

Refeeding syndrome

This syndrome sees a potentially fatal shift in fluid and electrolytes within the body that may occur in malnourished patients following a period of starvation (NICE 2018).

When trying to supplement a person's nutritional intake, caution must be taken to eliminate **refeeding syndrome**. This has possible fatal consequences leading to both metabolic and physiological changes in a person who has been malnourished. It is therefore imperative that fluid and electrolyte balances are monitored in individuals who receive supplementary dietary intakes, as this plays a key role in ensuring that the person receives optimal nutrition when the body is under insult of injury (BAPEN 2017).

See Willis (2015) for further reading of fluid and electrolyte balance. IV fluid does not provide nutrition for individuals, and it merely provides hydration, which is crucial for life. Chapter 10 includes a section on IV fluid administration, focusing on the medicine administration aspects.

Box 5.51 Children and young people practice points: nasogastric tube insertion

Nasogastric tube insertion is invasive and traumatic for children and parents. As with adults, it is essential to check that the nasogastric tube position is correct prior to administering medication or feeds; see NPSA's publications (2011a); Reducing the harm caused by misplaced nasogastric feeding tubes in adults, children and infants. Available from: http://www.gbukenteral.com/pdf/NPSA-Alert-2011.pdf

For details on nasogastric tube insertion and feeding, see:

Howe, R., Forbes, D. and Baker, C. 2010. Providing optimum nutrition and hydration. In: Glasper, A., Aylott, M. and Battrick, C. (eds.) *Developing Practical Skills for Nursing Children and Young People.* London: Hodder Arnold, 203–9.

Brind, J. 2012. Nutrition and feeding. In: Macqueen, S., Bruce, E.A. and Gibson, F. (eds.) *The Great Ormond Street Hospital Manual of Children's Nursing Practices.* Chichester: Wiley-Blackwell, 488–91.

Summary

- Enteral feeding is required when nutritional needs cannot be sufficiently met through the oral route.
- NGT insertion and gastrostomy insertion are invasive procedures with potential complications. There must be good rationale for their instigation.
- NGT insertion must be carried out carefully and skilfully, and practitioners must follow national guidance about confirming gastric tube position prior to any fluid administration, and checks thereafter. Insertion can be a difficult procedure for people to tolerate, and they need psychological support.
- Medicine administration via the enteral route must be carried out safely and in liaison with the pharmacist.
- If enteral feeding is not possible, parenteral feeding can provide nutrition. Intravenous fluid administration can maintain hydration and electrolyte balance.

CHAPTER SUMMARY

This chapter has highlighted throughout the importance of nutrition and hydration for the maintenance of health. Healthcare workers are in an excellent position to screen people for nutritional risk as part of their assessment and should work collaboratively with other healthcare professionals to identify and implement strategies to meet the differing nutritional needs of individuals. Nutrition and hydration should be considered at all times when caring for a person as adequate nutrition and hydration can improve well-being, thus improving outcomes. This chapter has included general principles that apply across a range of ages and settings. However, nutrition is a vast subject; you are encouraged to undertake further reading to enhance your knowledge and skills.

FURTHER READING RECOMMENDATIONS REGARDING INDIVIDUAL CHOICES IN LATER LIFE

To further advance your understanding of fluid and nutritional needs and how you make an impact on care, (National Nurses Nutrition Group, 2016www.nnng.org.uk) who offer an online forum to review good practice guidelines, also educational resources, conferences and online study courses.

BAPEN www.bapen.org.uk, continue to offer the BAPEN Principles of Good Practice to draw together existing guidelines and evidence-based information and review best practices as a continuous process. They offer decision trees to enable practitioners to review this ever-changing field of practice.

Recommended summary plan for emergency care and treatment (ReSPECT).

ReSPECT is a process that creates personalised recommendations for a person's clinical care in a future emergency in which they are unable to make or express choices. Includes preferences for care and Do Not Attempt Cardio Pulmonary

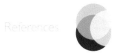

Resuscitation (DNACPR) from pre-hospital and hospital care, it enables the person to think ahead with individuals about realistic care options using a person-centred approach, see Resuscitation Council (UK) (2019) at www.resus.org.uk and www.respectprocess.org.uk

www.mariecurie.org.uk include guidance regarding hydration and nutrition when changes in eating and drinking occur, support for significant others and carers, how to approach people who have difficulty in swallowing, what to consider in the last few days of life, supported nutrition and fluids in end-of-life care and further resources for education.

www.pinnt.com enteral and parenteral tube feeding advice, people who are receiving intravenous and nasogastric treatment support, is available via my TUBE, http://mymnd.org.uk/ offer public support and guidance for placement of tubes, fitting, living with and caring for someone with a feeding tube.

For information on clinically assisted nutrition and hydration (CANH), www.bma.org.uk offer new guidance regarding decisions to start, restart, continue or stop nutritional and hydration support. CANH can be useful for adults who lack capacity to make decisions for themselves. CANH offer a decision-making tree to ensure that clinical practitioners consider lifestyle factors when assisting individuals to make choices about tube feeding, PEG, or parenteral nutrition.

REFERENCES

Age Concern. 2006. *Hungry to Be Heard: The Scandal of Malnourished Older People in Hospital.* London: Age Concern.

Age UK. 2017. *Still Hungry to Be Heard: The Scandal of People in Later Life Becoming Malnourished in Hospital.* London: Age UK

Age UK. 2020. Healthy eating –health and wellbeing. Available from: www.age.uk.org.uk (Accessed on 10 February 2021).

Alzheimer's Society. 2020. This Is Me Leaflet. Available from: http://www.alzheimers.org.uk/site/scripts/documents_info.php?documentID=1290 (Accessed on 10 February 2021).

Aneurin Bevan Health Board. 2013. *Guidelines for the Treatment of Under Nutrition in the Community Including Advice on Oral Nutritional Supplement (SIP Feed) Prescribing.* Available from: http://www.wales.nhs.uk/sites3/Documents/814/TreatmentOfMalnutrition%5BCommunity%5D-ABHBguidelinesJune2013.pdf. (Accessed on 10 February 2021).

Antwi-Ahima, L. 2020. An easy way to ensure good health. Available from: www.stmarys-treatmentcentre.nhs.uk. (Accessed on 10 February 2021).

Association of Dietician. 2018. Malnutrition – Food Fact Sheet. Available from: www.bda.uk.com (Accessed on 20 April 2020).

British Association for Parenteral and Enteral Nutrition (BAPEN). 2016 *Artificial Nutrition Support in the UK 2005–2015 Adult Home Parenteral Nutrition and Home Intravenous Fluids.* Available from: www.bapen.org.uk (Accessed on 10 February 2021).

British Association for Parenteral and Enteral Nutrition (BAPEN). 2018 *Drug Administration via Enteral Feeding Tubes: A Guide for General Practitioners and Community Pharmacists.* BAPEN. Available from: http://www.baben.org.uk (Accessed on 10 February 2021).

British Association of Parenteral and Enteral Nutrition (BAPEN). 2020. Malnutrition Universal Screening Tool (MUST). Available from: www.bapen.org.uk (Accessed on 10 February 2021).

British Association of Parenteral and Enteral Nutrition (BAPEN).2020. Principles of good nutritional practice – decision trees. Available from: www.bapen.org.uk (Accessed on 10 February 2021).

British Dieticians Association (BDA). 2020. Nutritional recovery and rehabilitation after critical illness. Available from: https://www.bda.uk.com/resource/critical-care-dietetics-guidance-covid-19.html (Accessed on 10 February 2021).

British Medical Association. 2020. Clinically assisted nutrition and hydration and the decision – making process. Available from: www.bma.org.uk (Accessed on 10 February 2021).

Campbell, N. 2014. Recognising and preventing dehydration amongst patients *Nursing Times* 110(46): 20–1.

Care Quality Commission (CQC). 2017. Regulation 14: Meeting nutritional and hydration needs – Available from: www.app.croneri.co.uk (Accessed on 10 February 2021).

Carers UK. 2020. *Carers and nutrition.* Available from: http://www.carersuk.org/help-and-advice/care-with-nutrition (Accessed on 16 April 2020).

Department of Health (DH). 1990. Food Safety Act, DH. Available from: www.legislation.gov.uk (Accessed on 10 February 2021).

Department of Health (DH). 2008. *Weaning: Starting Solid Food.* London: DH. Available from: www.legislation.gov.uk (Accessed on 10 February 2021).

Great Britain. 2005. Mental Capacity Act 2005. Available from: https://www.legislation.gov.uk/ukpa/2005/9/pdfs/ukpa_20050009_en.pdf (Accessed on 1 March 2021).

Hollis, S. 2011. Using red jugs to improve hydration. *Nursing Times* 107(28): 21.

Malhi, H. 2018 Assessing and managing malnutrition in adults in hospital. Nursing Standard doi: 10.7748.2018e11180

Malnutrition Advisory Group (MAG). 2017. *Malnutrition Universal Screening Tool.* Available from: http://www.bapen.org.uk/pdfs/must/must_full.pdf (Accessed on 10 February 2021).

Malnutrition Advisory Group (MAG). 2003. A consistent and reliable tool for malnutrition screening. *Nursing Times* 99 (46): 26–27.

Malnutrition Pathway. 2017. Managing Adult Malnutrition. Available from; www.malnutritionpathway.co.uk (Accessed on 10 February 2021).

Martindale, R., Patel, J., Taylor, B. et al. 2020. Nutrition therapy in the patient with COVID-19 disease requiring ICU care American Society for Parentral and Enteral Nutrition Society of Critical Care Medicine. Available from: https://www.sccm.org/getattachmnet/Disatster/Nutrition-TherpayCOVID-19-SCCM-ASPEN.pdf?lang=en=US (Accessed on 10 February 2021).

McIntyre, L., Munir, F. and Walker, S. 2012. Intelligent fluid management bundle to support practitioners to ensure patient get adequate hydration. *Nursing Times* 108(28): 18–20.

Murphy, J., Holmes, J. and Brooks, C. 2017. Nutrition and dementia care: Developing an evidence based model for nutritional care in nursing homes BMC Geriatric 17:55. Available from: www.ncbi.nlm.nih.gov (Accessed on 10 February 2021).

Najafi, M. 2021. *Improving the Safety of Nasogastric Tube Insertion by the SORT Maneuver during the Novel Coronavirus Pandemic (COVID 19). Patient Safety in Surgery 15 no 4.*

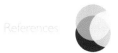

National Health Service England. 2015. Guidance – Commissioning excellent nutrition and hydration 2015–2018 Available from: www.england.nhs.uk. (Accessed on 9 February 2021).

National Institute for Health and Care Excellence (NICE). 2018. NICE CG 32 Refeeding Guidelines: Retrospective audit dietetic and medical practice of vitamin prescriptions, blood checks and K+. PO43 and Mg 2+ replacement including discharge medications. Available from: www.evidence..nhs.uk (Accessed on 10 February 2021).

National Institute for Health and Clinical Excellence (NICE). 2018. Eating Disorders Quality standard (QS 175) – Core *Investigations in Treatment and Management of Anorexia Nervosa, Bulimia Nervosa and Related Eating Disorders.* Clinical Guidelines 9. Available from: www.nice.org.uk (Accessed on 10 February 2021).

National Institute for Health and Clinical Excellence (NICE). 2017. Nutrition support for adults: Oral nutrition support, enteral tube feeding and parenteral nutrition. CG 32. Available from: www.nice.org.uk.uk (Accessed on 10 February 2021).

National Nutritional Nurses' Group. 2016. *Good Practice Guideline Safe Insertion and Ongoing Care of Nasogastric (NG) Feeding Tubes in Adults.* Available from: https:// nutrition2me.com/wp-content/uploads/2012/05/www.nnng_.org_.uk_wp-content_ uploads_2017_04_Nasal-Retention-Device-Good-Practice-Guidance (Accessed on 11 February 2021).

National Patient Safety Agency (NPSA) 2007. Promoting safer measurement and administration of liquid medicines via oral and other enteral routes. Available from: http:// www.nrls.npsa.nhs.uk/resources/?entryid45 = 59808 (Accessed on 10 February 2021).

National Patient Safety Agency (NPSA) 2016 Naso gastric tube misplacement: Continuing risk of death and severe harm www.improvement.nhs.uk/resources/patient-safety-alerts. Available from: www.improvment.nhs.uk (Accessed on 9 February 2021).

National Patient Safety Agency (NPSA). 2011a. Patient Safety Alert NPSA/2011/PSA002: Reducing the harm caused by misplaced nasogastric feeding tubes in adults, children and infants: Supporting information. Available from: http://www.nrls.npsa.nhs.uk/reso urces/?entryid45=129640&q=0%c2%acnasogastric+tube%c2%ac (Accessed on 10 February 2021).

National Patient Safety Agency (NPSA). 2011b. Nasogastric feeding tubes – decision tree Adults. Available from: http://www.nrls.npsa.nhs.uk/resources/?entryid45=129640&q =0%c2%acnasogastric+tube%c2%ac (Accessed on 10 February 2021).

National Patient Safety Agency (NPSA). 2016. Naso gastric tube misplacement: Continuing risk of death and severe harm, 22 July 2016. Available from: https://www.england. nhs.uk/2016/07/nasogastric-tube-misplacement-continuing-risk-of-death-severe-harm/ (Accessed on 1 November 2021).

National Patient Safety Agency (NPSA). 2018. Patient safety alert: Reducing the harm caused by misplaced nasogastric feeding tubes. Available from: http://www.nrls.npsa. nhs.uk/resources/?EntryId45=59794 (Accessed on 10 February 2021).

National Patient Safety Agency (NPSA). 2018. *The Never Events Policy and Framework.* London: DH.

NHS Choices. 2020. Signs of dehydration. Available from: http://www.nhs.uk/Conditions/dehydration/Pages/Introduction.aspx (Accessed on 16 April 2020).

NHS improvements. 2020. Nutrition and hydration. Available from www.improvments. nhs.uk (Accessed on 10 February 2021).

Nursing and Midwifery Council (NMC). 2018a. *Standards for Pre-registration Nursing Programmes*. Available from; www.nmc.org.uk (Accessed on 10 February 2021).

Nursing and Midwifery Council (NMC). 2018b. *Standards for Pre-registration Nursing Associate Programmes*. Available from: www.nmc.org.uk (Accessed on 10 February 2021).

Onder, A., Kapan, M. and Bilsel, B. 2012. Percutaneous endoscopic gastrostomy: Mortality and risk factors for survival. *Gastroenterology* Feb. 5(1): 21–27.

Public Health England. 2021. Independent high risk AGP panel summary of recommendations arising from evidence reviews to date. Available from: www.gov.uk (Accessed on 10 February 2021).

Resuscitation Council (UK). 2019. A quantitative and qualitative evaluation of the ReSPECT (Recommended Summary Plan for Emergency Care and Treatment Process in Forth Valley Scotland's first ReSPECT pilot: A case for change. April 2019. Available from: www.resus.org.uk (Accessed on 10 February 2021).

Roland J. 2019. What is the average (and ideal) percentage of water in your body? Available from: www.healthline.com (Accessed on 10 February 2021).

Royal College of Nursing (RCN) 2021. Nutrition essentials. Available from: https://www.rcn.org.uk/clinical-topics/nutrition-and-hydration/nutrition-essentials (Accessed on 26 October 2021).

Royal College of Nursing (RCN) 2020. Nutrition essentials Available from: https://www.rcn.org.uk/clinical-topics/nutrition-and-hydration/cpd/nutrition-for-vulnerable-groups (Accessed on 10 February 2021).

Royal College of Nursing (RCN). 2012. *Supporting and Assisting People*. Available from: http://www.rcn.org.uk/development/practice/cpd_online_learning/supporting_peoples_nutritional_needs/supporting_and_assisting_people (Accessed on 10 February 2021).

Royal College of Psychiatrists (RCP). 2012. *Eating Disorder Guidelines*. Available from: www. rcpsych.ac.uk (Accessed on 10 February 2021).

Sanaie, S., Mirzalou, N., Shadvar, K. et al. 2020. A comparison of naso gastric tube insertion by SORT 9 sniffing position, NGT orientation, contralateral rotation and twisting movement) versus neck flexion lateral pressure in critically ill patients admitted in critically ill patients admitted to ICU: A prospective randomized clinical trial *Annals of Intensive Care* 10, article 79.

Scanlon, V.C. and Sanders, T. 2018. *Essentials of Anatomy and Physiology*, 8th edn. Philadelphia: F.A. Davis Co.

Smith, A., Santa Ana, C., Fordtran, J. and Guileyardo, J. 2018. Deaths associated with insertion of naso gastric tubes for enteral nutrition in the medical intensive care unit: clinical and autopsy findings www.doi.org/10.1080/08998280 (Accessed on 10 February 2021).

Sprake, E., Russell, J., Cecil, J. et al. 2018. Dietary patterns of university students in the UK: A cross sectional study *Nutrition Journal* 17: 90.

Stratton, R., Smith, T. and Gabe, S. 2018. Managing malnutrition to improve lives and save money. Available from: www.bapen.org.uk (Accessed on 10 February 2021).

Stroke Association. 2012. Taste changes after stroke, Factsheet 39. Available from: http://www.stroke.org.uk (Accessed on 10 February 2021).

Stroke Association. 2020. Healthy eating and stroke. Available from: https://www.stroke.org.uk/resources/healthy-eating-and-stroke (Accessed on 26 October 2021).

Todorovic, V., Russell, C., Stratton, R., et al. 2003. *The MUST Explanatory Booklet*. Redditch: BAPEN.

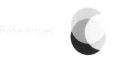

Wanten, G. 2011. Managing adult patients who need home parenteral nutrition. *British Medical Journal* 34: d1447.

Willis, L. 2015. *Fluids and Electrolytes Made Incredibly Easy*, 6th edn. London: Lippincott Williams and Wilkins.

World Health Organization. 2019. Integrated care for older people (ICOPE) guidance for person centred assessment and pathways in primary care. Available from: www.who.int (Accessed on 10 February 2021).

Meeting personal needs: elimination

Rachel Busuttil Leaver

INTRODUCTION

Elimination of urine and faeces is an essential bodily function that we usually become independent in within the first few years of life, continence being an important milestone in a child's development (Slater-Smith 2010). Elimination is then usually a private function, but disability or physical or mental health problems often affect independence in elimination, and nurses then play an important role in preventing problems and maintaining comfort. Wherever possible, the aim will be to return to independent elimination, although some people will need ongoing support with elimination, particularly where long-term, progressive conditions affect elimination. Promoting dignity and privacy is integral to meeting people's elimination needs; it requires great skill and sensitivity to carry out this care while preserving the individuals' self-esteem. Many other chapters in this book are relevant to care related to elimination, particularly Chapter 2, which focuses on communication, and Chapter 12, which focuses on preventing cross-infection. The Department of Health's (DH 2010) *Essence of Care Benchmarks* includes benchmarks for 'bladder, bowel and continence care', which are recommended as a resource.

This chapter includes the following topics:

- Assisting with elimination: Helping people use the toilet, bedpans, urinals and commodes
- Urinalysis
- Collecting urine and stool specimens
- Caring for people who have urinary catheters
- Preventing and managing constipation
- Stoma care
- Promoting continence and managing incontinence.

DOI: 10.4324/9781003020660-6

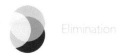

Table 6.1: Recommended biology reading

The following questions will help you to focus on the biology underpinning this chapter's skills. Use your recommended textbook to find out:

- What are the components of the urinary system?
- Within the kidney, blood is filtered. What forces are involved in filtration?
- Where does filtration occur? Which substances are not filtered out and why?
- What is the role of the juxtaglomerular apparatus?
- What happens to the glomerular filtrate as it passes along the nephron?
- How and why does the concentration of urine vary?
- What factors affect renal function?
- Urine is stored in the bladder. How does the bladder expand as it fills up?
- What is micturition and how does it occur?
- What is cystitis? Why is it generally more common in females than in males?
- How can urinalysis be used to assess health?
- What factors can increase the risk of UTI?
- What are the signs of UTI?
- What are the different regions of the digestive tract and their functions?
- How does food move through the digestive tract?
- How are peristalsis and segmentation distinguished?
- What is the consequence of increased gut motility? When might this occur?
- What is the gastro colic reflex?
- What do stools/faeces consist of?
- How do we defaecate?
- What is constipation?
- What factors increase the risk of constipation?
- How does the digestive tract respond to local infection or irritation?
- How does stress affect the digestive tract?

PRACTICE SCENARIOS

The following scenarios illustrate situations where assistance with elimination is needed, and this chapter will refer to these scenarios throughout.

Adult

Jean is a 68-year-old woman who was diagnosed with cancer in the large bowel. Jean has **rheumatoid arthritis** and she has difficulty mobilising. She uses a motorised wheelchair and is cared for by her husband who is 75 years. He is well but has problems with his sight as he has cataracts. They live in a ground-floor council flat that has been adapted to enable her to be as independent as possible. Jean is able to transfer unaided. Jean has been admitted for surgery to have the tumour removed and a **stoma** formed. She is distressed that she has cancer and is concerned about undergoing surgery. She is worried that she will not cope afterwards and does not want to be 'more of a burden' on her husband.

The stoma care specialist spends time with Jean to reassure her and answer her questions. The nurse also marks the site on Jean's abdomen for stoma placement. Jean has a total large bowel resection with formation of an **ileostomy**. On return to the ward, Jean has a stoma bag over the newly formed stoma and a urinary catheter in her bladder. The discomfort from the abdominal wound means that Jean has trouble moving and is incapable of transferring herself independently. Due to her lack of mobility, it is decided that the catheter should be left in the bladder until she regains the ability to transfer to the toilet. She develops a urinary tract infection (UTI), which is treated with antibiotics.

Once she has recovered from surgery, Jean and her husband start to learn how to care for her stoma. She will not be discharged until she is able to do this, but she is finding it difficult to get used to the change and her progress is slow.

Learning disability

Mark is 28 years old and has a syndrome that includes a learning disability, impaired renal function and deteriorating sight. He eats with some assistance and walks short distances. He has very limited verbal communication, and he also has frequent UTIs and bowel disturbances – both constipation and diarrhoea. He is cared for by his mother, who manages his physical health needs. Mark is usually continent but requires prompting and support, due to his visual impairment. When he is ill or in new surroundings, he can become incontinent of both urine and faeces and wears continence pads at these times. His mother, who is Mark's **health facilitator**, has contacted the community learning disability nurse (CLDN) as she has noticed blood in his urine, which he is infrequently passing even though she is encouraging fluids. Mark is also not eating, has a raised temperature and his mother believes he is in pain. The nurse arranges to take samples of both urine and faeces, liaises with the general practitioner (GP) and renal consultant, who decide to admit Mark to hospital for further investigations. Mark's mother completes a 'hospital passport' (provided by the local hospital on their website) with him, which includes essential information to help hospital staff care for him.

Mental health

Bob is 58 years old. He has a long history of psychosis. During an acute psychotic episode, while admitted to an acute psychiatric ward, he was prescribed an atypical antipsychotic drug, clozapine, which is licensed for treatment of resistant schizophrenia only, due to its known side effects. These include effects on white blood cell levels, causing vulnerability to infection. After 6 weeks, there was a marked improvement in Bob's mental state, but he developed urinary incontinence at night (nocturnal enuresis). He found this extremely embarrassing and distressing, never having been incontinent before. Unfortunately, urinary incontinence is known to be another side effect of clozapine, the exact reasons for which are unknown. A urinalysis performed on admission had shown no abnormalities.

ASSISTING WITH ELIMINATION: HELPING PEOPLE USE THE TOILET: BEDPANS, URINALS AND COMMODES

Box 6.1 Learning outcomes

By the end of this section, you will be able to:

1. identify why a person might need help with elimination and what equipment you could use to give assistance;
2. discuss important principles for assisting with elimination.

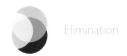

Learning outcome 1: identify why a person might need help with elimination and what equipment you could use to give assistance

Box 6.2 Activity: help with elimination

Reflect back on your practice experiences and write down all the reasons as to why a person might need help with elimination.

There are many situations where a person might need help with elimination. A person's assessment should include elimination issues and assistance needed. For example, someone who is temporarily confined to bed following orthopaedic surgery, or people who are very weak or confused need help with elimination. Mark will need assistance as the hospital is an unfamiliar environment and he has impaired eyesight.

Whenever possible, a person should be helped to reach the toilet and so sufficient and accessible toilets should be available. The toilet is a more familiar environment for elimination (helpful for people with dementia, or who are disorientated or, like Mark, have a learning disability). The toilet is also more private; to eliminate in a ward, behind closed curtains, may not feel very private as noise and smell may be obvious. This potential embarrassment can lead to individuals ignoring the need to defaecate, leading to constipation. You might need to accompany the person, sometimes with sticks, a walking frame or crutches (see Chapter 11, section on 'assisting with mobilisation and preventing falls'). If a person is unable to walk, you could take them to the toilet in a wheelchair.

If the person cannot leave the bedside, you can use equipment to help them.

Box 6.3 Activity: equipment to assist with elimination

What equipment could assist with elimination? There may be examples of equipment in the skills laboratory or within your practice setting.

The commode

If someone is very ill or weak, or has a great deal of invasive equipment attached to them, it may be safer to eliminate by the bedside. When making these decisions, check their care plan and seek advice if you are unsure. If a person can get out of bed, a commode is preferable to a bedpan, as it promotes a more conducive, comfortable position for elimination. A commode has a pan underneath, which is removed after use and either macerated (if disposable) or cleaned in the washer–disinfector, if reusable.

Bedpans/urinals

Some people must stay in bed for medical reasons, so they require bedpans or urinals. There are standard bedpans, which the person sits up on, and flat 'slipper' pans, which the person rolls on to – suitable when someone has to remain flat. There are both male and female urinals. Men sometimes find it difficult to urinate in seated or lying positions, so they may need assistance to stand, if their medical condition allows. Female urinals are useful for women lying flat (e.g. following back surgery) or where changing position is difficult, perhaps due to pain.

Box 6.4 Activity: principles of care when assisting with elimination

ACTIVITY

If you are assisting someone with elimination, what do you think would be important principles of care?

Learning outcome 2: discuss important principles for assisting with elimination

Box 6.5 lists the principles that you could have identified; these are discussed next.

Approachability and communication

People needing help with elimination often describe this as embarrassing and even distressing. The author has known people who admit to reducing their fluid intake, thus increasing their risk of complications such as a UTI, so that they need not ask for help so often. Some people have urinary symptoms such as frequency and others have urgency – where they cannot 'hold on' for very long. Elstad et al. (2010) identified a stigma associated with urgency and frequency with people experiencing embarrassment and shame, and Wareing (2005) found that men who experienced severe urgency described how 'having to hold on' was accompanied by panic and embarrassment. If a nurse does not appear approachable, then people may not feel comfortable asking for help and may experience emotional and physical discomfort, incontinence, retention of urine or constipation.

If people have communication difficulties, nurses must observe for non-verbal cues (e.g. restlessness or agitation). Sometimes a picture board (with a picture of a toilet) can be used to help communicate. Considering the scenario, Mark's hospital passport should include information about how Mark communicates that he needs to go to the toilet, which may be through a signing system, including gestures as often people will use their own personalised signs or indications of need. If the nurses ask Mark whether he needs to go to the toilet, they should give him enough time to answer, as processing information may take longer for people with learning

Frequency

Passing urine more frequently than about 7 times in 24 hours. A common symptom arising from conditions such as enlarged prostate and UTI.

Box 6.5 Principles to follow when assisting with elimination

- Approachability and communication
- Privacy and dignity
- Promptness
- Prevention of cross-infection
- Observation
- Prevention of accidents
- Promotion of independence
- Promotion of hygiene and comfort

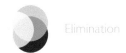

disabilities. While assisting individuals with elimination, nurses can build their relationship through conversation, which should help put the person at ease. Nurses should speak privately and quietly when assisting with elimination; using non-verbal communication may reduce the verbal communication needed, with less risk of others overhearing.

Privacy and dignity

If privacy and dignity are not addressed, people may feel embarrassed, degraded and experience a loss of self-esteem. Always ensure that bedside curtains are pulled, shut properly, or the toilet door closed, and that the individual is covered up while on the bedpan or commode. The British Geriatrics Society's (BGS) (2006) campaign to ensure that vulnerable people can use the toilet in private in hospitals and care homes has produced a best practice toolkit. The standards addressed accessibility, timeliness, equipment, safety, choice, privacy, cleanliness, hygiene and respectful language. The importance of treating the person with dignity when using the toilet is also emphasised in their guidelines. Nurses should be person-centred and approach each person as an individual, being sensitive and aware of the effect of cultural norms and religious beliefs (Heath 2009). For example, some people may prefer a nurse of the same sex to help them, and modesty within South Asian cultures is particularly important (Holland and Hogg 2010).

Promptness

People with certain types of incontinence (urge incontinence) will not be able to wait to pass urine (see the 'Promoting continence and managing incontinence' section). Resnick et al. (2006) found that care home staff contributed to residents' incontinence by not attending to them quickly enough. Clearly, such a situation is unacceptable as incontinence is distressing for people. If the individual cannot attempt to open their bowels when they feel the need, faeces are pushed back into the sigmoid colon or remain in the rectum, where water continues to be reabsorbed. Thus, faeces become harder, more painful and difficult to pass, which may lead to constipation. Nurses should prioritise meeting elimination needs as individuals are in a powerless position, dependent for help with this basic need. When the person has finished eliminating, nurses should respond promptly, to avoid discomfort and maintain safety. The individual should be given their call bell and shown how to use it.

Prevention of cross-infection

People in hospital are often particularly vulnerable to infection owing to their medical conditions (see Chapter 12 for more information), so measures to prevent cross-infection must be scrupulously applied. These include careful hand washing and application of personal protective equipment – non-sterile gloves and aprons – to prevent hands and uniform being contaminated (Pratt et al. 2007). Hands must be decontaminated after glove removal (National Institute for Health and Clinical Excellence [NICE] 2017). Equipment used to assist with elimination must be cleaned effectively. Disposable bedpans and urinals are disposed of in macerators. Non-disposable urinals and bedpans should be disinfected by thermal disinfection (exposure to hot water or steam), and supports for disposable bedpans should be washed after use, with a chlorine-releasing agent, if contaminated with faeces (Fraise and Bradley 2009). The seat and frame of commodes should be cleaned after use with particular attention to the arms, and if the seat is soiled, or used by an individual with an enteric infection, it should be disinfected with a chlorine-releasing agent, rinsed and dried (Fraise and Bradley 2009). However, Bucior and Cochrane (2010) found that commodes were not always cleaned adequately.

Urine was thought to be normally sterile but more recent studies now show that urine may actually harbour bacteria that are necessary to maintain normal urine homeostasis (Akerman and Chai 2019). It is also often contaminated while voiding, by bacteria present around the urethral opening (Gould 1994). Urine provides an excellent medium for bacterial growth, especially Gram-negative bacteria (*Pseudomonas*, *Klebsiella*, *Escherichia coli*, *Proteus*), which can survive only when water and inorganic ions are present (Gould 1994). Urine passed into a bedpan or urinal should therefore be disposed of quickly, as standing at room temperature allows any bacteria present to divide rapidly, doubling approximately every 30 min (Gould 1994), thus becoming a reservoir of infection.

When someone has diarrhoea that could be infective, cross-infection measures needed are prompt and careful disposal of the faeces, use of non-sterile gloves and aprons, scrupulous hand washing and source isolation (see Chapter 12). When caring for people with diarrhoea caused by *Clostridium difficile*, alcohol hand rub is ineffective against the spores produced, so wearing non-sterile gloves, with hand washing following glove removal, is essential.

Observation

There are many useful observations you can make when assisting with elimination, such as assessing the person's ability to move, or about the condition of their skin (see Table 6.2). If the person's urine output is measured, the jug used must be disposed of or cleaned in the bedpan washer, and a fluid chart will be used to record fluid balance. Chapter 5 provides a detailed description of fluid balance measurement. The Bristol stool chart can be used to record stool type (see Figure 6.1).

Box 6.6 Activity: monitoring input and output

When next in placement, look at any charts used for monitoring urine output and stools. What are the types of fluids listed for input and output? Does the stool chart incorporate the Bristol stool chart, as shown in Figure 6.1?

Prevention of accidents

Highlighting the hazardous nature of elimination, Thompson's (2007) falls and continence audit found that 36.8% of falls were related to toileting or incontinence. A moving and handling risk assessment should be carried out (see Chapter 11 for more

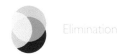

Type 1		Separate hard lumps, like nuts (hard to pass)
Type 2		Sausage-shaped but lumpy
Type 3		Like a sausage but with cracks on its surface
Type 4		Like a sausage or snake, smooth and soft
Type 5		Soft blobs with clear-cut edges (passed easily)
Type 6		Fluffy pieces with ragged edges, a mushy stool
Type 7		Watery, no solid pieces, entirely liquid

Figure 6.1: Bristol stool chart. [Reproduced with kind permission from Taylor & Francis Ltd. (www.tandf.co.uk/journals). From Lewis, S.J. and Heaton, K.W. 1997. Stool form scale as a useful guide to intestinal track time. Scandinavian Journal of Gastroenterology, 32, 920–4.]

information), and the moving and handling care plan should specify the equipment needed and the number of staff required. If a person is using a bedpan in bed, you must ensure that they do not topple over. Balancing on a bedpan can be difficult, so it may be safer to raise the bed or trolley rails for support. The National Patient Safety Agency (NPSA 2007) recommended that organisations should have a policy about bedrail use – a risk assessment form may be required as they can be hazardous. You must be sure about your reasons for using them (i.e. not using them as a form of restraint).

Table 6.2: Observations to make when assisting with elimination

Observation	explanation/examples
Emotional well-being	The person's mood and ability to cope with a situation.
Cognitive functioning	The person's memory of what to do, ability to retain information and follow instructions.
Mobility	The individual's ability to move on to a bedpan, to transfer on to a commode or toilet or stand to use a urinal.
	Whether any apparent discomfort/pain, breathlessness or weakness when moving.
Skin condition	Redness or broken areas on sacrum or buttocks; soreness of groins, perineum, penis or vulva.
Self-care ability	Physical/mental ability to remove or adapt clothing, before and after elimination, and to carry out hygiene afterwards.
Amount and frequency of urine output	A fluid input/output chart may be maintained if there are concerns about fluid balance.
	Urine will be measured in a jug and recorded in millilitres. Pads can be weighed: 1 g = 1 mL.
	Poor urine output (oliguria) could occur in dehydration or shock.
	No urinary output (anuria) could mean retention of urine.
	Frequent small amounts of urine might indicate a UTI.
	Monitoring of frequency and amount may be part of a bladder re-education programme.
Appearance of urine	See urinalysis, the next section.
	Very dark, concentrated urine might indicate dehydration, and smoky, offensive urine might indicate UTI.
	Presence of blood may be due to kidney trauma or disease.
Appearance of stools	Consistency and frequency of stools; hard and infrequent stools could indicate constipation, or frequent and loose stools could indicate diarrhoea, which could be infected.
	A stool chart to record frequency, appearance and consistency might be maintained: the Bristol stool chart is often used so that descriptions of stools are reliable (see Fig. 6.1).
	If infection is suspected, a stool specimen will be collected and sent.

Using the commode by the bedside is potentially hazardous. You should ensure that brakes are secure and that there are no fluids or slippery substances on the floor. You must assess whether the person is safe to leave: are they confused and likely to try to stand up alone and fall? Privacy is a very important principle when assisting people with elimination but has to be balanced against safety. A falls risk-assessment scale can help identify people who are at risk of falls (see Chapter 11).

PROMOTION OF INDEPENDENCE

Stroke

Stroke is cerebral damage caused either by decreased blood flow or by haemorrhage. Effects vary, but a stroke often causes paralysis down one side of the body (hemiplegia), speech and swallowing difficulty, and elimination difficulties.

While assisting with elimination, you should assess ability and promote independence while also maintaining hygiene and safety. Learning how to use the toilet unaided,

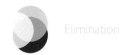

after a **stroke**, for example, may take some time, and both short- and long-term goals may be necessary (Kawanabe et al. 2018). The study by Clark and Rugg (2005) highlighted the importance of gaining independence in using the toilet for people following stroke to prevent decreased self-esteem. Nurses can liaise with occupational therapists to facilitate a return to a person's normal methods and if that is not possible, they can advise on how to assist the individual to adjust. Education could include teaching people how to manage transfers safely (e.g. from wheelchair to toilet), how to remove clothing or how to walk to the toilet on crutches.

To promote independence for people with learning disabilities, orientate them to their environment well, showing them where the toilet is and take them to the same toilet by the same route each time. These steps could also be helpful for people who have dementia. Ideally, Mark's bed would be situated near the toilet. The ward nurses could show Mark where the toilet is and how the facilities work. For example, Mark may be used to a toilet with a pull handle and separate taps, while the ward might have a toilet with a button to press for flushing and a mixer tap. Mark's mother will know the best way of explaining this to him. Time and repetition may be needed to explain and demonstrate how the toilet and sink work. Consistency in approach is important, and a regular prompt to go to the toilet, with appropriate support, may be needed to promote continence. The additional time required could be seen as a 'reasonable adjustment' (Equality Act 2010) that is required to enable people access appropriate care. Someone with a severe learning disability would not necessarily have an anatomical cause for their incontinence, although this must be considered. Their ability to control their bladder and bowels may take longer to develop and the challenges of their underlying disability and any co-morbidities means they may need specialist continence support to help them become continent (NICE 2019b).

A toilet door that has a different texture and colour to the wall, with an embossed picture of a toilet on, will help people with visual impairments and those with dementia.

PROMOTION OF HYGIENE AND COMFORT

For people whose elimination needs are met by their bedside, you must assist with hygiene. Within some cultures, which emphasise cleanliness, people are required to cleanse the perineal area with running water after using the toilet (Heath 2009). When you take people to the toilet, ensure that they can wash their hands at the sink afterwards. Always ensure access to toilet tissue, and if people cannot wipe themselves, then do it for them, or give assistance to people who are learning or relearning this skill. With females, always wipe the vulval area from front to back to prevent transmission of bowel bacterial flora (such as *E. coli*) from the anal area to the urethra. Females have a short urethra (4 cm), which can easily become contaminated by such bacteria. In Asia, the left hand is traditionally reserved for washing underneath after using the toilet, the right hand being used for eating and other activities (Holland and Hogg 2010). Make sure that the individual does not become cold during

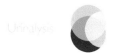

elimination, by covering their legs with a blanket. Ensure that anyone using a bedpan is comfortably supported with pillows. You will promote psychological comfort by your attitude and communication (see Chapter 2 for more information).

Box 6.7 Children and young people: practice points – nappy-changing

Infants and small children normally wear nappies until they are toilet-trained, usually by 3 years of age. Some children who have not yet reached successful toilet training or who have developmental delay may require nappies. Nappy-changing practice is described in detail in:

Himsworth, J. 2010. Caring for personal hygiene needs. In: Glasper, A., Aylott, M. and Battrick, C. (eds.) Developing Practical Skills for Nursing Children and Young People. London: Hodder Arnold, 188–202.

Macqueen, S., Bruce, E.A. and Gibson, F. 2012. Personal hygiene and pressure ulcer prevention. In: The Great Ormond Street Hospital Manual of Children's Nursing Practices. Chichester: Wiley-Blackwell, 167–220.

Summary

- Many health problems lead to people needing help with elimination.
- Various items of equipment are available to assist people who are unable to get to the toilet. Nurses must assess with which one is appropriate for each individual.
- There are important principles that must be followed when helping people with elimination to ensure that care is dignified, effective and safe.

URINALYSIS

Urinalysis is the testing of urine for the presence of various substances. This simple, non-intrusive test provides useful information about an individual's renal and urinary function (Beynon and Nicholls 2004).

You should be able to access urinalysis equipment either in the skills laboratory or in your practice setting.

ACTIVITY

Box 6.8 Learning outcomes

By the end of this section, you will be able to:

1. understand the process of urinalysis;
2. show insight into the meaning of urinalysis results and what action to take if abnormal results are obtained;
3. identify in what situations urinalysis should be performed.

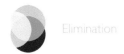

Learning outcome 1: understand the process of urinalysis

Box 6.9 Activity: reagent strips

Look at the reagent strips that are used to test urine in the skills laboratory or in a practice placement. Find the expiry date and note the substances that are tested for and the timings for reading the results on the side of the bottle.

Reagent strips must be in date, and stored and used properly, otherwise results may not be accurate. Public Health England (PHE) (2020) advises that the strips are used and stored as per the manufacturer's instructions to ensure accurate readings. The full range of substances that can be tested during a urinalysis are leucocytes, nitrite, urobilinogen, protein, pH, blood, specific gravity, ketones, bilirubin and glucose. The reagent strips that you looked at may include this full range, but there are also strips available that test for only a selection or even just one substance such as blood. It is worth noting that urine dip strips are less accurate in people over 65 years. This is because older age groups are more likely to have asymptomatic bacteria in their urine without infection, which will still show as positive. Treating with antibiotics is not needed in this group and may be harmful (PHE 2020).

Conducting a urinalysis

Figure 6.2 summarises key points for conducting a urinalysis, with some additional explanatory notes and rationale given below.

Urine for analysis should be collected in a clean, dry, preservative-free container, and infection control aspects should be adhered to throughout the procedure (PHE 2020). First-voided morning urine is best for a urinalysis as it is most concentrated. Ideally, the urine should be tested immediately or within 4 hours. Otherwise, you can refrigerate the specimen, but you must let it return to room temperature before testing. It is particularly important to use fresh urine when testing for bilirubin and urobilinogen as these compounds are relatively unstable when exposed to room temperature and light. When testing for nitrite, use a first morning sample if possible so that the urine will have been in contact with bacteria, if present, for at least 3 hours.

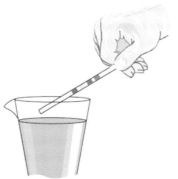

Requirements
- Reagent strip and bottle
- Freshly voided urine in a clean (preferably sterile) container

Procedure
- Observe urine for colour, consistency and smell
- Immerse all reagent areas in fresh urine and remove immediately
- Run the edge along the rim of the container to remove excess urine
- Hold the strip horizontally to prevent mixing of the chemicals from adjacent areas and prevent soiling of hands with urine
- Compare the test areas with the corresponding colour chart at the specified time or analyse in electronic reader following reader's instructions

Figure 6.2: Conducting a urinalysis: key points.

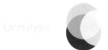

Jaundice

Jaundice is a condition characterised by the yellowness of skin, whites of eyes, mucous membranes and body fluids due to the presence of bile pigment resulting from excess bilirubin in the blood.

When testing urine, always observe the appearance of the urine sample first. Normal fresh urine is pale to dark yellow or amber in colour, and clear. If the urine is red or red–brown, this could be from consuming a food dye, beetroot or a drug and/or due to the presence of haemoglobin. If there are many red blood cells present, the urine will be cloudy as well. A strongly yellow sample could indicate jaundice.

The smell of the urine should also be noted; freshly voided, non-infected urine should be virtually odourless, but if infected, urine may smell offensive.

The strips must be read accurately as per the timings given on the bottle. Nurses on a busy ward may not wait the correct amount of time before reading the result, and lighting and colour vision may affect readings. If coloured charts are used for reading results, they must be stored away from direct sunlight to prevent fading, and the strip must be read at the correct time in good light. There are also electronic readers available, which can help to minimise reader error, leading to greater uniformity and consistency in readings. These readers also print the results, include the time and date, and indicate abnormal readings. Readers should be maintained and cleaned correctly and checked regularly; only strips validated for use with this device should be used.

Learning outcome 2: show insight into the meaning of urinalysis results and what action to take if abnormal results are obtained

If you look on the side of the urinary reagent bottle, you will find the key as to what each colour is testing for, the normal results, and abnormal results, which should be reported. Table 6.3 indicates the significance of abnormalities and suggests some possible actions. A nursing dictionary will help you with some of the technical terms included.

When to collect a urine specimen for microscopy and culture

A urinalysis can help in determining whether to send a urine specimen for microscopy, culture and sensitivity (MC&S). In this laboratory test, the urine is examined under the microscope, and the urine is cultured to see whether bacteria grow and what antibiotics the bacteria are sensitive to. The presence of nitrite in urine is particularly indicative of UTI as over 90% of urinary pathogens can reduce urinary nitrate to nitrite if they are in contact with urine in the bladder for a minimum of 3 hours (Panagamuwa et al. 2004). A positive test for leucocyte esterase (an enzyme within white blood cells) can also indicate infection.

The British Infection Association (BIA) and Health Protection Agency (HPA) (2011) provide a detailed and evidence-based flow chart for diagnosing UTI and when to send urine for culture. They recommend that with older people who have a positive urinalysis but are asymptomatic of a UTI, urine should not be sent for culture routinely, and that two or more UTI symptoms (especially dysuria, pyrexia over 38 degrees or new incontinence) should be present before sending off urine for culture.

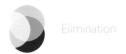

Table 6.3: Clinical significance of test results

Significance of positive results	Commonest causes of abnormalities and possible action to be taken
Glucose	
Not normally detectable in urine Found when its concentration exceeds the renal threshold	• In people with raised blood glucose concentration: diabetes mellitus or glucose infusion • In people without raised blood glucose concentration: pregnancy or renal glycosuria Action: If positive, a blood glucose measurement should be performed, and further action may follow
Bilirubin	
Presence in urine indicates an excess of conjugated bilirubin in plasma Note that stale urine may give a false-negative result	• Liver cell injury: e.g. viral or drug-induced hepatitis, paracetamol overdose, late-stage cirrhosis • Biliary tract obstruction: e.g. by gall stones, carcinoma of the head of pancreas Action: Should always be reported as further investigations will be needed
Ketones	
Indicates accumulation of acetoacetate secondary to excessive breakdown of body fat Some drugs (e.g. L-dopa) may give a false-positive result	• Fasting, particularly with fever and/or vomiting • Diabetic ketoacidosis Action: Urgent action is needed if the person is known or suspected to have diabetes
Specific gravity	
A measure of total solute concentration in urine In health, varies widely according to the need to excrete water and solutes	• High values found in dehydration, or in impaired kidney function (e.g. chronic renal failure) • Low values found in people with intact renal function and high fluid intake, diabetes insipidus, chronic renal failure, hypercalcaemia, hypokalaemia Action: Depends on likely cause and results of other investigations
Blood	
May be haematuria (intact blood cells) or haemoglobinuria (free haemoglobin, excreted from plasma or liberated from red cells in the urine)	Haematuria: • Due to kidney disorders (e.g. glomerulonephritis, polycystic kidneys, tumour) • Due to urinary tract disorders (e.g. stones, tumour, infection, benign prostatic enlargement) Haemoglobinuria: • Severe haemolysis (e.g. sickle cell disease crisis) • Breakdown of red cells in urine (especially when urine is dilute and testing is delayed) Action: Should be reported; follow-up will depend on other tests and the clinical picture
pH	
In health, the pH of uncontaminated urine ranges from 4.5 to 8.0 A high pH will be found if testing stale urine, so such specimens should not be used	• Low values found in acidaemia as in diabetic ketoacidosis; also starvation or potassium depletion • High values found in stale urine, alkalaemia (except when due to potassium depletion), for example, due to vomiting and consumption of large amounts of antacids, renal tubular acidosis, UTI with ammonia-forming organisms Action: Depends on other test results

(Continued)

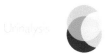

Table 6.3: (Continued)

Significance of positive results	Commonest causes of abnormalities and possible action to be taken
Protein	
A range of proteins can be detected but the reagent is most sensitive to albumin, so a negative result does not rule out presence of other proteins	· Albuminuria may be found in acute and chronic glomerulonephritis, UTI, glomerular involvement in systemic lupus erythematosus, nephrotic syndrome, pre-eclampsia, fever, heart failure and postural (orthostatic) proteinuria
	Action: Transient results are seldom important but persistent positive results need investigating for underlying cause
	Other test results and clinical picture should be considered
Urobilinogen	Increased secretion:
Urinary excretion of urobilinogen reflects the combined effects of conversion of bilirubin to urobilinogen in the gut and reabsorption into the bloodstream	· May be due to increased production (e.g. in red blood cell disorders such as sickle cell disease), or due to decreased uptake by the liver (e.g. in viral hepatitis and cirrhosis)
	Decreased secretion:
Note that false-negatives are found in stale urine	· May be due to biliary tract obstruction (e.g. gallstones, carcinoma of pancreas), or due to sterilisation of the colon by unabsorbable antibiotics (e.g. neomycin), which prevents bacterial conversion of bilirubin to urobilinogen
	Action: Urgent investigation is needed
Nitrite	
Most organisms which infect the urinary tract contain an enzyme system that catalyses the conversion of dietary nitrate, which is normally present in urine, to nitrite, which is not found in urine unless there is a urinary tract infection	· Presence indicates UTI due to nitrite-producing organisms · However, absence does not exclude infection, as some organisms are unable to convert dietary nitrate to nitrite · False-negatives are also found if there is insufficient dietary nitrate, or urine has not been in the bladder long enough (4 h is ideal) for the conversion to take place
	Action: Specimen should be sent for microscopy and culture
Leucocytes	
Will be present when some of the leucocytes that have entered inflamed tissue from the blood are shed in the urine	· Indicates a UTI, especially when it is accompanied by acute inflammation of the urinary tract
	Action: Specimen should be sent for microscopy and culture

Source: Adapted from Bayer. 1997. *Urine Analysis: The Essential Information.* Newbury: Bayer; Bayer. 1998. *A Practical Guide to Urine Analysis.* Newbury: Bayer.

Older people, especially women and people with urinary catheters, may have bacteria present in their urine (termed 'bacteriuria') without an infection being present (Nazarko 2009). For people aged under 65 years who have mild UTI symptoms and cloudy urine, a urinalysis should be performed and if nitrite is present, a UTI is likely. However, if urine is negative to nitrite but positive to leucocytes, a UTI diagnosis is possible though not definite and sending urine for culture is appropriate to assist diagnosis (BIA and HPA 2011).

The National Institute for Health and Clinical Excellence (NICE 2019a) recommends that all women with urinary incontinence should have a urinalysis performed, and if it is

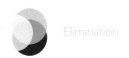
positive to leucocytes and nitrites, and symptomatic of UTI, a midstream specimen (see the next section) should be sent for MC&S. It is worth noting that typical symptoms of UTI, such as pain on micturition (dysuria), frequency, fever and sometimes loin or suprapubic pain may not be present in older people (Midthun et al. 2004; Woodford and George 2009).

Learning outcome 3: identify in what situations urinalysis should be performed

ACTIVITY

> **Box 6.10 Activity: urinalysis**
>
> For each person in the scenarios at the start of the chapter, identify why a urinalysis would be appropriate.

A urinalysis gives many clues about a person's health and well-being, so a nursing assessment of a newly referred or admitted person should always include a urinalysis. Urinalysis is also performed for other people at risk of developing health problems that can be indicated through a urinalysis, for example, after an abdominal injury (to screen for blood, which might indicate renal damage).

When Bob was first admitted, a urinalysis could have been performed as part of a general health screen. He should have been reassured that it is routine and there is nothing to be worried about and given a clean container in which to collect urine the morning after admission. When he developed urinary incontinence, he should have been asked for a further morning specimen to rule out UTI, which can predispose to, or compound, urinary incontinence. Remember that taking clozapine has rendered him more vulnerable to infection.

Mark is known to have a renal impairment and frequent UTIs. The CLDN has already collected a urine specimen. On admission to the ward, a urinalysis will give immediate information about his renal function and indicate whether he could have a UTI. Jean's urine would have been tested on admission to hospital as part of her general health assessment, including the likelihood of a UTI preoperatively. Postoperatively, Jean has a urinary catheter, which is accompanied by a risk of UTI, which the scenario states did occur. If Jean were symptomatic of a UTI, a catheter specimen of urine (CSU) (see Box 6.15) would be obtained to test her urine initially before sending a sample for culture.

> Box 6.11 Children and young people: practice points – urinalysis
>
> UTI symptoms in infants and small children are often non-specific, so NICE (2018a) guidelines advise conducting a urinalysis for those with an unexplained temperature of 38 degrees or higher, as well as for children and infants with UTI symptoms.

Box 6.12 Pregnancy and birth: practice points – urinalysis

Pregnant mothers must have their urine tested at each antenatal assessment. Protein in the urine, in conjunction with oedema or hypertension, could indicate pre-eclampsia, a potentially serious complication of pregnancy or infection. Glucose in the urine could indicate gestational diabetes, a type of diabetes that affects pregnant mothers. See www.nice.org.uk/guidance/ng3

Summary

- Urinalysis is a non-invasive and frequently performed practical skill that can provide very useful information about people's health status.
- To obtain an accurate result, the steps in a urinalysis must be carried out carefully with an appropriately collected specimen.
- It is important to understand the significance of abnormal results and the subsequent plan of action.

COLLECTING URINE AND STOOL SPECIMENS

In this section, common types of urine specimen and the collection of a stool (faeces) specimen are discussed. It is often necessary to obtain specimens such as these from individuals in your care as they can provide important diagnostic information, which impacts on their management. General principles of specimen collection are considered in Box 6.14.

Box 6.13 Learning outcomes

By the end of this section, you will be able to discuss the collection of:

1. a CSU;
2. a MSU;
3. a 24-hour specimen of urine;
4. a stoma urine specimen;
5. a stool specimen.

Learning outcome 1: discuss the collection of a catheter specimen of urine

A CSU is often taken for bacteriological examination to find out if treatment is required when symptoms of a UTI are present in a person who is catheterised. However, a person with a catheter may not display these symptoms, and in an older and/or confused person, the symptoms can be still less apparent. As discussed earlier in the chapter, a CSU may have to be collected from Jean if a UTI is suspected. The risk of infection increases by 5–8% each day of catheterisation (Maki and Tambyah 2001), so the longer the catheter is left in place, the more likely the person will have bacteriuria. Bacteria prefer to live on surfaces rather than in a solution such as urine.

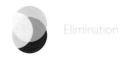

A catheter provides this surface and bacteria can coat it and form what is called a biofilm. Bacteria that live in a biofilm are more resistant to treatment, so that even if eliminated in urine by using antibiotics, the ones on the catheter will persist and recontaminate the urine (Saye 2007).

Box 6.14 Collection of specimens: key points

- Adherence to infection control standard principles (hand hygiene, personal protective equipment)
- Clear explanations
- Maintenance of the individuals privacy, dignity and comfort
- Avoidance of contamination of the specimen
- Prompt transportation to the laboratory, or retention in a designated specimen refrigerator for up to 24 hours
- Clear labelling
- Correct and comprehensive accompanying information
- Documentation in the persons notes of the date and time of the specimen collection

---

It is important to distinguish between bacteriuria and a 'clinical infection'. Bacteria can colonise the urinary tract without invading the surrounding tissues (bacteriuria), often not causing clinical symptoms, and not being susceptible to treatment. However, clinical infection involving invasion of surrounding tissues, often producing symptoms in infected people, requires treatment.

Whatever the classification of the infection, if a specimen is considered necessary, then nurses must use aseptic techniques and sterile equipment. This is to reduce the risk of further contaminating the specimen and potentially introducing different bacteria to those from the individual. This is particularly important since the treatment is based on the results of the bacteriological examination of the urine.

Urine should be obtained from the special sampling port on the drainage system; the catheter and drainage system should never be disconnected to take a specimen. You should adhere to manufacturers' instructions concerning the number of times the port may be punctured safely. Urine should never be taken from the catheter bag because the bag acts as a reservoir where microorganisms can multiply. It is thus likely to contain greater numbers of microorganisms than urine accessed via the port. The bag can also be heavily contaminated from environmental sources. Box 6.15 outlines the key principles to follow when taking a CSU.

Learning outcome 2: discuss the collection of a midstream specimen of urine

The midstream specimen of urine (MSU) is collected if a UTI is suspected in a non-catheterised individual, and it is obtained using a clean procedure. It is a useful aid in diagnosis and the aim is to collect the midstream specimen, which is not contaminated by microorganisms outside the urinary tract.

How MSUs should be collected has been the subject of much research but the evidence base for best practice remains unclear. People have often been asked to undertake perineal cleansing with sterile swabs and saline prior to giving an MSU to prevent contamination. However, a Canadian study concluded that contamination of urine specimens from women with acute dysuria who cleaned the perineal area prior to collection did not differ from those who did not (Blake and Doherty 2006). A study on toilet-trained children, however, found that those who did not clean their genital area did have a higher contamination rate than those who did (Vaillancourt et al. 2007). However, it is debatable whether results on children are transferable to adults. The Health Protection Agency (2012) recommends thorough peri-urethral cleaning but also states that the need for this has been questioned in both men and women. It is therefore good practice to assess the person's level of personal hygiene and follow local guidelines regarding peri-urethral cleaning when obtaining an MSU. It is theorised that the first part of the stream flushes away microorganisms from the first part of the urethra, and that the urine does not flow over the perineum as long as there is sufficient urine in the bladder to produce a good stream. If there is insufficient urine in the bladder, the specimen should be collected later. The equipment required and key points of the procedure are listed in Box 6.16.

Box 6.15 Collection of a catheter specimen of urine: equipment and key points

Equipment

- Alcohol swab, receiver, specimen pot, request form, syringe (20 mL) and a needle (21 g bore), if the sampling port is not needleless.
- A gate clamp may be required.

Key points

- Adhere to general points outlined in Box 6.14
- Locate the sample port on the catheter bag tubing. Needleless sampling ports are preferable but some drainage bags have a latex port that requires a needle and syringe to aspirate the urine.

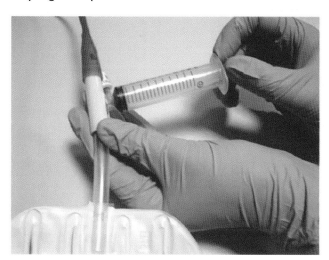

Figure 6.3: Needleless port.

(*Continued*)

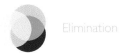
Box 6.15 (Continued)

- If there is no urine present in the catheter tubing, clamp the tubing below the sample port until sufficient urine collects. Never clamp the actual catheter, as this could damage it.
- Swab the sample port with alcohol swab and allow the port to dry.
- If using a needleless port, attach a syringe directly to the port to withdraw the urine.
- If the sampling port is not needleless, insert the needle into the port at an angle of 45 degrees to prevent going straight through the tubing.
- Withdraw the required amount of urine, remove the top from the specimen pot and fill the pot with urine. Dispose of the syringe (and needle if used) into a sharps box immediately. Replace the cap on the pot.

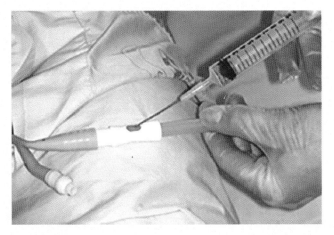

Figure 6.4: Needled port.

Box 6.16 Midstream specimens of urine: equipment and procedure

Equipment

A toilet/commode/bedpan/urinal as appropriate, specimen pot and request form, disposable gloves.

Procedure

- Adhere to key points in Box 6.14
- Follow local policy as regards meatal cleansing.
- Ask the person to start passing urine as usual, then catch some urine (about 20 mL: about 2.5 cm up the pot) in the specimen pot, and then finish voiding into the toilet or commode. Wear gloves and assist the person, if necessary.

If a urine specimen is being collected because of suspected tuberculosis (TB) or cancer of the urinary tract, then an early-morning specimen is preferable because it is more concentrated, and it is most likely to contain the tubercle bacillus or malignant cells (Beynon and Nicholls 2004). Usually, three consecutive early-morning specimens are required.

Box 6.17 Activity: practice scenarios

Read through Box 6.16. As you can see, the person's cooperation and understanding would be needed. Look at the practice scenarios: to what extent might you achieve understanding and consent from Bob and Mark?

You are more likely to gain informed consent and cooperation from anyone if you explain the procedure and its importance carefully and confidentially. You should respect the person's right to privacy and dignity throughout the whole episode of care. Remember that what may be a simple and routine procedure in your eyes may feel quite different to the person concerned. It is likely that Bob would be able to produce the specimen with little assistance. Mark may have become used to giving urine samples at his GP's surgery because of his frequent urine infections. One approach would be for his mother or a nurse to take him to the toilet about 30 min after a drink (assuming he is not being kept 'nil by mouth') and try to collect the specimen in a clean receptacle in the toilet or, if possible, catch the midstream in a pot for him, while wearing gloves. This approach can also be used for people who are confused.

It can be difficult to produce an MSU, especially if the individual is confined to bed. Adaptations will need to be made, for example, placing a waterproof pad beneath them to soak up any possible spillage, helping to diminish fears of wetting the bed. Allowing people plenty of time and not rushing is also important.

Learning outcome 3: discuss the collection of a 24-hour specimen of urine

Sometimes, it is necessary to collect the total volume of urine passed within a 24-hour period. This is then analysed within the laboratory so that the 24-hour excretion of a variety of key metabolites (e.g. protein, creatinine) can be assessed (Beynon and Nicholls 2004). Box 6.18 outlines the equipment needed and the procedure.

Box 6.18 Twenty-four-hour urine collection: equipment and key points

Equipment

A jug, a 24-hour urine collection container, gloves

Procedure

- Assess the person's ability to participate in the collection. When the person next passes urine, it is discarded. This marks the beginning of the 24-hour period for collection.
- Label the container with the person's details (name, ward and hospital number) and the time and date the collection started.

(Continued)

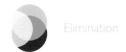

Box 6.18 (Continued)

- Put a sign on the bed or door of the room belonging to the person indicating that a 24-hour urine collection is in place, the date and time it started and when it will finish.
- Every time the person passes urine, it is collected and poured into the container. The person may be able to do this independently or may need assistance. Check their understanding and ability.
- Ask the person to empty their bladder just before the end of the 24-hour collection period.
- Advise that this ends the collection period.
- Remove the sign from the door or bed.
- Clean or discard the jug used.
- Record the completion time and ensure that the urine collection and laboratory request forms are dispatched correctly as soon as possible.

Note: If one sample of urine becomes contaminated or is accidentally discarded, the test must be discontinued and restarted.

Learning outcome 4: discuss the collection of a stoma urine specimen

In learning outcome 1, the importance of not obtaining a CSU from the drainage bag was stated. The same rationale applies to individuals who have had an ileal conduit (i.e. urinary stoma) formed (see section on 'Stoma care' later). If taken from the stoma bag, the urine will have multiple bacteria and may be contaminated.

The correct method of collecting a stoma urine is by passing a small intermittent catheter into the stoma (see Box 6.19). This is a sterile procedure. The catheter is introduced into the opening of the stoma and gently pushed in (2.5–5 cm deep only) until urine starts to flow down the catheter into the waiting collection pot (Fillingham and Fell 2004). Occasionally, this may be difficult as the stoma may be narrow or very long, or the person may not be able to tolerate a catheter being used. In these instances, a non-touch technique can be used with a sterile collecting pot held under the stoma, making sure that the rim does not touch the stoma or the surrounding skin. Urine should start to drip out of the stoma and into the pot. This may take a few minutes but should ensure the specimen is not contaminated. Alternatively, a clean new bag can be put onto the abdomen over the stoma and the urine collected within a few minutes. The bag is not sterile, but it will be clean and therefore there is less risk of contamination or multiple bacteria.

Box 6.19 Collection of a stoma urine specimen: equipment and key points

Equipment

Sterile pack containing gloves and sterile gauze, sterile single-use catheter (8–14 Ch), sterile specimen pot, disposable plastic apron, water or normal saline, clean stoma appliance (if required), disposal bag, incontinence pad or paper towel.

(Continued)

Box 6.19 (Continued)

Procedure

- Adhere to general points in Box 6.14.
- Prepare a new stoma bag, if this needs to be replaced after the procedure.
- Position an incontinence pad or paper towel under the person.
- Remove the stoma bag and dispose it. Alternatively unclip the bag from the flange on the person's abdomen and put aside (see the 'Stoma care' section).
- Cover stoma with sterile gauze.
- Wash and dry hands.
- Open sterile pack and prepare sterile field. Put on sterile gloves. Open sterile catheter and place on sterile field.
- Clean around stoma with sterile water or saline and gauze using strokes from the centre outwards. Dry the area.
- Insert the catheter tip into the stoma opening and gently push it in to a depth of 2.5–5 cm only. Wait for urine to start to drain out into the sterile container. A minimum of 2–5 mL is sufficient, though more is preferable.
- Remove catheter and seal specimen container.
- Clean around stoma again, if needed. Make sure skin is dry. Reapply a clean stoma bag or clip the stoma bag back onto the flange.
- Dispose of equipment as per local policy.

Learning outcome 5: discuss the collection of a stool specimen

Box 6.20 Activity: collecting a stool specimen

ACTIVITY

When do you think it might be necessary to collect a stool specimen?
Thinking about a 'normal' tool will help you begin to answer this question.

You may have identified that a stool specimen is collected if a person has complained of abnormal stools, or you have observed an abnormality (e.g. diarrhoea), which may be caused by gastrointestinal infection. Infection is particularly likely if the stool is offensive and has an abnormal colour such as green. In these instances, the stool is sent for MC&S, to detect the causative microorganism and identify any antibiotics to which it is sensitive.

Normal frequency of passing stools varies from person to person, but if frequency is altered, it can be a reason to collect a specimen. Altered consistency might also be a reason. For example, lots of mucus can indicate disease such as ulcerative colitis, whereas fatty, offensive-smelling and floating stools sometimes indicate gall bladder disease.

Stool specimens are sent for examination for occult (hidden) blood, if rectal bleeding is suspected but not obvious. If the colour of a stool is different from that normally seen, that too can be suggestive of disease, indicating that a specimen should be taken. Bright red, fresh blood must be reported and may indicate the presence of

Ulcerative colitis

Ulceration of the mucosa of the colon, causing offensive, watery stools with mucus and pus. Can cause haemorrhage and perforation.

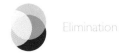

Haemorrhoids

Dilated blood vessels in the rectal mucosa. The common term is 'piles'.

haemorrhoids or other diseases. Stools that are black and tarry in consistency can indicate digested blood from the alimentary tract (termed melaena). Sometimes, stool specimens are sent for examination for parasites. In addition, if a person experiences pain or discomfort associated with defaecation, or flatus is a problem, then a stool specimen might be taken.

See Box 6.22 for key points on collecting a stool specimen. There are stool specimen collectors available that have a spoon attached to the lid. Although these are easy to use when collecting the specimen, they can be difficult for laboratory staff to handle without getting contaminated. Also, pots should not be overfilled as the contents may ferment and build up sufficient pressure to force off even a tight-fitting lid.

Box 6.21 Children and young people: practice points – urine and stool specimens

To obtain a urine sample from a child who is not toilet-trained, NICE (2018a) recommends collecting a 'clean-catch' sample (catching the urine in a clean container, that is, a potty washed in hot water – 60 degrees with washing-up liquid). If a clean-catch specimen is unobtainable, other non-invasive methods such as urine collection pads should be used, though they are less accurate. NICE (2018a) outlines criteria for sending urine off for culture, and UTI treatment, in children. Stool specimens can be collected from nappies in children not yet toilet-trained.

For further information, see

Macqueen, S., Bruce, E.A. and Gibson, F. 2012. *The Great Ormond Street Hospital Manual of Children's Nursing Practices*. Chichester: Wiley-Blackwell, Chapter 5 'Bowel Care' 87–101 and Chapter 14 'Investigations.' 353–4.

Willock, 2010. Elimination: Collecting, measuring and testing urine. In: Glasper, A., Aylott, M. and Battrick, C. (eds.) *Developing Practical Skills for Nursing Children and Young People*. London: Hodder Arnold, 259–76.

Summary

- Explaining the procedure and its importance carefully, while maintaining dignity, privacy and respect for people, is of prime importance when collecting specimens.
- It is essential to be certain about the purpose of collecting the specimen so that it is collected appropriately.
- Great care should be taken when collecting urine and stool specimens to prevent their contamination, which would in turn invalidate results.
- Precautions to prevent cross-infection must be adhered to when collecting urine and stool specimens.
- It is essential to label specimens accurately and to document their collection in persons' notes.

Box 6.22 Collection of a stool specimen: equipment and key points

Equipment

Bedpan, gloves, apron, sterile stool specimen pot or sterile specimen pot and spatula, specimen bag, laboratory request form.

Procedure

- Adhere to general points in Box 6.14.
- If possible, the person should be helped to a toilet rather than use a commode. A disposable bedpan can be placed under the toilet lid. Otherwise, a bedpan or commode is used to catch the specimen.
- When the stool is available, take the bedpan to the sluice, open the sterile container and using a spatula fill the container about a third full with faeces and then secure the lid.
- Place the specimen in a dedicated specimen refrigerator if it cannot go to the laboratory immediately. In infections, such as amoebiasis, the stool must be fresh and warm (Mead 1998), thus special arrangements for collection must be made with the laboratory.
- Remember to complete the stool chart if a record is being kept.

CARING FOR PEOPLE WITH URINARY CATHETERS

Urinary catheterisation involves the insertion of a hollow tube into the bladder for evacuating or instilling fluids. The catheter may be inserted intermittently or left *in situ* (termed 'in-dwelling'), and emptied intermittently via a catheter valve. In these instances, the bladder then retains its function as a reservoir. In many cases, an in-dwelling catheter continuously drains the bladder within a closed system into a bag, in which case only a small volume of urine will be present at the base of the bladder. This method was used as a temporary measure for Jean immediately after surgery.

Some people are taught to self-catheterise intermittently, termed 'intermittent self-catheterisation', often to manage incontinence or incomplete emptying in those with neurological disorders such as multiple sclerosis. Teaching a person to self-catheterise requires specific skills and knowledge (Getliffe and Fader 2007).

Urinary catheters are usually passed along the urethra, but sometimes a suprapubic catheter is passed directly through the mid-suprapubic region of the anterior abdominal wall into the bladder. This is a surgical procedure, performed under anaesthesia, and may be used for people who need a long-term urinary catheter or after certain surgical procedures and in pelvic/urethral trauma or disease. The principles of catheter care for people who have suprapubic catheters are the same as for those with urethral catheters (Colpman and Welford 2004). However, as the catheter is inserted into a tract into the skin, this can result in infection, bleeding and encrustation around the catheter site. Any secretions that form around the catheter site can be removed with soap and water. Most people prefer not to wear a dressing around this site, though some may prefer to do so to prevent staining of clothing.

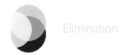
> **Box 6.23 Learning outcomes**
>
> By the end of this section, you will be able to:
>
> 1. identify the main indications for urinary catheterisation;
> 2. show awareness of equipment commonly used for catheterisation;
> 3. state the main complications associated with urinary catheterisation;
> 4. understand the principles underpinning urethral catheterisation;
> 5. discuss the care required for people who have an in-dwelling urinary catheter.

You may be able to access a urinary catheter in the skills laboratory. An opened one would be particularly useful. If not, see if you can look at equipment in your practice setting.

Nursing associates are expected to care and manage urinary catheters but not insert them. However, understanding the principles and what the skill entails will help them in the care they give to individuals with urinary catheters (see nursing-associates-proficiency-standards.pdf NMC 2018).

Learning outcome 1: identify the main indications for urinary catheterisation

> **Box 6.24 Activity: why are people catheterised?**
>
> Make a list of the reasons why people are catheterised. Thinking back to your practice experience will give you some clues.

ACTIVITY

It has been estimated that up to 25% of people in hospital have an in-dwelling catheter (Schumm and Lam 2010), with up to 28% of individuals residing in care homes and 4% in the community having long-term in-dwelling catheters (McNulty et al. 2003).

You may have identified the following reasons:

Neurogenic bladder

Commonly results from lesions of the central nervous system (e.g. spinal injury, multiple sclerosis). Effects include urinary retention, overactive, underactive or uncoordinated detrusor activity.

* to relieve retention of urine (e.g. because of enlarged prostate or neurogenic bladder);
* before pelvic surgery and certain investigations, to minimise the risk of damage to the bladder;
* to measure urine output accurately postoperatively and in very ill people (e.g. major trauma, shock) – Jean's urethral catheter was originally inserted for this reason;
* to empty the bladder during labour;
* to introduce fluids into the bladder for irrigation purposes;
* to introduce drugs as direct therapy (e.g. cytotoxic drugs);
* to facilitate bladder healing;
* following certain pelvic, urethral or bladder neck surgery.

Cytotoxic drugs

These are drugs that have a destructive effect on cells and are used to treat cancer.

(List adapted from Royal Marsden Hospital Manual of Clinical Nursing Procedures 2020)

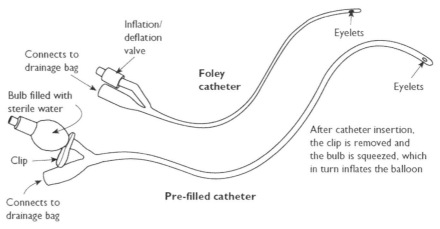

Inflation/
deflation
valve

Connects to
drainage bag

Bulb filled with
sterile water

Clip

Connects to
drainage bag

Foley
catheter

Eyelets

Eyelets

After catheter insertion,
the clip is removed and
the bulb is squeezed, which
in turn inflates the balloon

Pre-filled catheter

Figure 6.5: Examples of urinary catheters.

Incontinence is not given as a primary reason for catheterisation above because long-term catheterisation is rarely free of complications and should, therefore, only be considered when other options have failed, or are no longer appropriate. The major complications of catheterisation are considered in more detail later in this chapter.

Learning outcome 2: show awareness of equipment commonly used for catheterisation

> **Box 6.25 Activity: sterile or non-sterile urinary catheters**
>
> In the skills laboratory, there may be a sterile or non-sterile (for demonstration purposes) urinary catheter complete with packaging material. See Figure 6.5 for examples. Take note of the following:

- the manner in which it is packaged, batch number, expiry date
- size
- length
- balloon capacity
- the catheter material.

If you have access to a non-sterile catheter, try inflating and deflating the balloon using a syringe and water. Some catheters are manufactured pre-filled with water for inflation. Now read through the following points and relate them to your observations.

Packaging

Catheters are packaged to enable ease of insertion into the bladder. With the exception of self-catheterisation, a strict aseptic technique is employed. The way in which the catheter is packaged, including double wrapping, assists in maintaining sterility. There is a batch number and expiry date on the packaging that must be entered into the persons' documentation or digital records. Many packets have removable sticky labels printed with these details that are put on the individual's notes for future reference.

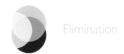

Catheter size

The catheter size is measured according to its external diameter and is measured in Charrière (Ch) or French gauge units (Fg). One Ch unit equals 0.3 mm, and the catheters range in size from 6 to 8 (for paediatric use) to 30 Ch. A size 12 Ch catheter is 4 mm in diameter and is usually adequate for urine drainage for both men and women. The key general rule to follow is that the smallest size catheter that will allow free urinary outflow should be used (Pratt et al. 2007). Large catheters are associated with complications including urethral irritation, urethral trauma, bladder spasm, urinary bypassing, pressure necrosis and increased risk of infection (Wilson 2012).

Catheter length

Catheters are usually manufactured in three lengths: standard catheters (sometimes referred to as 'male-length'), 40–44 cm in length; female catheters, 30–40 cm in length; and paediatric catheters, 30 cm in length (Wilson 2011). The standard catheter is often used for women, particularly if obese, because it allows easier access to the junction of the catheter and the drainage bag (Colpman and Welford 2004). Female catheters must never be used urethrally in males as they are too short for the male urethra and would not reach the bladder. If inflated in the urethra, the balloon may cause this to rupture and haemorrhage and may lead to severe trauma (Getliffe and Fader 2007).

Balloon

The Foley catheter is the design most frequently used for in-dwelling urethral catheterisation (Getliffe and Fader 2007). It has a rounded tip with two drainage eyes and an integral balloon, which, when inflated, holds the catheter *in situ*. There are two channels, one for drainage and the other for inflating the balloon. The balloon sits at the sensitive base of the bladder and can potentially cause irritation, spasm and mechanical damage to the bladder. Retention balloons come in various sizes: 10 mL is recommended for adults, but larger 30 mL balloons are sometimes used after some urological procedures (Pratt et al. 2007). Inflation valves are colour-coded according to the Charrière size (Yates 2012).

Catheters for intermittent use are usually a simple tube design and do not have an inflatable balloon as there is no requirement for them to be retained in the bladder. Some suprapubic catheters do not have a balloon but are secured by a flange and held in place by skin sutures.

Material

Catheters are available in various materials. The choice of which type to use depends on the clinical experience of the practitioner, individual assessment and the length of time it is envisaged the catheter will remain *in situ* (Pratt et al. 2007).

For short-term use, plastic, latex (up to 7–10 days) and Teflon-coated latex (up to 28 days) are commonly used; these materials are considerably cheaper than long-term catheter materials. Some people are allergic to latex, and screening is advisable if latex is to be used (Newman 2012; Wilson 2012). Plastic catheters have been found to exert low toxicity because of the inert nature of plastic. Also, the rate at which this material absorbs water is low and so the catheter retains the widest internal diameter, making these catheters a common choice for drainage of postoperative blood clots and debris. However, plastic catheters can remain rigid at body temperature and have been associated with bladder spasm, pain and leakage of urine (Wilson 2012). The DH (2003) recommends that in-dwelling catheters used for long-term use should have low allergenicity. Silicone, silicone-elastomer-coated latex and hydrogel-coated catheters are suitable products (Newman 2012; Wilson 2012; Yates 2012).

Recent research has focused on developing catheters with properties specifically intended to reducing infection incidence. These tend to have special coatings such as silver ions or aloe vera along their length. The aim is to either stop or limit formation of biofilms (Godfrey and Fraczyk 2005). These substances have been found to have anti-infection properties. However, a review found that very few trials have compared different types of catheter for long-term use and most were carried out on small numbers of individuals (Jahn et al. 2007). The reviewers concluded that the evidence was too weak to provide reliable evidence about which type of catheter is best for which individual. The cost of the catheter should not be the primary factor in the selection process, but nurses should be aware of the different costs when selecting.

Urine drainage bags and catheter valves

In-dwelling catheters are normally used in conjunction with an attached collection bag to allow periodic emptying. This is known as a closed system. Figure 6.6 shows a catheter attached to a leg bag, which would be secured to the person's leg with straps see Figure 6.8. Figure 6.7 shows a urinary catheter attached to a urine drainage bag supported on a stand, which is suitable for overnight use or for a person who has to remain in bed. A catheter valve (see Figure 6.9) may provide an alternative for some people, but an adequate bladder capacity is required. Unless a committed carer is available, the user requires good manual dexterity for manipulating the valve, and sufficient cognitive function to understand the need to release the valve regularly to prevent overdistension (Gibney 2010; Yates 2012). Catheter valves are also unlikely to be suitable if the person has uncontrolled detrusor overactivity, ureteric reflux or renal impairment (Gibney 2010) (Figure 6.7).

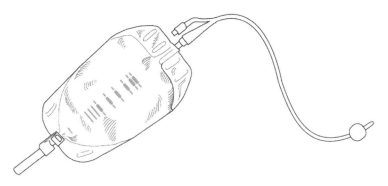

Figure 6.6: A urinary catheter attached to a leg bag.

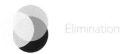

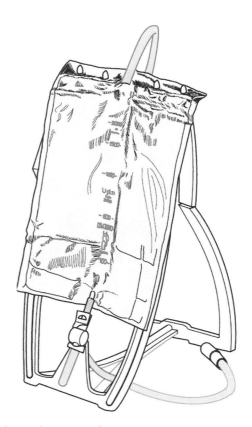

Figure 6.7: A urine drainage bag on a stand.

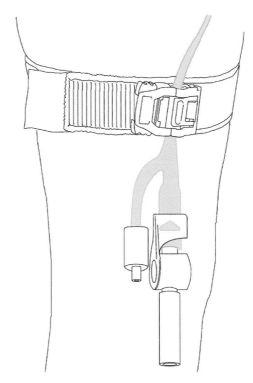

Figure 6.8: A urinary catheter strapped to the leg, with a valve in place, for emptying.

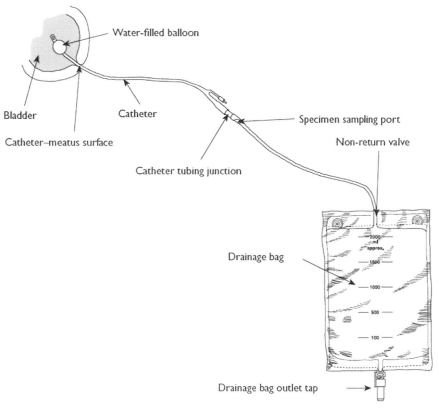

Figure 6.9: A closed urinary drainage system.

When selecting a bag, factors to consider are capacity, length of inlet tube and type of outlet tap for emptying. Bags vary in capacity from 350 to 750 mL and up to 2 L for use overnight or postoperatively. Some bags are specially designed for wheelchair users. Outlet taps are usually of a lever-type design or push-across mechanism, but other designs are also available. The manual dexterity of the person and their carers needs to be considered. There are catheter supports available for people with restricted mobility that aim to provide firm support to prevent tugging, without restricting movement or impeding drainage.

Whatever equipment is used, you must document details of the catheter and drainage system used in the person's records carefully. You should also provide the person with adequate information about the rationale for insertion, the insertion itself, and the maintenance and removal of catheter.

ACTIVITY

Box 6.26 Activity: drainage bag type

What sort of drainage bag might be suitable for Jean?

Following discussion with Jean, you may decide to use a leg bag (see Figure 6.8). The length of the inlet tube selected would depend on whether Jean found it most

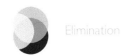

comfortable to position the bag on her thigh, knee or calf. At night, the nurses will be able to attach a night bag on a stand, directly to the leg bag. For most individuals, body-worn bags are preferable because their attachment to the person's leg or suspended from the waist allows maximum freedom and at the same time can be concealed beneath clothing. This reduces discomfort and promotes dignity for people like Jean who find themselves in the difficult and sometimes embarrassing situation of needing a urinary catheter *in situ*. A body-worn bag will help Jean as she begins to mobilise as she will not have to contend with carrying the bag or long trailing drainage tubes. Once she is comfortable moving and fully mobile, the catheter can be removed.

Did you know?

Prior to the use of closed drainage systems, almost all individuals developed UTIs within 96 h (Kass 1957, cited by Macauley 1997). As closed drainage systems have been shown to reduce this rate of infection, they are now accepted as good practice (Wilson 2011). However, many healthcare-associated infections are related to urinary catheterisation, causing significant morbidity and even mortality. Therefore, care for people with catheters must aim to prevent infection, as well as promote comfort and understanding.

Box 6.27 Bacteria entry

ACTIVITY

Figure 6.9 shows a diagram of a closed urinary drainage system. Where do you think bacteria could enter into the system?

The following are the potential ports of entry:

- the catheter tip during catheterisation
- the urethral meatus around the catheter
- the junction between the catheter and the tubing to the catheter bag
- the specimen sampling port
- the drainage outlet.

Bacteria are also believed to enter the bladder at the time of catheterisation via the peri-urethral space. Coagulase-negative staphylococci or micrococci can normally be found in the anterior urethra, and these are a common cause of infection immediately following catheterisation (Tlaskalová-Hogenová et al. 2004).

Some systems now have a tamper-evident seal at the junction between the catheter and the connection tube aimed at preventing bacteria from entering here.

Learning outcome 3: state the main complications associated with urinary catheterisation

Box 6.28 Activity: complications with catheterisation

ACTIVITY

Look back over this section and see whether you can name one major complication associated with catheterisation. Try to identify some other complications.

You probably identified that infection is a major complication of catheterisation. Encrustation and eventual blockage are also problems associated with urinary catheterisation (Wilson 2012). Other complications include urethral strictures, pressure necrosis, spasm, discomfort and pain (Yates 2012).

With a catheter *in situ*, the bladder's normal closing mechanism is obstructed and the natural flushing mechanism of micturition is lost. In addition, the close proximity of the catheter to the bowel presents a risk of infection, because bacteria can be mechanically transferred across skin surfaces from anus to urethral meatus (Tlaskalová-Hogenová et al. 2004). As discussed earlier, bacteria having entered the urinary system may cling to the surface of the catheter, which creates a living biofilm that is almost impossible to remove and one that is highly resistant to antibiotics (Getliffe 2002). The bacteria can cause the urine to become more alkaline than usual, leading to encrustation on the catheter surface, which can lead to blockage and then to retention of urine or to leakage and pain. These outcomes are distressing for individuals and can result in loss of comfort and dignity (Stickler 2008).

When tissue is invaded by bacteria, problems include local infection, which may result in foul-smelling urine, or systemic infection leading to pyrexia (raised body temperature). Catheterising someone places them in significant danger of acquiring a UTI, and the longer a catheter is in place, the greater the danger. Of people with a catheter-associated UTI, 1–4% develop bacteraemia and of these, 13–30% die (Pratt et al. 2007). Therefore, catheterisation is best avoided, if at all possible (Pratt et al. 2007), and catheters should be removed as soon as possible, if no longer needed.

Learning outcome 4: understand the principles underpinning urethral catheterisation

Catheterisation is a skilled aseptic procedure and should be carried out only by healthcare personnel who are trained and competent to carry it out (Pratt et al. 2007). Catheterisation is an invasive procedure and the effects on individuals may be many: physical, psychological and social.

ACTIVITY

Box 6.29 Activity: aseptic technique

Before reading the following section, refer to Chapter 12 for an explanation of the aseptic technique. These principles underpin the procedure of urinary catheterisation.

Appropriate and effective communication and sensitivity are essential when catheterisation takes place (see Chapter 2 for more information). Care should be taken to explain where the catheter is inserted, and why the procedure is necessary, ensuring that verbal consent is gained. This could be difficult with a person who is confused. Also, catheters should not be changed unnecessarily or as part of routine practice.

Box 6.31 outlines the equipment needed and the key points to be adhered to while undertaking female urethral catheterisation. In many NHS trusts, additional training

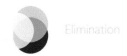

must be undertaken by trained nurses to perform male urethral catheterisation (see Box 6.32 for key points on male catheterisation) if proficiency in the skill has not previously been assessed and achieved during nurse training. This is because though many of the principles are synonymous with female urethral catheterisation, the male urethra is much longer (15–20 cm) and passes through the prostate gland before entering the bladder, so potentially there is greater risk of causing trauma on catheter insertion. Suprapubic catheterisation is usually a medical procedure and is not considered here.

Once the catheter has been inserted, dietary advice, including fluid intake and avoidance of constipation, is an important part of a person's education (European Association of Urological Nurses [EAUN] 2012). Further explanations and instructions concerning why and how the catheter has been inserted, its maintenance requirements and discussion of removal will be required if the person goes home with a urinary catheter *in situ*. Individuals and their carers should also be educated about techniques to prevent infection (NICE 2017). The district nurse will probably be involved.

Learning outcome 5: discuss the care required for people who have an in-dwelling urinary catheter

Box 6.30 Activity: care needed for Jean

What specific care might be needed in relation to catheter care for Jean?

You may have thought of:

* maintaining hygiene;
* emptying the catheter bag;
* appropriate positioning of the catheter bag;
* adequate fluid intake.

These pertinent issues will now be discussed.

Maintaining hygiene

The main aim of cleansing is to remove secretions and encrustation and prevent infection. Where possible, individuals should be encouraged to attend to their own meatal and perineal hygiene needs, thus reducing the risk of cross-infection while promoting self-care and dignity. Maintaining routine daily hygiene is all that is needed, with the meatus being washed with soap and water (Wilson 2011). However, for people unable to maintain their own hygiene, nurses should carry this out, wearing gloves, in a gentle and sensitive manner. Vigorous cleansing may increase the risk of infection (Pratt et al. 2007).

Cleansing of the perineum and the area surrounding the catheter–meatus junction is essential after faecal incontinence and should be carried out using clean wipes.

Box 6.31 Female urethral catheterisation: equipment and procedure

Equipment

- A catheterisation pack, if available, or a dressing pack and sterile receiver, sterile gloves, an appropriate catheter, sterile sodium chloride, catheter bag and stand or holder, sterile single-use lubricant or anaesthetic gel, syringe and sterile water of appropriate size to inflate the balloon (often included with catheter), disposable waterproof absorbent pad, specimen pot, if required, and a good light source.

Note: A second nurse may be needed to help position the individual, who needs to be preferably flat with legs apart to allow good access and visibility.

Procedure

- Aseptic technique should be strictly adhered to throughout (see Chapter 12 sections on 'Hand hygiene' and 'Aseptic technique').
- Explain the procedure and ensure consent.
- Maintain privacy and reassure the person throughout.
- Place the disposable pad under the person's buttocks.
- Open the catheter bag and arrange at the side of the bed, ensuring the attachment tip remains sterile.
- Open the catheterisation or dressing pack and open the catheter on to the sterile field but do not remove it from its internal wrapping.
- Draw up the sterile water to inflate the balloon (unless pre-filled syringe is supplied, or catheter is pre-filled).
- Pour sodium chloride into the gallipot.
- Open sterile gloves, wash hands and apply gloves.
- Place sterile towels over the person's thighs and between their legs.
- Cleanse the perineal area with sodium chloride, and then using non-dominant hand, separate labia minora and cleanse the meatus.
- Carefully locate the urethra and insert single-use lubricant gel to minimise urethral trauma and infection (NICE 2017). Some gels contain anaesthetic too. Inserting the gel directly into the urethra opens up and lubricates the length of the urethra. Lubricating the tip of the catheter only is ineffective as the lubricant is quickly wiped away on insertion. Wait for the time recommended by the manufacturer, usually 5 min.
- Place a receiver with the catheter on the sterile towel between the person's legs.
- Expose the tip of the catheter by pulling open the wrapper at the serrations.
- Hold the catheter so that the distal end remains in the receiver and gradually advance it out of its wrapper as you insert it into the meatus in an upward and backward direction along the line of the urethra.
- Advance the catheter 5–7 cm or until urine flows out of the catheter.
- Advance the catheter a further 5 cm. Never force the catheter. If resistance is encountered, stop and seek medical advice.
- Inflate the balloon with the correct amount of sterile water, generally 10 mL for adults (NICE 2017). Incorrectly filled balloons can inflate irregularly and irritate the bladder mucosa.
- Attach the urinary drainage bag and make the person comfortable.
- Send a urine specimen, if indicated, and measure and record the urine collected.
- Document the catheterisation in the individual's records including date of insertion, catheter size and amount of water used to inflate the balloon. The catheter packaging may have an adhesive label with the catheter's details, which can be used with paper records.

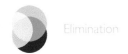
For females, you should clean from front to back to prevent possible movement of bacteria from the anal area and perineum to the catheter–meatus junction. The catheter should be gently wiped in one direction, away from the vulva. In males, the foreskin should be retracted before cleansing and the same principles of cleaning the catheter away from the catheter–meatus junction should be adhered to. The foreskin must be replaced afterwards. With a suprapubic catheter, once the wound has healed around the catheter, simple cleansing with soap and water is usually sufficient to maintain hygiene.

Box 6.32 Male urethral catheterisation: equipment and procedure

Equipment

- A catheterisation pack, if available, or a dressing pack and sterile receiver, sterile gloves, an appropriate catheter, sterile sodium chloride, catheter bag and stand or holder, sterile single-use lubricant or anaesthetic gel, syringe and sterile water of appropriate size to inflate the balloon (often included with catheter), disposable waterproof absorbent pad, specimen pot, if required, and a good light source

Note: The person needs to be preferably flat with legs slightly apart to allow the sterile receiver to be placed in the space in between.

Procedure

- Aseptic technique should be strictly adhered to throughout (see Chapter 12 sections on 'Hand hygiene' and 'Aseptic technique').
- Explain the procedure and ensure consent.
- Maintain privacy and reassure the individual throughout.
- Place the disposable pad under the person's buttocks.
- Open the catheter bag and arrange at the side of the bed, ensuring the attachment tip remains sterile.
- Open the catheterisation or dressing pack, and open the catheter on to the sterile field but do not remove it from its internal wrapping.
- Draw up the sterile water to inflate the balloon (unless pre-filled syringe is supplied or catheter is pre-filled).
- Pour sodium chloride into the gallipot.
- Open sterile gloves, wash hands and apply gloves.
- Place sterile towels over the person's thighs and between legs.
- Using your non-dominant hand, wrap a sterile gauze swab around the penis and if the person has a foreskin use this to retract it to expose the glans. Cleanse the meatus using sodium chloride.
- Still holding the penis in your non-dominant hand, extend the penis to straighten it so that it is almost at 90 degrees to the abdomen.
- Insert single-use lubricant gel to minimise urethral trauma and infection (NICE 2017). Some gels contain anaesthetic too. Inserting the gel directly into the urethra opens up and lubricates the length of the urethra. Wait for the time recommended by the manufacturer, usually five minutes, for the anaesthetic to take effect.
- Place a receiver with the catheter on the sterile towel between the person's legs.
- Expose the tip of the catheter by pulling open the wrapper at the serrations.

(Continued)

Box 6.32 (Continued)

- Still keeping the penis extended, grasp the catheter so that the distal end remains in the receiver and gradually advance it out of its wrapper as you insert it into the meatus and downwards along the line of the urethra.
- Advance the catheter 15–20 cm or until urine flows out of the catheter. You may feel some slight resistance at the level of the prostate. Ask the person to cough or take a deep breath to help relax the muscles in this area and allow you to advance the catheter until it reaches the bladder and urine starts to flow.
- Advance the catheter a further 5 cm. Never force the catheter. If resistance is encountered, stop and seek medical advice.
- Inflate the balloon with the correct amount of sterile water, generally 10 mL for adults (NICE 2017). Incorrectly filled balloons can inflate irregularly and irritate the bladder mucosa.
- Ensure the foreskin is replaced back into place.
- Attach the urinary drainage bag, and make the individual comfortable.
- Send a urine specimen, if indicated, and measure and record the urine collected.
- Document the catheterisation in the person's records including date of insertion, catheter size and amount of water used to inflate the balloon. The catheter packaging may have an adhesive label with the catheter's details, which can be used with paper records.

Emptying the catheter bag

Box 6.33 Activity: safely emptying a catheter bag

ACTIVITY

You may recall that microorganisms can be introduced into the drainage system at the junction between the catheter and the bag or via the drainage tap. Bearing this in mind, work out the equipment you would need, and how you would use it, to safely empty a catheter bag. Compare your answer with Box 6.34.

Unless hands are thoroughly washed between individuals and a clean container is used to collect the urine, microorganisms are readily transferred to the next person. Although disinfection of hands with 70% alcohol is rapid and effective, hands that are visibly soiled or potentially grossly contaminated with dirt or organic material must be washed with soap and water (see Chapter 12, section on 'Hand hygiene').

The urinary drainage bag should be emptied frequently enough to maintain urine flow and prevent reflux, and to prevent it from becoming so heavy that its weight pulls on the catheter and causes urethral trauma. There is no evidence that bags need to be changed at specific intervals though they should be changed when damaged or blocked with deposits. Bags should be changed when clinically indicated and/or in line with the manufacturers' recommendations (Pratt et al. 2007). But the key principle – and the way to prevent bacteria or other harmful organisms entering the system – is to leave the closed system alone as much as you can. NICE (2017)

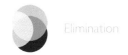

recommends that the connection between the catheter and the drainage system should not be broken except for sound clinical reasons.

Box 6.34 Emptying a catheter bag: equipment and procedure

Equipment

Non-sterile gloves and apron, a heat-disinfected or disposable container, for example, a urinal or jug, paper towel to cover and alcohol swabs.

Procedure

- Explain the procedure to the individual and ensure privacy.
- Wash hands and put on apron and gloves.
- If the drainage bag is on a stand, it may not need removing. If it is hanging on the bed, you may need to access it by removing the bag and placing it over the jug.
- Clean the outlet port with alcohol swab and allow it to dry.
- Open the port and drain the urine into the receptacle, ensuring that the port does not touch the side of the receptacle.
- Close the port and wipe with alcohol swab.
- Reposition bag.
- Cover the container and take to sluice for disposal. Measure the urine first if a fluid balance chart is being kept.
- The container should be disinfected, or macerated, if disposable.
- Remove gloves and apron and wash hands.

Jean has a leg drainage bag attached to her catheter, which can remain unchanged for up to a week as per the manufacturer's advice. A night drainage bag can be attached to the open tap of the leg bag for overnight drainage. This can be removed and discarded during the day as Jean goes back to draining into her leg bag. This process ensures that the closed drainage system is not broken. Disconnection of the catheter from the drainage bag significantly increases the risk of introducing bacteria into the system and should therefore be avoided, if possible (Wilson 2006). Someone with a catheter on drainage who live at home where the risks of cross-infection are low can reuse the night drainage bag for up to one week, if rinsed with water and allowed to dry between use. However, in hospital and other institutional settings, individuals should have a new night drainage bag each time as the risk for cross-contamination and infection is too great to allow reuse. Adding antiseptic or antimicrobial solutions into drainage bags is not recommended (Pratt et al. 2007).

Appropriate positioning of the catheter bag

Catheter bags should be positioned to avoid reflux and facilitate the use of gravity, and positioned clear of floors or other sources of contamination (NICE 2017). Drainage bags should always be positioned below the level of the bladder with the catheter and the inlet tubing secured in a downward position (Colpman and Welford 2004). This is because reflux urine is associated with infection, so bags must be positioned to prevent backflow of urine. When it is difficult to maintain the level of the bag below the bladder, for example, when moving the person, the drainage bag tube should be clamped and the clamp removed only on resumption of dependent drainage (Pratt et al. 2007). The catheter itself should never be clamped as this can easily be damaged.

The catheter should be secured to prevent movement of the catheter within the urethra, which may introduce infection (EAUN 2012). A variety of straps, 'net' sleeves, holsters and sporrans are available to suspend the drainage bag. Securing the catheter also ensures that it does not pull on the urethra and cause ulceration or cleaving where pressure from the tube can split the urethra. In extreme cases, the whole urethra may be split open and require surgical repair (Colpman and Welford 2004; EAUN 2012).

Adequate fluid intake

If the individual's condition allows, encourage oral fluids. This has traditionally been believed to result in dilute urine containing fewer nutrients, thus discouraging the growth of bacteria in the drainage bag and encrustation of components. It is believed that the larger volume of urine maintains a constant flow through the drainage system, making it more difficult for bacteria to multiply in the drainage bag (Wilson 2006). Getliffe and Fader (2007) identified that although there is no clear evidence that drinking large quantities of fluid will prevent infection, in practice it is sensible to promote good fluid intake to prevent dehydration and constipation.

Catheter removal

Box 6.35 Activity: preparing the patient for catheter removal

Think about how you would prepare Jean, or anyone else, for catheter removal.

A clear explanation should be given, emphasising that the procedure is not normally painful but that there may be a feeling of discomfort. Box 6.36 outlines equipment and key points for removing a catheter.

You should ensure that urine is passed satisfactorily after catheter removal and observe for problems such as incontinence, frequency and retention. A person who is confused may need prompting to pass urine (see section on 'Promoting continence'). Some people, particularly men who have had prostate surgery, should perform pelvic floor exercises to help them regain control (see the later section). People with long-term catheters for specific medical reasons will require periodic changing of the catheter depending on clinical need, such as any problems experienced, and/or in line with manufacturers' recommendations (Pratt et al. 2007).

Getliffe and Fader (2007) cover catheterisation in depth, so further reading from that source is recommended.

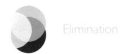

Box 6.36 Removal of a urethral catheter: equipment and procedure

Equipment

- Non-sterile gloves and apron, syringe of sufficient volume to remove the water from the balloon, disposable absorbent pad, receiver and waste bag. If a CSU is required: specimen pot, 20 mL syringe, needle and alcohol swab.

Procedure

- Give explanation, ensure privacy and position the person comfortably. For a female, the knees and hips should be slightly flexed and apart.
- Wash and dry hands and apply gloves and apron.
- Obtain a specimen of urine from the sampling port, if indicated (see Box 6.15).
- Place the disposable pad under the person's buttocks and then place the receiver between the thighs.
- Check the balloon volume and attach an appropriately sized syringe to the balloon port of the catheter. Withdraw the water from the balloon via the syringe.
- Ask the person to breathe in and out, and as they exhale, the catheter is gently withdrawn and placed in the receiver. If problems are encountered, stop and seek medical advice.
- Remove gloves and apron and wash hands.
- The individual should be made to feel comfortable and because increased frequency may be experienced, the nurse should ensure that a toilet or commode is close by.
- If the person needs help with mobility, ensure a call bell is nearby.
- Document the date and time of catheter removal in the clinical notes and record the amount of urine in the catheter bag.
- The individual may be encouraged to increase fluid intake to 'flush' out the bladder.
- Monitor whether the person is passing urine satisfactorily. A chart may be kept so that frequency and amount can be monitored. Also, ask the person to inform a nurse if any unusual symptoms are experienced, for example, dysuria (pain when passing urine).

 Box 6.37 Children and young people: practice points – catheterisation

To read about urethral catheterisation for children and related care, see Macqueen, S., Bruce, E.A. and Gibson, F. 2012. Urinary catheter care. In: *The Great Ormond Street Hospital Manual of Children's Nursing Practices*. Chichester: Wiley-Blackwell, 718–32.

Willock. 2010. Elimination: Collecting, measuring and testing urine. In: Glasper, A., Aylott, M. and Battrick, C. (eds.) *Developing Practical Skills for Nursing Children and Young People*. London: Hodder Arnold, 259–76.

Summary

- Urinary catheterisation is experienced by many individuals in care settings and may be a short-term or long-term measure.
- Catheterisation is an invasive procedure and there are many complications associated with it, infection being particularly common. Therefore, catheterisation should be performed only if there is a clear indication.
- Strict asepsis should be maintained, and the catheter should be removed as soon as possible, using the correct technique.
- Nurses should be aware of the different types of equipment available, and make appropriate choices regarding types of catheter and drainage bag.
- The closed system should not be broken except for good clinical reasons.
- Care should be taken to reduce physical and psychological discomfort for people with urinary catheters.

PREVENTING AND MANAGING CONSTIPATION

Faecal impaction

In very severe constipation, a large mass of faeces that cannot be passed accumulates in the rectum and can back up in the sigmoid colon or even higher (Kyle 2010).

Constipation is a common condition with multifactorial causes. People with constipation can experience various uncomfortable symptoms including headache, bloatedness, loss of appetite, nausea and vomiting (Kyle 2011a). Chronic constipation with faecal impaction is the most important cause of faecal incontinence in frail, older people as the bowel produces mucus to try to soften the hard mass of faeces causing overflow (Kyle 2010).

For some people constipation can be dangerous; Pellatt (2007) explains that if a person with a spinal cord injury above the sixth thoracic vertebra develops bowel distension due to constipation or impaction, they can develop autonomic dysreflexia (severe hypertension), which may lead to cerebral haemorrhage, seizures or cardiac arrest. Risk of constipation should be assessed so that preventative measures can be implemented, rather than waiting until constipation has developed. If constipation occurs, it should be managed effectively to relieve discomfort and prevent complications. Enemas and suppositories may be required to treat constipation, but they are also a means of medicine administration via the rectal route. Therefore, principles of medicine administration should be followed (see Chapter 10).

Box 6.38 Learning outcomes

By the end of this section, you will be able to:

1. identify how to assess risk of constipation;
2. discuss how to prevent and manage constipation;
3. understand key principles of administering suppositories and enemas.

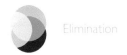

Learning outcome 1: identify how to assess risk of constipation

Box 6.39 Activity: risk factors for constipation

ACTIVITY

What are the likely risk factors for constipation? Think back to individuals you encountered in placement. Who was at risk of constipation?

There are many risk factors for constipation (see Kyle 2007a; Richmond and Wright 2004); some examples of people likely to become constipated will be discussed here. Candy et al. (2011) identified that constipation is common in palliative care and can generate considerable suffering due to the unpleasant physical symptoms. Constipation is more common in people with learning disabilities than the general population (Marsh et al. 2010), particularly if they are less mobile, have inadequate nutrition and fluid intake or are taking long-term medication that has constipation as a side effect (Royal College of Nursing (RCN) 2011). People who are in hospital often experience reduced exercise alongside a changed diet, increasing their risk of constipation. Psychological and environmental factors can also contribute to constipation in hospital. Constipation is a side effect of many medicines including antipsychotic medication (de Hert et al. 2011). Constipation is not an inevitable result of ageing (Holman et al. 2010), but it is common in older people (Gallagher et al. 2008; Kyle 2010; Woodward 2012).

Kyle (2007a, 2009) presents the Norgine risk-assessment tool for constipation (see Figure 6.10). The tool includes the main risk factors for constipation. The assessor ticks and adds up all that apply; the higher the score, the greater the risk. The tool is designed to be used with adults on admission, and alerts nurses to individuals' risk of constipation – leading to proactive preventative measures (Kyle 2007a).

Box 6.40 Activity: Norgine risk-assessment tool

ACTIVITY

Look back at Mark's scenario and, using the Norgine risk-assessment tool in Figure 6.10, assess his risk.

You will have found that the tool is quick and easy to use. Mark's score is 5. Under 'Medical condition', you should have ticked 'History of constipation' and 'Impaired cognition'. For 'Toileting facilities', you should have ticked 'Supervised use of lavatory/commode', and for 'Mobility', you should have identified 'Walks with aids/assistance'. For 'Nutritional intake', Mark 'Needs assistance to eat'. If Mark is prescribed any of the medications listed, these would add to his risk. If Mark's fluid intake is inadequate, his risk increases further.

Norgine® Risk Assessment Tool for Constipation

NORGINE

Medical Condition	
Cancer	
Clinical depression	
Diabetes	
Haemorrhoids, anal fissure, rectocele, local anal or rectal pathology	
History of constipation	
Impaired cognition/dementia	
Multiple sclerosis	
Parkinson's disease	
Postoperative	
Rheumatoid arthritis	
Spinal cord conditions (injury, disease or congenital)	
Stroke	

Current Medication	✓
Aluminium antacids	
Anticholinergics	
Anti-Parkinson drugs	
Antipsychotic drugs	
Calcium channel blockers	
Calcium supplements	
Diuretics	
Iron supplements	
Non-steroidal anti-inflammatory drugs (NSAIDs)	
Opioids	
Tricyclic antidepressants	
Polypharmacy (more than 5 drugs including ones not on this list)	

Toileting Facilities	✓
Bedpan	
Commode by bed in hospital/care home/home	
Supervised use of lavatory/commode	
Commode/raised toilet seat at home (without foot stool)	

Mobility	✓
Restricted to bed	
Restricted to wheelchair/chair	
Walks with aids/assistance	
Walks short distances but less than 1/3 mile (0.5km)	

Nutritional Intake	✓
At nutritional risk as identified by local nutritional screening tool	
Fibre intake 6 g or less per day	
Difficulty in swallowing/chewing	
Needs assistance to eat	

Daily Fluid Intake (see below for calculation table)	✓
Minimum fluids not achieved	

Fluid Requirement Calculation
30 mL fluid per 1kg of body weight

Patients minimum fluid intake should be:

Weight in kg=   × 30 mL=

Patients actual fluid intake is:

PATIENT'S NAME	
PATIENT'S DATE OF BIRTH	
PATIENT'S NHS NUMBER	

INSTRUCTIONS

1. Tick all relevant categories in each table.
2. There may be more than one tick in a table.
3. Add all the ticks together.
4. Fill in the number of ticks in the box below.
5. Date and sign.

DATE	TOTAL NO. OF TICKS	SIGNATURE

Figure 6.10: Norgine risk-assessment tool for constipation. (Reproduced with kind permission from Gaye Kyle, senior lecturer, Thames Valley University; Phil Prynn, continence services manager, Berkshire West PCT; and Terri Dunbar, advanced nurse practitioner, Berkshire West PCT. © 2006 Norgine Pharmaceuticals Ltd.)

Box 6.41 Action to take when risk of constipation is identified

- Complete full bowel assessment using locally approved care pathway.
- Monitor and record bowel movements daily using the Bristol stool chart (see Figure 6.1) and bowel record chart.
- For stool type 1 or 2 on the Bristol stool chart, prescribe appropriate laxative therapy.
- Advise on toileting position.
- Review medication, including over-the-counter medicines.
- Advise on ways to improve mobility.
- Encourage individuals to achieve at least minimum fluid intake.
- Improve nutrition according to nutritional intake score.

Source: Reproduced with kind permission from Gaye Kyle, Senior Lecturer, Thames Valley University; Phil Prynn, Continence Services Manager, Berkshire West PCT; and Terri Dunbar, Advanced Nurse Practitioner, Berkshire West PCT. © 2006 Norgine Pharmaceuticals Ltd.

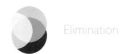

People who, like Mark, score more than four on the Norgine risk-assessment tool should have further assessment leading to appropriate actions (see Box 6.41).

Learning outcome 2: discuss how to prevent and manage constipation

The first section in this chapter included many aspects relevant to preventing constipation in hospital: ensuring that people felt able to ask for assistance, encouraging them to go to the toilet when the 'call to stool' occurs (often early in the morning or about 30 min after a meal), attending to them promptly giving assistance to go out to the toilet when required, ensuring that they are comfortable and well-supported, and giving them unhurried time and privacy.

As regards the correct position to open the bowels, you should advise individuals to:

* sit with the knees higher than the hips;
* lean forward with elbows on knees;
* bulge out the abdomen and straighten the spine.

A footstool may be needed to assist someone into this position. Anyone who can use the toilet or commode can be advised to use this position, unless there are contraindications owing to their medical condition.

Adequate fluid intake is important and dietary fibre should be increased gradually alongside increased fluid intake to prevent bloating. Intake of high-fibre foods, fruits and vegetables should be encouraged according to people's preference. For example, if Mark likes biscuits, he could be encouraged to eat flapjacks, oatcakes, digestive biscuits or fig rolls. Depending on the risk factors, referrals to other health professionals and specialists may be helpful (e.g. doctor, continence adviser, dietician, dentist, physiotherapist, occupational therapist, speech and language therapist and pharmacist). The community nurse for learning disabilities can work with Mark and his mother to ensure that Mark has appropriate multidisciplinary support.

NICE (2007, 2014) advised that people with faecal loading need rectally administered treatment to clear the bowel – which may need to be repeated daily for a few days. If these do not work satisfactorily, oral laxatives should be given and a plan developed to prevent recurrence. The main groups of laxatives are bulking agents (e.g. Isogel, regulan), stimulants (e.g. senna, bisocodyl), stool softeners and lubricants (liquid paraffin, ducoset sodium) and osmotic agents (e.g. lactulose); see the British National Formulary for more details (www.bnf.org). Although laxatives may be necessary to prevent and manage constipation, they are preferable only as a short-term measure. The RCN (2011) identified that, for people with learning disabilities, there has been an overreliance on laxatives rather than promoting adequate nutrition and fluid intake. Where feasible, medicines that predispose to constipation should be avoided particularly in those who are at risk. Exercise should be increased, if possible.

A digital rectal examination (DRE) might be carried out to check for faecal impaction, and for abnormalities such as blood, pain or obstruction. DRE involves observing the perianal area and inserting a gloved and lubricated finger into the rectum (Kyle 2007b). You will also see DREs carried out during abdominal examinations of individuals and for screening for rectal or prostate cancer, or prostate enlargement (Steggall 2008). Digital removal of faeces (DRF) (using a lubricated, gloved finger) is an invasive procedure only conducted after individual assessment, but it can be part of the bowel management regime for some individuals, for example those with spinal cord injuries (RCN 2019). DRE and DRF can be carried out only by registered nurses who can demonstrate competence in these skills, but they can also delegate these procedures to carers or individuals' in their care if their competence has been assessed (RCN 2019). These procedures are invasive and require consent of the individual; the RCN (2019) discusses these procedures and consent issues. There are contraindications to these procedures and potential risks, and many organisations have developed their own policies. Steggall and Cox (2009) explain the DRE procedure in detail.

In some instances, suppositories or enemas may be needed to treat constipation – these are considered in learning outcome 3.

Learning outcome 3: understand key principles of administering suppositories and enemas

An enema is a liquid that is inserted into the rectum, whereas a suppository is a medicated solid formulation, usually torpedo-shaped, that is inserted into the rectum, where it dissolves at body temperature. An enema that should be retained following administration is termed a 'retention enema' and is primarily used for its local effect. For example, a steroid enema may be administered to people with ulcerative colitis for its anti-inflammatory effect. An 'evacuant enema' is given to initiate bowel emptying and is used for constipation or to empty the bowel prior to surgery or investigations of the gastrointestinal tract. Suppositories are often administered for evacuant purposes, but they are also often used to administer medication and may be administered as a local treatment, as for haemorrhoids.

> **Box 6.42 Activity: rectally prescribed drugs**
>
> Drugs commonly prescribed rectally include paracetamol (for its analgesic and/or antipyretic effect) and anticonvulsants. What are the advantages and disadvantages of this route of drug administration?

ACTIVITY

You might have thought of the following advantages:

- The rectum is an alternative route for when people cannot take oral medication because they are vomiting, unable to swallow or are 'nil by mouth' (e.g. preoperatively).
- Drugs administered rectally are absorbed into the bloodstream and bypass the liver (Greenstein 2009). For example, a person who is having a seizure cannot take oral medication, and rectal administration is safer and more rapid than intramuscular injections. As faecal impaction can inhibit rectal drug absorption, constipation should be prevented in people who might require emergency rectal medication.

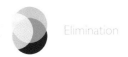

Disadvantages include:

- Suppository and enema administration is more invasive and embarrassing than oral administration and involves some discomfort, undressing and moving into the correct position.
- Traumatic and even fatal side effects of enemas, including inflammation, electrolyte imbalance and perforation of the colonic mucosa have been reported (Schmelzer and Wright 1996). Newer, small, pre-packaged enemas aim to prevent such problems. However, enemas should only be used if there is no other alternative.

Prior to administering an enema or suppository, the nurse should carefully assess the appropriateness of this route.

Box 6.43 Activity: contraindications

Can you think of any physical problems that might be contraindications?

ACTIVITY

Anal fissure

A painful crack in the mucous membrane of the anus, generally caused by hard faeces.

Rectal prolapse

A protrusion of rectal mucosa through the anus.

ACTIVITY

Contraindications might include recent colorectal or gynaecological surgery, malignancy or other pathology of the perineal area, and a low platelet count, as this predisposes to bleeding. Thus, the nurse should check with both the person and the case notes for any previous anorectal surgery or abnormalities. Further visual inspection should also be made immediately before administration. The perianal region should be checked for abnormalities, including haemorrhoids, anal fissure and rectal prolapse.

Box 6.44 Activity: enemas and suppositories

Find out what types of enemas and suppositories are available to evacuate the bowel. There may be examples in the skills laboratory, or you can look at them in your practice setting.

When giving an enema or suppositories for evacuation purposes, there can be a choice of products.

Suppositories may be of the type that will simply soften the stools, or they may have a stimulant effect. Greenstein (2009) recommends that glycerol suppositories are satisfactory and other types offer no advantage. There are microenemas available containing only 5 mL of solution that can act as a colon stimulant. For more vigorous bowel cleansing (e.g. prior to a bowel investigation), a larger phosphate enema may be used. Phosphate enemas work through osmosis – by extracting water from the bowel to draw into faeces, thus increasing the faecal mass (Bowers 2006). Bowers asserts that there is a lack of evidence to support use of phosphate enemas for constipation above other products, but that they are an effective way of clearing the colon prior to flexible sigmoidoscopy. Complications of phosphate enemas are rare but can be serious. People with severe constipation often have other underlying

Flexible sigmoidoscopy

The sigmoid colon is examined with a lighted scope, usually for bleeding, non-cancerous growths (polyps) or colorectal cancer.

conditions that may make them more at risk of complications. It is important to check the manufacturer's instructions when administering a phosphate enema. There are a number of contraindications, and the RCN (2019) advises that they may be contraindicated for older or debilitated individuals and people with renal impairment. The systematic review of sodium phosphate enema administration by Mendoza et al. (2007) identified that side effects (mainly water and electrolyte disturbances) were rare, mainly occurring in the very young (under 5 years) or people older than 65 years. Individuals suffering side effects often had conditions such as neurological, gastrointestinal or renal disorders.

Box 6.46 provides guidance for safe administration of suppositories/enemas based on the evidence available.

Box 6.45 Children and young people: practice points – constipation

Constipation within childhood is a very common problem (Gordon et al. 2012) and NICE (2010a) has produced detailed guidelines. For further reading, see

Macqueen, S., Bruce, E.A. and Gibson, F. 2012. Bowel care. In: *The Great Ormond Street Hospital Manual of Children's Nursing Practices.* Chichester: Wiley-Blackwell, 87–101.

Slater-Smith, S. 2010. Promoting children's continence B) Childhood constipation. In: Glasper, A., Aylott, M. and Battrick, C. (eds.) *Developing Practical Skills for Nursing Children and Young People.* London: Hodder Arnold, 229–41.

Box 6.46 Administration of enemas and suppositories: equipment and procedure

Equipment

An absorbent underpad, tissues, lubricating gel, the enema or suppository/ies, gloves and apron. Ensure that a good light source is available and that privacy can be maintained.

Procedure

- Local medicine policy should be followed (see Chapter 10). Check the expiry date of suppositories/enema.
- Explain the procedure and gain consent (by using communication methods that ensure the person understands and is able to provide informed consent). If the person is known to regularly require rectal anticonvulsants, consent should be obtained in advance and documented.
- Some people can insert a suppository themselves; if so, carefully explain the procedure.
- Ensure privacy, dignity and sensitivity throughout the procedure.
- Maintain infection control procedures throughout: hand hygiene, use of gloves and aprons, correct waste disposal (see Chapter 12).
- Give explanations, encouragement and reassurance.
- Some enemas should be warmed before administration – check the manufacturer's instructions. Warm by placing the enema in a jug of warm water. The temperature should be slightly higher than body temperature, feeling warm to the wrist (Schmelzer and Wright 1996).

(Continued)

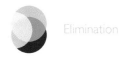

Box 6.46 (Continued)

- Position the person on the left side to allow easy flow of the fluid into the rectum by following the individual's anatomy. Place the underpad under the person's buttocks, and ask them to lie at the edge of the bed with knees flexed, and covered by a blanket. This position aids the passage of the nozzle of the enema through the anal canal. This position may need adapting for someone with a physical disability.
- Examine the area around the anus (see discussion on contraindications).
- **Enemas**: Remove the enema cap, expel any air from the enema container (if introduced into the colon this can cause distension and discomfort). Lubricate the nozzle of the enema (some enemas have a pre-lubricated tip). Part the buttocks and gently insert into the anal canal. Squeeze the fluid gently into the rectum from the base of the container to prevent backflow. Some enemas include one-way valves that prevent backflow. Then slowly withdraw the container nozzle to avoid reflux emptying of the rectum.
- Clean the perianal area and make the person comfortable.
- **Suppositories**: Lubricate the end of the suppository with the gel. There is conflicting evidence about which end should be inserted first (Bradshaw et al. 2009). Abd-el-Maeboud et al. (1991) suggested that inserting the blunt end first allowed the contracting sphincter to close tightly around the anus, aiding retention. However, most manufacturers suggest the pointed end is inserted first; follow the manufacturer's advice unless local policy advises otherwise. If there is stool present in the rectum, introduce the suppository around the side of the stool, so that it is in contact with the bowel mucosa; avoid embedding it in the stool, which will be ineffective (Bradshaw et al. 2009). Wipe the person's perianal area.
- If the enema or suppository/ies were given to empty the bowel, ask the person to retain it inside for as long as possible (Schmelzer and Wright 1996). The individual may find it more comfortable to remain lying down. However, an enema can be very difficult to hold on to for long as the effect is likely to be rapid.
- The person should be assisted to the toilet or other receptacle as necessary.
- Medication administered as a suppository should be retained by the person. With a retention enema, the individual should remain lying down for the amount of time prescribed on the manufacturer's instructions.
- A call bell must be near at hand.
- Document that the enema/suppository/ies have been administered in the nursing notes or prescription chart of a medication.
- If the enema or suppositories were given to empty the bowel, you will need to note the result using the Bristol stool chart (see Figure 6.1).

 Box 6.47 Pregnancy and birth: practice points – constipation

Constipation is very common in late pregnancy possibly due to circulating progesterone causing slower gastrointestinal movement (Jewell and Young 2009). Dietary supplements of fibre, such as bran or wheat fibre, are likely to be helpful, but if the problem persists, stimulant laxatives are recommended (Jewell and Young 2009).

Summary

- Constipation is a common condition that can cause considerable discomfort. The causes are multifactoral and a risk-assessment tool can help nurses to identify people at risk.

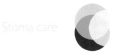

- Prevention of constipation involves adequate fibre and fluid intake, exercise and avoiding constipation-inducing medicines, if possible. Laxatives can be used but should be a short-term measure.
- Suppositories or enemas may be given to administer medication or to evacuate the bowel. Careful assessment should precede administration as there are contraindications.
- Preparation of the individual should include explanation and gaining consent, correct choice of enema/suppositories and other equipment, maintenance of dignity and privacy, and correct positioning of the person to prevent damage to the wall of the rectum.

STOMA CARE

Some people have to cope with major changes to the way they empty their bladder or bowels. In some cases, the only remedy is the removal of the malfunctioning or diseased bladder or intestine. A stoma is formed (see example, Figure 6.11), and the person wears an appliance that attaches to the abdomen to collect and dispose of the elimination products.

There are three main types of stoma:

- *Ileal conduit* – formed to drain urine into the stoma bag, if the bladder is removed or bypassed.
- *Ileostomy* – formed when the whole of the large bowel is removed (liquid stool is collected by the stoma bag).
- *Colostomy* – formed when only part of the large bowel is removed (faeces are usually more formed and solid or semi-solid).

Colostomies are the most common types of stoma with more than 11,000 formed a year, compared with approximately 6,500 ileostomies and just over 2000 ileal conduits (Coloplast 2010).

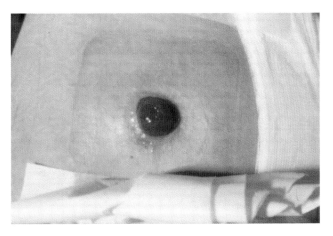

Figure 6.11: An example of a stoma.

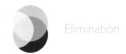

This surgery requires careful planning and major inputs by stoma care nurses and other members of the multidisciplinary team. Their roles are meant to ensure that the individual is able to recover and reintegrate into society and the family and cope with everyday life (Parascandolo and Doughty 2001). Not all surgery can be planned, and sometimes a stoma is formed after emergency surgery. These individuals therefore have no preparation or stoma nurse involvement prior to surgery, making it more difficult for them to come to terms with the changes and learn to look after their stoma (Erwin-Toth 2003; Richbourg et al. 2007). Whether planned or not, caring for this group of individuals is always a challenge (Erwin-Toth 2003). This section focuses on key aspects of nursing care. Other specialist textbooks should be consulted for further details.

Box 6.48 Learning outcomes

By the end of this section, you will be able to:

1. identify the main indications for stoma formation;
2. show awareness of the range of equipment commonly used for the different types of stoma;
3. discuss the care required for people who have a stoma.

Learning outcome 1: identify the main indications for stoma formation

Box 6.49 Activity: diseases of the bladder or bowel

Make a list of some diseases that may lead to someone's bladder or small or large bowel having to be removed or bypassed, resulting in stoma formation.

ACTIVITY

Different types of stoma and the reasons for their formation are discussed below.

Ileal conduit

This is formed when the person's lower urinary tract is malfunctioning. The most common cause is bladder cancer, where the bladder is removed. However, ileal conduits are also an option for individuals with intractable incontinence or post-pelvic trauma. The ureters are attached to a segment of small bowel (ileum), which is brought to the surface of the body forming a stoma, and draining into a urostomy bag. It is usually sited in the right iliac fossa or, though rarely, on the left.

Ileostomy

This can be formed for cancer of the bowel but most commonly for individuals with inflammatory bowel disease such as ulcerative colitis. When the disease progresses to the point when the pain and diarrhoea and urgency become debilitating and interferes with quality of life, then sometimes an ileostomy is recommended. The stoma is usually in the right iliac fossa. The stoma is made of the small bowel. Nowadays, some individuals opt to have an ileoanal pouch formed instead of having

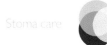

a permanent ileostomy. In this case, a temporary ileostomy is usually formed first. An ileoanal pouch is an internal reservoir made of bowel in which faecal matter collects and is emptied out by a catheter inserted into a continent stoma. The ileostomy is formed to allow the pouch to heal before being reversed and allowing faecal matter to move into the pouch (Black 2012).

Colostomy

Partial resection of the large intestine means that the stoma is formed of the person's large bowel. Colon cancer may result in partial bowel resection and stoma formation. Unlike the ileostomy or the ileal conduit, this stoma can be positioned in different parts of the abdomen, depending on the part of the colon that is being removed. The stoma can be placed in either the sigmoid, descending, ascending or transverse colon. This can be a permanent stoma (called a 'permanent end-colostomy') or a temporary one. A temporary colostomy is used when the bowel is not being resected but may need time to heal. Collecting faeces in the stoma bag rather than allowing it to move down the colon promotes this healing. The bowel is partially opened and both ends are brought through the stoma still attached on one side. A plastic 'bridge' is fixed in place under the bowel stoma to stop it slipping back into the abdomen. The stoma is reversed when the two sections of bowel are reattached to each other and pushed back into the abdomen before closing the wound.

Learning outcome 2: show awareness of the range of equipment commonly used for the different types of stoma

Box 6.50 Activity: stoma appliances

In the skills laboratory, there may be sterile or non-sterile (for demonstration purposes) stoma appliances complete with packaging material. See Figure 6.12 for examples. If you can access 'real' equipment, take note of the following:

- the manner in which it is packaged, batch number, expiry date
- the difference between one- and two-piece bags and emptying devices
- the different materials forming the baseplate or flange and how these affect the flexibility of the appliance

There are a huge number of appliances available for individuals to choose from. Most bags are made specifically to cope with the output of a particular type of stoma. They come in one- or two-piece format:

- The **one piece** (Figure 6.12a and d) has the bag and flange or baseplate (i.e. the flat part that sticks to the person's abdomen) attached to each other. To change the bag, the whole appliance is peeled off the abdomen and replaced by a new one.
- The **two piece** (Figure 6.12b and c) has a separate bag that clicks on to the baseplate (similar to a Tupperware lid) (Figure 6.12e). In some products, a locking

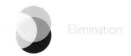

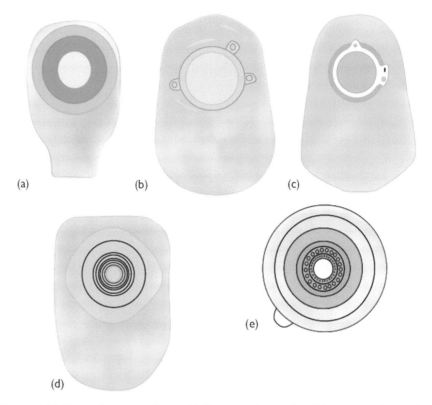

Figure 6.12: Types of stoma appliances. (a) One-piece drainage bag; (b) two-piece drainage bag; (c) two-piece non-drainable bag; (d) one-piece non-drainable bag; (e) flange/baseplate for fitting with two-piece systems, for example, (b) and (c).

system can be activated to ensure greater security. If the bag needs changing, it can simply be clicked off and replaced by a new one. As the baseplate remains in place rather than being peeled off the skin each time, it is kinder to the skin. If a person has to change bags more than once a day (e.g. for religious reasons), then a two-piece appliance allows them to do this without compromising the skin by having to change the baseplate each time.

The baseplate is usually made of a hydrocolloid (natural or artificial) with an integral adhesive area. This can have an extra taped area surrounding it for extra security. This taped area is also more flexible than the hydrocolloid area and can fit to the body's contours more easily (Black 2012). The bags can be clear plastic or flesh coloured.

Bags may be drainable or non-drainable:

- **Drainable bags** (Figure 6.12a and b). As ileal conduit and ileostomy stomas produce constant liquid output, bags are used, which can be emptied via a tap (if urine) or via an opening device like a clip (if stool; see Figure 6.12a and b). This means individuals do not need to change their bags each time, especially if they choose to wear a one-piece bag. Bags should be able to hold a reasonable capacity to avoid individuals constantly having to empty the bags. Bags come in different sizes – from paediatric (holding as little as 100 mL) to adult (holding anything up to 750 mL). If the colostomy is in the ascending or hepatic flexure of the transverse colon, then the output is semi-solid and a drainable bag should be used.

- **Non-drainable bags** (Figure 6.12c and d). These are used for the more formed output of colostomies sited in the descending or sigmoid colon. The person simply must change the bag once they have had their bowels open and dispose of it with its contents. Some companies now produce biodegradable colostomy bags that can be flushed down the toilet. Many individuals can anticipate when they are going to have their bowels open because, if regular, most people have them open at a certain time of day (e.g. morning, before or after breakfast) and usually only once a day. Thus, bags need not be large or bulky as the person can anticipate when a larger bag is warranted.

Some people prefer not to wear a colostomy bag. They wear a small pouch or cap to cover the stoma. To ensure they do not have their bowels open unexpectedly, they opt to perform a washout or irrigation of the bowel. This is similar to a rectal washout but performed via the stoma instead. Ensuring the bowel is clean in this way means that elimination is predictable and most individuals achieve complete continence in between washouts. The whole procedure can take 30–60 min, though experienced individuals can complete it in 15 min (Collett 2002; Karadag et al. 2005).

Use of suppositories or enemas with stomas

If a person becomes constipated, then suppositories or an enema can be inserted down the stoma to either lubricate or stimulate the bowel to pass a motion (Collett 2002). However, specific techniques are required as there are no sphincters to control motions in stomas (see Williams 2012). Suppositories should not be inserted into ileostomies as these do not become constipated and lack of output is likely to be a blockage (Williams 2012).

Learning outcome 3: discuss the care required for people who have a stoma

Box 6.51 Activity: stoma surgery care

ACTIVITY

Try to put yourself in the place of a person who has to have stoma surgery. What feelings or fears do you have? What skills do you think you will have to learn to be able to care for yourself once you recover?

Preoperative preparation

Effective preoperative preparation is essential and individuals should therefore be referred to a stoma care nurse specialist well in advance. There may be psychological issues such as coping with a change in body image. Meeting a person who has already had a stoma can help individuals to see what living life with an appliance is really like. Bowel preparation is necessary only if the person is impacted with faeces, which cannot be cleared by restricting food intake and only allowing fluids to drink.

Siting the stoma is an extremely important consideration. The stoma care nurse specialist will address both physical and social aspects during assessment, ensuring that

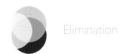
the bag will not hinder the person's daily activities. It is also important to ensure the individual is not allergic to the adhesive or hydrocolloid in the baseplate, the plastic material or cover of the drainage bag, so a patch test should be carried out.

Postoperative care

The most vital part of the postoperative care is to ensure that the stoma is viable and healing well. Besides the usual postoperative care after major abdominal surgery, the stoma should be checked to ensure it is pink and warm and it should adhere to the abdominal wall. The stoma should not look blue or black, or feel cold as this means that the circulation is compromised and if allowed to deteriorate, the stoma may become sloughed, black and necrotic. The output should be checked; if it is an ileal conduit, then the output should be urine; if it is a colostomy, then there may be flatus though not necessarily stool; and an ileostomy should have some liquid faecal matter.

Sometimes, there is a delay in the stoma becoming active and producing faeces. Any prolonged delay should be reported as the person may need more surgery. Diet following stoma formation needs consideration, both postoperatively and in the long term (see Floruta 2001).

Teaching self-care

Ideally, people are discharged from hospital only when they have learnt how to care for their stoma. Usually, individuals are ready to start learning how to empty and change the bags after the first week following surgery. The person must also learn what a normal stoma looks like, how it should function and what complications to look out for, as well as how to clean the stoma area and how to safely dispose of the output and the appliances. Ideally, the individual should have the support of district nurses or community stoma care nurses on returning home to help adjust to living with a stoma in a non-hospital environment (Richbourg et al. 2007). People with learning disabilities may require additional time to learn about the care requirements and may need longer-term assistance, this can sometimes be from paid carers or family who can assist either through prompting or direct care.

Managing the appliance

The stoma is usually swollen postoperatively, but it slowly shrinks to a more normal size as the person recovers. The baseplates that adhere to the abdomen need a central aperture cut out to fit around the stoma. These baseplates are usually all one size but are made such that the hydrocolloid area varies in size, allowing it to be cut to fit all sizes of stoma. The nurse specialist will provide a template of the correct size that the person can use to cut out a hole in the centre of the baseplates. This must fit snugly around the stoma without being too tight or cutting off circulation to the stoma. Correct fitting ensures that the skin under the baseplate is protected from the effluent produced by the stoma, which otherwise may cause excoriation and leakage and result in the bag not adhering securely and falling off. As the stoma shrinks, this template may have to be altered.

Stoma appliances are available on prescription and are provided free of cost to individuals with a stoma in the United Kingdom. They can be obtained from pharmacies, though many individuals prefer to use supply companies who deliver the

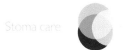

appliances in discreet packages directly to their homes. Delivery in most cases is within 24 h of placing an order, and many companies provide extras such as cleaning wipes and disposal bags at no extra cost. If the person finds it difficult to cut the template openings, then these companies also provide a cutting service using a personalised template that the person can send in or that the nurse specialist can fax to the company.

Box 6.52 Activity: when to change an appliance

What equipment do you think you will need to change an appliance?

The materials needed to change a stoma appliance are as follows:

- a new appliance
- wipes for cleaning and drying skin
- warm water
- a waste disposal bag (at home the individual may use a nappy sac)
- scissors (if the baseplate is not pre-cut)
- measuring guide, to measure the size of stoma and cut out correct size in template for baseplate
- gloves and apron

Once the old baseplate and bag are removed, the skin and stoma are cleaned using warm water and a soft wipe. The skin around the stoma is dried thoroughly to ensure the new baseplate sticks to the abdominal skin securely. Applying gentle but firm pressure over the baseplate helps this process. If the baseplate cannot lie flat on the abdomen, then there are products (e.g. stoma paste) and appliances that can help – the stoma care nurse specialist can advise.

Someone with ileal conduits may wish to clip a larger drainage bag to the tap at the bottom of the stoma bag at night. Once the tap is open, urine will drain out of the stoma bag into the larger drainage bag. This ensures that the stoma bag will not leak or come off if it becomes too full of urine when the person is in bed.

Colostomy bags come with built-in flatus outlets to let gas out as it builds up in the bag. This allows the bag to lie flat under clothes and not come off or leak because of the build-up.

Box 6.53 Activity: emptying a stoma bag

What steps would you follow to teach Jean to empty her stoma bag?

Jean should be encouraged to do this by herself as soon as possible following recovery from the effects of surgery. She should be supervised as she goes through the following steps:

- Encourage her to find the best position, such as sitting on the toilet or kneeling or standing beside it.
- Put toilet paper in the toilet bowl to avoid splashback.

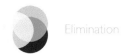

- Open the tap/clip/Velcro end of the bag and drain into the toilet bowl.
- Squeeze out all the contents.
- Close and clean the tap/clip/Velcro on the outside to avoid staining clothing.
- Flush the toilet and wash her hands (Stoma Care 2007).

Box 6.54 Activity: disposal of stoma equipment

ACTIVITY

How should you dispose of used stoma equipment in a hospital? How would Jean dispose of used stoma equipment at home?

In hospital, hand hygiene and use of gloves and apron are necessary (see Chapter 12), and the equipment should be disposed of in the infective waste bag unless local policy advises otherwise. The DH (2006) advised that, in the community, stoma care waste can be disposed of in the black-bag waste stream. Accordingly, Stoma Care (2007) advises that disposal at home does not require any special arrangements and suggests that, after emptying, the appliance can be wrapped in newspaper, put in a nappy sac and disposed of in normal household refuse. However, if when at home Jean developed any type of gastrointestinal infection or the site became infected, her bag must be disposed of as infectious waste – the community nurse should advise her about this.

Most bags can stay on for up to 3 days as long as the person is comfortable. Some people may prefer to change the bags daily, so regimes must be tailored to individuals (Erwin-Toth 2003). If the skin becomes sensitive there are specially developed non-greasy lotions to sooth it and protect it from the adhesive. There are also lotions or wipes that dry on application to the skin forming a plastic barrier layer to protect the skin under the baseplate.

Teaching individuals how to change bags and care for the stoma can be time-consuming. Someone with a learning disability or physical problems with dexterity or eyesight may need a lot of time and input from nurses and carers. If Jean, the person in our scenario, cannot change the bag and care for the stoma herself, her husband may have to do it instead. Even if Jean is successful, she will need his help and support as someone will have to take over this part of her care should she become ill and unable to cope. This may be problematic for her husband who has problems with his sight. It is imperative, therefore, that Jean learns how to care for this herself no matter how much time it takes for her to become confident and competent. People should not be rushed; support and continued teaching should ideally continue after discharge.

All stomas present similar management problems for people. Individuals should be followed up regularly by the stoma nurse to continue supporting the person and to identify and deal with any problems. Richbourg et al. (2007) found that people who had been counselled by nurses both before and after surgery suffered fewer complications – or at least found they coped with them more effectively. Individuals who had their stoma sites marked preoperatively and were assessed by a stoma nurse also suffered fewer problems with sore skin and badly fitting appliances (Parascandolo

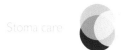

and Doughty 2001; Ratliff et al. 2005). However, complications such as stenosis, prolapse, incisional or bowel hernias or disease progression could not be predicted or avoided by nursing intervention.

Nurses should be aware of other complications that often occur, including sexual dysfunction (e.g. after cystectomy for bladder cancer), problems with body image, decrease in social activities and interaction, isolation, anxiety and depression (Ratliff et al. 2005), and have strategies in place to help individuals cope. This may include counselling or regular visits to nurse clinics to reinforce teaching and offer support. The likelihood of long-term complications (e.g. upper urinary tract changes in people with an ileal conduit) increases the longer the person has a stoma (Madersbacher et al. 2003).

Caring for individuals with a stoma who have dementia

There are different types of dementia that produce similar symptoms that may progress and be treated differently (Nazarko 2011). One of the main problems for people with dementia is memory loss, which can occur early at the onset of the disease and has significant impact on the ability to learn and retain new information or experiences (Milwain 2010). Learning how to care for a stoma has a huge impact on anyone and for someone with dementia, this may be even more challenging. Many people (who have a stoma) with dementia do not acknowledge that they even have a stoma, so teaching them to care for it presents challenges for healthcare professionals and carers alike, for example, inappropriate disposal of stoma bags.

People with dementia need more time to acclimatise to the ward environment before surgery, and their discharge should be delayed until they are able to take care of themselves (Black 2011). Nurses teaching these individuals should take the time to get to know the person and identify their specific needs such as what causes them anxiety or triggers challenging behaviour. Any care should be tailored to the needs of individuals and their carers (Scottish Intercollegiate Guidelines Network [SIGN] 2006). Black (2011) advocates individualised learning programmes that take into consideration the person's memory, communication and understanding problems. She also advises that how and where the person is taught may also impact on the eventual outcome, for example, teaching self-care in small steps and in an environment that is quiet and has fewer distractions. Using repetition and ensuring continuity also helps.

However, being completely independent in caring for the stoma may be beyond some individuals' abilities no matter how much time and care is invested. Ultimately, having a stoma may result in someone with dementia going into residential care because relatives and carers cannot cope with the extra stress of a stoma (Black 2011). Healthcare professionals therefore face an ethical dilemma when it comes to performing this surgery in individuals with dementia as it can have a far-reaching impact on the quality of life of both the person and their carers.

Caring for young people with a stoma

If possible, the young person should be offered an alternative surgery to avoid them having a permanent stoma. However, this may not always be appropriate or feasible. Nurses who care for individuals of this age group need to have an understanding of

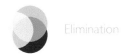

adolescent physical and cognitive development and what young people want from the hospital experience and those who care for them. Ideally, they should be cared for in special units that have specific facilities and staff trained to support young people.

During adolescence, the young person is developing both physically and cognitively, and it is during this period that they address issues around their sexual development, self-esteem and body image. So, having stoma care surgery at this time could impact greatly on normal development and their ability to build relationships and reach maturity (Busuttil Leaver and Leach 2004). Communication is key to building a rapport. Nurses should develop active listening skills, be non-judgemental, straightforward in approach, use clear language and ensure privacy (Deering and Cody 2002). Nurses should be prepared to offer alternatives and allow for compromise when setting limits. The way a young person copes with illness, hospitalisation, disability and the family dynamics should also be assessed especially in long-term illness. Physical and psychological care should go hand in hand to help the young person cope.

Summary

- Having stoma surgery is life-changing and can have serious psychological consequences for individuals such as problems with body image.
- Planned, individualised preoperative preparation, and postoperative care and teaching minimise complications and help people cope and achieve self-care.
- Understanding these problems and having a good knowledge of stoma appliances and accessory products will help nurses offer acceptable solutions to individuals and in some cases avoid further surgery.
- However, complications cannot always be anticipated and tend to increase the longer a person has a stoma.
- Continued support of the person and/or carer and long-term follow-up will help ensure the individual continues to have a good quality of life and ultimate survival.
- Special consideration should be given to supporting people with dementia or young people who have stomas formed, and how adjustment and self-care can be facilitated.

PROMOTING CONTINENCE AND MANAGING INCONTINENCE

The DH (2010) defines continence as: 'people's control of their bladder and bowel function' (p. 7). Urinary incontinence is the inability to control the leakage of urine and is a common and distressing problem (Wallace et al. 2009). Faecal incontinence is defined as the involuntary passage of faecal material through the anal canal (Deutekom and Dobben 2012). This section focuses on understanding the causes and effects of incontinence and practical issues of management, but not specialist interventions. Continence is a huge topic to which whole books are devoted; for example, Getliffe and Dolman (2007) cover all aspects in detail.

Box 6.55 Learning outcomes

By the end of this section, you will be able to:

1 discuss the causes and effects of urinary and faecal incontinence;
2 explain principles of assessment relating to incontinence;
3 identify interventions for promoting urinary continence;
4 discuss appropriate nursing interventions for promoting faecal continence and managing faecal incontinence;
5 explain the nursing management of incontinence.

Learning outcome 1: discuss the causes and effects of urinary and faecal incontinence

Continence is a complex skill and relies on being able to recognise the need to eliminate faeces and/or urine, identify an appropriate place in which to eliminate and being able to wait until arriving there. When any of these fail, incontinence occurs.

Box 6.56 Activity: what causes urinary and faecal incontinence

ACTIVITY

Reflect back on individuals you have been in contact with and consider what causes urinary and faecal incontinence?

Urinary incontinence

Causes are diverse and varied and you may see different classifications in different texts. The main types are as follows:

Urge incontinence: leakage of urine when a person is unable to control the strong desire to pass urine (void) (Wallace et al. 2009) as a result of overactivity of the detrusor (bladder) muscle (overactive bladder syndrome) (Pellatt 2012).

Stress urinary incontinence: the involuntary leakage of urine on effort or exertion, for example, on sneezing or coughing, presumably due to raised abdominal pressure; contributing factors include: obesity, high-impact sport and severe constipation (Billington 2010).

Mixed urinary incontinence: where there is involuntary urine leakage associated with both urgency and exertion, effort, sneezing or coughing (NICE 2019a).

Functional incontinence: the inability to get to the toilet in time due to mobility or other functional difficulties such as dexterity.

Although urinary incontinence can be an isolated condition, it also occurs in the context of other health problems, particularly those that affect activity (Chiarelli and Weatherall 2010). Some medicines can contribute to incontinence; Bob's incontinence was probably caused by clozapine. Studies have indicated an association between urinary incontinence and diabetes (Jackson et al. 2005; Lewis et al. 2005). As the central and peripheral nervous systems regulate bladder function, neurological conditions, such as multiple sclerosis, often affect continence (see NICE 2012 for a detailed consideration). Bar and Sowney (2007) identified that incontinence rates are often higher among people with learning disabilities due to accompanying physical

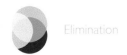

disabilities and impaired mobility. People with learning as well as a physical disability may not be able to communicate that they need to be taken to the toilet, especially if staff are not familiar with their method of communicating this need, which may be through signing or symbols. People with dementia may develop functional incontinence due to difficulties in finding the toilet, memory problems, poor manual dexterity, impaired cognition or reduced mobility (Hägglund 2010). The unfamiliarity of the hospital environment may increase these difficulties for all individuals. For prevalence of urinary incontinence, see Box 6.57.

Box 6.57 Estimated prevalence of urinary incontinence

Women living at home

15–44 years: between 1 in 20 and 1 in 14

45–64 years: between 1 in 13 and 1 in 7

Aged 65 years plus: between 1 in 10 and 1 in 5

Men living at home

15–64 years: over 1 in 33

Aged 65 years plus: between 1 in 14 and 1 in 10

Both sexes living in institutions

One-third of those in residential homes

Nearly two-thirds of those in nursing homes

One-half to two-thirds in wards for older people, or older people with mental health problems

Source: Department of Health (DH). 2000. *Good Practice in Continence Services.* London: DH.

Faecal incontinence

NICE (2007) identifies that faecal incontinence is a sign or symptom, not a disease. High-risk groups for faecal incontinence include: people who are old and frail, have loose stools/diarrhoea from any cause, have a neurological or spinal disease/injury, have severe cognitive impairment, urinary incontinence, pelvic organ prolapse or rectal prolapse following colonic resection or anal surgery, people with learning disabilities and women following obstetric injury in childbirth (NICE 2007). NICE (2007) asserted that faecal incontinence is largely a hidden problem due to its social stigma but estimates that up to 10% of adults are affected by faecal incontinence and between 0.5% and 1% of adults have regular faecal incontinence affecting their quality of life.

Establishing accurate prevalence figures for incontinence in the population can be problematic as people do not always seek help for continence issues.

Box 6.58 Activity: not seeking help for continence problems

ACTIVITY

Consider: why might people not seek help for continence problems?

There are two main reasons for non-reporting of incontinence: embarrassment, and the belief that nothing can be done to help. MacDonald and Butler (2007) identified the isolation of women with incontinence who did not talk to anyone about it as they felt it was not a socially acceptable topic of conversation and that it was untreatable. Wells and Wagg (2007) found that Bangladeshi women saw bladder weakness as a loss of self-control and a personal problem rather than a medical problem, so they did not seek professional help. People's definitions of incontinence vary, so they may not interpret their problem as incontinence. Studies have found that older people with urinary incontinence consider it to be an inevitable part of ageing (Avery et al. 2006; Palmer and Newman 2006) and even some nursing staff share this view with individuals and relatives (Kristiansen et al. 2011). However, urinary incontinence is not a disease or a normal result of ageing, but a symptom of an underlying condition.

You read in the scenario that Bob was distressed and embarrassed about his urinary incontinence.

Box 6.59 Activity: effects of incontinence

How might incontinence affect people: physically, psychologically and socially?

The many possible effects include physical (e.g. increased falls, skin problems, dependency), social (e.g. impact on relationships, sexuality, employment and leisure) and psychological (e.g. embarrassment, lack of self-esteem). Kristiansen et al. (2011) identified that urinary incontinence led to increased vulnerability, loss of independence and a feeling of being a burden. Faecal incontinence is a particularly distressing condition with significant medical, social and economic implications (Norton and Cody 2012). Faecal incontinence is also a common reason for older people to need nursing home care (Brown et al. 2013).

To accurately assess the underlying cause and suggest possible ways of managing incontinence, a thorough assessment is necessary (see learning outcome 2).

Learning outcome 2: explain principles of assessment relating to incontinence

As people are often too embarrassed to report incontinence to health professionals, staff should provide opportunities for people to discuss any concerns about their bladder or bowel functions during consultations and offer an initial bladder and bowel continence assessment, as indicated (DH 2010). As discussed under learning outcome 1, there are many possible underlying causes of incontinence. Temporary causes of urinary incontinence, such as UTI, confusion, medication, faecal impaction, impaired mobility and depression, should be identified. In Bob's case, staff investigated further the side effects of clozapine and discovered that incontinence was a recognised side effect, but it was also important that their assessment included a urinalysis.

Box 6.60 Activity: assessment of urinary incontinence

Assessment includes interviewing, observation and measurement. Keeping these in mind, consider how a nurse might initially assess a person's urinary incontinence.

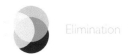

Box 6.61 identifies some key points, and these are expanded on below.

When using interviewing skills to assess incontinence, approach and terminology used need careful consideration. Stewart (2010) suggests that assessment needs to be undertaken by an empathetic, sensitive practitioner who uses easily understandable language and avoids technical medical jargon. For example, when assessing nocturia, the person should be asked, 'how many times do you get up to go to the toilet at night?' rather than 'do you suffer from nocturia?' Similarly, an individual can be asked how often they pass water rather than being asked if they have frequency. Palmer and Newman (2006) identified that questions should be worded carefully (e.g. 'Do you lose water when you don't want to?') rather than asking if they are incontinent. Rassin et al. (2007) found that women often did not perceive they had incontinence but described 'leaking'. If a person has a cognitive impairment, involvement of the carer to obtain a history is particularly important. Likewise, observation while assisting the person to go to the toilet will be very helpful (see Box 6.61). As regards measurement, NICE (2019) recommends bladder diaries should be completed for a minimum of 3 days to more accurately assess urinary frequency and incontinence episodes. Use of 'Word Swaps' should be considered, using the words and phrases familiar to the person rather than the medical terminology, for example 'pee' instead of 'urinate', but this has to be personalised for each individual.

Box 6.61 Assessment of urinary incontinence: key points

Interviewing

- Sensitive, empathetic approach
- Careful and appropriate use of language
- Involvement of carers

Observation

- Physical factors, for example, obstructive symptoms, hesitancy, intermittent stream, dribbling after voiding and straining to void, urgency, difficulty in undressing
- Psychological factors, for example, confusion, fear
- Environmental factors, for example, access to the toilet

Measurement

- Urinalysis
- Charting frequency and amount

NB: Referral to a continence adviser may be required. Use of an assessment tool will promote a systematic approach.

NICE (2007) recommends that healthcare professionals should ask people in high-risk groups for faecal incontinence sensitively about symptoms. Smith (2010) suggests that nurses should initially seek to identify each individual's risk factors for developing faecal incontinence during the initial assessment process, as some will be modifiable. These risk factors range from reduced dietary and fluid intake to the complex symptoms associated with long-term conditions. NICE (2007) recommends that a baseline assessment for people with faecal incontinence should comprise relevant medical history, a general examination, an anorectal examination and a cognitive assessment, if appropriate.

The RCN (2011) has warned that incontinence may be attributed to a person's learning disabilities rather than other causes, including ill-health. This is termed diagnostic overshadowing, where signs and symptoms are attributed to the learning disability rather than investigating for other causes. Bar and Sowney (2007) recommend that when assessing a person with a learning disability, the nurse should observe what the person is able to do, and ask questions such as 'How do you get on with using the toilet?', or ask a carer 'How does he manage with the toilet?' Closed negative questions asking whether the person is incontinent should be avoided. People with a physical disability and a communication difficulty may know when they want to go to the toilet, but carers will not be able to recognise this need if a method of communication has not been established.

Some people with urinary and/or faecal incontinence require a more specialised assessment and should be referred to the continence service, to see a continence specialist nurse, for example. Specialist investigations are sometimes necessary.

> ### Box 6.62 Activity: how referrals are made
>
> When next in practice:
>
> 1 Find out how referrals are made to a continence adviser in your area of practice.
> 2 Investigate whether any specific assessment documents are used in practice for assessment of incontinence.

Many practice settings have a specific continence assessment tool that will help to identify both the cause and possible management of incontinence. The DH (2010) advises that assessment tools are evidence-based and adapted for specific groups.

For people with neurological conditions, NICE (2012) outlines a detailed and evidence-based assessment.

Mark's CLDN should work with him and his mother to empower him to access continence services and could carry out a joint assessment with a continence adviser. Mark's continence should be addressed in his health action plan. Smith and Smith (2007) examine continence training for people with learning disabilities in detail.

Learning outcome 3: identify interventions for promoting urinary continence

How urinary continence is promoted obviously depends on the underlying cause, which is why an understanding of causes and careful assessment is important.

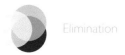
Box 6.63 Activity: methods to promote confidence

Think back to people you have encountered who had urinary continence problems. What methods have you seen being used to promote continence for them in practice settings?

The methods you have seen should have been chosen to address the type of incontinence, based on the person's assessment. You might have seen lifestyle advice (e.g. fluid intake, weight loss) being given, pelvic floor muscle (PFM) training being taught (for stress or mixed incontinence), or have assisted with bladder training (for urge or overactive bladder syndrome) or voiding programmes. Following a systematic review, Chiarelli et al. (2009) recommended addressing inter-related factors associated with both falls and incontinence. Risk factors that could be modified include: mobility and transfer impairments, visual impairment, cognitive decline, poly-pharmacy, environmental hazards, and orthostatic hypotension (Chiarelli et al. 2009). To reduce functional incontinence, physiotherapists can help with mobility and balance, enabling quicker transfers; and occupational therapists help in making the environment and dressing and undressing easier, for example, with clothing adaptations. Vickerman (2003) asserts that many people are rendered incontinent by a poorly adapted environment and advises that the heights of chairs, beds and toilets should be assessed and adjusted, as well as considering lighting, signs, floor coverings, grab rails and provision of commodes and hand-held urinals. You may also have seen medical interventions that can include pharmacology (Rigby 2007) or surgery (when conservative measures have failed). According to Alzheimer's Society (2009), nurses and carers identified concerns related to continence of people with dementia. In response, Alzheimer's Society developed some 'Top tips'. Box 6.64 includes some of these additional points.

Box 6.64 Promoting continence for people with dementia: top tips for nurses

1. Check whether the person with dementia can get to the toilet without any problems. They may want to use the toilet but be unable to find it.
2. Make sure the person knows where the toilet is by showing them.
   A picture of a toilet on the door can act as a visual reminder. Make the image bright and easy to see by positioning it at eye level.
3. Remove any obstacles in the way such as awkwardly placed furniture or doors that are hard to open.
4. Remind the person to go to the toilet, or take them there, at regular intervals (see sections on prompted voiding and timed voiding).
5. Observe for signs that the person wants to go to the toilet such as fidgeting, getting up and down or pulling at their clothes.
6. Encourage others to keep the toilet door open when not in use so it is obvious when the toilet is vacant. However, ensure that the door is fully closed when in use.
7. A coloured toilet that contrasts with the pan can make it easier to see as bathroom facilities that are all the same colour can be disorientating to people with dementia.
8. Ensure that clothing can be quickly removed and unfastened. For example, Velcro fastenings may be easier to use than zips or buttons.

Source: Adapted with permission from original information produced by Alzheimer's Society alzheimers.org.uk

NICE (2019) recommends that, at initial assessment of women, urinary incontinence should be categorised as either 'stress urinary incontinence', 'mixed urinary incontinence' or 'urge/overactive bladder syndrome', so that appropriate interventions can be planned. NICE (2019) provides algorithms for each type of incontinence.

Some of the measures for promoting urinary continence will be explained in more detail.

Pelvic floor muscle training

Pelvic floor muscle training involves the PFMs being squeezed and lifted, then relaxed, several times in a row, up to 3 times a day (Herderschee et al. 2011). The exercises can help strengthen the muscles and improve their endurance and coordination, so that the muscle squeezes hardest when the risk of leaking is greatest (e.g. with a cough) (Herderschee et al. 2011).

PFM training is the most commonly used physical therapy for women with stress urinary incontinence and is sometimes advised for mixed and, less commonly, for urge urinary incontinence (Hay-Smith et al. 2011). NICE (2019) suggests a trial of supervised PFM training for at least 3 months as the first-line treatment for women with stress or mixed urinary incontinence, which should involve at least 8 contractions performed 3 times a day. Women receiving regular (e.g. weekly) supervision are more likely to report improvement than women doing PFM training with little or no supervision (Hay-Smith et al. 2011). Weighted vaginal cones can be inserted into the vagina and the pelvic floor is contracted to prevent them from slipping out (Herbison and Dean 2009). Biofeedback can be used to teach contraction of the correct muscles and when and how to contract the muscle to prevent leakage (Herderschee et al. 2011). Biofeedback uses a vaginal or anal device to measure the muscle squeeze pressure or the electrical activity in the muscle and gives feedback as a sound or visual display (Herderschee et al. 2011).

In men, stress incontinence may occur following prostatectomy, for whom NICE (2015) advises PFM training for at least 3 months before considering other options. Dorey (2007) details exercises that can be taught to men to perform at home in different situations and positions, but states that they should be taught by a specialist to ensure that they are performed correctly.

Bladder re-education

Bladder re-education involves re-educating the bladder to an improved pattern of voiding and has several variations, suitable for different client groups. All staff should be fully aware and motivated towards these programmes, so that they are implemented consistently. Roe et al. (2006) explained that bladder training is used for cognitively and physically able adults, while prompted voiding, habit retraining and timed voiding – collectively known as voiding programmes – are generally used for people with cognitive or physical impairments in institutional settings. NICE (2012) recommends that for people with neurogenic lower urinary tract dysfunction, a behavioural management programme (e.g. timed voiding, bladder retraining or habit retraining) can be used but only after assessment by a healthcare professional

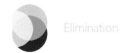

trained in the assessment of people with neurogenic lower urinary tract dysfunction and combined with education about the lower urinary tract function for the person and/or their carers.

Bladder training

Based on limited evidence, bladder training may be helpful for the treatment of urinary incontinence (Wallace et al. 2009). Bladder training aims to increase the interval between voids so that continence might be regained and is widely used for the treatment of urinary incontinence (Wallace et al. 2009). For example, the person might initially be asked to go to the toilet every hour. This is then gradually extended by half an hour at a time. NICE (2019) recommends that, for women with overactive bladders, with or without urge incontinence, bladder training for a minimum of 6 weeks should be offered. Education of individuals and carers, use of a continence chart and continuous encouragement are all important elements. Carers need to praise to build up confidence and reinforce behaviour and they should be patient and understanding.

Voiding programmes

Timed voiding

Timed voiding is also referred to as scheduled, fixed, routine or regular toileting/voiding. The main feature is voiding to a fixed time pattern; for example, two-, three- or four-hourly. Timed voiding is promoted for people with urinary incontinence who cannot participate in independent toileting and is commonly assumed to represent current practice in residential care settings for older people (Ostaszkiewicz et al. 2011). It is often used for people with a neurogenic bladder, such as those with spinal cord lesions, and for people with a physical or mental disability. It can include techniques to trigger voiding such as tapping over the suprapubic region or running water. However, there is currently little evidence about the effects of timed voiding on the management of urinary incontinence (Ostaszkiewicz et al. 2011).

Habit retraining

Habit retraining involves the identification of a person's natural voiding pattern and the development of an individualised toileting schedule, which pre-empts involuntary bladder emptying (Ostaszkiewicz et al. 2010). A record of voiding and incontinent episodes is kept so that the schedule can be adjusted, with voiding intervals lengthened if the person is dry, and reduced if incontinence occurs. NICE (2012) recommends that habit retraining is particularly suitable for people with cognitive impairment.

Prompted voiding

Prompted voiding is a behavioural therapy, which aims to improve bladder control for people with or without dementia using verbal prompts and positive reinforcement (Eustice et al. 2009). Prompted voiding programmes have been recommended for women who have urinary incontinence and cognitive impairment (NICE 2019a) and other people with cognitive impairment (NICE 2017). Prompted voiding has been used with people with learning disabilities too and could be an appropriate strategy for Mark, in our scenarios. Ostaszkiewicz (2006) found that prompted voiding was more sustainable than habit retraining or timed voiding, but it needed more resources to implement. Although there is evidence of short-term benefits of prompted voiding, it is not known if these persist (Eustice et al. 2009).

Learning outcome 4: identify appropriate nursing interventions for promoting faecal continence and managing faecal incontinence

Faecal incontinence is a distressing disorder with high social stigma (Deutekom and Dobben 2012). NICE (2007, 2014a) includes a comprehensive flow chart for managing faecal incontinence in adults. Underlying conditions should be addressed and, if faecal incontinence continues, people should be referred for specialised management. Anal sphincter exercises (PFM training) and biofeedback therapy have been used to treat the symptoms of people with faecal incontinence (Norton and Cody 2012). Other measures include PFM training, bowel retraining, specialist dietary assessment and management, and electrical stimulation or rectal irrigation. Some interventions recommended are discussed below.

Diet

There should be a balanced nutrient intake and at least 1.5 L of fluid intake daily for people with hard stools or those who are dehydrated (unless contraindicated). Hansen et al. (2006) found that diet modification was central to managing faecal incontinence: restricting foods that exacerbated faecal incontinence, avoiding gas-producing foods, and limiting portion or meal size.

Bowel habit

Predictable bowel emptying should be promoted by encouraging bowel emptying after a meal, ensuring toilet facilities are private, comfortable and safe, allowing sufficient time, encouraging people to adopt a sitting/squatting position and avoiding straining. Akpan et al. (2006) highlighted that many older people, especially those who were dependent, lacked privacy during bowel movements.

Toilet access

Staff can help the person to access the toilet by ensuring that the location is clear to them, provide equipment to assist access, and advise them about easily removable clothing. A home/mobility assessment may be necessary.

Medication

Alternatives to those contributing to faecal incontinence should be considered. Anti-diarrhoeal drugs (e.g. loperamide) may be appropriate.

Coping strategies

These include continence products (disposable body-worn pads, bed pads, anal plugs and faecal collectors), skin care, odour control, laundry advice and support. Learning outcome five addresses incontinence pads and skin care. Anal plugs aim to

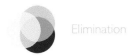

block the loss of stool (Deutekom and Dobben 2012). Though they can be difficult to tolerate, they can be effective; they are available in different designs and sizes and plug selection can affect performance (Deutekom and Dobben 2012). Palmieri et al. (2005) studied the use of a bag to collect stools in faecal incontinence and found no adverse reactions. The bag was well tolerated and it was not painful to remove or apply. The 'Flexi-Seal faecal management system' is a temporary containment device, consisting of a soft, flexible silicone catheter with a low-pressure balloon that is filled with water or saline to aid retention. The device is inserted into the person's rectum and attached to a catheter bag. It can collect liquid or semi-liquid stools and is most suitable for bed-bound individuals, for example, in critical care. In the evaluation of this system by Padmanabhan et al. (2007), skin condition was maintained or improved in most individuals. Along with diverting faeces from the skin, the system also assists with infection control and allows more accurate fluid balance monitoring.

Education and support

Targeted education improved bowel dysfunction symptoms in the study by Harari et al. (2004). Chelvanayagam and Stern (2007) found that group therapy facilitated by experienced therapists improved both physical and psychological well-being of people with faecal incontinence.

Learning outcome 5: explain the nursing management of incontinence

Incontinence should be managed in a manner that is unobtrusive, reliable and comfortable. If incontinence cannot be prevented, then a suitable containment method is needed, for example, pads, or, for a man with urinary incontinence, possibly a penile sheath. As mentioned in the previous section, for faecal incontinence there are also anal plugs, faecal collection bags and systems. Incontinence aids should preserve hygiene, dignity, psychological and social comfort.

Transanal irrigation can reduce the severity of constipation and incontinence. However, it may not be ideal for all types of bowel dysfunction and may take a few weeks for a person to become comfortable using this treatment. Fluid is introduced into the rectum and sigmoid colon via a rectal tube and pump device such as Peristeen® that washes out all faecal matter when the fluid is drained out. NICE (2018b) recommends this as an option when offered with specialist training and support and when effective can improve quality of life and promote dignity and independence.

Urethral catheterisation is rarely appropriate for managing urinary incontinence as it may lead to catheter-related problems such as UTI (see the 'Caring for people with urinary catheters' section). However, NICE (2019) recommends that catheterisation should be considered for women with persistent urinary retention that causes incontinence, symptomatic infections or renal dysfunction that cannot be corrected. NICE (2019) suggests that the risks and benefits should be discussed considering urine contamination of skin wounds, pressure ulcers, irritation, distress and disruption caused by bed and clothing changes, and women's preferences. Intermittent urethral catheterisation is another option that can be taught to the person or their carer.

NICE (2019) recommends that absorbent products (pads) should not be considered a treatment option for urinary incontinence in women and should only be used to help individuals who are waiting for treatment, as an adjunct to other therapies, and for long-term management, if other treatments have failed. Similarly, for men, NICE (2010a) recommends use of temporary containment products (e.g. pads or collecting devices) to achieve social continence until a diagnosis and management plan have been established.

ACTIVITY

> ### Box 6.65 Activity: priorities of care
>
> If you find that a person has been incontinent, what would your priorities of care be?

Priorities are to assist the person quickly, to prevent skin damage, relieve discomfort and restore dignity. Many of the principles discussed earlier related to dealing with a person's elimination needs are relevant, in particular: approachability and communication, privacy and dignity, promptness, prevention of cross-infection, observation, hygiene and comfort. The nurse's approach when dealing with incontinence is crucial to the level of distress experienced. Nurses dealing with Bob's urinary incontinence should be discreet and matter-of-fact in changing his bed while reassuring him that the cause would be investigated. In faecal incontinence, in particular, prompt changing of soiled pads or clothing is essential to help to prevent odours and skin excoriation, and reduce the risk of cross-infection.

Skin care

Ersser et al. (2005) identified that urinary incontinence is an important cause of skin vulnerability and that older people are a high-risk group for skin damage as their skin is more permeable, enabling external moisture to infiltrate epidermal layers and increasing the friction coefficient at the skin's surface. Incontinence-associated dermatitis can develop, which is an inflammatory condition of the skin that is associated with faecal or urinary incontinence (Wolfman 2010). Ersser et al. (2005) explained that incontinence leads to skin problems because:

- wetness of the skin encourages maceration, disrupting the skin barrier leading to breakdown;
- decomposition of the urinary urea by microorganisms' releases ammonia, forming the alkali ammonium hydroxide, thus altering the skin's pH (the pH of normal skin ranges from 5.4 to 5.9, providing an acid mantle);
- chemical irritation of the skin arises from urine, the rise in alkalinity and bacterial proliferation;
- the presence of faecal urease results in breakdown of the urinary urea causing increase in pH, increasing activities of faecal proteases and lipases.

Candida albicans is the most common fungus found on the skin, and as it prefers a moist environment, this fungus can proliferate in people with incontinence leading to fungal infection and skin breakdown (Beldon 2012).

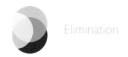

Skin care following incontinence is very important; see Box 6.67 for some key points.

ACTIVITY

Box 6.66 Activity: skin care following incontinence

Compare Box 6.67 to skin care following incontinence that you have seen in practice.

Box 6.67 Skin care after incontinence: key points

- Ensure prompt action, with privacy, dignity and sensitivity.
- Observe infection control: hand hygiene, gloves and apron, correct waste disposal.
- Use skin cleanser rather than soap (Bale et al. 2004; Bliss et al. 2006; Hodgkinson et al. 2007; Nix and Ermer-Seltun 2004). Wash gently, avoiding friction.
- Cleanse from front to back, and least soiled area to most soiled area.
- Start with the labia with females, and the tip of the penis with men.
- Cleanse the anal area last.
- Observe the skin condition.
- Dry skin carefully to avoid maceration and undue cooling, maintain comfort and permit dressing. Pat rather than rub to reduce friction (Ersser et al. 2005).
- Apply barrier cream, or for moderate/severe incontinence dermatitis, barrier film (Baatenburg de Jong and Admiraal 2004; Bale et al. 2004; Beldon 2012).

Soap and water is not advised for skin cleansing following incontinence; soap removes the skin's natural oils, causing dryness and could alter the pH from its natural acid state (Ananthapadmanabhan et al. 2004). Skin cleansers have evaluated well in several small studies (Bale et al. 2004; Bliss et al. 2006). Barrier creams can help prevent skin damage caused by incontinence. Barrier creams are protective products, designed to form an occlusive barrier between the skin and noxious substances, not to be confused with emollients that moisturise the skin (Voegeli 2008). Beeckman et al. (2010) recommend that optimal skin care should be provided according to a structured perineal skin care programme, including a skin cleanser, moisturiser and skin protectant. A barrier cream that contains dimethicone can provide an almost invisible barrier, and it will not affect the absorbency of body-worn continence pads (Beldon 2012).

Containment of incontinence: pads

Super-absorbent pads aim to prevent mixing of urine and faeces by keeping skin dry. Pads are produced for all situations, ranging from light to severe and night-time use. Light urinary incontinence is defined as urine loss that can be contained within a small absorbent pad (Fader et al. 2009a). A practical definition of moderate–heavy incontinence is urine or faecal loss that requires a large absorbent pad (typically with a total absorbent capacity of 2000–3000 g) for containment (Fader et al. 2009b).

Box 6.68 Activity: incontinence pads

ACTIVITY

Find out what incontinence pads are available in your practice setting.

There is a wide range of incontinence pads available: all-in-one body-worn products, pads worn with elasticated pants or insert pads. Under-pads are also available but should be used only as a procedure pad when a clean (not sterile) field is needed, for extra chair/bed protection, for example, after administration of an enema, or where a body-worn pad is not practical or possible as with a very obese person, or for persistent diarrhoea in bed, which cannot be contained with alternative methods (e.g. faecal collector). The systematic review by Hodgkinson et al. (2007) identified that disposable body-worn pads may prevent deterioration of skin condition better than non-disposable under-pads or body-worns. Box 6.69 summarises key points in the choice and use of incontinence pads.

Kristiansen et al. (2011) found that individuals, close relatives and nursing staff all expressed that a good urinary incontinence aid had good absorption capacity, shape and comfort level, and suited the individual. Differently shaped pads are available for men and women. It is important to read the manufacturers' instructions as correct fitting of pads is essential to contain urine and faeces, and it will reduce skin contact with excreta to the minimum. As urine is broken down into its constituents – ammonia and urea – on contact with air, close-fitting pads ensure that urine and air are not mixed. Kristiansen et al. (2011) evaluated the use of an alarmed pad at night and found that the person affected, their close relatives and nursing staff all viewed the alarmed pad system as a good complement to ordinary care. It improved the quality of the individuals' nightly rest as staff did not have to wake them to check if it was necessary to change their pad. However, there were some concerns that the design needed improvement, that there should not be overreliance on the alarm and that the alarm's sound might be confusing for people with dementia.

Box 6.69 Choice and use of incontinence pads: key points

Choice of pad

- Disposable, super-absorbent pads are preferable.
- Body-worn pads (either all-in-ones, or pad and pants) should be used rather than under-pads.
- Choose the correct pad for the individual person, considering gender, size, and extent and frequency of incontinence.

Fitting

Always follow the manufacturer's instructions for fitting, but the following general principles normally apply:

- Maintain privacy, dignity and prevention of cross-infection during pad changes.
- If using pants, ensure the seams are on the outside and pull up to mid-thigh.
- Fold the pad lengthways and create a cupped shape.
- Place the pad from front to back with largest area at the back.
- Ensure pad is smoothed out both front and back, and fitted into the groin well.
- If using pants, pull up; or if all-in-ones, seal the tapes firmly. Lower tapes should be sealed first.
- Check if the pad is as close to the body as possible.

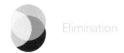

When changing a pad, never refer to it as a 'nappy', which is demeaning. Nurses should take care not to show annoyance or embarrass the person and should use discreet communication (see Chapter 2). It is important to ensure that people have a clean pad at mealtimes and before going out anywhere. When changing the pad, maintain privacy by shutting curtains, and change any wet or soiled clothing. To prevent cross-infection, use of gloves and aprons; hand hygiene and correct waste disposal are essential (see Chapter 12).

Fader et al. (2004) found that incontinence pads had an adverse effect on pressure redistribution properties on mattresses, with pad folds contributing to this effect. Thus, individuals who are incontinent and wearing pads may be at increased risk of pressure damage, but smoothing out the folds reduced interface pressures.

Getliffe and Fader (2007) address absorbent products for containment in detail, fully illustrated; further reading from that source is recommended. A detailed evaluation of different types of pads can be found in Cochrane reviews by Fader et al. (2009a, 2009b).

Penile sheaths

Penile sheaths (also referred to as 'condom catheters') (see Figure 6.13) consist of a soft, flexible sleeve that fits over the penis with an anti-reflux bulbous end leading to a short tube that attaches to any standard urinary drainage system (Kyle 2011b). They can provide a reliable form of containment for men with unresolvable urinary incontinence or as a temporary measure, but they should not be used for people with urinary retention. NICE (2015) suggests that penile sheaths should be offered to

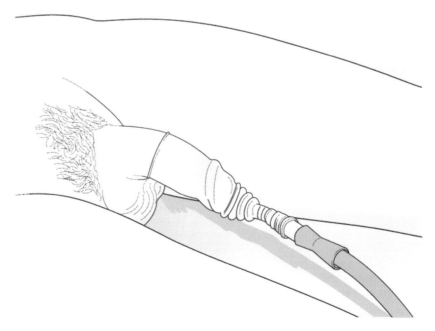

Figure 6.13: Penile sheath.

men, prior to considering in-dwelling catheterisation. They avoid the complications of long-term in-dwelling urethral catheters and, by diverting urine into a bag, prevent odour and contact of urine on skin (Pemberton et al. 2006). In the study by Saint et al. (2006), urinary sheaths reduced adverse outcomes, such as infection, and individuals reported that they were comfortable and less painful than catheters. In many cases, people can manage the system themselves or carers can be taught to do so but manual dexterity will be necessary.

ACTIVITY

> ### Box 6.70 Activity: individuals for whom urinary incontinence methods may be unsuitable
>
> Can you think of any individuals for whom this method of dealing with urinary incontinence might be particularly unsuitable?

Someone with any skin soreness of the penis should not have a sheath applied. People with cognitive impairment may pull the device off, causing trauma (Williams and Moran 2006). Penile length is another important factor; there should be at least 1.5 inches (3.8 cm) of penile length available (Kyle 2011b). For men with significant retraction, a urinary sheath is unlikely to be successful as it will roll off the shaft of the penis. Kyle (2011b) advises that if the penile length is very short, an external device (the Clinimed Bioderm®) that fixes just to the glans of the penis can be used. The Bioderm is made of hydrocolloid, so it is hypoallergenic and latex-free, and it can be attached to any urinary drainage system.

If a person is considered suitable for a penile sheath, selection of equipment should next occur with consideration to:

Material: A silicone sheath can be used if there is a history of latex allergy. A clear sheath as opposed to an opaque one allows observation of the penile skin.

Choice of one piece or two piece: The two-piece sheath requires application of an adhesive strip to the penis in a spiral manner, before rolling the sheath on, while the one-piece sheath has an integral adhesive coating.

Correct size: Dwivedi et al. (2012) report on a person who developed a urethral diverticulum as a complication of wearing a sheath, and they stress the importance of avoiding over tight application and careful sizing. You should measure the circumference of the penis at its widest point and measure the length. If the sheath is too big, there will be leakage as urine will seep under the sheath and loosen the adhesive, causing the sheath to slip off. Sheaths that are too small could cause sores and discomfort. Sheaths are available in a variety of widths (20–40 mm) and lengths (50–80 mm) and each manufacturer has a defined size range and provides their own measurement guide, which must be used together (Williams and Moran 2006).

Box 6.73 outlines how to apply a penile sheath and subsequent care.

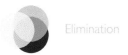

Support for people with continence problems

People with continence problems can benefit from support and advice, but they may often be unaware of what support is available, and where it can be accessed. Nurses should be aware of the resources available so that they can advise people with continence issues. There are many local self-help support groups that can be very beneficial to participants and these give people the opportunity to meet informally and share ideas and experiences. The DH (2010) advises that best practice is for people with continence problems, and their carers, to be able to access other people and carers with similar problems to gain support. Bladder and Bowel UK (www.bbuk.org.uk) provides information and support to people affected by bladder and bowel problems. Other organisations have also developed information leaflets for people who have continence problems, for example, the Alzheimer's Disease Society (www.alzheimers.org.uk).

 Box 6.71 Children and young people: practice points – continence

In some situations, children who are usually toilet-trained may need to wear incontinence pads due to special needs or health conditions such as neuropathic bladder or congenital malformation. This can be upsetting for them so great sensitivity is needed. For changing an incontinence pad in a child, see

Himsworth, J. 2010. Caring for personal hygiene needs. In: Glasper. A, Aylott, M. and Battrick, C. (eds.) *Developing Practical Skills for Nursing Children and Young People.* London: Hodder Arnold, 188–202.

Children who are anxious or fearful may regress to day or night wetting. Bedwetting is a widespread and distressing condition that can have a deep impact on a child or young person's behaviour, emotional well-being and social life. It is also very stressful for the parents or carers (NICE 2010b). NICE (2014b) provides detailed guidelines for managing this distressing condition.

For further reading, see

Glasper, A., Aylott, M., and Battrick, C. (eds.). 2010. *Developing Practical Skills for Nursing Children and Young People.* London: Hodder Arnold, Chapter 14 Promoting children's continence, 220–41.

See also:

ERIC – Enuresis Website: http://www.eric.org.uk/

Box 6.72 Pregnancy and birth: practice points – continence

There is an established association between urinary incontinence and pregnancy and childbirth (Herbruck 2008). The physiological changes occurring during pregnancy and the processes of childbirth have a detrimental effect on the structure and function of the muscles, nerves and connective tissue that make up the pelvic floor complex. Dysfunction of the pelvic floor complex can result in a wide range of symptoms including urinary or anal incontinence. PFMs and their associated structures are at risk of becoming weakened during pregnancy or of experiencing trauma and damage during delivery. PFM training should be offered to women in their first pregnancy as a preventative strategy for urinary incontinence. There is evidence that pelvic floor muscle training used during a first pregnancy reduces the likelihood of postnatal urinary incontinence (NICE 2019a).

Box 6.73 Application of penile sheath and subsequent care: key points

Preparation

- Carefully select the person for suitability, explain the procedure and gain consent.
- Gather equipment (correctly sized sheath, urinary drainage system).
- Conduct hand hygiene and wear non-sterile gloves and apron.
- Ensure privacy during the procedure.

Procedure

- If provided, use the manufacturer's pubic hair guard over the penis to keep hair away from the adhesive. If necessary pubic hair can be trimmed but must not be shaved.
- Ensure the penis is clean and dry – avoid powder, cream or sprays.
- If using a two-piece sheath, apply the adhesive strip in a spiral fashion around the penis.
- Roll the sheath over the penis: leave a small space (1–2 cm) between the end of the penis and the outlet of the sheath. If the person is uncircumcised, ensure that the foreskin remains over the glans and is not retracted.
- Gently squeeze the sheath to ensure adhesion.
- Attach the urine drainage bag and place it on a stand.
- Make the person comfortable.
- Remove and dispose of gloves and apron and wash hands.

Subsequent care

- Ensure that the catheter tubing does not kink, to allow collection of urine and prevent pressure on the sheath, weakening the adhesive.
- Remove the sheath daily by gently rolling it off (preferably in the bath), and wash and dry the skin before reapplying.
- Observe the penile skin for any problems. Note that an individual with reduced or absent sensation will not be able to feel if the sheath is too tight or a sore is developing, so observe carefully for problems and teach the person and/or carers to do so too.

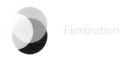

Summary

- Nurses within almost any setting are likely to encounter people with continence issues, so an understanding of the underlying causes and the wide-ranging effects on people is important.
- Nurses should have knowledge about specialised services, such as the continence adviser and support organisations, so that they can advise and refer people accordingly.
- Promoting continence and managing incontinence requires careful assessment of each individual, and knowledge about appropriate strategies and products. Care for people with continence problems should be based on the best evidence available.

CHAPTER SUMMARY

This chapter has focused on assisting people with elimination, emphasising that quality care requires a sensitive and empathetic approach, effective communication skills and a sound, evidence-based knowledge. Implementing measures to prevent cross-infection, while assisting people with elimination, are also paramount. Urinalysis and specimen collection are very common investigations, but if not carried out with care, they can lead to misleading results and inappropriate treatment. Constipation is a common problem and preventing and managing constipation was addressed. Urinary catheterisation is invasive and potentially harmful but is nevertheless often necessary as a short- or long-term measure. An understanding of this procedure, and particularly how potential complications can be reduced, is also important. Nurses may encounter people with stomas in a range of acute and long-term settings and key aspects of stoma care were considered.

Continence is a huge topic and may require specialist involvement. Here, the practical skills in dealing with continence have been explored; students wishing to extend their knowledge should access the referenced material. To conclude, nurses need to value the care given in relation to a persons' elimination needs, which, if effective, can do much for comfort, well-being and self-esteem.

REFERENCES

Abd-el-Maeboud, K.H. et al. 1991. Rectal suppositories and mode of insertion. *The Lancet* 338: 798, 800.

Akerman, A.L. and Chai, T. (2019) The bladder is not sterile: An update on the urinary microbiome. *Current Bladder Dysfunction Reports*. https://doi.org/10.1007 14: 331–41.

Akpan, A., Gosney, M.A. and Barrett, J. 2006. Privacy for defecation and fecal incontinence in older adults. *Journal of Wound, Ostomy and Continence Nursing* 33(5): 536–40.

Alzheimer's Society. 2009. *Counting the Cost: Caring for People with Dementia on Acute Hospital Wards*. London: Alzheimer's Society.

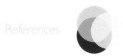
Ananthapadmanabhan, K.P., Moore, D.J., Subramanyan, K. et al. 2004. Cleansing without compromise: The impact of cleansers on the skin barrier and the technology of mild cleansing. *Dermatological Therapy* 17(Suppl 1): 16–25.

Avery, J.C., Wilson, I. and Braunack-Mayer, A.J. 2006. Beliefs and barriers about seeking help for incontinence. *Australian and New Zealand Continence Journal* 12(1): 6.

Baatenburg de Jong, H. and Admiraal, H. 2004. Comparing cost per use of 3M Cavilon no sting barrier film with zinc oxide oil in incontinent patients. *Journal of Wound Care* 13(9): 398–400.

Bale, S. et al. 2004. The benefits of implementing a new skin care protocol in nursing homes. *Journal of Tissue Viability* 14(2): 44–50.

Bar, O. and Sowney, M. 2007. Inclusive nursing care for people with intellectual disabilities using urology services. *International Journal of Urological Nursing* 1(3): 138–45.

Bayer. 1997. *Urine Analysis: The Essential Information.* Newbury: Bayer.

Bayer. 1998. *A Practical Guide to Urine Analysis.* Newbury: Bayer.

Beeckman, D., Defloor, T., Verhaeghe, S. et al. 2010. What is the most effective method of preventing and treating incontinence associated dermatitis? *Nursing Times* 106(38): 22–5.

Beldon, P. 2012. Incontinence-associated dermatitis: Protecting the older person. *British Journal of Nursing* 21(7): 402–7.

Beynon, M. and Nicholls, C. 2004. Urological investigations. In: Fillingham, S. and Douglas, J. (eds.) *Urological Nursing*, 3rd edn. Edinburgh: Baillière Tindall, 25–42.

Billington, A. 2010. The management of stress urinary incontinence. *British Journal of Nursing* 19(Continence Care, Suppl. 18): S20–5.

Black, P. 2011. Caring for the patient with a stoma and dementia. *Gastrointestinal Nursing* 9(7): 19–24.

Black, P. 2012. Choosing the correct stoma appliance. *Gastrointestinal Nursing* 10(7): 18–25.

Blake, D.R. and Doherty, L.F. 2006. Effect of perineal cleansing on contamination rate of midstream urine culture. *Journal of Pediatric and Adolescent Gynecology* 19(1): 31–4.

Bliss, D.Z. et al. 2006. Incontinence-associated skin damage in nursing home residents: A secondary analysis of a prospective, multicenter study. *Ostomy/Wound Management* 52(12): 46–55.

Bowers, B. 2006. Evaluating the evidence for administering phosphate enemas. *British Journal of Nursing* 15(7): 378–81.

Bradshaw, E., Collins, B. and Williams, J. 2009. Administering rectal suppositories: preparation, assessment and insertion. *Gastrointestinal Nursing* 7(9): 24–8.

British Geriatrics Society. 2006. *Dignity: Supporting Toilet Access and Use in Frail Older People.* Updated 2018. Available from: https://www.bgs.org.uk/resources/dignity-supporting-toilet-access-and-use-in-frail-older-people (Accessed on 10 November 2020).

British Infection Association and Health Protection Agency. 2011. *Diagnosis of UTI: Quick Reference Guide for Primary Care.* Available from: http://www.hpa.org.uk/webc/HPAwebFile/HPAweb_C/1194947404720 (Accessed on 6 January 2012).

Brown S.R., Wadhawan, H. and Nelson, R. 2013. Surgery for faecal incontinence in adults. *Cochrane Database of Systematic Reviews* 7. Art. No.: CD001757. doi: 10.1002/14651858.CD001757.pub4.

Bucior, H. and Cochrane, J. 2010. Lifting the lid: A clinical audit on commode cleaning. *Journal of Infection Prevention* 11(3): 73–80.

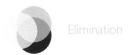

Busuttil Leaver, R. and Leach, C. 2004. Psychological effects of urological problems. In: Fillingham, S. and Douglas, J. (eds.) *Urological Nursing*. Edinburgh: Baillière Tindall, 305–20.

Candy, B., Jones L., Goodman, M.L., et al. 2011. Laxatives or methylnaltrexone for the management of constipation in palliative care patients. *Cochrane Database of Systematic Reviews* 19(1) Art. No.: CD003448. doi: 10.1002/14651858.CD003448.pub3.

Chelvanayagam, S. and Stern, J. 2007. Using therapeutic groups to support women with faecal incontinence. *British Journal of Nursing* 16(4): 214–18.

Chiarelli, P.E. and Weatherall, M. 2010. The link between chronic conditions and urinary incontinence. *Australian and New Zealand Continence Journal* 16(1): 7–14.

Chiarelli, P.E., Mackenzie, L.A. and Osmotherly, P.G. 2009. Urinary incontinence is associated with an increase in falls: A systematic review. *Australian Journal of Physiotherapy* 55: 89–95.

Clark, J. and Rugg, S. 2005. The importance of independence in toileting: The views of stroke survivors and their occupational therapists. *British Journal of Occupational Therapy* 68(4): 165–71.

Collett, K. 2002. Practical aspects of stoma management. *Nursing Standard* 17(8): 45–52, 54.

Coloplast. 2010. *High Impact Actions for Stoma Care. High Impact Action Steering Group*. Peterborough: Coloplast Ltd.

Colpman, D. and Welford, K. 2004. Urinary drainage systems. In: Fillingham, S. and Douglas, J. (eds.) *Urological Nursing*. Edinburgh: Baillière Tindall, 67–92.

Deering, C.G. and Cody, D.J. 2002. Communicating with children and adolescents: Children are all foreigners. *American Journal of Nursing* 102(3): 34–41.

de Hert, M. et al. 2011. Prevalence and severity of antipsychotic related constipation in patients with schizophrenia: A retrospective descriptive study. *BMC Gastroenterology* 11: 17.

Department of Health (DH). 2000. *Good Practice in Continence Services*. London: DH.

Department of Health. 2003. *Winning Ways: Working Together to Reduce Healthcare Associated Infection in England*. London: Department of Health. Available from: http://webarchive.nationalarchives.gov.uk/20130107105354/http://www.dh.gov.uk/prod_consum_dh/groups/dh_digitalassets/@dh/@en/documents/digitalasset/dh_4064689.pdf (Accessed on 25 November 2020).

Department of Health (DH). 2006. *Environment and Sustainability: Safe Management of Healthcare Waste*. Health Technical Memorandum 07-01. London: DH.

Department of Health (DH). 2010. *Essence of Care 2010: Benchmarks for Bladder, Bowel and Continence Care*. Gateway Reference 14641. London: The Stationery Office, DH.

Deutekom, M. and Dobben, A.C. 2012. Plugs for containing faecal incontinence. *Cochrane Database of Systematic Reviews* 4. Art. No.: CD005086. doi: 10.1002/14651858.CD005086.pub3.

Dorey, G. 2007. Why men need to perform pelvic floor exercises. *Nursing Times* 103(26): 40–6.

Dwivedi, A.K., Singh, S. and Goel, A. 2012. Massive urethral diverticulum: A complication of condom catheter use. *British Journal of Nursing* 21(Urology, Suppl 9): S20–2.

Elstad, E.A. et al. 2010. Beyond incontinence: The stigma of other urinary symptoms. *Journal of Advanced Nursing* 66(11): 2460–70.

Ersser, S.J. et al. 2005. A critical review of the interrelationship between skin vulnerability and urinary incontinence and related nursing intervention. *International Journal of Nursing Studies* 42: 823–35.

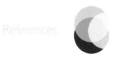
Erwin-Toth, P. 2003. Ostomy pearls: A concise guide to stoma siting, pouching systems, patient education, and more. *Advances in Skin and Wound Care* 16(3): 146–52.

European Association of Urological Nurses (EAUN). 2012. *Catheterisation: Indwelling Catheters in Adults. Evidence-Based Guidelines for Best Practice in Urological Health Care.* EAUN Guidelines. Available from: http://www.uroweb.org/fileadmin/EAUN/guidelines/EAUN_Paris_Guideline_2012_LR_online_file.pdf (Accessed on 20 December 2012).

Eustice, S., Roe, B. and Paterson, J. 2009. Prompted voiding for the management of urinary incontinence in adults. *Cochrane Database of Systematic Reviews* 2. Art. No.: CD002113. doi: 10.1002/14651858.CD002113.

Fader, M., Bain, D. and Cottenden, A. 2004. Effects of absorbent incontinence pads on pressure management mattresses. *Journal of Advanced Nursing* 48(6): 569–74.

Fader, M., Cottenden, A.M. and Getliffe, K. 2009a. Absorbent products for moderate-heavy urinary and/or faecal incontinence in women and men. *Cochrane Database of Systematic Reviews* 4. Art. No.: CD007408. doi: 10.1002/14651858.CD007408.

Fader, M., Cottenden, A.M. and Getliffe, K. 2009b. Absorbent products for light urinary incontinence in women. *Cochrane Database of Systematic Reviews* (2). Art. No.: CD0014067408. doi: 10.1002/14651858.CD001406.pub2.

Fillingham, S. and Fell, S. 2004. Urological stomas. In: Fillingham, S. and Douglas, J. (eds.) *Urological Nursing.* Edinburgh: Baillière Tindall, 207–26.

Floruta, C.V. 2001. Dietary choices of people with ostomies. *Journal of Wound, Ostomy and Continence Nursing* 28(1): 28–31.

Fraise, A.P. and Bradley, C. 2009. Decontamination of equipment, the environment and the skin. In: Fraise, A.P. and Bradley, C. (eds.) *Ayliffe's Control of Healthcare-Associated Infection*, 5th edn. London: Hodder Arnold, 107–49.

Gallagher, P.F., O'Mahony, D. and Quigley, E.M.M. 2008. Management of constipation in the elderly. *Drugs Aging* 25(10): 807–21.

Getliffe, K. 2002. Managing recurrent urinary catheter encrustation. *British Journal of Community Nursing* 7: 574–80.

Getliffe, K. and Dolman, M. (eds.) 2007. *Promoting Continence: A Clinical and Research Guide*, 3rd edn. Edinburgh: Baillière Tindall.

Getliffe, K. and Fader, M. 2007. Catheters and containment products. In: Getliffe, K. and Dolman, M. (eds.) *Promoting Continence: A Clinical and Research Guide*, 3rd edn. Edinburgh: Baillière Tindall, 259–308.

Gibney, L.E. 2010. Offering patients, a choice of urinary catheter drainage system. *British Journal of Nursing* 19(15): 954–8.

Godfrey, H. and Fraczyk, L. 2005. Preventing and managing catheter-associated urinary tract infections. *British Journal of Community Nursing* 10(5): 205–12.

Gordon, M. et al. 2012. Osmotic and stimulant laxatives for the management of childhood constipation. *Cochrane Database of Systematic Reviews* 7. Art. No.: CD009118. doi: 10.1002/14651858.CD009118.pub2.

Gould, D. 1994. Controlling infection spread from excreta. *Nursing Standard* 8(33): 29–31.

Greenstein, B. 2009. *Trounce's Clinical Pharmacology for Nurses*, 18th edn. Edinburgh: Churchill Livingstone.

Hägglund, D. 2010. A systematic literature review of incontinence care for persons with dementia: The research evidence. *Journal of Clinical Nursing* 19: 303–12.

Hansen, J.L., Bliss, D.Z. and Peden-McAlpine, C. 2006. Diet strategies used by women to manage fecal incontinence. *Journal of Wound, Ostomy and Continence Nursing* 33: 52–62.

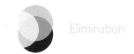

Harari, D. et al. 2004. Treatment of constipation and fecal incontinence in stroke patients: Randomized controlled trials. *Stroke* 35(11): 2549–55.

Hay-Smith, E.J.C. et al. 2011. Comparisons of approaches to pelvic floor muscle training for urinary incontinence in women. *Cochrane Database of Systematic Reviews* 12. Art. No.: CD009508. doi: 10.1002/14651858.CD009508.

Health Protection Agency. 2012. UK standards for microbiology investigations: Investigation of urine. *Bacteriology* B41 (7.1).

Heath, H. 2009. The nurse's role in helping older people to use the toilet. *Nursing Standard* 24(2): 43–7.

Herbison, G.P. and Dean, N. 2009. Weighted vaginal cones for urinary incontinence. *Cochrane Database of Systematic Reviews* 7. Art. No.: CD002114. doi: 10.1002/14651858. CD002114.pub2.

Herbruck, L.E. 2008. Urinary incontinence in the child bearing woman. *Urologic Nursing* 28(3): 163–71.

Herderschee, R. et al. 2011. Feedback or biofeedback to augment pelvic floor muscle training for urinary incontinence in women. *Cochrane Database of Systematic Reviews* 7. Art. No.: CD009252. doi: 10.1002/14651858. CD009252.

Hodgkinson, B., Nay, R. and Wilson, J. 2007. A systematic review of topical skin care in aged care facilities. *Journal of Clinical Nursing* 16: 129–36.

Holland, K. and Hogg, C. 2010. *Cultural Awareness in Nursing and Health Care: An Introductory Text*, 2nd edn. London: Arnold.

Holman, C., Roberts, S. and Nichol, M. 2010. Preventing and treating constipation in later life. *Nursing Older People* 20(5): 22–4.

Jackson, S.L. et al. 2005. Urinary incontinence and diabetes in postmenopausal women. *Diabetes Care* 28(7): 1730–8.

Jahn, P. et al. 2007. Types of indwelling urinary catheters for long-term bladder drainage in adults. *Cochrane Database of Systematic Reviews* 3. Art. No.: CD004997. doi: 10.1002/14651858.CD004997.pub2.

Jewell, D. and Young, G. 2009. Interventions for treating constipation in pregnancy. *Cochrane Database of Systematic Reviews* 2. Art. No.: CD001142. doi: 10.1002/14651858. CD001142.

Karadag, A., Mentes, B. and Ayaz, S. 2005. Colostomy irrigation: Results of 25 cases with particular reference to quality of life. *Journal of Clinical Nursing* 14(4): 479–85.

Kawanabe, E. et al. 2018. Impairment in toileting behaviour after a stroke. *Geriatrics & Gerontology International* 18: 8.

Kristiansen, L. et al. 2011. Urinary incontinence and newly invented pad technique: Patients' close relatives' and nursing staff's experiences and beliefs. *International Journal of Urological Nursing* 5(1): 21–30.

Kyle, G. 2007a. Norgine risk assessment tool for constipation. *Nursing Times* 103(47): 48–9.

Kyle, G. 2007b. Bowel care. Part 5: A practical guide to digital rectal examination. *Nursing Times* 103(46): 28–9.

Kyle, G. 2009. Common bowel problems: Constipation risk assessment. *Nursing & Residential Care* 11(2): 76–9.

Kyle, G. 2010. The older person: Management of constipation. *British Journal of Community Nursing* 15(2): 58–64.

Kyle, G. 2011a. Constipation: Symptoms, assessment and treatment. *British Journal of Nursing* 20(22): 1432.

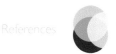

Kyle, G. 2011b. The use of urinary sheaths in male incontinence. *British Journal of Nursing* 20(6): 338.

Lewis, C.M. et al. 2005. Diabetes and urinary incontinence in 50–90 year-old women: A cross-sectional population-based study. *American Journal of Obstetrics and Gynaecology* 193(6): 2154–8.

Macauley, M. 1997. Urinary drainage systems. In: Fillingham, S. and Douglas, J. (eds.) *Urological Nursing*, 2nd edn. London: Baillière Tindall, 90–130.

MacDonald, C. and Butler, L. 2007. Silent no more: Elderly women's stories of living with urinary incontinence in long-term care. *Journal of Gerontological Nursing* 33(1): 14–20.

Madersbacher, S. et al. 2003. Long-term outcome of ileal conduit diversion. *Journal of Urology* 169(3): 985–90.

Maki, D.G. and Tambyah, P.A. 2001. Engineering out the risk for infection with urinary catheters. *Emerging Infectious Diseases* 7(2): 342–7.

Marsh, L. et al. 2010. Management of constipation. *Learning Disability Practice* 13(4): 26–8.

McNulty, C. et al. 2003. Prevalence of urinary catheterisation in UK nursing homes. *Journal of Hospital Infection* 55(2): 119–23.

Mead, M. 1998. Stool culture. *Practice Nurse* 16(3): 170.

Mendoza, J. et al. 2007. Systematic review: The adverse effects of sodium phosphate enema. *Alimentary Pharmacology and Therapy* 26(1): 9–20.

Midthun, S.J., Paur, R. and Lindseth, G. 2004. Urinary tract infections: Does the smell really tell? *Journal of Gerontological Nursing* 30(6): 4–9.

Milwain, E. 2010. The brain and person centred care. 4. Memory, belief, emotion and behaviour. *Journal of Dementia Care* 18(3): 25–9.

National Institute for Health and Clinical Excellence (NICE). 2007. *Faecal Incontinence: The Management of Faecal Incontinence in Adults*. Clinical Guidelines 49. London: NICE.

National Institute for Health and Clinical Excellence (NICE). 2010a (Updated 2017). *Constipation in Children and Young People: Diagnosis and Management of Idiopathic Childhood Constipation in Primary and Secondary Care*. Clinical Guidelines 99. London: NICE.

National Institute for Health and Clinical Excellence (NICE). 2010b. *Nocturnal Enuresis – The Management of Bedwetting in Children and Young People*. Clinical Guidelines 111. London: NICE.

National Institute for Health and Clinical Excellence (NICE). 2012. *Urinary Incontinence in Neurological Disease. Management of Lower Urinary Tract Dysfunction in Neurological Disease*. Clinical Guidelines 148. London: NICE.

National Institute for Health and Clinical Excellence (NICE). 2014a. *Faecal Incontinence in Adults*: Quality statement QS54.

National Institute for Health and Clinical Excellence (NICE). 2014b. Bedwetting in Children and Young People. Quality Standard QS70. London: NICE.

National Institute for Health and Clinical Excellence (NICE). 2015 *Lower urinary tract symptoms in men: Management*. Clinical Guideline CG97. London: NICE.

National Institute for Health and Clinical Excellence (NICE). 2017 Healthcare-associated infections: prevention and control in primary and community care. https://www.guidelines.co.uk/infection/nice-healthcare-associated-infections-guideline/453383.article (Accessed on 10 November 2020).

National Institute for Health and Clinical Excellence (NICE). 2018a. Urinary tract infection in under 16s: diagnosis and management. Clinical guidelines [CG54] published 22 August 2007. Updated 31 October 2018. London: NICE.

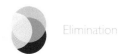

National Institute for Health and Clinical Excellence (NICE). 2018b Peristeen transanal irrigation system for managing bowel dysfunction. Medical Technologies Guidance MTG36. London: NICE.

National Institute for Health and Clinical Excellence (NICE). 2019a. *Urinary Incontinence and Pelvic Organ Prolapse in Women: Management* NICE guideline NG123. https://www. nice.org.uk/guidance/ng123

National Institute for Health and Clinical Excellence (NICE) (2019b) Learning Disability: Behaviour that Challenges. Quality Statement https://www.nice.org.uk/guidance/ qs101

National Patient Safety Agency (NPSA). 2007. *Using Bedrails Safely and Effectively.* London: NPSA.

Nazarko, L. 2009. Urinary tract infection: Diagnosis, treatment and prevention. *British Journal of Nursing* 18(19): 1170–4.

Nazarko, L. 2011. Understanding dementia: Diagnosis and development. *British Journal of Healthcare Assistants* 5(5): 216–20.

Newman, D.K. 2012. *Indwelling Urinary Catheters in Acute Care: A Step-by-Step Clinical Pathway for Nurses.* Available from: http://verathon.ca/portaW0/Uploads/ProductMaterials/_bsc/CAUTI/0900–2813–02–84.pdf (Accessed on 13 December 2012).

Nix, D. and Ermer-Seltun, J. 2004. A review of perineal skin care protocols and skin barrier product use. *Ostomy/Wound Management* 50(12): 59–67.

Norton, C. and Cody, J.D. 2012. Biofeedback and/or sphincter exercises for the treatment of faecal incontinence in adults. *Cochrane Database of Systematic Reviews* 7. Art. No.: CD002111. doi: 10.1002/14651858.CD002111.pub3.

Nursing and Midwifery Council (2018) Standards of proficiency for nursing associates. Available from: nursing-associates-proficiency-standards.pdf (nmc.org.uk) (Accessed on 10 December 2020).

Ostaszkiewicz, J. 2006. The clinical effectiveness of systematic voiding programmes: Results of a meta study. *Australian and New Zealand Continence Journal* 12(1): 5–6.

Ostaszkiewicz, J., Johnston, L. and Roe, B. 2010. Habit retraining for the management of urinary incontinence in adults. *Cochrane Database of Systematic Reviews* (2). Art. No.: CD002801. doi: 10.1002/14651858.CD002801.pub2.

Ostaszkiewicz, J., Johnston, L. and Roe, B. 2011. Timed voiding for the management of urinary incontinence in adults. *Cochrane Database of Systematic Reviews.* (1). Art. No.: CD002802. doi: 10.1002/14651858.CD002802.pub2.

Padmanabhan, A. et al. 2007. Clinical evaluation of a flexible fecal incontinence management system. *American Journal of Critical Care* 16(4): 384–93.

Palmer, M.H. and Newman, D.K. 2006. Bladder control: Educational needs of older adults. *Journal of Gerontological Nursing* 32(1): 28–32.

Palmieri, B., Benuzzi, G. and Bellini, N. 2005. The anal bag: A modern approach to fecal incontinence management. *Ostomy/Wound Management* 51(12): 44–52.

Panagamuwa, C., Glasby, M.J. and Peckham, T.J. 2004. Dipstick screening for urinary tract infection before arthroscopy: A safe alternative to laboratory testing? *International Journal of Clinical Practice* 58(1): 19–21.

Parascandolo, M.E. and Doughty, D. 2001. Multiple ostomy complications in a patient with Crohn's disease: a case study. *Journal of Wound, Ostomy and Continence Nursing* 28(5): 236–43.

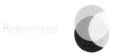
Pellatt, G. 2007. Clinical skills: Bowel elimination and management of complications. *British Journal of Nursing* 16(6): 351–5.

Pellatt, G.C. 2012. Non-containment management options of urinary continence. *Nursing & Residential Care* 14(2): 68–73.

Pemberton, P. et al. 2006. A comparative study of two types of urinary sheath. *Nursing Times* 102(7): 36–41.

Pratt, R.J. et al. 2007. National evidence-based guidelines for preventing healthcare-associated infections in NHS England. *Journal of Hospital Infection* 65(Suppl 1): S1–64.

Public Health England. 2020. Diagnosis of urinary tract infection: A quick guide for primary care. Available from: https://assets.publishing.service.gov.uk/government/uploads/system/uploads/attachment_data/file/927195/UTI_diagnostic_flowchart_NICE-October_2020-FINAL.pdf (Accessed 10 November 2020). PHE publications gateway number: GW-1263.

Rassin, M. et al. 2007. Levels of comfort and ease among patients suffering from urinary incontinence. *International Journal of Urological Nursing* 1(2): 64–70.

Ratliff, C. et al. 2005. Descriptive study of peristomal complications. *Journal of Wound, Ostomy and Continence Nursing* 32(1): 33–7.

Resnick, B. et al. 2006. Nursing staff beliefs and expectations about continence care in nursing homes. *Journal of Wound, Ostomy and Continence Nursing* 33(6): 610–18.

Richbourg, L., Thorpe, J.M. and Rapp, C.G. 2007. Difficulties experienced by the ostomate after hospital discharge. *Journal of Wound, Ostomy and Continence Nursing* 34(1): 70–9.

Richmond, J.P. and Wright, M.E. 2004. Review of the literature on constipation to enable development of a constipation risk assessment scale. *Clinical Effectiveness in Nursing* 8(1): 11–25.

Rigby, D. 2007. Medication for continence. In: Getliffe, K. and Dolman, M. (eds.) *Promoting Continence: A Clinical and Research Guide*, 3rd edn. Edinburgh: Baillière Tindall, 239–58.

Roe, B. et al. 2006. Systematic reviews of bladder training and voiding programmes in adults: A synopsis of findings from data analysis and outcomes using metastudy techniques. *Journal of Advanced Nursing* 57(1): 15–31.

Royal College of Nursing (RCN). 2011. *Meeting the Health Needs of People with Learning Disabilities*. London: RCN.

Royal College of Nursing (RCN). 2019. *Bowel Care: Management of Lower Bowel Dysfunction, Including Digital Rectal Examination and Digital Removal of Faeces*. London: RCN.

Royal Marsden Hospital Manual of Clinical Nursing Procedures. 2020. 10th edn. Wiley-Blackwell.

Saint, S., Kaufman, S.R., Rogers, M.A.M., et al. 2006. Condom versus indwelling urinary catheters: A randomized trial. *Journal of the American Geriatrics Society* 54(7): 1055–61.

Saye, D.E. 2007. Recurring and antimicrobial resistant infections: considering the potential role of biofilms in clinical practice. *Ostomy/Wound Management* 53(4): 46–52.

Schmelzer, M. and Wright, K.B. 1996. Enema administration techniques used by experienced registered nurses. *Gastroenterology Nursing* 19: 171–5.

Schumm, K. and Lam, T.B.L. 2010. Types of urethral catheters for management of short-term voiding problems in hospitalised adults. *Cochrane Database System Review* 2. Art. No.: CD004013. doi: 10.1002/14651858.CD004013.pub3.

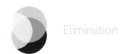
Scottish Intercollegiate Guidelines Network (SIGN). 2006. *Management of Patients with Dementia*. Available from: http://www.sign.ac.uk/pdf/sign86.pdf (Accessed on 1 September 2012).

Slater-Smith, S. 2010. Promoting children's continence. B) Childhood constipation. In: Glasper, A., Aylott, M. and Battrick, C. (eds.) *Developing Practical Skills for Nursing Children and Young People*. London: Hodder Arnold, 229–41.

Smith, B. 2010. Faecal incontinence in older people: Delivering effective, dignified care. *British Journal of Community Nursing* 15(8): 370–4.

Smith, P. and Smith, L. 2007. Continence training in intellectual disability. In: Getliffe, K. and Dolman. M. (eds.) *Promoting Continence: A Clinical and Research Resource*, 3rd edn. Edinburgh: Baillière Tindall, 173–202.

Steggall, M. and Cox, C. 2009. A step-by-step guide to performing a complete digital rectal examination. *Gastrointestinal Nursing* 7(2): 28–32.

Steggall, M.J. 2008. Digital rectal examination. *Nursing Standard* 22(47): 46–8.

Stewart, E. 2010. Treating urinary incontinence in older women. *British Journal of Community Nursing* 15(11): 526, 528, 530–2.

Stickler, D. 2008. Bacterial biofilms in patients with indwelling urinary catheters. *Nature Clinical Practice Urology* 5: 598–608.

Stoma Care. 2007. *An Educational Resource for Stoma Care Nursing,* DVD. Cambridgeshire: Burdett Institute of Gastrointestinal Nursing and Dansac Ltd.

Thompson, J. 2007. Falls and incontinence: Evaluation of a quality management project. *Australian and New Zealand Continence Journal* 13(1): 18, 20–1.

Tlaskalová-Hogenová, H. et al. 2004. Commensal bacteria (normal microflora) mucosal immunity and chronic inflammatory and autoimmune diseases. *Immunology Letters* 93: 97–108.

Vaillancourt, S. et al. 2007. To clean or not to clean: Effect on contamination rates in midstream urine collections in toilet-trained children. *Pediatrics* 119: e1288–93.

Vickerman, J. 2003. The benefits of a lending library for female urinals. *Nursing Times* 99(44): 56–7.

Voegeli, D. 2008. Skin care and incontinence in the elderly. *Nursing and Residential Care* 10(10): 487–92.

Wallace, S.A. et al. 2009. Bladder training for urinary incontinence in adults. *Cochrane Database of Systematic Reviews* (1). Art. No.: CD001308. doi: 10.1002/14651858.CD001308. pub2.

Wareing, M. 2005. Lower urinary tract symptoms: A hermeneutic phenomenological study into men's lived experience. *Journal of Clinical Nursing* 14: 239–46.

Wells, M. and Wagg, A. 2007. Integrated continence services and the female Bangladeshi population. *British Journal of Nursing* 16: 516–9.

Williams, D. and Moran, S. 2006. Use of urinary sheaths in male incontinence. *Nursing Times* 102(47): 42–5.

Williams, J. 2012. Inserting suppositories and enemas into a colostomy. *Gastrointestinal Nursing* 10(1): 13–14.

Wilson, J. 2006. *Infection Control in Clinical Practice,* 3rd edn. Edinburgh: Baillière Tindall.

Wilson, M. 2011. Addressing the problems of long-term urethral catheterisation: Part 1. *British Journal of Nursing* 20(22): 1418–24.

Wilson, M. 2012. Addressing the problems of long-term urethral catheterisation: Part 2. *British Journal of Nursing* 21(1): 16–25.

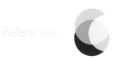
Wolfman, A. 2010. Preventing incontinence-associated dermatitis and early-stage pressure injury. *World Council of Enterostomal Therapists Journal* 30(1): 19–24.

Woodford, H.J. and George, J. 2009. Diagnosis and management of urinary tract infection in hospitalized older people. *Journal of the American Geriatrics Society* 57: 107–14.

Woodward, S. 2012. Assessment and management of constipation in older people. *Nursing Older People* 24(5): 21–6.

Yates, A. 2012. Management of long-term urinary catheters. *Nursing and Residential Care* 14(4): 172–8.

Meeting personal needs: hygiene

Moira Walker

Assisting people to meet their fundamental hygiene needs has always been at the forefront of nursing care. The importance of personal hygiene is reinforced by its inclusion in the Department of Health's (DH) *Essence of Care 2010* benchmarks (DH 2010). The Chief Nursing Officer's review of mental health nursing, *From Values to Action*, also highlighted personal and physical care as being important skills for mental health nurses (DH 2006). This has now been reinforced by the inclusion within the Nursing and Midwifery Council's (NMC) (2018a) 'Future nurse: Standards of proficiency for all registered nurses' and NMC's (2018b) 'Standards of proficiency for nursing associates'.

The ability to maintain one's own personal hygiene is a skill generally learnt early in life and affects a person's self-esteem, confidence and health. It is important to understand what is involved in personal care that includes activities such as bathing, washing the hair, brushing the teeth, and perineal care. These activities eliminate the sources of most preventable infections and has a marked impact on an individual's sense of self (Sener et al. 2019). However, sometimes disability and/or physical and mental health problems lead to people needing assistance on either a temporary or a permanent basis. Meeting hygiene needs greatly contributes to comfort and well-being, and for those who lack the ability to care for themselves, provides the opportunity to build up a trusting therapeutic relationship (Cowdell 2010). As with any other skill/procedure, hygiene needs must be discussed fully with the person beforehand and verbal consent obtained so it is tailored to their individual's needs (NMC 2018a&b).

The principles of care (e.g. observation, comfort, communication, safety and prevention of cross-infection) discussed in this chapter are generally relevant to anyone but how they are carried out for each individual varies with privacy and dignity being at the forefront of that care. It is also important to consider the religious and cultural needs of individuals when meeting hygiene needs.

This chapter includes:

- Rationale for meeting hygiene needs and potential hazards
- Bathing a person in bed (includes hair-washing in bed)
- Bathing and showering in the bathroom
- Shaving
- Oral hygiene

DOI: 10.4324/9781003020660-7

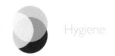

RECOMMENDED READING

You should revise the layers of the skin. In addition, these questions will help guide you to understand the biology/physiology underpinning this chapter's skills. Use your recommended textbooks to find out:

- The skin and oral cavity host a range of microorganisms. Which of these are potentially pathogenic?
- What is saliva composed of? Where is it produced, and what is its role in maintaining a healthy mouth?
- What protective mechanisms do eyes have that prevent them from infection?
- Distinguish between transient and resident bacteria found on the skin. Which of these cannot be removed by handwashing? Chapter 12 will help you with this.
- How does skin maintain its waterproof properties?
- Why does the skin of the palms of the hands and soles of the feet wrinkle when soaked in water?
- How does ageing affect the skin?
- What part does nutrition play in maintaining a healthy skin, hair and nails?
- Why do we sweat and what does sweat contain?
- Why does stale sweat smell?
- What is the 'acid mantle' and how can it be destroyed?

How important it is to a person, do you think, is the touch, smell and look of their skin/mouth when interacting with others?

What does the complexion of the person tell you about a person's health, both physical and mental?

PRACTICE SCENARIOS

The following practice scenarios are referred to throughout this chapter in relation to meeting hygiene needs.

Adult

Metastases

Secondary deposits of cancer that have spread from the primary site, either directly or via blood or lymph.

William Newton, who likes to be called 'Bill', is a retired accountant aged 73. He is terminally ill with a history of oesophageal cancer and metastases in his lungs. He is cared for by his wife at home with the support of community nurses and the Macmillan nurse. He is taking regular oral morphine for pain control. He has a very low haemoglobin and has been admitted for a blood transfusion. He is weak, breathless and his general condition is poor. He has a **body mass index (BMI)** of 16. He can swallow only very small amounts of liquidised food and drink. He has some of his own teeth but also a partial denture that he likes to wear although it is now ill-fitting. His tongue appears coated, and his mouth is dry.

Learning disability

Ellen Grey is a 47-year-old woman with a learning disability. She lives in sheltered accommodation in her own flat. There is a communal lounge. She has always managed her own personal hygiene adequately. However, recently she has developed an unpleasant smell and other residents have begun to avoid her because of this. The community nurse for learning disabilities has been asked to assess the situation and find out what has changed. She identifies that Ellen's personal hygiene has become compromised because of the recent development of nocturnal incontinence. As well as her bed linen being wet, the situation has disrupted Ellen's usual hygiene routine.

Mental health

Miss Smith, aged 83 years, was admitted to an inpatient assessment unit for older people following concerns from her social worker and GP about her inability to cope at home due to severe depression. She lives on her own with only her pet dog for company. As she can no longer climb her stairs she has been sleeping in an armchair downstairs. Her poor mobility also prevented her from reaching the bathroom. Although Miss Smith is in reasonable physical health her clothing has obviously not been changed for many months and is encrusted with dirt and excrement. Her hair is badly knotted and matted and her skin is in poor condition. She also has poor oral hygiene, which she has obviously neglected for some time. Miss Smith was initially distrusting of staff and resisted all attempts to help her have bath and clean clothes. Eventually she agreed to do this but remained hostile towards staff, accusing them of stealing her dog and her house. However, nurses explained that her dog had been taken to the local RSPCA kennels and was in good health. Gradually Miss Smith became more accepting of her new surroundings and began to engage nurses in conversation without her previous hostility or suspicion.

RATIONALE FOR MEETING HYGIENE NEEDS AND POTENTIAL HAZARDS

Box 7.1 Learning outcomes

By the end of this section you will be able to:

1. explain why facilitating people to meet their hygiene needs is a beneficial nursing action;
2. discuss possible hazards and problems associated with meeting hygiene needs.

Learning outcome 1: explain why facilitating people to meet their hygiene needs is a beneficial nursing action

Box 7.2 Activity: nurse assistance with hygiene needs

ACTIVITY

Why is it important for nurses to assist with hygiene needs? Consider how you might feel if you were incapacitated mentally or physically and unable to meet your hygiene needs.

Feeling clean and comfortable is an important social need for most people; to feel well-groomed and not offensive to others can help maintain self-esteem. Thus, for

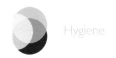

Ellen to be aware that she has an unpleasant odour which others are discussing could cause her some distress. Miss Smith's poor mobility has prevented her maintaining her hygiene and this is probably upsetting for her. Being unkempt can at times also mask the deterioration of an illness (Gústafsdóttir 2011) either physical or mental so it is important to understand the reasons behind the decline. Psycho-dermatology links the way someone is physically displaying changes to a process within the body whether that is psychological or physiological in nature (Jafferany, Roque Ferreira and Patel 2020).

- Cleanliness is important within many cultures and religions (see later discussion). For example, for Muslims, cleanliness has both a spiritual and physical dimension (Rassool 2000). A study of older South Asian people's experiences of culturally sensitive care highlighted that maintaining their hygiene was essential for dignity (Clegg 2003). Some cultures consider some aspects of bodily functions as unsavoury or 'dirty', so it is important to understand social and cultural background the individual is from (Priya 2019).
- The act of assisting people with personal hygiene needs allows nurses to build up a trusting relationship (Stonehouse 2016). It is a private time where communication may be facilitated. Brawley (2002) points out that for people living in care homes, bath time may be one of the only opportunities for individual attention. It is also important to realise that care is personal to the individual and to the caregiver, it can be considered their job. This in turn impacts the relationship and ease in which the receiver (person receiving care) feels displaced as that care to them might no longer be private (Sundström et al. 2018).
- Valuable observations can be made, for example the condition of the skin (Cowdell 2010). This will be important for all the people in this chapter's scenarios.
- Cleansing the skin removes potentially harmful microorganisms and also sweat, dead skin cells and the bacteria that produce body odour. This is especially important with regard to the genitalia of both men and woman as they are prime sources for the build-up of harmful microorganisms due to urinary or faecal incontinence (NHS Choices 2018).
- Washing can have a number of positive attributes from stimulating the circulation, aiding in relaxation of physical and mental agitation, allows time out from having to be with others in a place that is considered private (Kottner and Surber 2016).

For some people, being washed or bathed by others can be humiliating so nurses must protect self-esteem and dignity as far as possible by adhering to individual wishes (DH 2010). As identified above, observant nurses can learn a great deal about people when assisting with their hygiene needs.

Box 7.3 Activity: observations while assisting someone with hygiene

ACTIVITY

What could you observe while assisting a person with hygiene? Looking at the scenarios may give you some clues.

- Condition of the skin. Is there redness or bruising, and are there breaks in the skin? Is there any skin infection? Are there any old scars? This is important for Bill because of advancing disease, but is also relevant to Ellen and Miss Smith.
- Hydration and nutrition. Does the skin feel dry, loose or oedematous? Any of the people in this chapter's scenarios could become dehydrated due to poor fluid intake and their skin could become dry.
- Mental state. Is the person anxious, calm, restless, depressed, de-motivated, cheerful, lethargic or confused?
- Physical ability. How much can the person do? Do they require prompting? With Ellen, the nurse will be able to assess how much she can do for herself, what aspects she requires assistance with and what aids she might require. Does the activity cause breathlessness or fatigue? These will affect Bill's ability to care for himself.
- Condition of wounds, drains, intravenous sites (IV): these could apply to Bill, for example, inflammation of his IV site.

Oedematous

Swelling caused by the accumulation of fluid in the interstitial spaces

Learning outcome 2: discuss the possible hazards and problems associated with meeting hygiene needs

As discussed above, meeting a person's hygiene needs should be a therapeutic intervention, yet there are several potential complications or difficulties.

Box 7.4 Activity: hazards or problems associated with hygiene needs

Consider: what hazards or problems could be associated with meeting hygiene needs?

ACTIVITY

Review the points below and reflect on the questions raised:

- **Access**. The person might be unable to get into a bathroom or the shower owing to mobility issues. *Can you think what those mobility issues might be?*
- **Environment**. People can become cold if left exposed for too long. There are health and safety aspects in relation to wet floors, and water being too hot/cold. *How does skin exposure affect the temperature control of a child/adult/older person who is unwell?*
- **Cross-infection**. Some studies have shown that there were more bacteria on a person's skin after a bed bath than before (Parker 2004). *Can you think of the possible cause for the increase of the bacteria on the skin and how this could be minimised?*
- **Damage to skin**. The person might have allergies to particular soaps, or over-washing may remove essential oils. *What other factors could impact on the skin, while meeting hygiene needs?*
- **Fatigue**. For example, meeting Bill's hygiene needs could exhaust him. *What is it about Bill's illness that might have an impact on his energy levels?* Is there a long distance to get to the bathroom or toilet? Is the room on the same floor or is it upstairs or downstairs from where the person spends most of their time? What aspect might impact on Bill making the effort to go to the bathroom?

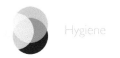

• **Embarrassment**. People may have a fear of their bodies being seen naked by others. Cultural or religious beliefs need to be considered. *What might you do to help maintain the dignity of the individual you are helping?*

Box 7.5 Activity: cultural and religious considerations

Consider further the cultural and religious beliefs of the people you care for. What particular aspects are you aware of?

The list that follows gives some examples but take care not to make assumptions and find out about individuals' wishes.

• African – Caribbean. Hair type requires regular moisturising. The hair and scalp should be moistened every other day at least and the skin moistened once or twice a day (Christmas 2002). In some African/American cultures, it is rude to ask if they are wearing a wig so broaching the subject of cleaning their hair or touching their head must be done with sensitivity (Rowe 2019).

• Rastafarian. The person might wear hair natural and uncut in obedience to God, who told the Nazarenes (a group of ancient Israelites) to do so. Some Rastafarians keep their hair covered. Modesty in dress is important. Hospital gowns may be viewed as immodest for women (Baxter 2002).

• Sikhism. Personal hygiene is very important. Hands and face must be washed and teeth brushed before eating. It is also really important that you adhere to the individual's preferred timings or rituals with regard to their own hygiene habits (Queensland Health 2011).

• Islam. A very high standard of hygiene is required (Rassool 2000). Muslims must wash before they pray (Holland and Hogg 2010).

• Hinduism. Handwashing is essential before and after eating. Washing in running water is very important for Hindus (Holland and Hogg 2010).

Assessment and discussion with people on how they would like their hygiene needs met are key for this procedure to be therapeutic and will ensure any individual cultural/religious needs are met. The Essence of Care (DH 2010) emphasises the need for assessment and re-assessment to maintain their optimum levels of hygiene.

Summary

● Assisting people with meeting their hygiene needs can greatly increase comfort and provide an excellent opportunity for observation and assessment.

● Nurses must remember that not all people will enjoy the experience of being washed. They should therefore consider the key principles of care and comfort, so care is delivered therapeutically.

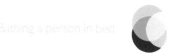

BATHING A PERSON IN BED

Bathing a person in bed is necessary when people are unable to get out of bed for medical reasons (e.g. after certain surgery or injuries), or when they are too unwell or weak to be able to get out of bed. Bill may need this option at present. The procedure described in this section – bed-bathing – involves washing a person's body while they are in bed, using a bowl of water and cloths or alternatives such as emollients.

While this section focuses on bathing in bed, some people who are unable to wash in the bathroom can sit out in a chair to wash, using a bowl. Nurses need to give assistance according to individual needs that have been jointly decided on as well as being based on assessment of the individual at that time; the principles discussed in this section can be adapted to each situation.

Box 7.6 Learning outcomes

By the end of this section, you will be able to:

1 discuss ways of maintaining dignity and enhancing comfort when bathing a person in bed.
2 describe the procedure for carrying out bed-bathing and hair-washing in bed.

Learning outcome 1: discuss ways of maintaining dignity and enhancing comfort when bathing a person in bed

---

Box 7.7 Activity: maintaining a person's dignity and comfort

How might you maintain a person's dignity and comfort while undertaking a bed bath?

Points you may have considered include:

- ensuring that you have all necessary equipment before starting, to avoid leaving the person during the procedure;
- ensuring privacy by drawing the curtains and informing other members of staff of what you are doing to limit interruptions;
- ensuring windows are closed to avoid draughts;
- encouraging the person to do as much as possible, allowing them the time to do this;
- asking the person how they normally wash, what do they use for cleaning;
- covering the person with a towel, only exposing areas of the body when necessary;
- using your communication skills – the atmosphere and relationship the nurse builds with the person will do much to promote dignity;
- being aware that clothing may have special significance within some religions (Holland and Hogg 2010).

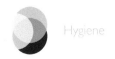

Learning outcome 2: describe the procedure for carrying out bed-bathing

Before commencing the bathing of a person in bed, you must assess the individual.

> ### Box 7.8 Activity: items that should be included in your assessment
>
> Using one of the scenarios as a guide, what items should you include in your assessment?

Compare your list with the following.

- What is the person's normal hygiene routine? When do they normally wash/ bathe? Can that be facilitated while they are in hospital/ care facility?
- Does the person have capacity to consent to have a bed bath and what best interest decisions need to be made? Particularly consider what decisions the person made if they had capacity to make them. Family, friends and carers may be able to provide insight into this.
- What toiletries do they use? Are they available?
- How does the person feel today? Do they want a full wash or the bare minimum? This may change on a daily basis depending on how the person is feeling.
- Does any care need to be given prior to the wash? For example, if the person is due to have any bowel medication rectally, it would be preferable to administer this prior to the wash.
- Does the person require any analgesia prior to the bed bath to ensure comfort when moving and turning?
- How much assistance is required? How much can the person do? Does the nurse need to be present to prompt and guide, or does the person want to be left alone to undertake some aspects?
- Does the person want a family member to be involved in providing care? If yes, have they been asked? What is that person willing to do?
- How much time is needed to undertake this activity for this particular person? What else is happening to the person today: X-ray, theatre?
- How many staff are needed to undertake this activity for a particular person?
- Are other healthcare professionals involved in the person's care: occupational therapist, physiotherapist? Do they need to be involved to make a needs assessment?

Equipment

It is important to gather everything required prior to starting, to avoid having to leave the person unattended; this will enhance privacy, dignity and comfort. Box 7.9 lists the equipment that you are likely to need, but you must always consider the person's own individual requirements.

Box 7.9 Preparing to bathe a person in bed: equipment required

- Person's own washing bowl
- Soap, skin cleanser
- Person's own flannel or disposable flannel
- Towels
- Comb and/or brush
- Toiletries as required, and may include shaving foam, razor, antiperspirant, moisturiser
- Clean bed linen and bed clothes
- Linen bags and waste bag
- Plastic apron and disposable gloves

Procedure

Listed below is a suggested procedure for bathing a person in bed that is likely to maintain comfort and prevent the person from becoming cold. A sensitive and empathetic approach should be maintained throughout. It is also important that the nurse does not impose their idea of what is cleanliness but respects what the person feels as a level of hygiene that is appropriate for them (Downey and Lloyd 2008). Ensure that you have introduced yourself to the person, and that you use the bed bath as an opportunity to build further rapport. People may be pleased to engage in conversation, but they may feel too weak and wish for a minimum of interaction, so be sensitive to non-verbal cues.

- Wash your hands and put on the plastic apron (and gloves if needed – see Chapter 12).
- Fill the bowl with comfortably warm water.
- Remove the top bedclothes, leaving the person covered by a blanket, sheet or towels.
- Remove the pyjama jacket or nightdress. If the person has a weak arm or has an intravenous infusion attached (as has Bill), remove this arm from the clothing last.

Box 7.10 Activity: removing a jacket with impaired arm mobility

ACTIVITY

Practice with a friend or colleague, removing a jacket or cardigan from each other, while pretending that one arm's mobility is impaired. Now try replacing it, inserting the affected arm first.

- Can the person wash their own face? Even quite unwell people often like to do this for themselves. Otherwise, wash the person's face, using soap if wanted. Never poke inside ears. Rinse off soap, if used, and pat dry carefully. With eyes, take care to wash from the inner to outer corner of the eye, thus reducing the risk of contamination. Make sure there is little or no soap on the cloth as this can be extremely painful if it gets into the eyes. Always approach any care relating to eyes with gentleness and cleanliness to avoid risk of trauma or cross-infection.

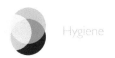
- People who are unconscious or semi-conscious are at risk of their eyes becoming dry. Eyes need to be assessed regularly for signs of irritation, corneal drying, abrasions and oedema (Geraghty 2005).
- Find out about the eye care policy in your current care setting.

ACTIVITY

Box 7.11 Activity: washing/drying faces

With a friend or colleague, practice washing and drying each other's face. How did it feel? Is there a difference in feeling of being pat dried or rubbed dry?

People with sensitive skin such as babies, toddlers or those who have had radiation treatment for cancer might find rubbing of the skin extremely uncomfortable. Can you think of who else might have sensitive skin?

ACTIVITY

Box 7.12 Activity: practising washing and drying an arm

With a friend or colleague, practise washing and drying on an arm. Leave the soap on the skin and let it dry. Note what it looks like and how does it feel to you touching the skin but more importantly the person whose skin it is. Does it feel uncomfortable/itchy/patchy? Think how this would feel for your patient who might have sensitive skin?

- Having completed your person's face wash, the bathing procedure should continue.
- Place a towel under the arm furthest away from you, and wash from the hand to the axilla. Rinse off the soap and pat dry thoroughly, taking care not to dislodge any cannulae or dressings. Repeat with the other arm.
- Uncover the chest and abdomen and wash and dry this area in the same way, again taking care not to dislodge dressings or attachments. Work gently but quickly to prevent the person from becoming chilled. Pay special attention to skin folds and under the breasts, as these areas may be moist through sweat and therefore heavily colonised with microorganisms. When cleaning under the breasts, use the back of your hand gently to lift as you are trying to maintain their dignity by not grabbing or holding the flesh. Cover the chest and abdomen once this is completed.
- Toiletries such as antiperspirant or body spray can be applied as wished by the person. If a person is sweating excessively, putting gauze under the breasts or between the folds can help to prevent heat rash and help to keep the area dry. The areas must be closely monitored for any abrasions or rashes.
- Change the water at this point, or at any time if it feels cool or becomes excessively soiled. If water is not changed and the same washcloth is used for the whole body, the water can become full of bacteria and be a potential hazard to people with breaks in their skin (Ayliffe et al. 2001).
- Now remove any lower body clothing including anti-embolism stockings, cover the leg nearest you, and place the towel under the opposite leg. Wash the leg from toes to groin, rinse and dry. Apply moisturising lotion if the skin appears dry over the shins or feet. Repeat with the other leg.

Box 7.13 Activity: observations while washing arms, body and legs

What observations should you be making while washing arms, body and legs?

Your observations should include condition of the skin, checking for dryness, colour, bruises, abrasions, rashes, swelling or oedema. Nurses should apply skin moisturisers as needed (Kottner & Surber 2016). You should also note any tenderness in the limbs, particularly the calves, which might indicate a deep vein thrombosis (see Chapter 11).

For some people, attention to foot care is particularly important. Those at risk of foot problems include older people and people with diabetes, peripheral vascular disease or peripheral neuropathy (Nazarko 2017). Foot problems in people with diabetes are discussed in detail elsewhere (e.g. Howell and Thirlaway 2004; NICE 2019a, 2011); see also Chapter 13 in this book. Patient education about foot care may reduce foot ulceration and amputations, especially in high-risk people (Nazarko 2017) and doing this through personal care is an optimum time to do that. When people are unable to self-care, nurses must carry out the foot care and observation required, and report any concerns immediately. Box 7.14 outlines the key principles in footcare. Some people find it comforting to soak their feet in warm water for a while. This can be done easily by sitting them in the chair (if they are able) and putting their feet into a bowl of warm water but be aware that there is evidence that this is contraindicated with someone who is diabetic (Nazarko 2017). Make sure that when you dry the feet you pay particular attention to drying in between the toes as this area can often harbour bacteria and fungi.

Box 7.14 Advice about foot care for people with diabetes (adapted from NICE 2004)

- Wash feet daily, drying them carefully and thoroughly, particularly between the toes.
- Examine feet daily for problems (colour change, swelling, breaks in skin, pain or numbness). If they occur, report them to a healthcare professional. People with a foot care emergency (new ulceration, swelling, discoloration) should be seen by a multidisciplinary foot care team within 24 hours. Check the top of the foot, the sole of the foot (people can be taught to use a mirror to do this), between the toes and pressure areas, i.e. tips of toes and heels.
- Check for signs of redness around nail areas, and ensure nails do not cut into adjacent toes. Cut immediately after bathing when nails are soft, following the shape of the toe and not down into tissue. If nails are thick and brittle, **do not** attempt to cut – refer to podiatrist. Note: Follow local policies regarding nail-cutting.
- Make sure that shoes and hosiery fit well.
- Ensure that feet are assessed at least annually by trained personnel.

(Continued)

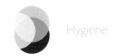

Box 7.14 (Continued)

In addition, people at increased or high risk of foot ulcers (neuropathy, and/or absent pulses or other risk factor) should:

- Have feet reviewed by a foot protection team every 3–6 months.
- Never walk barefoot.
- Realise that any break in the skin is potentially serious.
- Check bath temperatures carefully (numb feet cannot assess temperature).
- Avoid hot water bottles, electric blankets, foot spas and sitting with feet too close to fires.
- Get help to deal with calluses and corns (avoid over-the-counter remedies).
- Regularly inspect footwear for rough areas, ripped linings, etc.

The bathing procedure should continue:

- Using a disposable washcloth, wash the genitals and perineal area, working from front to back to prevent contamination of the urethra and/or vagina with faecal matter. Catheter care may be required at this point (see Chapter 6, section on 'Caring for people who have urinary catheters'). Change the water now – remember the rationale for this (see the previous section, learning outcome 2).

  Phimosis

  Tight foreskin will not retract over the glans of the penis.

  Paraphimosis

  Once retracted, a tight foreskin gets stuck behind the glans.

  Note: when cleaning the penis, the foreskin needs to be drawn back from the glans and the area gently cleaned. It is essential that the foreskin is then brought back over the glans after cleaning otherwise a phimosis or paraphimosis can develop. In boys up to the age of 17–19, the foreskin is still attached and should not be forced down the glans as this could cause pain and damage (Wilson et al. 2009)

- When cleaning the labia in women, it is important that the soap is properly rinsed from the area as any soap residue can cause extreme irritation and itching.

  Note: Cleaning the genital area must be conducted with sensitivity as this particular area is extremely private and the person could feel very embarrassed. Be sure to ask permission and if possible encourage the person to do much of the care themselves to reduce their feelings of vulnerability, although some people will be too physically or mentally impaired. Although Bill is weak, he might be able to do this for himself with some help.

- At this point, you need to assess how you can wash the person's back. You can either sit the person forward or lie them on their side. Sitting Bill forward to wash his back would be best as he might become breathless if lying on his side for long, you can ask/assist him to lean forward, wash, rinse and dry his back, using a clean washcloth. The pillowcases can be changed, and he can be assisted into a clean pyjama jacket. For a woman, a clean nightdress can be put on at this point.

- To wash a person's back if they cannot sit forward, and to wash a person's buttocks, you need to turn them on their side; you may require assistance to do this. The bottom sheet can be changed at this time. You can insert a slide sheet to assist with turning and then moving the person up the bed after completing the wash. If you feel assistance is not required, you need to raise the opposite bed rail to provide security for the person when rolling on to their side. Assist the person to roll over, using the log roll method and putting a pillow under their top knee to make it more comfortable and preventing them going onto their front. Roll up the soiled bottom sheet lengthways, close to the person. Place a towel along the person's back, wash, rinse and dry the back and buttocks, noting any skin problems as previously outlined.

Box 7.15 Activity: areas of the skin you should pay most attention to

Which areas of skin do you think you should pay most attention to, while the person is on their side?

You should observe the area's most at risk from pressure damage. These include the sacrum, trochanters, elbows and shoulder tips, base of the skull and heels. See Chapter 11 section on 'Pressure ulcer risk assessment' for more details; Box 11.5 outlines categories of pressure ulcer.

- Now assist with putting on pyjama trousers or adjusting a nightdress. Some people prefer to wear underwear in bed, so then ensure you help them with this. Replace the anti-embolism stockings if worn and change the bottom sheet. To do this, roll or concertina fold a clean sheet close to the person, taking care not to contaminate the clean sheet with the soiled one. Assist the person to roll back towards you, and support them while your assistant removes the soiled sheet, pulls through the clean one and secures it.

Box 7.16 Activity: infection control issues when disposing soiled linen

What might be the infection control issues when disposing of the soiled sheet?

Look back to the principles of preventing cross-infection outlined in Chapter 12. Used linen (soiled and foul) should be disposed of in white or off-white bags. Infected linen should be placed into a water-soluble bag and then into a red bag (or according to local policy).

Box 7.17 Activity: assessing vulnerability when changing a sheet

You will need two friends/colleagues for this exercise, and access to a bed in the skills laboratory. Practise changing the bottom sheet, taking it in turns to be the 'patient'. Consider whether you felt vulnerable during this. What reassured you?

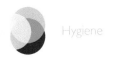

- Using safe moving and handling methods, assist the person into an appropriate and comfortable position, according to their condition and care plan.
- Brush or comb the person's hair into their preferred style. Carry out any other hair care needed at this stage – check the person's personal requirements and what assistance they need.
- Assist with make-up if required and with oral hygiene (see later section).
- Place the locker and call bell within reach.
- Wash and dry the bowl, and dispose of soiled equipment appropriately (see Chapter 12, section on 'Waste disposal'). Washbowls should be stored upside down to reduce colonisation by microorganisms, which prefer horizontal surfaces. Also, if washbowls are not dried properly and are stacked together, bacteria multiply in the moisture trapped between the bowls; contaminated washbowls have been implicated in infection outbreaks, Gram-negative bacteria being most likely to be found (Ayliffe et al. 2001).
- People's own washcloths need to be washed thoroughly after use and stored so that they can dry. They should not be wrapped around the soap (Parker 2004).
- Document any observations made, and the care given, in the care plan or nursing notes.

Box 7.18 Washing hair in bed: equipment and procedure

Equipment

Large jug or bowl of hand-hot water, empty bowl, shampoo guard if available, plastic sheeting if available, small jug, shampoo and conditioner (according to the person's wishes), towels and flannel, brush/comb and hairdryer, plastic apron

Procedure

- Remove the head of the bed and assist the person to lie flat. **NB:** For people who cannot lie flat, hair can be washed over a bowl on a bed table.
- Place the empty bowl on a chair/bed table at the head of the bed, at a lower level. Arrange the plastic sheet to protect the mattress and a towel to protect the person's shoulders.
- Move the person, using a slide sheet, so that their head is over the bowl.
- Check the water temperature and wet the hair using the small jug. The person may like to protect their eyes with a clean flannel.
- Apply shampoo, massage gently into the scalp, and rinse off, repeat if desired, and then apply conditioner and rinse until the hair feels clean. Empty the bowl at intervals, before it gets too full.
- Wrap the person's hair in a clean towel and move the bowl out of the way.
- Slide the person back on to the bed, and remove the plastic sheet. Check the bottom sheet is not damp; replace if necessary.
- Replace the head of the bed, and assist the person to sit up if able, using a safe moving and handling technique.
- Empty the bowl of water, once the person is comfortable, wash and dry the bowls and jug, and dispose of all equipment safely.
- Towel the hair dry, and style the hair as desired, using a hairdryer if necessary. Take care with the hairdryer: ensure that it is not too hot and avoid trailing flexes.
- Leave the person comfortable, with bed table, locker and call bell within reach. Document the care given in the care plan or nursing notes.

People whose health condition requires them to stay in bed for more than a few days are likely to need their hair washed while in bed, to promote their comfort and well-being. Box 7.18 summarises equipment and procedure used.

> ## Box 7.19 Children and young people: practice points – Involving parents in meeting hygiene needs
>
> Parents and children themselves may wish parents to meet the child's hygiene needs. The wishes of the child and family should be ascertained and respected, with offers of support from nurses. It is equally important to respect privacy, dignity and prior levels of independence for children as adults. Effective hand hygiene is essential when changing nappies for parents, as is use of gloves and aprons and effective hand hygiene by nursing staff.
>
> It is important however that the nurse teaches the parents what they need to observe with regard to skin integrity, for example. Depending on the child's condition, they may also need help with moving and handling. For detailed discussion of caring for personal hygiene needs in infants and children, including 'topping and tailing' infants, bathing infants and umbilical cord care, see:
>
> Himsworth (2010) Caring for personal hygiene needs. In Glasper, A., Aylott, M. and Battrick, C. (eds.) *Developing Practical skills for Nursing Children and Young People.* London: Hodder Arnold, 188–202.

Summary

- It is important to assess the suitability of a bed bath for the individual person, and negotiate involvement by the person and their family, as desired.
- Respect for the individual's privacy and dignity, and maintenance of comfort, should be promoted.
- Adherence to infection control procedures and safe moving and handling techniques is vital.

BATHING AND SHOWERING IN THE BATHROOM

If people are able to visit the bathroom to meet their personal hygiene needs, this is usually preferable for various reasons. For some people, actually going in the bath or shower may not be possible, but they may be able to at least sit and wash at the sink, which is usually preferable to washing in, or by, the bed. It is important to remember to attend to the feet and lower legs, as they are often overlooked when people are taken to the sink for a wash.

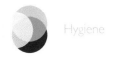

Learning outcome 1: explain the particular benefits and possible problems of meeting hygiene needs in the bathroom rather than at the bedside

ACTIVITY

All should be able to at some stage, but as previously mentioned, Bill may be too weak, tired or in pain to do so at present. Miss Smith will be able to visit the bathroom but will require mobility aids. Ellen will carry out her hygiene care in her own bathroom, but the nurse must revisit her knowledge and skills and reinforce the importance of good hygiene and a bathing routine. Underlying causes of her incontinence must be investigated using a specific tool that addresses physical, psychological and environmental dimensions. The nurse can support Ellen in accessing the necessary services (e.g. continence adviser). The aim should be for Ellen to regain continence and her ability to maintain her hygiene so her **Health Action Plan** should be amended to address these issues. The nurse should broach the subject sensitively; it is important to ensure that this short-term problem does not impact on her social integration and relationships in the longer term. Perhaps a carer could visit in the mornings and evenings, to help Ellen structure her day and ensure that her hygiene needs are being met.

Ellen will probably not require physical assistance in the bathroom, but she needs prompting, encouragement and praise for success in meeting her hygiene needs plan. As she re-establishes her skills, support can reduce until Ellen is self-caring once more.

The presence of a surgical wound is not a contraindication to a shower or bath, as long as the skin edges of the wound are sealed (Copland-Halparin et al. 2020) and it is at least 48 hours after surgery (NICE guidelines 2019). It has been advised that complete immersion such as in a bath is not advised until day 10–14 days after surgery. However, a shower is preferable to a bath for a person with a wound as there is less risk of cross-infection from a previous user (Gilchrist 1990). People with chronic wounds can bathe or shower according to preference. If there is no wound infection present, cleaning of the bath with normal detergent is adequate but if the wound is infected, the bath should be cleaned with hypochlorite solution (see Chapter 13).

Box 7.22 Activity: bathroom vs bedside

Why might it be preferable for hygiene needs to be met in the bathroom if possible, rather than at the bedside?

- The bathroom is a more familiar environment for hygiene, which is important for someone who is confused, or who is preparing for a discharge home. Ellen's teaching programme to meet her hygiene needs will be more effective if carried out in her own familiar bathroom. The bathroom is the most appropriate environment for Miss Smith to re-establish a routine of hygiene care.
- Privacy can be more easily maintained in a bathroom than behind curtains at the bedside.
- There is a continuous supply of water, which may be desirable for cultural and/or religious reasons. For example, in Hinduism, washing in running water, as a shower or by pouring water from a jug, is very important (Holland and Hogg 2010). This is easier to achieve in the bathroom.
- For older people, getting into a bath is a familiar activity. Some people, for example those with muscle spasm, find a bath relaxing and enjoyable.

Box 7.23 Activity: problems carrying out hygiene in the bathroom

While there are good reasons why people can better carry out hygiene in the bathroom, you may be able to think of some possible problems.
List these.

- People can become chilled if a suitable temperature cannot be maintained. It can also be exhausting for people with few reserves of strength, like Bill. There are various health and safety hazards; these are discussed later.
- A bathroom may cause problems for a person whose condition is unstable – physically and mentally. Unless a nurse stays with the person, observation is more difficult in bathrooms, than when behind curtains in the ward.
- Alzheimer's Society (2015) suggests that being calm, ordered and relaxed helps those with dementia, particularly if they have a visual or hearing impairment. Planning out the needs of the individual before you get them in the rooms can help lessen the anxiety they might have especially if you can create a familiar environment for them. Other ways this can be minimised will be discussed later; see Box 7.25.

The Essence of Care (DH 2010) emphasised the importance of providing an appropriate environment for hygiene needs to be met in the benchmark of best

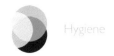

practice. People with impaired mobility, like Miss Smith, have special moving and handling requirements and need suitable equipment to enable them to access baths or showers. Nurses must maintain sound moving and handling practices within bathrooms to prevent injury to patients/residents and themselves. Appropriate risk assessments must be done to ensure the space is safe for both the patient and the carer to provide care (HSE 2020). Occupational therapists can advise on equipment. There are shower trolleys available, which can be useful for people with spinal injuries or other neurological conditions such as cerebral palsy. There is a wide range of other equipment available to assist with bathing and showering.

Learning outcome 2: discuss the procedure for assisting with bathing/showering in the bathroom, including health and safety issues

As with washing a person in bed, you should introduce yourself and build a rapport prior to assisting with personal care. Miss Smith was initially resistant to going to the bathroom, but as a relationship with the staff was established, she became more accepting of their help. Nurses should be patient and understanding in such situations. Assisting with hygiene in the bathroom provides opportunities to further the relationship with the person, as it involves one-to-one interaction in a private environment.

The carers of some adults might wish to continue to be involved in bathing. A person with dementia, for example, may be more comfortable if their usual carer assists. This involvement in care should be negotiated by nurses and not taken for granted, as some informal carers may be exhausted and might appreciate a break. Involving families in bathing can be important preparation for discharge, particularly where a person has a new disability. Nurses can teach families about use of equipment and skin observation and care for example.

Equipment
As always, it is important to plan ahead, gathering all equipment likely to be needed. Having to leave the bathroom to fetch items when the person is undressed could lead to chilling and exposure, and if a person is unsafe to leave, the nurse would have to ring the call bell and wait for help to arrive. The toiletries required vary between individuals, so always ask about preferences, which some people may indicate through non-verbal rather than verbal communication. You are likely to need towels, soap/shower gel or other cleansing agent, shampoo/conditioner (if hair-washing is to be carried out), clean clothing (of the person's choice), brush/comb, toothbrush and toothpaste, and flannel/disposable washcloths. Some people are prescribed specific skin care agents for use in the bath or afterwards.

Preparing the bathroom
After assembling the equipment, check that the bathroom is free, warm, and has been cleaned after any previous user. You also need to ensure that any equipment that you will be using, such as a hoist, is in good repair and is following the HSE (2020) risk assessment guidelines.

Box 7.24 Activity: checking on a person in the bathroom

Why is it necessary to check the bathroom prior to taking a person there?

Apart from any physical soiling, you should consider cross-infection risk. As earlier mentioned, normal detergent can be used to clean baths/showers but apply hypochlorite solution after use by a person with an infection or adhere to local infection control policy. You should also check that the floor is not wet or slippery, and that any extra equipment, such as a hoist or shower stool, is available and in safe working order. Also check the temperature of the bathroom, as some people are susceptible to the cold, particularly if underweight like Bill or older people like Miss Smith. Warm the bathroom first if necessary.

Bathing or showering procedure

The following steps provide a suggested procedure that will maintain comfort and safety. As with bed-bathing, nurses must be sensitive and respectful when assisting with hygiene in the bathroom.

- If bathing, fill the bath with warm water, using your elbow or a bath thermometer to check the temperature.
- Assist the person to the bathroom, offering them the opportunity to use the toilet first.
- Consider people who have sensory impairment. People with visual impairment can find bathrooms difficult as there are often white walls and white bathroom suite, making it difficult to locate the sink or bath. Therefore, always take time to orientate them to the environment, showing them where everything is. You should also consider people who are neuro-diverse and find the environment difficult to manage.
- Assist with undressing, maintaining dignity and comfort and avoiding unnecessary exposure by using towels.
- If the person has a urinary catheter in situ, a shower is preferable. However, if a bath is used, then the catheter should be clamped if the catheter has to be lifted above bladder level (e.g. when assisting the person in and out of the bath), to prevent reflux of urine back into the bladder (Pratt et al. 2007).
- If bathing, check the bathwater temperature again and allow the person to check for themselves if they are able. Remember: some people have impaired sensation in their feet and will not be able to feel the temperature accurately.
- Using suitable equipment if necessary, help the person into the bath, or on to the shower chair. If the shower is being used, check the temperature before allowing the person to be wet by the spray.
- Promote independence by supporting/enabling people to wash themselves as far as possible. Miss Smith's independence should be encouraged to rebuild her

neuro-diverse

displaying or characterised by autistic or other neurologically atypical patterns of thought or behaviour; not neurotypical

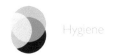

confidence in meeting her hygiene needs. Ellen will need prompting without being patronising.

- As with bathing in bed, particular attention should be given to skin creases, and areas susceptible to becoming sore – for example under breasts, palms of hands which are fixed in tonic flexion. Remember from the earlier section 'Bathing a person in bed', the importance of foot care for some people, particularly those with diabetes. Check Box 7.14, to remind yourself of the essential observations and care. Miss Smith's feet could be in a poor condition as she might not have been able to reach them for some time. She may need to be referred to a podiatrist.

- You should only leave a person alone in the bath or shower if you have assessed that it is safe to do so. For example, people who have epilepsy should not be left alone and neither should people who are confused. Always check with the registered nurse, if unsure. If it is safe to leave a person, ensure that the call bell is within reach, and working, before leaving.

- Remember, skin condition can be specifically observed, as well as psychological and physical condition – for example, any pain or breathlessness on movement, level of motivation to assist. These will all be important observations when assisting Miss Smith.

- If hair-washing is required, as for Miss Smith, use clean water in a washbasin or bowl, and a jug, or shower attachment (while ensuring that the water is at a temperature that is comfortable). Wet the hair, allowing the person to protect their eyes with a flannel. Apply shampoo, and massage gently into the scalp. Rinse and repeat, if necessary, and apply conditioner, as needed. Rinse again, and dry with a clean towel.

- Before assisting the person out of the bath, it may be easier to let some water out, and dry the upper body. This minimises the time for the person to become chilled. Assist the person out of the bath or shower, using equipment as necessary, and assist with drying as needed, again thinking about maintaining comfort and dignity by avoiding unnecessary exposure. Toiletries can be applied at this point.

- Assist the person to dress in clean clothes, clean teeth (see oral hygiene section) and brush/style hair as desired. Once again, assess the person's ability to participate in these activities. Both Miss Smith and Ellen may need verbal encouragement and reinforcement. A structured approach may help carers advise what her normal routine and support needs are. She may also have a 'Hospital Passport' or 'All About Me', which may provide additional information on this.

- Dispose of used equipment in accordance with waste disposal policy, and leave the bathroom clean and ready for the next user.

- Document the care given in the care plan or nursing notes.

Alzheimer's Society developed some 'Top tips' for care of those with dementia and helping with washing and dressing. Box 7.25 includes some of these additional points.

> ## Box 7.25 Washing and bathing for people with dementia: top tips for nurses (summarised from Alzheimer's Society)
>
> - Talk to the person about how they would prefer you to do things or ask their carer about preferences. Ask about their normal routine and encourage them to continue with these routines by providing support as needed.
> - Some people may be worried by deep water. You can reassure them by making sure the bath water is shallow or set up a bath seat for their use.
> - People with dementia sometimes lose the ability to judge temperature so check the water temperature is not too hot or too cold.
> - An overhead shower's rush of water can be frightening or disorientating, particularly when hitting the head. It may be preferable to use a hand-held shower or a bath.
> - While most people like having their hair washed regularly, others do not enjoy this. If the process is distressing for the person with dementia, stop.
> - Give gentle reminders about washing but think about the timing of your request and how you phrase it.
> - Use the time to chat and reassure the person with dementia, explaining what you are doing or about to do.
>
> Make the experience as pleasant and stress-free as possible, using pleasant toiletries, relaxing music or singing.

Summary

- Meeting hygiene needs in the bathroom is preferable for many reasons, for example privacy and the availability of running water.
- When assisting with hygiene in the bathroom, always assemble all equipment beforehand, to avoid leaving people alone.
- The bathroom is potentially hazardous. It is important to take active steps to avoid accidents, such as falls or scalding, and only leave people alone if you have assessed that it is safe to do so.
- Maintain privacy and dignity throughout, and promote independence.

SHAVING

> ## Box 7.26 Learning outcomes
>
> On completion of this section, you will be able to:
>
> 1. discuss the rationale for shaving people who are unable to do this for themselves;
> 2. identify the equipment needed and describe the procedure for shaving.

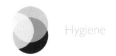

Learning outcome 1: discuss the rationale for shaving people who are unable to do this for themselves

Facial hair has important social and cultural meanings. In some religions, for example, Sikhism, neither facial hair nor hair on the head may be cut. In many Western European cultures, a wide variety of facial hair is socially acceptable, and contributes to maintaining self-esteem. While facial shaving is usually associated with men, some females (particularly older women) have unwanted facial hair that they prefer to remove. This is important to their body image. If a woman requests assistance with shaving or using tweezers, always approach this sensitively and matter-of-factly. Some younger women might also want their underarms and legs shaved as this is an important part of their own body image.

Box 7.27 Activity: inability to shave

ACTIVITY

Talk to a male relative or friend who is usually clean shaven. Ask him how he would feel if unable to shave himself.

For many men, being clean shaven is important and being unable to self-care in this way would be distressing. In addition, families visiting can be upset to find the person unshaven if they are usually clean shaven, and would view such a lack of care as neglectful, leading to a loss of confidence in staff. For some people shaving may be hazardous. For example, individuals receiving anti-coagulant or chemotherapy medication can be at risk of bleeding from minor cuts, so it is safer to use an electric razor rather than carrying out a wet shave.

Learning outcome 2: identify the equipment needed and describe the procedure for shaving

Equipment
You need:

- either a razor, with shaving soap/foam and shaving brush, or the person's own electric razor (communal razors pose a high risk of cross-infection);
- towel and flannel/disposable washcloth;
- bowl of hand-hot water;
- aftershave, if desired.

Consider using moisturiser, if the skin is dry or excoriated from use of soap, especially if shaving others areas of the body.

Procedure
Assemble the equipment and assist the person to sit up if possible. Protect the person's chest with a towel. Assess to what extent the person can assist. For some men, careful positioning, provision of a shaving mirror and having all equipment to hand may enable them to be independent with shaving. Shaving requires very fine motor control, so it is important to assess the person's capability. The individual's care plan should clarify this and any particular precautions needed.

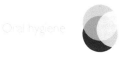

Wet shaving

- Wet the brush and apply the soap to the face, or use the foam, working up a good lather.
- Work in the direction of the hair growth, starting with the cheeks and moving on to the neck and around the mouth.
- Hold the skin taut and avoid any sores or moles. The person may be able to help by tightening his facial muscles. However, this would not be possible for all men, for example if facial weakness is present.
- For some men, the facial skin can be hypersensitive and therefore take great care.
- Rinse the razor after each stroke.
- When you have finished, rinse the face with clean water and dry by patting, apply aftershave if used. Dispose of used equipment safely. Document your care in the care plan or nursing notes.

Dry shaving

- The skin should be clean and dry; a little talcum powder may help. Work with circular strokes, keeping the skin taut as for wet shaving.
- Assist the person to rinse his face when finished, apply aftershave if desired, and clean the razor ready for the next occasion. Document your care in the care plan or nursing notes.

Box 7.28 Activity: practising a wet and dry shave on a friend/colleague

ACTIVITY

Find a willing male friend, relative or colleague and practise both a wet shave and a dry shave. Even if you shave yourself, you may find this more difficult than you expect. Ask your 'patient' to comment on your technique.

Summary

- Facial shaving is important to many people. Nurses should assist if people are unable to self-care, thus maintaining self-esteem.
- A gentle and careful technique should be used, using the person's preferred equipment.

ORAL HYGIENE

Maintaining oral hygiene is an important aspect of nursing care, which can do much to enhance quality of life and promote health. A high standard of oral hygiene should also be promoted in people who can self-care. The *Essence of Care 2010*'s (DH 2010) benchmark on 'Personal hygiene' explicitly includes mouth hygiene which it defines

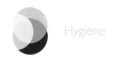
as: *the effective removal of plaque and debris to ensure the structures and tissues of the mouth are kept in a healthy condition* (p. 7). The WHO (2020) defined oral health as

> a state of being free from chronic mouth and facial pain, oral and throat cancer, oral infection and sores, periodontal (gum) disease, tooth decay, tooth loss, and other diseases and disorders that limit an individual's capacity in biting, chewing, smiling, speaking, and psychosocial well-being.

Public Health England (2017) has developed a tool kit to help professionals explore how they can help support their patients from how to brush their teeth to the best nutrition and lifestyle changes we can support them to make to improve their oral care.

Box 7.29 Learning outcomes

By the end of this section you will be able to:

1 reflect on the rationale for maintaining good oral hygiene;
2 explain factors that increase vulnerability to poor oral hygiene, and consider how those at risk can be identified;
3 discuss how oral hygiene can be carried out safely and based on best evidence.

Learning outcome 1: reflect on the rationale for maintaining good oral hygiene

Oral hygiene aims to maintain a healthy oral mucosa, teeth, gums and lips, by using toothpaste, brush or other cleansing agents. It is also important to realise maintaining good oral care can also help prevent infections and some types of disease.

Box 7.30 Activity: poor oral hygiene

ACTIVITY

What problems may arise if oral hygiene is poor, as in Miss Smith's case?

You may have considered:

- poor oral function/hygiene and chronic oral problems can lead to systemic ill health and can be life-threatening if not treated properly (Martin et al. 2020);
- mouth and gum infections may develop, such as candidiasis ('thrush'), which is a fungal infection;
- inability to eat may result, leading to malnutrition (Archer et al. 2020);
- halitosis leading to social withdrawal;
- infection risk, particularly in people who are immuno-compromised or for those who have difficulty in swallowing;
- low self-esteem (Huff et al. 2006);
- discomfort and distress.

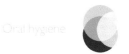

Martin et al. (2020) explore the connection between oral health with general health with impact on increasing haematological inflammatory markers to adverse diabetic control and the development of cardiovascular disease. Malnutrition is another marker of poor oral health as it can already exacerbate any existing issues leading to mucositis, oral ulceration, tongue alterations and can ultimately impact on the flow of saliva into the mouth (Delwal et al. 2018).

Learning outcome 2: explain factors that increase vulnerability to poor oral hygiene, and consider how those at risk can be identified

ACTIVITY

Box 7.31 Activity: reasons for poor oral hygiene and associated risks

You already know that Miss Smith's oral hygiene is poor. What might be the reasons for this? Now consider the other people in this chapter's scenarios. Do you think any of them are at risk of poor oral hygiene too?

Miss Smith's poor mobility has affected her ability to carry out her usual hygiene care as she cannot get to the bathroom. Although she could clean her teeth at the kitchen sink, she might not have been able to adapt her routine in this way, perhaps because of her depression. She may not have been able to access a dentist or buy the necessary equipment to carry out oral hygiene. Her poor oral hygiene might have led to poor oral intake of food and fluids, thus worsening her mouth condition.

Bill is at risk of oral hygiene problems. He has an ill-fitting denture; he can drink only small amounts and he is generally debilitated and thus at risk of developing an oral *Candida* infection.

Ellen may be maintaining good oral hygiene but the community nurse for learning disabilities could check that she is coping with her oral hygiene. Phadraig et al. (2020) discussed that it was important to understand three factors when reviewing someone with neurodiversity and their oral hygiene needs. Frequency and duration of teeth brushing, the tools applied (e.g. type of toothbrush, floss and toothpaste) and the technique used are important to monitor, for any one of these can have a lasting effect on the oral health of the individual. Some people with learning disabilities can have oral hypersensitivity, making it uncomfortable to clean their teeth. The Royal College of Nursing (2011) highlights that people with learning disabilities are more likely to have various mouth and dental problems, including:

tooth decay, loose teeth and gum disease, which may be due to poor diet, poor dental hygiene or a lack of access to oral health promotion. The **health facilitator** should provide support in overcoming these problems and regular visits to the dentist must be included in Ellen's **Health Action Plan**. Tooth decay would adversely affect her quality of life, leading to pain, the need for dental treatment and poor food intake.

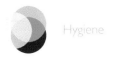

There are many factors that can lead to poor oral hygiene (see Table 7.1). Looking at this table might prompt you to identify further risk factors for the people in the scenarios, for example, Bill is taking morphine, which causes mouth dryness. Alzheimer's Society (2019) explains how dementia can affect oral health at different stages of dementia and provides a detailed factsheet with useful advice.

People's ability to self-care for oral hygiene can change quickly, so nurses should regularly reassess this and other risk factors.

Box 7.32 Activity: assessing oral hygiene needs

What aspects would you consider when assessing oral hygiene needs?

You may have thought of the following:

- condition of the teeth – plaque, cavities;
- condition of the tongue – coated, clean;
- condition of the lips;
- ability to undertake oral care;
- ability to eat;
- whether people have their own teeth or plates/dentures;
- whether they are able to breathe on their own or require some form of ventilation and the impact this might have on the mouth and the throat.

Doing an initial Oral Health Risk Assessment (OHRA) can help you to understand if there are any problems with the person's oral cavity such as dry mouth/tongue, infections, any sores, broken teeth or broken or ill-fitting dentures (British Society

Table 7.1: Factors predisposing to mouth problems

Drugs	• Cytotoxic drugs (reduce autoimmune response)
	• Corticosteroids (affect tissue healing)
	• Antibiotics (alters oral bacterial balance, allowing infection by *Candida albicans*)
	• Antihistamines, antispasmodics, anticholinergics, psychotropics, antidepressants and tranquillisers (reduce salivary production)
	• Diuretics (increase fluid loss)
	• Morphine (causes mouth dryness)
Treatments	• Radiotherapy of head/neck (causes localised inflammation, affects ability to eat/drink normally)
	• Oxygen therapy, particularly if given unhumidified at high flow rates (dries oral mucosa)
	• Suction (can damage oral mucosa)
	• Restricted oral intake, such as 'nil by mouth' pre- or post-op (potential for dehydration and dry mouth)
Mental or physical health	• Diseases: diabetes, thyroid dysfunction, oral disease/trauma, problems or disability, cerebrovascular disease, swallow dysfunction
	• Mental health problems: confusion, depression
	• Terminal illness
	• Acute/chronic breathing problems
	• Unconsciousness
	• Lack of manual dexterity

Adapted from Thurgood (1994).

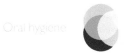

of Gerodontology 2010). Assessment tools can be helpful for assessing the need for, and frequency of, mouth care. They incorporate scoring systems indicating levels of risk (Public Health England 2020). Factors commonly included are current mouth condition, nutritional status and special risk factors, like those in Table 7.1 (e.g. certain medication, oxygen therapy).

Box 7.33 Activity: oral assessment tools in your clinical area

Find out whether an oral assessment tool is used in your current clinical area and, if so, look at the aspects included and ensure you understand any scoring systems used.

Learning outcome 3: discuss how oral hygiene can be carried out safely and based on best evidence

As with any other nursing practice, best available evidence should be used for oral hygiene. A variety of equipment may be needed, depending on the care identified as appropriate for the individual. Possible items are listed in Box 7.34.

Box 7.34 Equipment for oral care

- Spatula and pen torch (to inspect the oral cavity)
- Small, soft-bristled toothbrush (for teeth cleaning)
- Mouthwash, e.g. chlorhexidine (to prevent dental plaque) or water (for teeth cleaning)
- Toothpaste – if poor swallow reflex, use low-foaming toothpaste to limit aspiration
- Container for dentures, if needed
- Lip lubricant, e.g. non-petroleum based (especially if on oxygen), to prevent dry lips
- Beaker and receiver (for mouth rinsing)
- Disposable gloves and plastic apron
- Towel, tissues.

Rationale for choice of equipment

A small, soft-bristled toothbrush is the most effective agent for removing plaque and debris from the mouth, teeth and tongue (British Society of Gerodontology 2010). A trial comparing the ability of foam swabs and toothbrushes in removing plaque confirmed that toothbrushes perform substantially better (Pearson and Hutton 2002). Fluoridated toothpaste should be used (NHS QIS 2005) and for people with swallow reflex problems, a low-foaming toothpaste is important (British Society of Gerodontology 2010).

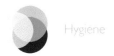

Jones (1998) advises that toothpaste has a generally drying effect so it should be used sparingly – about the size of a pea. Most antiseptic mouthwashes have a very transient effect, so they are of limited value (Jones 1998). However, those containing chlorhexidine gluconate, for example Corsodyl, if used for one minute, can reduce bacterial counts by up to 80% (Schiott et al. 1970, cited by Jones 1998). Its use is therefore worthwhile in very vulnerable people, for example immune-compromised, very sick or frail older people. Mouthwash is also useful in areas that are hard to reach (Xavier 2000).

Jones (1998) advises that, for cleansing and moistening oral mucosa, pH-balanced swab sticks are preferable; but if foam swab sticks are used, they are best when coated with Corsodyl gel, which is gentler to the delicate oral mucosa. Avoid using a foam mouth swab if the person might bite down on it as if the foam head detaches, it can be a choking hazard (Medicine and Healthcare products Regulatory Agency [MHRA] 2012). If foam mouth swabs are used, always check that the foam head is firmly attached to the stick before using and do not soak it before use as this can reduce the strength of the attachment (MHRA 2012). There are also saliva substitutes available for people with dry mouths. It has been shown in diabetic research that the use of saliva substitutes actually helps in maintaining the immune defence (Montaldo et al. 2010).

> ### Box 7.35 Activity: drawing on practice experience
>
> Drawing on your practice experience, how could nurses approach promoting oral hygiene for each of the people in this chapter's scenarios?

ACTIVITY

Bill may be able to carry out his own oral hygiene if equipment is placed within his reach. Perhaps he could sit at a sink to carry out his oral care, which will include cleaning his teeth and dentures. Due to his mouth's current poor condition, and if his condition worsens, he may need regular oral hygiene carried out in between teeth cleaning. This is discussed later.

Ellen can be verbally encouraged and supported in carrying out her own oral hygiene in the bathroom. For Miss Smith, equipment for oral hygiene will need to be provided and nurses should support her and encourage her to re-establish teeth cleaning, which can be done in the bathroom at the sink. She should be approached sensitively about visiting a dentist.

Teeth cleaning should be carried out twice daily (Public Health England 2017). Cleaning of dentures should be carried out at least daily but ideally after meals too. If people are unable to carry this out independently, nurses must provide the necessary equipment and assistance. Some people, who are more dependent and debilitated, require nurses to carry out oral hygiene on a regular basis by the bedside. The use of the Mouth Care Matters Toolkit for Improving Mouth Care in Hospitals has an outline of what to look for and helps you to assess oral health. It also contains an outline on how best to clean a mouth and dentures for optimum care (HEE 2019a).

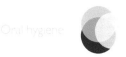

The frequency of oral care should be determined on an individual basis. This care, which may be necessary for Bill, is described below.

Oral hygiene procedure: key points

- After explaining the procedure and gaining consent, the person should be assisted into a sitting position or, if unconscious, on their side to prevent inhalation of solutions or secretions.
- Protect the person's chest with a towel, or the bed with the waterproof sheet. Provide a receiver for spitting.
- Assemble the equipment. Any mouthwash solution should be freshly prepared, and renewed after 24 hours.
- Wash your hands and put on gloves and apron, if required. Kilkenny (2019) recommend that gloves should be worn as some infectious agents (e.g. herpes, hepatitis B) can be present in the mouth or saliva and it is important to take universal precautions when dealing with any form of body fluid. However, oral hygiene is a hygienic procedure rather than an aseptic one; it does not breach body defences but instead enhances them (Ayliffe et al. 2001). Therefore, gloves need not be sterile.
- Lip crusting can be removed by gently sponging with warm water (Jones 1998). Observe for any breaks in the skin or signs of Herpes simplex (cold sore), which would require treatment.
- Remove the person's dentures, if worn. They should be brushed well to remove debris using denture paste – ordinary toothpaste is too abrasive – and rinsed well. Box 7.36 lists key points for effective denture care.

If the person has their own teeth, they should be brushed using the toothbrush and paste. Box 7.37 explains how teeth cleaning should be carried out, and Figure 7.1 illustrates teeth cleaning. If people can clean their own teeth, it is better to facilitate this.

Box 7.36 Denture care adapted from HEE 2019a

- Wash hands and wear gloves.
- Remove dentures (noting any damage) into a container and rinse to remove loose debris.
- Use the person's special denture brush, scrubbing all surfaces, using denture paste or a little soap, to remove all debris.
- Rinse thoroughly.
- When dentures are not being worn, store in a marked container filled with clean water.
- Soaking plastic dentures 2–3 times per week in dilute sodium hypochlorite will help to prevent oral candidiasis. Always rinse thoroughly before replacing in the mouth.
- Dentures with a metal portion should be soaked in dilute hypochlorite for only about 20 min, because of the danger of corrosion.

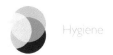

Box 7.37 Teeth cleaning (adapted from Jones 1998)

- Explain the procedure and gain consent.
- Wash hands, wear gloves and maintain privacy.
- It may be best to work at the side of the person, cradling the head.
- Remove any partial dentures into a bowl.
- Start at the front of the mouth in the upper jaw.
- Use a soft brush with a small amount of toothpaste pressed into the surface (to avoid it dislodging into the mouth and possible aspiration). Use toothpaste that has limited foam.
- Place the brush sideways against the teeth overlaying the gum edges with bristles pointing towards the teeth roots.
- Use a side-to-side motion, moving the brush head just a fraction of an inch at a time, using light pressure to squeeze the gum tissue against the teeth.
- Move around the upper teeth, replacing the brush section by section against the teeth.
- Try to use the same action inside the upper jaw.
- Repeat for the outer and inner surfaces of the lower jaw.
- Finally, scrub the chewing surfaces of the upper and lower teeth with a forward and backward motion.
- Teeth should be cleaned for a minimum of 90 s.
- Ask the person to rinse the mouth with warm water to remove debris, paste, etc., or use foam sticks moistened with water to gently sweep away the debris and toothpaste.
- Wash toothbrush well and leave it to dry in the air. Do not store in a sponge bag or container. Toothbrushes should be replaced every 6–12 weeks.

- Assist the person to rinse the mouth thoroughly with the chosen mouthwash solution, or use a rinsed toothbrush to do this if they are unable. Suction can be used to remove excess fluid from the mouth if they are unconscious, or have dysphagia (swallowing difficulty), as it is essential to prevent choking or aspiration of fluid (Jones 1998). A conscious person who is nursed flat, for example, after a spinal injury, can use a straw to suck fluid into the mouth to rinse and to spit through afterwards.
- Replace any dentures, top set first. Some people use denture fixative.
- Apply lip lubricant, if lips are dry. Use tissues to blot any excess water or lubricant.
- Leave the person comfortable, and dispose of equipment according to waste disposal policy. Document the care given in the care plan or nursing notes (Kilkenny 2019).

Box 7.38 Activity: taking turns to clean each other's teeth

ACTIVITY

With a friend or colleague, take turns to clean each other's teeth, using your own toothbrushes and the instructions in Box 7.37 and Figure 7.1.

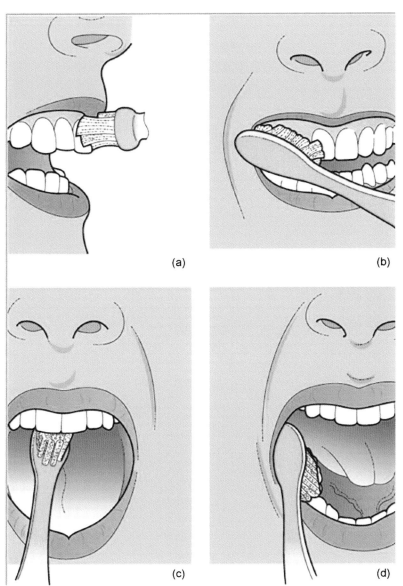

Figure 7.1: How to clean teeth.

🛁 Box 7.39 Children and young people: practice points – mouth care.

For information about children's teeth and dental care see: Mini Mouth Care Matters: A guide for hospital healthcare professionals (HEE 2019b).

For oral hygiene for children see:

Himsworth (2010) Caring for personal hygiene needs. In: Glasper, A., Aylott, M. and Battrick, C. (eds.) Developing Practical Skills for Nursing Children and Young People. London: Hodder Arnold, 196–7.

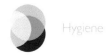
Summary

- Effective oral care makes an important contribution to people's physical, psychological and social well-being.
- Nurses should ensure that best evidence is used as a basis for assessing and implementing oral care.

CHAPTER SUMMARY

Giving personal care, with attention to the individual's dignity, privacy and personal needs, is a fundamental and essential skill for nurses, and this extends to the care of a person's body after death. Further key principles include cultural sensitivity and prevention of cross-infection. It is important to assess carefully how hygiene needs can be met for each individual, maintaining and promoting independence where possible. People with physical and mental health problems may be able to regain self-care skills with appropriate aids, encouragement and support. Teaching people to manage personal hygiene and dressing can be an important part of rehabilitation, and should involve the multidisciplinary team for an individualised approach.

REFERENCES

Alzheimer's Society. 2015. Washing and Dressing. Fact Sheet 504LP. Available from: https://www.alzheimers.org.uk/get-support/daily-living/understanding-issues-around-washing-and-bathing#content-start (Accessed on November 2020).

Alzheimer's Society. 2019. Dental care and oral health. Fact sheet 448LP. Available from: https://www.alzheimers.org.uk/sites/default/files/2019-09/448lp-dental-care-and-oral-health-190521.pdf (Accessed on November 2020).

Archer, N., Martin, K. and Johnston, L. 2020. Oral conditions in the community patient: Part 1. *British Journal of Community Nursing* 25(10): 490–5.

Ayliffe, G.A.J., Babb, J.R. and Taylor, L.J. 2001. *Hospital-acquired Infection: Principles and Prevention*, 3rd edn. London: Arnold.

Baxter, C. 2002. Nursing with dignity. Part 5: Rastafarianism. *Nursing Times* 98(13): 42–3.

Brawley, E.C. 2002. Bathing environments: How to improve the bathing experience. *Alzheimer's Care Quarterly* 3: 38–41.

British Society of Gerodontology. 2010. *Guidelines for the Oral Healthcare of Stroke Survivors* Available from: https://www.gerodontology.com/content/uploads/2014/10/stroke_guidelines.pdf (Accessed on November 2020).

Christmas, M. 2002. Nursing with dignity. Part 3: Christianity 1. *Nursing Times* 98(11): 37–9.

Clegg, A. 2003. Older South Asian patient and carer perceptions of culturally sensitive care in a community hospital setting. *Journal of Clinical Nursing* 12: 283–90.

Cowdell, F. 2010. Promoting skin health in older people. *Nursing Older People* 22(10): 21–6.

Delwel S, et al. 2018. Oral hygiene and oral health in older people with dementia: A comprehensive review with focus on oral soft tissues. *Clinical Oral Investigations* 22: 93–108. https://doi.org/10.1007/s00784-017-2264-2

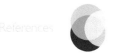

Department of Health. 2006. *From Values to Action: The Chief Nursing Officer's Review of Mental Health Nursing.* Gateway reference 6140. London: DH.

Department of Health. 2010. *Essence of Care 2010 Benchmarks for Personal Hygiene.* Gateway reference 14641. London.

Downey, L. and Lloyd, D.L. 2008. Bed Bathing Patients in Hospital. *Nursing Standard* 22(34): 35–40.

Geraghty, M. 2005. Nursing the unconscious patient. *Nursing Standard* 20(1), 54–64.

Gilchrist, B. 1990. Washing and dressing after surgery. *Nursing Times* 86(50): Suppl, 71.

Gústafsdóttir, M. 2011. Keeping up health promotion in specialized day care units for people with dementia. *American Journal of Alzheimer's Disease and Other Dementias* 26(6): 437–42.

Health Education England [HEE]. 2019b. Mini mouth care matters: A guide for hospital healthcare professionals. Available from: http://mouthcarematters.hee.nhs.uk/wp-content/uploads/sites/6/2020/01/MINI-MCM-GUIDE-2019-final.pdf (Accessed on 2019).

Health Education England [HEE]. 2019a. Mouth care matters: Toolkit for improving mouth care in hospitals. *Mouth Care Matters.* Available from: http://mouthcarematters.hee.nhs.uk/wp-content/uploads/sites/6/2019/12/MCM-toolkit-2019-V9.pdf (Accessed on November 2020).

Health and Safety Executive [HSE]. 2020. What you need to do - Moving and handling. *Health and Safety Executive* https://www.hse.gov.uk/healthservices/moving-handling-do.htm (Accessed on November 2020).

Himsworth, J. 2010. Caring for personal hygiene needs. In Glasper, A., Aylott, M. and Battrick, C. (eds.) *Developing Practical Skills for Nursing Children and Young People.* London: Hodder Arnold, 188–202.

Holland, K. and Hogg, C. 2010. *Cultural Awareness in Nursing and Health Care*, 2nd edn. London: Arnold.

Howell, M. and Thirlaway, S. 2004. Integrating foot care into the everyday clinical practice of nurses. *British Journal of Nursing* 13(8): 470–3.

Huff, M. et al. 2006. Self-esteem: a hidden concern in oral health. *Journal of Community Health Nursing* 23(4), 245–55.

Jafferany, M., Roque Ferreira, B. and Patel, A.2020. *The Essentials of Psychodermatology.* Springer International publishing.

Jones, C.V. 1998. The importance of oral hygiene in nutritional support. *British Journal of Nursing* 74: 76–8, 80–3.

Kilkenny, N. 2019. Oral care in adults. *British Journal of Nursing* 28(16): 1054–5.

Kottner, J. and Surber, C. 2016. Skin care in nursing: A critical discussion of nursing practice and research. *International Journal of Nursing Studies* 61: 20–28.

Mac Giolla Phadraig, C. et al. 2020. The complexity of tooth brushing among older adults with intellectual disabilities: Findings from a nationally representative survey. *Disability and Health Journal* 13: 1936–6574. Available from: https://doi.org/10.1016/j.dhjo.2020.100935 (Accessed on 27 May 2021).

Martin, K., Johnston, L. and Archer, N. 2020. Oral conditions in the community: Part 2 – systemic complications of poor oral health. *British Journal of Community Nursing* 25(11): 535–6.

Medicine and HealthCare Products Regulatory Agency [MHRA]. 2012. Medical device alert Ref: MDA/2012/020. Oral swabs with a foam head, all manufacturers. Available from: http://www.mhra.gov.uk/Publications/Safetywarnings/MedicalDeviceAlerts/CON149697 (last accessed November 2020).

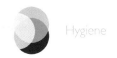

Montaldo, L. et al. 2010. Effects of saliva substitutes on oral status in patients with Type 2 diabetes. *Original Article: Treatment. Diabetic Medicine: A Journal of The British Diabetic Association* Nov. 27(11): 1280–3.

National Institute for Health and Clinical Excellence (NICE). 2004. *Type 2 Diabetes: Prevention and Management of Foot Problems*. Clinical Guideline 10. London: NICE.

National Institute for Health and Clinical Excellence (NICE). 2011. *Diabetic foot Problems: Inpatient Management of Diabetic Foot Problems*. Clinical Guideline 119. London.

National Institute for Health and Clinical Excellence (NICE). 2016. Oral health for adults in care homes. Available from: https://www.nice.org.uk/guidance/ng48 (Accessed on November 2020).

National Institute for Health and Clinical Excellence (NICE). 2019a. Diabetic foot problems: Prevention and management (NG19) NICE guideline. Available from: https://www.nice.org.uk/guidance/ng19 (Accessed on March 2021).

National Institute for Health and Clinical Excellence (NICE). 2019b. Surgical site infections: prevention and treatment. (NG125). NICE guideline. Available from: www.nice.org.uk/guidance/ng125 (Accessed on March 2021).

Nazarko, L. 2017. Diabetes series, 6. Prevention and management of diabetic foot problems. *British Journal of Healthcare Assistants* 11(05): 218–23.

NHS Choices. 2018. *How to Wash a Penis*. Available from: http://www.nhs.uk/Livewell/penis-health/Pages/how-to-wash-a-penis.aspx (Accessed on March 2021).

NHS Quality Improvement Scotland. 2005. *Working with Dependent Older People to Achieve Good Oral Health*. Edinburgh: NHS QIS.

Nursing and Midwifery Council. 2018a. Future nurse: Standards of proficiency for registered nurses. Available from: www.nmc.org.uk

Nursing and Midwifery Council. 2018b. Standards of proficiency for nursing associates. Available from: www.nmc.org.uk

Parker, L. 2004. Infection control: Maintaining the personal hygiene of patients and staff. *British Journal of Nursing* 13(8): 474–8.

Pearson, L.S. and Hutton, J.L. 2002. A controlled trial to compare the ability of foam swabs and toothbrushes to remove dental plaque. *Journal of Advanced Nursing* 39: 480–9.

Pratt, R.J., Pellowe, C., Wilson, J.A. et al. 2007. National evidence-based guidelines for preventing healthcare-associated infections in NHS England. *Journal of Hospital Infection* 65, Suppl: S1–64.

Pryia, B., Kumari, A. and Meena, J. 2019. A study to assess the knowledge on menstrual hygiene among adolescent girls in selected schools, Mangalagiri, Guntur District, Andhra Pradesh. *International Journal of Nursing Education* 11(4): 35–8.

Public Health England. 2017. *Delivering Better Oral Health: An Evidence-based Toolkit for Prevention*, 3rd edn. PHE publications. Available from: https://assets.publishing.service.gov.uk/government/uploads/system/uploads/attachment_data/file/605266/Delivering_better_oral_health.pdf (Accessed on November 2020).

Public Health England. 2020. *Delivering Better Oral Health: Guideline Development Manual*. PHE publications. Available from: https://assets.publishing.service.gov.uk/government/uploads/system/uploads/attachment_data/file/853643/DBOH_Guideline_Development_Manual_2019.pdf (Accessed on November 2020).

Queensland Health. 2011. Health care providers' handbook on Sikh patients. Division of the Chief Health Officer, Queensland Health Brisbane. Available from: https://www.health.qld.gov.au/__data/assets/pdf_file/0019/156043/hbook-sikh.pdf (Accessed on March 2021).

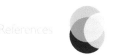

Rassool, G.H. 2000. The crescent and Islam: healing, nursing and the spiritual dimension. Some considerations towards an understanding of the Islamic perspectives on caring. *Journal of Advanced Nursing* 32: 1476–84.

Rowe, K.D. 2019. "Nothing else mattered after that wig came off": Black women, unstyled hair, and scenes of interiority. *The Journal of American Culture* 42(1): 21–36.

Sener, D.K., Aydin, M. and Cangur, S. 2019. Evaluating the effects of a personal hygiene program on the knowledge, skills, and attitudes of intellectual disabilities teenagers and their parents. *Journal of Policy and Practice in Intellectual Disabilities* 16(3): 160–70. doi:10.1111/jppi.12277

Stonehouse, D. 2016. HCAs and APs building a therapeutic relationship. *British Journal of Healthcare Assistants* 10(09): 460–3.

Sundström, M., Blomqvist, K., Edberg, A. and Rämgård, M. 2018. The context of care matters: Older people's existential loneliness from the perspective of healthcare professionals—A multiple case study. *International Journal for Older People Nursing* 14: e12234. https://doi.org/10.1111/opn.12234 (Accessed on November 2020).

Thurgood, G. 1994. Nurse maintenance of oral hygiene. *British Journal of Nursing* 3(7): 351–3.

Wilson, N.J. et al. 2009. Penile hygiene: Puberty, paraphimosis and personal care for men and boys with an intellectual disability. *Journal of Intellectual Disability Research* 53(2):106–14.

World Health Organisation. 2020. Oral health: Overview. Available from: https://www.afro.who.int/health-topics/oral-health (Accessed on November 2020).

Xavier, G. 2000. The importance of mouth care in preventing infection. *Nursing Standard* 14(18): 47–51.

8

Promoting comfort and sleep

Scott Elbourne

Comfort is a fundamental concept in nursing practice. The term 'comfort' originates from the Latin 'confortare', which means 'become strong, comfort or encourage' (Pinto et al. 2017). Individuals in all healthcare settings experience discomfort, whether it is physical, emotional or spiritual. The seminal work of Morse and Kolcaba is widely recognised amongst the different theories that have analysed the theme of comfort. Morse defines comfort as a product of holistic nursing interventions and describes the idea of comfort as a process inherent in the act of comforting (Pinto et al. 2017). The studies of Kolcaba are based on the well-known theory of comfort that considers the four contexts of holistic human experience: physical, psychospiritual, sociocultural and environmental (Kolcaba 1995).

Discomfort can impact many aspects of individuals' lives including sleep. Around one in three of the UK population suffer from problems related to falling asleep, staying asleep, waking early and feeling unrefreshed when they do wake up (NHS 2018). Pain and discomfort are among the factors that disturb sleep. Understanding the consequences of poor sleep and how to improve sleep are further key components of nursing. This chapter aims to help you understand how nursing skills may be used to promote comfort and sleep.

This chapter includes the following topics:

- Promoting comfort – the nature of comfort care, using presence and developing relationships, touch, verbal interactions, physical actions and integrating comfort care skills in practice.
- Promoting sleep – normal sleep physiology across the age range, restorative versus non-restorative sleep, hints and tips for sleep at home and discussion of how these can be applied in hospital and residential settings.

DOI: 10.4324/9781003020660-8

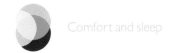

The questions below will help you to focus on the biology underpinning the skills used in sleep management. Use your recommended textbook and web resources to find out:

- What is sleep?
- How much sleep do children, teenagers, adults and older people need?
- What are the different types and stages of sleep?
- How long does each stage last in a young adult and what is its purpose?
- What is a sleep cycle?
- What factors can lead to sleep deprivation?
- How quickly do we become sleep deprived?
- What happens in sleep deprivation?

PRACTICE SCENARIOS

The following scenarios illustrate when promoting comfort and sleep may be needed. They will be referred to throughout this chapter.

Adult

William Newton, who likes to be called 'Bill', is a retired accountant aged 73. He is terminally ill with a history of oesophageal cancer and metastases in his lungs. He is cared for by his wife at home with the support of community nurses and the Macmillan nurse. He is taking regular oral morphine for pain control. He has a very low haemoglobin and has been admitted for a blood transfusion. He is weak, breathless and his general condition is poor. He has a **body mass index** of 16. He can swallow only very small amounts of liquidised food and drink. He has some of his own teeth but also a partial denture, which he likes to wear, although it is now ill-fitting. His tongue appears coated, and his mouth is dry.

Metastases: The process whereby cancerous cells from a tumour migrate and spread from their original site and proliferate in distant sites (Cook et al. 2019).

Haemoglobin (Hb): Haemoglobin is a large, complex molecule consisting of a pigmented iron-containing complex called haem and a globular protein called globin (Waugh and Grant 2018).

Learning disability

Maria is a 58-year-old woman with a moderate learning disability who has been living in a group home for the last five years. She has long-standing diabetes mellitus treated with insulin and has recently developed painful diabetic neuropathy. She has pain in both legs below the knees, which she finds particularly distressing when she is walking and during the night; her sleep is disturbed. She is in the care of both her GP and the diabetic team at her local hospital. Maria's mother, who is 85 years old and recently widowed, visits on a weekly basis and is concerned about Maria's

Diabetes mellitus

Diabetes is a chronic, life-long condition of glucose metabolism in which the body responds abnormally (insulin resistance) or does not produce a sufficient amount of insulin to control the blood glucose level (Cook et al. 2019).

Painful diabetic neuropathy

Peripheral neuropathy in people living with diabetes is common, affecting around 50% of the population. Signs and symptoms of peripheral neuropathy can be motor, sensory or autonomic in nature. Pain or painful neuropathy can interfere with activities of daily living, work and sleep and can have a significant effect on the quality of life of its sufferers (Diabetes UK 2020).

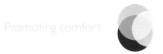

distress. Her Community Learning Disability Nurse would like to understand more about how he can support Maria, her mother and the group home staff on how to manage Maria's pain and increase her comfort.

Mental health

Violet Davies, aged 76 years, has moderate Alzheimer's disease. She has been admitted to a care home for respite as her husband is physically and emotionally exhausted and needs a break. He has refused help in the past as he has been determined to look after his wife, but he has now agreed to take a holiday, visiting friends. Violet is physically well, but she is also known to have osteoarthritis in her right hip and knee. She looks permanently worried and is agitated; she keeps repeating the same phrase over and over. Mr Davies looks shaky and tearful at the thought of leaving his wife for a week.

PROMOTING COMFORT

People can usually promote their own comfort, but when they are unwell, physically or mentally, particularly when outside their own environment, their usual ways of seeking comfort may not be possible. Promoting comfort is closely aligned with empathy and compassion as it requires nurses to recognise and respond to a person's distress by taking action to alleviate discomfort and promote comfort.

Box 8.2 Learning outcomes

By the end of this section, you will be able to:

1. discuss the nature of comfort care;
2. reflect on how presence and developing relationships can provide comfort;
3. consider how touch can be used in comfort care;
4. explore how verbal interactions can be used to promote comfort;
5. select physical actions that can be used to promote comfort;
6. integrate comfort care skills in different circumstances.

Learning outcome 1: discuss the nature of comfort care

There are many situations where comfort care is necessary.

Box 8.3 Activity: discomfort scenarios

Review the scenarios at the start of this chapter. What discomfort might these people experience and why?

- Violet appears to be suffering discomfort, which might be emotional due to her change of environment and her mental condition. However, she might also have physical discomfort as she could be in pain due to her osteoarthritis, or she may

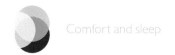
need to pass urine but be unable to express this verbally. She could be too hot or too cold, or hungry or thirsty. It is important not to make assumptions about the reasons underlying discomfort.

- Bill is suffering physical discomfort from the pain associated with the cancer. Additionally, he is also likely to be experiencing discomfort from his ill-fitting dentures, the thrush infection on his tongue and dry mouth. It should also be appraised that Bill may be experiencing emotional discomfort such as anxiety and fear from the breathlessness and the need for the urgent blood transfusion. It is not uncommon for people needing palliative care to experience anxiety and depression with a life-limiting illness.
- Maria obviously has discomfort due to the pain caused by her peripheral neuropathy. She is likely to have emotional discomfort due to this new complication, and associated anxiety.

Comfort is central to person-centred care and experience and is an essential skill that all nurses need to develop. However, the nature of comfort care is often poorly defined. Wensley et al. (2017) argue that promoting comfort is often confined to physical aspects of reliving pain or physical distress, and often emotional comfort measures such as empathy and compassion are overlooked leading to frustration, stress and anxiety. The nature of comfort is multidimensional and is experienced not only by the relief of physical discomfort, such as pain, but as an integration of positive emotions that include feeling safe, feeling cared for, valued and having a sense of control of the situation. A study undertaken by Wensley et al. (2017) found that individual descriptions of comfort vary across the lifespan and are dependent on the person's current situation; for example, older adults with a life-limiting illness described comfort in terms of feeling at ease or at peace; adult people receiving general care, described comfort in terms of feeling safe, cared for and able to relax, and lastly, children described comfort in terms of feeling better, safe and not sad.

Box 8.4 Activity: relating these examples to Bill, Violet and Maria

ACTIVITY

How might these examples relate to Bill, Violet and Maria in their scenarios?

Comfort care involves actions to promote comfort; for some people, total comfort may not be possible, due to the effects of illness or surgery, so the aim is then to promote comfort as far as possible using different approaches. Kolkaba (1995, 2003) has developed theories of comfort and applied these to care in different settings. She asserts that when comfort care is successful, people feel well cared for and comforted because the care was efficient, individualised and holistically targeted to the whole person. Kolkaba (2003) gives examples of comfort existing in three forms: *relief, ease* and *transcendence*, for example, (1) the *relief* of postoperative pain by administering prescribed analgesia, (2) addressing the anxiety of an individual by comforting them to feel content and at *ease* and (3) supporting an individual to *transcend* or rise above their challenges, e.g. an individual who is involved in physical therapy or a rehabilitation programme.

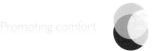

Box 8.5 Activity: using personal qualities when comforting someone

Reflect on a situation where you comforted someone in distress: what personal qualities did you use?

The qualities of staff that promote comfort include kindness, empathy and compassion (Wensley et al. 2017). Furthermore, Wensley et al. (2020) found that competent staff, who display ability and confidence, promoted emotional comfort by helping people to feel secure. An individualised and holistic approach is necessary for promoting comfort. For example, Coelho et al. (2016) found that a comprehensive approach with recognition of emotional, spiritual, psychosocial and family needs, along with physical needs, helped to provide comfort for people receiving palliative care.

Box 8.6 Activity: comfort in practice

Reflect on a practice situation where a person needed comfort.

1 What did you do to find out what would provide comfort for the person as an individual?
2 What did you do to help the person to feel that you were interested in them as an individual?

Using effective communication skills, particularly listening and questioning skills, is key to understanding what will be comforting to an individual person and to help people to feel that you are interested in them; Chapter 2 addresses these skills in detail.

Box 8.7 Activity: distressing pain

Maria's scenario mentions that she experiences distressing pain during the night. What could the staff do to promote Maria's comfort?

The staff could try to be with Maria as much as possible – 'being there' or 'presence' is well recognised as a comfort strategy. The unit staff will have an established relationship with Maria, which she should derive comfort from; they will also know how best to comfort Maria, for example, they may know that she finds touch comforting. The staff could talk to Maria and explain why her legs are painful. The community healthcare team will therefore need to educate the care home staff about peripheral neuropathy and how they can best explain this to Maria. The staff should administer prescribed analgesics and use other non-pharmacological pain-relieving strategies (see Chapter 9 and 10) and monitor the effect of these. Any care should be detailed in a plan that carers can follow consistently. The staff should promote Maria's general physical comfort, ensuring that she is in a comfortable position, and check whether she has any other needs, such as a drink. Thus, in promoting comfort for Maria, staff would use:

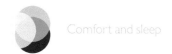

- presence and their relationship with her
- touch
- verbal interactions
- physical actions.

The next sections look at each of these ways of promoting comfort in more detail.

Learning outcome 2: reflect on how presence and developing relationships can provide comfort

Presence is about 'being there' with someone who is in distress and needs comfort. Nursing presence has been described as a holistic and reciprocal exchange between the nurse and the person that involves a sincere connection and sharing of the human experience through active listening, attentiveness, intimacy, therapeutic touch, spiritual exploration, empathy, caring and compassion (Hessel 2009). Kornhaber et al. (2016) give a similar description of presence but describes this as the development of 'therapeutic interpersonal relationships.' Such relationships are defined and perceived as caring, supportive, non-judgemental behaviour, which is embedded in a safe environment during an often-stressful period.

Studies in various care settings have confirmed that the presence of nurses is a source of comfort. Fatemeh et al. (2017) found that people felt more secure when they perceived that assistance was available to them when it was needed. For Maria, her carers could be the source of this assistance providing they understand need and that there is a consistent care plan. Although some people benefited from care provided by family's members, this did not replace the 'feeling of peace' given that while nurses are present, they can monitor their condition, observing and checking their mental and/or physical condition, asking about symptoms and assessing for pain. Mottram (2009) found that trust in the health professional promoted comfort for those having day surgery and she described 'befriending', conveyed through empathic understanding and practical support, from which people received emotional comfort and reassurance. Conversely, Bundgaard and Nielsen (2011) found that for those undergoing endoscopy, a lack of nursing presence was associated with feelings of insecurity and discomfort. Williams and Irurita (2006) found that staff promoted emotional comfort through spending time with individuals, getting to know them as people and making frequent contact. In a day surgery-based study, Mottram (2009) highlighted that presence needs to be not just physical but actual engagement with the person – listening and showing interest. While some people preferred a constant presence of the nurse, others were content with a nurse being close by. People identified that the presence of nurses was a therapeutic, comforting experience and some appreciated continuity of the nurse during their day surgery stay (Mottram 2009).

Alonzo (2017) discusses the importance of staff getting to know residents with dementia. Understanding the needs of residents with dementia and developing care strategies focusing on their comfort, can make a considerable difference to their quality of life. Alonzo (2017) recognises that comfort is unique to the individual, but there are considerations that can help nursing homes adopt and embed comfort through staff practice and individualised routines. The care home staff will need to get to know Violet as a person so that they can promote her comfort during her stay. Alzheimer's Society (2017) has developed a second edition of a leaflet 'This is me', which when completed by the person with dementia and their family, provides a useful communication tool for staff to quickly find out about a person with dementia and their preferences. The care home staff could invite Mr Davies to complete 'This is me' with Violet.

ACTIVITY

Box 8.8 Activity: reacting to distress

Think about when you have been sitting with someone who was distressed, either in the healthcare setting or in everyday life. Were you comfortable doing this or was it difficult in any way?

It is not always easy to be with someone who is in distress, particularly if you are unable to fully relieve their discomfort. If someone has received bad news, perhaps about a serious diagnosis or death of a loved one, nothing you can say or do can take that away. The home staff may find it quite distressing to sit with Maria during the night if she is in pain. Nurses often feel more comfortable when they can 'put things right': relieve mental distress, pain, vomiting or breathlessness. If they are unable to do this, being present with a person who, despite medication and other measures, continues to express feelings of hopelessness and is in pain, vomiting or acutely breathless, can engender feelings of helplessness. Nevertheless, nurses should be aware that their presence will be comforting for the person, even though it may be an uncomfortable situation for the nurse. The presence of a relative or friend (rather than a nurse) can be the best source of comfort and when relatives or friends are providing comfort by being present, nurses should then support them to be with their loved one, remembering that they may find it difficult to be there.

During the COVID-19 pandemic, those at the end of their lives were faced with dying in hospitals without the comfort of their loved ones by their side. It has been reported that families were denied access to their relatives dying from COVID-19. Some hospitals allowed one visitor who was asymptomatic to be with the person at the end of their life, providing they wore appropriate personal protective equipment; however, not all hospitals allowed this (Yardley and Rolph 2020). Although discussion of death and dying is often a taboo subject in modern Britain, many would agree that a person dying alone is considered a societal wrong (Bailey and Walter 2016). Unfortunately, health professionals have borne witness to the absence of family and friends, and in their stead, have expanded their reserves of emotional labour to comfort those who are dying alone. Yardley and Rolph (2020) assert that this is due to our collective belief in the need for humanity for those approaching the end of life, and that it was highly valued by many families in an unprecedented pandemic situation. End of life care is discussed further in Chapter 15.

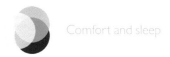

Learning outcome 3: consider the use of touch in comfort care

The value of touch to comfort is well supported by research (Connor and Howett 2009; Bales et al. 2018; Jagan et al. 2019). There are two main types of touch used in nursing care: instrumental (or procedural) touch and comforting touch:

> ***Instrumental touch*** is used while carrying out nursing actions such as repositioning someone or undertaking physical assessment such as recording their pulse manually. This type of touch is diminishing as care increasingly uses technology, for example, electronic blood pressure measurement equipment (Dion-Nist et al. 2020).
>
> ***Comforting touch or interpersonal touch*** is used intentionally to comfort a person through putting an arm around their shoulder or holding their hand. Connor and Howett (2009) describe interpersonal touch as inherent in the nurse–patient relationship. It is used to give comfort, communicate needs, reduce stress and demonstrate compassion. Comforting touch is described as a need that is essential across the lifespan from neonates in the ICU to older adults at the end of their life (Connor and Howett 2009). In Bundgaard and Nielsen's (2011) study, people found that comforting touch helped in developing trust and confidence in the nurse and helped individuals to feel secure; one person said, 'I need to know that someone is watching over me, I may need a hand to hold, so that I feel their presence and know that they will take care of me' (p. 37).

Dion-Nist et al. (2020) suggest that nurses can use touch in a variety of ways. This could be procedural and part of instrumental care, e.g. hydration, elimination and hygiene. Conversely, touch can also support psychosocial care, e.g. respect and dignity, and relational care, empathy and compassion, e.g. hand-holding. Touch can also be combined with assessment and monitoring of a person's condition; for example, if Bill was in distress, the nurses looking after him could observe his breathing while holding his hand, to comfort him. In Bundgaard and Nielsen's (2011) study, nurses described how, while holding the person's hands, they were monitoring responses. For example, they could feel anxiety or calmness.

ACTIVITY

Box 8.9 Activity: using touch when comforting someone

- Think back to a recent experience when you were comforting someone: did you use touch? If so, how did you use it? Reflect on how comfortable you feel about using touch to comfort.
- Now, ask three close family members or friends: how would they feel about nurses using touch to comfort them. Compare their responses.

People vary in how comfortable they feel about using and receiving touch; some people are much more 'touchy' than others. Some nurses use touch a great deal and feel comfortable to use touch in a variety of ways, while others shy away from using touch. Indeed, in the study by Picco et al. (2010), some nurses reported that they rarely used touch to comfort. Dion-Nist et al. (2020) suggest that society gives nurses and other health professionals permission to touch as it is perceived as inherent in their role as caregivers. Conversely, Picco et al. (2010) argue that nurses may not be comfortable touching people outside of the instrumental context. Pedrazza et al. (2018) suggest that nurses may differ in their 'attachment style' and this may influence their willingness to touch, particularly if they are anxious or worried to use touch for emotional support. While many people respond well to touch to comfort them, nurses should be sensitive to any non-verbal cues that indicate the person does not want to be touched. In some care situations, use of touch could be misconstrued, and some people might view touch as an invasion of privacy and personal space. Touch has cultural significance and has different meanings and rules according to the gender of those involved. In Gleeson and Higgins's (2009) study, mental health nurses emphasised the importance of respecting clients' personal space, thereby taking care in using touch with people whom the nurses did not know, clients who were experiencing psychosis and those from different cultural backgrounds. Gleeson and Higgins (2009) suggest that mental health nurses need to be careful in the use of touch; for example, being sensitive to how male nurses touching female clients might be perceived. Maria's carers will know how she responds to touch as a means of comfort. Violet's husband can explain to care home staff how best to comfort Violet and whether she responds well to touch. Since Bill has just arrived on the medical ward, you will need to spend some time getting to know his personal preferences of touch through verbal and non-verbal cues.

As with any care, you should evaluate the effect, so observe for responses to touch. For example, if a nurse attempts to use comforting touch with Violet, does she become calmer or more agitated? Does she grasp the nurse's hand tightly or snatch her hand away? In some situations, it is appropriate to ask: 'Would you like to hold my hand during this (procedure)?'

Learning outcome 4: explore how verbal interactions can promote comfort

Kornhaber et al. (2016) found that nurses' interpersonal approach to individuals was central in promoting comfort and as discussed in Chapter 2, interpersonal skills comprise verbal and non-verbal communication.

Box 8.10 Activity: verbal interactions when comforting someone

ACTIVITY

Reflect on a situation in practice where you comforted a person in your care or a family member. What verbal interactions did you use?

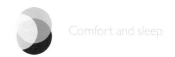

Consider your responses, as you continue to read this section: what type of interactions did you use?

Hawley (2000) identified four types of comforting talk which those admitted to an emergency unit described nurses using:

- **Reassuring talk** – phrases like 'Don't worry, we'll take care of you';
- **Coaching talk** – helps people to stay in control and cope with pain and anxiety;
- **Explanatory talk** – giving information about what is happening and answering questions;
- **Empathetic talk** – conveys understanding and caring, for example, 'I understand this is really hard for you – I am so sorry'.

A pattern of talk – 'comfort talk' – has been identified (Morse and Proctor 1998), which nurses use to help people to get through difficult situations or painful procedures. This appears to be what Hawley (2000) referred to as 'coaching'. Comfort talk is slow and rhythmic, with short simple sentences and uses phrases such as 'We're almost there, 'You're doing well' along with other emotionally supportive statements (Proctor et al. 1996; Wensley et al. 2020). Wensley et al. (2020) suggest that comfort talk helps people endure the situation, allows an information exchange and communicates a sense of caring. They emphasised that nurses' comfort talk is accompanied by being face-to-face with the person, holding their hand and focusing on their eyes.

The comforting effect of appropriate verbal interactions is supported by several studies. Palliative care nurses expressed that to promote comfort care, they were attentively present and dedicated to listening to individual needs (Sekse et al. 2018). The study concluded that the essential personal characteristics of palliative care nurses included, interpersonal skills and qualities such as kindness, warmth and compassion (Sekse et al. 2018). Wensley et al. (2020) found that person-centred comfort from holistic care was enhanced when delivered by nurses who gave attention to 'engagement and commitment'. It was suggested that these two qualities included, making an effort to connect, providing reassurance, encouragement and responding to their discomfort or distress.

Williams and Irurita (2006) found that explaining openly and honestly about what to expect and being encouraging provided emotional comfort, as did 'chit-chat' and social conversation. The Royal College of Nursing (2017) highlights that the way explanations are given can be as important as the content, so you should be aware of the tone used during your verbal communication. Techniques to promote relaxation, such as guided imagery and distraction are discussed in Chapter 9: Assessing and managing pain.

Learning outcome 5: select and apply physical actions for promoting comfort

Appropriate physical actions play an important role in comfort as highlighted in several research studies. Bergstrom et al. (2018) found that, to achieve physical

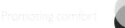

comfort, the relief of physical symptoms (especially pain) is necessary. Roche-Fahy and Dowling (2009) identified that in palliative care, physical comfort was important, and it was promoted through actions such as repositioning, personal hygiene and pain control. The way in which physical comfort measures are carried out will affect how they are perceived, and physical actions can be combined with other aspects of comfort care: presence, touch and verbal interactions (Ellingsen et al. 2018; Wensley et al. 2020; Dion-Nist et al. 2020).

Box 8.11 Activity: physical actions to promote comfort

ACTIVITY

What physical actions have you used in practice, or seen used, to promote comfort?

There are a wide range of physical actions that can help promote people's comfort.

- *Administering medicines.* Obvious examples include analgesics (see Chapter 9, Assessing and managing pain), anti-emetics (to prevent nausea and vomiting), antipyretics (to reduce high temperature) and bronchodilators (via nebulisers or inhalers) to reduce dyspnoea. However, many other prescribed medicines also reduce discomfort from unpleasant symptoms. Examples include drugs to regulate the heart rate and rhythm, thus stopping palpitations, and antibiotics which relieve fever-related symptoms such as headache, aching and malaise by treating infection.
- *Repositioning.* Assisting a breathless person into a sitting position well supported by pillows or in a chair, turning people to provide relief from pressure and positioning limbs to prevent contractures are all examples of using repositioning to promote comfort. Positioning for both Bill and Maria will be important in relieving physical discomfort.
- *Providing a comfortable bed.* For a person who is in bed for all or part of the day, a comfortable bed and appropriate bedding are fundamental. A comfortable, pressure-relieving mattress should be provided (see Chapter 11). Clean, unwrinkled bedlinen covers that are not too hot, too heavy or too cold, and sufficient supportive pillows are all essential.
- *Assisting with hygiene.* Dion-Nist et al. (2020) found that people were comforted by being helped with hygiene care. Chapter 7 covers all aspects of this in detail, and attention should be paid to mouth care, hair care and shaving, as well as the skin. Hygiene is an important comfort measure for people who are vomiting. Teeth cleaning, mouthwashes, hand and face washes, and changing of clothes can help people feel more comfortable. Assistance with hygiene may be required for the people in this chapter's scenarios – Chapter 7 covers the concerns regarding Bill's mouth care.
- *Assisting with elimination.* Incontinence causes both physical and psychological discomfort. Chapter 6 looks in detail at assisting people with elimination and promoting continence and managing incontinence in ways that promote comfort.
- *Providing food and drink.* Hunger and thirst cause discomfort, as you will almost certainly have experienced yourself. Chapter 5 looks in detail at how to assist

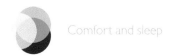

people with eating and drinking. Wilby (2005) found that people were comforted by being helped with eating. For people who are 'nil by mouth', it is important to explain why they cannot eat and drink and to offer mouthwashes to reduce the discomfort of a dry mouth.

- *Modifying the environment*. You need to observe whether the environment is too hot or too cold for the people you are caring for and modify the temperature where possible. Remember, those who lack mobility can quickly become cold and may need a blanket around them while sitting. Nurses should reduce excessive or unpleasant noise, for example, avoid banging waste bin lids. Music can be comforting (Mondanaro et al. 2017; Poulsen and Coto 2018), as can a pleasant décor, plants and pictures. For Violet, having some familiar items from home, such as framed photos, could be comforting. The psychological environment in which care takes place is also important for comfort; a calm, confident and relaxed atmosphere where there is good teamwork can all engender comfort for individuals.

In many instances, people may not request the physical actions listed above owing to communication difficulties or because they feel unable to ask, so nurses must be proactive in assessing people's needs for these comfort measures.

Learning outcome 6: integrate comfort care skills in different circumstances

The previous sections discussed different skills to promote comfort, but integrating skills is often more effective in comfort care. Competent physical actions are fundamental aspects of a nurse's role, but to provide comfort, these need to be integrated with presence, touch and verbal interactions. These latter measures are the ones that nurses often feel they do not have time for, but the art of comfort care is about smoothly integrating comfort during other nursing actions.

One way in which comfort care can be integrated is through 'intentional rounding'.

Intentional rounds ('care rounds', 'comfort rounds')

'Intentional rounding', also known as 'care rounds' or 'comfort rounds', is a way of promoting individual comfort (Harris et al. 2017). Intentional rounds involve a nurse going to each person every 1 or 2 h to check on four key elements – the four Ps: *Positioning* – making sure the person is comfortable and assessing pressure ulcer risk; addressing any *Personal needs*, such as taking them to the toilet; *Pain assessment*; and *Placement* – making sure they can reach everything they need (Harris et al. 2017). 'Care rounds' are not a new nursing concept and have been undertaken for many years; however, the concept of intentional rounding was highlighted in the Francis Inquiry, further endorsed by the Prime Minister and was given a formal structure (protocol) for nurses to follow to improve and monitor the care (Department of Health 2013; Harris et al. 2017).

Elements of intentional rounds are that: the nurse starts with an introduction that puts the person at ease; assesses the care environment, for example, the temperature, any fall hazards; asks 'Is there anything else I can do for you before I go?'; and informs when the next round is. The nurse must document the round: what time it took place, and any actions taken. In some settings, depending on local protocols, a student nurse, nursing associate or assistant practitioner may carry out these rounds, and they must report any necessary follow-up actions, such as the need for analgesics, to a registered nurse (Bartley 2011).

ACTIVITY

Box 8.12 Activity: intentional rounding

From the description above, reflect on your practice experience: have you seen intentional rounding being used? If so, what were responses to intentional rounding? What benefits might there be, both for individual comfort and care quality?

From the evidence available, Kings College London (2012) identified possible benefits of 'intentional rounding' as: better pain management, decreased falls, reduction in pressure ulcers and increased satisfaction for people in hospital care. In relation to comfort, the regular presence of a nurse, the interactions and the potential to build up a relationship will promote comfort as well as the direct actions to promote physical comfort.

ACTIVITY

Box 8.13 Intentional rounding to comfort Bill

Bill has been admitted to a medical ward for a blood transfusion due to his low Hb, how might intentional rounding make him more comfortable?

If the admitting nurse explains to Bill when a nurse will be coming round to check if he is comfortable has any personal needs and can reach everything he needs, he is likely to feel reassured that although there will not be a nurse there all the time, a nurse will attend to him regularly. Remember the four Ps of comfort rounds and to follow the intentional rounding protocol for your clinical setting.

Summary

- Promoting comfort is a key role of nurses in many different settings and is fundamental to a caring approach.
- Promoting comfort requires a holistic approach and the integration of presence and building a relationship, touch, verbal interactions and physical actions, encompassing a range of skills and knowledge, as applicable for each individual.

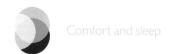

> ### Box 8.14 Children and young people: practice points – comfort
>
> Durations of stay in hospital for children and young people are usually kept as short as possible because of the recognition of the potentially harmful effects of the stress caused. Parents (or usual carers) are the most important presence for children and know how best to comfort their child. They are encouraged to stay with their child in hospital if possible; care should be family-centred with nurses supporting the whole family and providing comfort during what is likely to be an anxious, stressful time, including ensuring parents feel they can have breaks from the ward environment. Cantrell and Matula (2009) found that children and young people with cancer were comforted by being treated as individuals with interests, not only people with cancer; simply being asked how they were doing was comforting. Providing choices where possible helps children and young people to have some sense of control, as does keeping both the children and parents fully informed of developments. Play and involvement of play specialists can help to reduce fears and anxieties. Parents need to be given up-to-date information regarding safe sleeping positions and current views on bed-sharing with babies and infants (Peter et al. 2020).
>
> For further information, see:
>
> Ångström-Brännström, C. and Norberg, A. 2014. Children undergoing cancer treatment describe their experiences of comfort in interviews and drawings. *Journal of Pediatric Oncology Nursing*, 31: 135–46. doi:10.1177/1043454214521693
>
> Cantrell, M. and Matula, C. 2009. The meaning of comfort for pediatric patients with cancer. *Oncology Nursing Forum* 36(6). doi:10.1188/09.ONF.E303-E309
>
> Lerwick, J. 2016. Minimizing paediatric health care induced anxiety and trauma. *World Journal of Clinical Pediatrics* 5(2): 143–50. doi:10.5409/wjcp.v5.i2.143
>
> Peter, S., Blair, I., Helen, L. et al. 2020. Bedsharing and breastfeeding: The academy of breastfeeding medicine protocol #6, revision 2019. *Breast Feeding Medicine* 15(1). doi:10.1089/bfm.2019.29144.psb

PROMOTING SLEEP

Sleep is a state of rest during which our eyes close, muscles and nerves relax, and our mind becomes unconscious. It is something that we all need, no matter what our age, colour or creed. It can also be something we crave. Sleep deprivation causes a detrimental effect on our health, which can lead to acute and chronic physical and mental health illnesses.

Box 8.15 Learning outcomes

By the end of this section, you will be able to:

1 reflect on the importance of sleep for health;
2 examine factors that may affect sleep for people with acute and long-term health conditions;
3 apply a range of strategies to promote sleep for people with health needs.

Learning outcome 1: reflect on the importance of sleep for health

Box 8.16 Sleep satisfaction scale

ACTIVITY

On a scale of 0–10, how happy are you with your sleep? (Figure 8.1)

Through your biology reading, you will have learned that there are different types and stages of sleep. For us to be satisfied with our sleep, each type and stage needs to be experienced in full during a sleep cycle. Sleep cycles last 90–120 min, and we will have several of them during each period of normal sleep. Table 8.1 shows how the stages of sleep follow each other during a single sleep cycle.

You may have found in your reading that the stages were talked of as 1, 2, 3 and 4, with stage 2 being called light sleep; however, these were reclassified as in Table 8.1 in 2007 (Iber et al. 2007; Nasca and Goldberg 2017).

Sleep can be either restorative when the person wakes feeling rested and refreshed, or non-restorative. Although the usual definition of non-restorative sleep refers to light, restless, poor quality sleep, in the chronic pain syndrome fibromyalgia, there

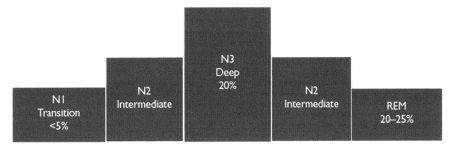

Figure 8.1: Sleep cycle showing the different stages.

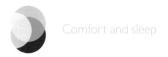
Table 8.1: Sleep cycle stages

N1 (Transition)	Is the transition period from being awake to falling to sleep. You will be drifting off to sleep but may still have awareness of your surroundings and can easily be aroused back to wakefulness.
N2 (Intermediate)	During this stage, your heart rate and breathing will gradually slow. We will spend around half of our sleep time in stage N2 throughout the entire sleep cycle (see Figure 8.1).
N3 (Deep)	Referred to as slow wave sleep due to slow brain waves. This is the period of sleep where the body regenerates and repairs itself. This stage normally lasts around 45–90 min. Subsequent episodes of N3 or slow wave sleep have shorter time periods as the night progresses.
REM (4)	Occurs after 90–120 min of sleep and then repeats approximately every 90 min thereafter. REM periods often increase in length later in the night. It is during REM that we dream, the body creates chemicals that temporarily paralyse us from acting out our dreams. During REM, our brains are highly active, and our eyes, although closed, move rapidly as if we were awake.

Adapted from Nasca and Goldberg (2017).

is evidence that individuals can appear to sleep well, having fallen asleep within a reasonable time and maintained their sleep for many hours. However, they wake unrested and unrefreshed (Roth et al. 2016).

It is not unusual to wake for a few moments at the end of each sleep cycle. We are often not aware of doing so, unless there is something disturbing us – such as the noise of clinical equipment that might disturb Bill on the hospital ward, the pain and associated distress that Maria is experiencing, the worry and anxiety that is affecting Mr Davies and the concerns that you might be experiencing regarding your next course assignment. Waking is of itself not an issue; the speed of falling back asleep and the degree of restoration are more important.

It is often said that the average adult needs 7½–8 h sleep. However, optimum sleep is related to the circadian rhythm and needs to occur at the 'right' time. Sleep needs also vary greatly at different ages and between different individuals.

Box 8.17 Activity: sleep across the lifespan

ACTIVITY

Ask your family and friends across different ages (child, teenage, young adult, mature adult, older person) how much sleep they think they get and how much they think they need. It might also be worth asking whether they feel rested and refreshed on waking.

You may find that, as an example, a 40-year-old family member says that he is in bed from 23.00 to 06.30, wakes frequently and wishes he could sleep like he did as a teenager. Yet when you ask him if his sleep refreshes him, he says, 'yes'. A 40-year-old gets half the deep sleep of a 20-year-old and is more likely to have family worries, perhaps children 'to keep an ear out for', and to believe that he should be sleeping as he used to.

The Royal College of Psychiatrists (RCP) website offers a number of useful leaflets including one on sleep 'Sleeping well' (RCP 2015). They suggest that:

- Babies sleep around 17 h each day.
- Older children sleep for 9 or 10 h each night.

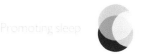

- Adults sleep around 8 h each night.
- Older people often have only one period of deep sleep during the night, usually in the first 3 or 4 h. After that, they wake more easily.

Adults' individual sleep requirements in fact vary from perhaps 3 or 4 h up to 11 h. However, the amount we sleep can affect how long we live, with 6–7 h per night proving optimal and much more than this being linked to increased mortality (Akerstedt et al. 2017).

In 2007, a longitudinal survey involving 10,308 civil servants showed that those who had reduced their sleep from 7 h in 1985–88 to 5 h by 1992–93 had a 1.7-fold increase in mortality overall and twice the risk of dying from cardiovascular disease as those who had not reduced their sleep (Ferrie et al. 2007). Similarly, a systematic review found that the risk of cardiovascular disease in children and adolescents has increased due to inadequate sleep (Fobian et al. 2018). Losing 1 h of sleep per night for 1 week can leave you feeling sleepy and irritable the following day; reactions are slower, concentration is poor, heart rate increases, and you feel cold. Everything is an effort and by the time you go to bed you either fall asleep immediately or lie awake worrying whether you will get to sleep. Figure 8.2 summarises some of the effects of sleep deprivation on the body and mind.

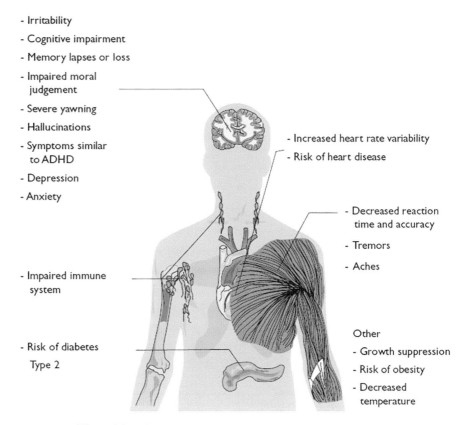

- Irritability
- Cognitive impairment
- Memory lapses or loss
- Impaired moral judgement
- Severe yawning
- Hallucinations
- Symptoms similar to ADHD
- Depression
- Anxiety

- Increased heart rate variability
- Risk of heart disease

- Decreased reaction time and accuracy
- Tremors
- Aches

- Impaired immune system

- Risk of diabetes Type 2

Other
- Growth suppression
- Risk of obesity
- Decreased temperature

Figure 8.2: Effects of sleep deprivation.

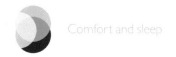

Speigel et al. (2005) found significant alterations in glucose metabolism, with decreased glucose tolerance and insulin sensitivity, in a group of healthy young adults. The study relates to a recent review of the literature undertaken by McHill and Wright (2017) that there is increasing evidence that short sleep duration is associated with diabetes and obesity.

It is possible that Maria had a history of poor sleep predating the onset of her diabetes. Daytime napping and sleep disturbance have been found to be associated with an increased cognitive decline and risk of dementia (Shi et al. 2017; Stone et al. 2019). Again, it is possible that Violet has a history of less night-time sleep and daytime napping preceding the onset of her Alzheimer's disease.

McFarlane et al. (2019) cite several studies examining sleep disturbance on acute medical wards. Bill was admitted to a medical ward for treatment of his anaemia. Sleep disruption is common in these environments with sleep fragmentation, frequent arousal and loss of deep and rapid eye movement (REM) sleep. Other barriers to sleep on medical wards also include the need to urinate, pain, light and noise.

Learning outcome 2: examine factors that may affect sleep for people with acute and long-term health conditions

> ### Box 8.18 Activity: factors affecting sleep
>
> What factors do you think might be affecting:
>
> * Bill's sleep on the medical ward?
> * Maria's sleep?
> * Violet and her husband's sleep?

The sleep of those with acute pain is frequently disturbed by the intensity of their pain and anxiety. In the case of Bill, his sleep on the medical ward may also be disturbed by environmental noise. A study undertaken by McFarlane et al. (2019) found that the mean duration of overnight sleep for inpatients was 4.6 h. Xie et al. (2009) list staff conversations and alarms as the most disturbing noises in ICU. The WHO recommends that noise levels in hospital wards are kept below 30dBA (Sheild et al. 2016), while the Environmental Protection Agency suggests 35dBA during sleeping hours and 45dBA in waking hours. Noise levels in inpatient environments have been found to be at 50–61dBA during the day and 41–51dBA at night-time (Sheild et al. 2016). It is not surprising that environmental sound is thus disturbing the sleep of many people in the hospital setting, leading to daytime tiredness that inhibits medical rehabilitation, can lead to hyperalgesia, nurtures delirium and is related to poor quality of life following acute episodes of illness (McFarlane et al. 2019).

At the age of 58, Maria may be menopausal, which is likely to disturb her sleep. As she has diabetes mellitus, alterations in blood sugar may also rouse her. Her painful diabetic neuropathy is likely to interfere with sleep quantity and quality. Husack and

Blair (2020) found that people with chronic pain feel tired all the time due to sleep disturbance and this can lead to an exacerbation of pain and other comorbidities such as depression. Finally, because of the natural ageing process, Maria will be having less deep sleep than she did when she was younger; the factors listed above are therefore even more likely to interfere with her sleep.

Violet's husband is exhausted. The USA National Sleep Foundation (2020) highlights that Alzheimer's disease and senile dementia are often characterised by frequent sleep disturbance, both for those diagnosed and their caregivers. Many caregivers cite sleep disturbances, which may include night wandering and confusion, as the reason for institutionalising their elderly relatives.

Sleep patterns can alter in a number of ways for people with dementia; they tend to wake more often and stay awake for longer at night, while being drowsy during the day. Some 20% also experience late afternoon/early evening restlessness and agitation, which has been termed 'sundowning'. Alzheimer's Society (2017) provides coping strategies for sleeping issues and sundowning. Some of these will be discussed later under learning outcome 3.

Insomnia is a significant issue in the United Kingdom and affects around a third of the population (Hartescu and Morgan 2018). In today's society, many individuals operate a voluntary sleep restriction programme going to bed late and getting up early. This may be for school, work, family or social reasons; it frequently becomes a difficult habit to break. Bedrooms have become living room extensions with televisions, sound systems, computers and telephones all designed to stimulate the individual.

Doghramji and Choufani (2011) and Frank et al. (2017) list the following dietary and lifestyle issues as potential factors affecting sleep:

- Caffeine and alcohol consumption before bedtime
- Nicotine (both smoking and cessation)
- Large meals or excessive fluid intake within 3 h of bedtime
- Exercising within 3 h of bedtime
- Utilising the bed for non-sleep activities (work, telephone, Internet)
- Staying in bed while awake for extended periods
- Activating behaviours up to the point of bedtime
- Excessive worrying at bedtime
- Clock-watching before sleep onset or during nocturnal awakenings
- Exposure to bright light before bedtime or during awakenings
- Keeping the bedroom too hot or too cold
- Noise
- Behaviour of a bed partner (e.g. snoring, leg movements)

While many of these may not be directly relevant to the hospital setting, people may be admitted to hospital after having developed these habits. Many of them will be applicable in primary and community care settings. The next section moves onto consider strategies for promoting sleep.

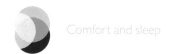

Learning outcome 3: apply a range of strategies to promote sleep for people with health needs

Establishing a bedtime routine and good habits creates the right associations for sleep. We invest time helping young children establish a pattern that fits with the family way of life. As we get older, changes in lifestyle and circumstances alter these patterns. Unfortunately, bad habits and poor routines can develop. Recognising unhelpful patterns and creating helpful associations is the first step in identifying what needs to be changed to improve sleep; see Box 8.20 for questions about sleep.

ACTIVITY

Box 8.19 Activity: reflecting on responses to questions about sleep

Review Box 8.20. Can you think of any other relevant questions to add to this list? Complete the list of questions, first for yourself and then with a friend or family member. Compare the responses and reflect on the differences.

Box 8.20 Questions about sleep

Sleep pattern

1 What time do you usually go to bed?
2 Do you go off to sleep straight away? If not, why not?
3 Do you wake during the night? If so, how often and why?
4 What time do you usually wake up in the morning?
5 How do you feel when you wake up in the morning?

Sleep hygiene

6 What time do you eat your evening meal?
7 How do you spend your time most evenings?
8 What is your routine prior to going to bed?

Sleep environment

9 How old is your mattress? What is it made of?
10 Is it soft, medium or hard?
11 How many pillows do you use and what are they made of?
12 What position do you sleep in?
13 Do you find your bedroom a relaxing and pleasant place to go? If not, why not?
14 Is your room noisy or quiet?
15 Do you watch television in bed?
16 Is your room at a comfortable temperature for you?

Sleep anxieties

17 Do you look forward to bedtime?
18 Do you spend time thinking about the things you have to do the following day or worrying about things at night?
19 Do you 'try' to sleep?

Sleep pattern

Much of sleep is a habit; we should go to bed when we are tired, but we frequently stay up, for example, to watch the 22.00 news, which may then stimulate us and delay sleep onset. There are some parameters that are essential when thinking of sleep pattern; see Table 8.2. Sleep specialist centres will also measure non-REM and REM sleep stage percentages and the time taken to the first period of REM when analysing individuals' sleep profiles (Fedorova et al. 2020). A further parameter is how restorative sleep is perceived by the individual.

There are a number of sleep assessment tools available; however, they tend to be used by sleep specialists. Asking Maria and her carers about her sleep and perhaps maintaining a sleep diary may provide additional insight into how her pain is interfering with her sleep pattern.

Sleep hygiene

Sleep is the opposite of arousal. Unfortunately, in today's 24/7 society, there is much to maintain arousal at a time of day when our circadian rhythm is synchronised to sleep.

Light is the strongest environmental stimulus to the sleep/wake cycle in humans (Ambrogetti 2005; Blume et al. 2019). During daylight hours, melatonin production is suppressed and cortisol, which promotes wakefulness, is released. As darkness falls, melatonin is released to cause a fall in body temperature and a slightly hypnotic state (Bartlett and Ambrogetti 2005; Blume et al. 2019). Turning lights down in the evening and reducing light stimulation from electronic devices will aid sleep.

Napping after 15.00 will reduce sleep debt and interfere with night-time sleep. Large meals should be eaten several hours before bedtime, although a carbohydrate snack or malted milk drink, half an hour before bedtime, may promote the release of tryptophan, which is a precursor to increasing melatonin levels. Exercise needs to cease, to allow the body to cool down, 5 h before bedtime, if it is vigorous, and 1 to 2 h for gentle exercise, such as walking (Bartlett and Ambrogetti 2005). Warm baths should be taken at least an hour before bedtime for the same reason. Nicotine, caffeine and alcohol all affect sleep and should be avoided before bedtime as should other stimulants (Sharine et al. 2020) (Table 8.3).

Another important factor is a signal or cue that it is time for sleeping. We often associate two things together, such as tea and biscuits, bread and cheese, sun and

Table 8.2: Parameter of sleep

Parameter	Accepted abbreviation	Definition
Sleep latency	SL	Amount of time required to fall asleep
Wakefulness after sleep onset	WASO	Amount of time awake after initial sleep onset
Time in bed	TIB	Time spent in bed
Total sleep time	TST	Actual time spent in bed
Sleep efficiency	SE	Ratio between TIB and TST

Source: Castronovo, V 2005. Basic concepts of polysomnography. In: Ambrogetti, A., Hensley, M.J. and Olson, L.G. (eds.) *Sleep Disorders: A Clinical Textbook.* Chapter 7. London: Quay Books, 211–76.

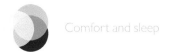
Table 8.3: Sleep hygiene hints and tips check list ©Dee Burrows

Sleep hygiene hints and tips that I could use	Tried but no longer doing ✓	I always do this ✓	I will try this for two to four weeks ✓
Aim to wake at the same time each day – set your alarm!			
Make sure you are exposed to bright light during the day.			
Exercise daily physically and mentally – but not late at night.			
Limit day time napping – unless you are Mediterranean!			
Limit caffeine, nicotine and alcohol – unless you are having the same amount now that you were before you developed sleep problems.			
Consider a busy brain journal – to dump your worries and overactive brain.			
Proteins for lunch, carbohydrates for supper (4 h before bedtime) and a milky Horlicks or Ovaltine as you start winding down really can help.			
Start relaxing 2 h before bedtime – a warm bath with candles and smellies; a relaxation or mindfulness technique; soothing music and soft lighting.			
Shut down 1 h before bedtime – including turning off televisions, radios, computers and even mobile phones.			
Valerian, St John's Wort, Vitamin B6 and other supplements can help – but must not be taken with prescription medication without medical advice.			
Keep a tidy bedroom – used only for sleep.			
Go to bed only when you are sleepy.			
The bedroom should be dark – perhaps blackout blinds?			
The bedroom should be cool, with the bed comfortable and warm.			
Mattresses and pillows need to be supportive and right for you.			
Try orange blossom, rather than lavender.			

sand. Creating an association between time and sleepiness and with bed and sleep can be very helpful.

Sleep environment

Bedrooms should be dark and cool, with the bed being cosy. All electronic devices should be turned off to reduce noise and light and to decrease the frequency and length of time awake after initial sleep onset (Lastella et al. 2020). People who do not draw their curtains, who have the television or radio on in their bedrooms and who complain of poor sleep can improve sleep by attention to these environmental factors (Desjardins et al. 2018).

Mattresses should be supportive of body curves, neither too hard nor too soft; mattress toppers may be useful to promote comfort, particularly for people with pain and insomnia (Desjardins et al. 2018). Pillows should be sufficient to fill the area between the edge of the shoulder and neck so as to maintain cervical posture when lying on the side. A bolster pillow under the top arm and firm pillow between

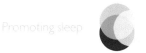

the knees and ankles can help maintain spinal alignment. Tidy, relaxing bedroom environments will help to decrease brain stimulation.

Sleep anxieties

People who are anxious about their sleep are more likely to have disturbed sleep. Bartlett and Ambrogetti (2005) comment:

> Watching the clock at night tends to increase anxiety about sleep. Good sleepers see 2.00 am on the clock when they wake and think 'Wonderful, four more hours in bed'. Poor sleepers see the same and think 'Disaster – I am never going to get back to sleep'.
>
> (p. 244)

There is no evidence that the poor sleepers will not get back to sleep, unless perhaps having had the same thought the night before, resulting in no further sleep. Catastrophic thinking – trying to get to sleep and worrying about sleep – disrupts sleep, which requires mental and physical relaxation, e.g. mindfulness meditation (Huang et al. 2020).

People who spend the night planning or worrying about the following day should consider 'brain dumping' 2–4 h before bedtime; make your list of work priorities at work, do the shopping list when cooking supper, plan your weekend over the meal, dump your worries in a journal for attention the following day; after all, there is little one can do about them during the night hours.

The Sleep Hygiene Hints & Tips Check List (Table 8.3) was developed by Dee Burrows the previous author of this chapter (4th edition) in her work with people with chronic pain.

ACTIVITY

Box 8.21 Activity: strategies that would be applied in a hospital setting

- Complete the checklist for yourself and then complete it with someone you know (e.g. relative, friend) who has difficulty sleeping.
- Pick two of the strategies this person will try for the next 2–4 weeks and look up the evidence base.
- Next make a list of which strategies you might try with Maria whose sleep is disturbed by painful diabetic neuropathy.
- Finally, think about which, if any, of the strategies could be applied in a hospital setting. Is there any difference between what could be offered in a mental health unit, an acute hospital ward or community setting such as a nursing home or the person's own home?

For Maria, you might have thought of a pictorial busy brain journal for her to dump her worries in and a relaxation technique such as an assisted relaxed bedtime routine. You may also need to undertake a bedroom environment assessment.

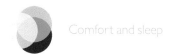

For Bill, a crucial sleep-enhancing strategy is to reduce noise and light stimulation. Bill is in a strange environment and a strange bed; he is attached to an intravenous blood transfusion and possibly other technical devices. He is likely to be drowsy from the low Hb and exhausted form having shortness of breath, but potentially hyper-aroused by noise and light. Xie et al. (2009) and Van Rompaey et al. (2012) both advocate the use of sound-masking, rather than sound-absorbing techniques. Sound-masking includes white noise, such as ocean sounds. Xie et al. (2009) found that sound-masking improves sleep by 42.7%, while earplugs did so by 25.3%.

The Alzheimer's Association provide some hints and tips for sleep and sundowning management.

ACTIVITY

Box 8.22 Alzheimer's association

Visit the Alzheimer's Association website (http://www.alz.org/care/alzheimers-dementia-sleep-issues-sundowning.asp) and read through their suggested strategies for sleep issues and sundowning. Consider:

- Which of these strategies to improve sleep might you discuss with Violet's husband?
- How do these suggested strategies differ from advice given to people who do not have dementia? (discussed in this chapter)

The strategies to reduce pain (see Chapter 9) and promote comfort, discussed earlier in this chapter, will be important additions to enhance the quality and quantity of sleep. Some of them, such as relaxation techniques, can have a direct impact on sleep by reducing hyper-arousal. Recognising tension is the first step followed by relaxation practice during the daytime until the individual feels competent and confident to try it at night. Imagery relaxation is one example. This approach is about creating pictures, or images, in our minds (Afshar et al. 2018). These can be based on fantasy, such as being on a beautiful island; on a real event, such as a holiday or on visualising the actual problem and the desired outcome. Imagery can either be guided by another or involve self-visualisation where the individuals make up their own. If the latter approach is adopted, it is worth writing the imagery down so that it can be practised as a prescribed technique. As many of the senses as possible should be involved. In developing one's own imagery, you can experiment with sight, sound, touch, smell and taste. Vividness and clarity can be enhanced by colours, shapes and thoughts. The imagery should be as real and involving as possible. Guided imagery can contain an element of risk if the facilitator creates an image that is unpleasant for the listener. For instance, if the fantasy was based on a walk through a garden and the individual has a poor recollection of pink roses, they may tense up and come out of the imagery. For these reasons, guided imagery can sometimes be generalised, leaving the individual to imagine their favourite flower and perfume.

Pharmacological management of sleep should not be commenced without a detailed sleep assessment and diagnosis. Drugs used for sleep include hypnotics, benzodiazepines, antidepressants, anticonvulsants and beta blockers. Some drugs, such as opioids, can make us drowsy. This may prompt relaxation and aid time taken to get to sleep. Reducing pain during sleep may improve sleep quality. The impact of daytime drowsiness as a consequence of medication side effects may or may not be an issue. For instance, Bill may be encouraged to nap during his hospital stay, whereas early morning drowsiness for the school run or travel to work is less advisable. Drugs like amitriptyline can leave people feeling drowsy and spaced out in the morning. Conversely, there is evidence that pregabalin has a positive impact on sleep quality as may the class of drugs called serotonin-norepinephrine reuptake inhibitors (SNRI). These drugs may therefore be useful for Maria whose sleep is disturbed by pain and discomfort.

Poor sleep will enhance perceptions of pain and discomfort, while managing pain and promoting comfort will aid sleep. However, other factors also impact sleep, and a biopsychosocial approach that takes into account individual patterns and behaviours is crucial to managing sleep.

Summary

- Sleep deprivation will affect physical, mental and social health.
- Promoting sleep is a key role of nurses in many different settings and is fundamental to caring.
- Promoting sleep requires an understanding of normal sleep and insight into the individual's usual sleep pattern and any factors that may be contributing to poor sleep.
- A holistic approach to sound sleep hygiene and sleep management is crucial for health.

CHAPTER SUMMARY

Throughout this book, practical nursing skills are contextualised within a philosophy of caring. This chapter has focused on some fundamental aspects of nursing, promoting comfort and sleep and has emphasised a caring approach, including compassion, competence and effective communication. Nurses have an important role in promoting comfort, a role recognised by Florence Nightingale, who wrote in 1854:

> The benefits which this Institution [hospital] ought to afford to the sick are perhaps best seen when we are enabled to give comfort in the time of danger and to lessen the agony of death.
>
> (Quoted in McDonald 2009, p. 108)

Promoting comfort and sleep require nurses to integrate a range of skills, with an appropriate attitude and a sound underpinning knowledge base.

REFERENCES

Afshar, M., Abbas, M., Gilsasi, H. and Sadegi-Ganomani, H. 2018. The effects of guided imagery on state and trait anxiety and sleep quality among patients receiving hemodialysis: A randomized control trial. *Complementary Therapies in Medicine* 40: 37–41.

Akerstedt, T., Ghilotti, F., Grotta, A. et al. 2017. Sleep duration, mortality and the influence of age. *European Journal Epidemiology* 32: 881–91.

Alonzo, T. 2017. Hope for Person with dementia: Why comfort matters. *American Society on Aging: Generations* 41(1): 81–5.

Alzheimer's Society. 2017. This is me. Available from: https://www.alzheimers.org.uk/sites/default/files/2020-03/this_is_me_1553.pdf (Accessed on 17 August 2020).

Alzheimer's Society. 2020. Alzheimer's disease? Available from: https://www.alzheimers.org.uk/about-dementia/types-dementia/alzheimers-disease (Accessed on 4 March 2013).

Ambrogetti, A. 2005. Neuroanatomy and pharmacology of sleep: Clinical implications. In: Ambrogetti, A., Hensley, M.J. and Olson, L.G. (eds.) *Sleep Disorders: A Clinical Textbook*. Chapter 7. London: Quay Books, 211–76.

Bailey, T. and Walter, T. 2016. Funerals against death. *Mortality*, 21 (2): 149–66.

Bales, K.L., Witczak, L.R., Simmons, T.C. et al. 2018. Social touch during development: Long-term effects on brain and behaviour. *Neuroscience & Biobehavioral Reviews* 95: 202–19.

Bartlett, D. and Ambrogetti, A. 2005. Insomnia. In: Ambrogetti, A., Hensley, M.J. and Olson, L.G. (eds.) *Sleep Disorders: A Clinical Textbook*. Chapter 7. London: Quay Books, 211–76.

Bartley, A. 2011. The King's Fund Hospital pathways programme. Making it happen: intentional rounding London: The King's Fund and the Health Foundation. Available from: https://www.kingsfund.org.uk/audio-video/annette-bartley-making-intentional-rounding-happen. (Accessed on August 2020).

Bergstrom, A., Warren-Stomberg, M. and Bjersa, K. 2018. Comfort theory in practice – nurse anaesthetists comfort measures and interventions in a preoperative context. *Journal of Peri Anesthesia Nursing* (33)2: 162–71.

Blume, C., Garbazza, C. and Spitschan, M. 2019. Effects of light on human circadian rhythms, sleep and mood. *Somnologie* 23: 147–56. *British Medical Journal Open* (7)1.

Bundgaard, K. and Nielsen, L.B. 2011. The art of holding hand: A fieldwork study outlining the significance of physical touch in facilities for short-term stay. *International Journal for Human Caring* 15(3): 34–41.

Castronovo, V. 2005. Basic concepts of polysomnography. In: Ambrogetti, A., Hensley, M.J. and Olson, L.G. (eds.) *Sleep Disorders: A Clinical Textbook*. Chapter 7. London: Quay Books, 211–76.

Coelho, A., Parola, V., Escobar-Bravo, M. 2016. Comfort experience in palliative care: A phenomenological study. *BMC Palliative Care* 15(71). doi 10.1186/s12904-016-0145-0.

Connor, A. and Howett, M. 2009. A conceptual model of intentional comfort touch. *Journal of Holistic Nursing* 27(2): 127–35.

Cook, N., Shepherd, A., Boore, J. and Dunleavy, S. 2019. *Essentials of Pathophysiology for Nursing Practice*. London: SAGE.

Department of Health. 2013. Report of the Mid Staffordshire Foundation NHS Trust public inquiry, vol. 1–3. HC-898-I-III. London: The Stationery Office.

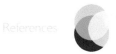

Desjardins, S., Desaulniers, J., Lapierre, S. and Desgagné, A. 2018. Sleep environment and insomnia in elderly persons living at home. *Journal of Aging Research* 15(1): 2217–27.

Diabetes UK. 2020. Diabetic neuropathy. Available from: https://www.diabetes.org.uk/guide-to-diabetes/complications/nerves_neuropathy (Accessed on 15 August 2020).

Dion-Nist, M., Tondi, M., Harrison, T., Robinson, A. et al. 2020. Losing Touch. *Nursing Inquiry* 27: 3. https://doi.org/10.1111/nin.12368

Doghramji, K. and Choufani, D. 2011. Taking a sleep history. In: Winkelman, J. and Plante, D. (eds.) *Foundations of Psychiatric Sleep Medicine*. Cambridge. MA: Cambridge University Press, 95–110.

Fatemeh, M., Foroozan, A., Soroor, P. and Meimanat, H. 2017. An explanatory study on the concept of nursing presence from the perspective of patients admitted to hospitals. *Journal of Clinical Nursing* 26 (24–24): 4313–24.

Fedorova, T., Knudsen, K., Sommerauer, M., Svendsen, K., Otto, M. and Borghammer, P. 2020. A screening-based method for identifying patient with REM sleep behaviour disorder in a Danish community setting. *Journal of Parkinson's Disease* 10(3): 1249–53.

Ferrie, J.E., Shipley, M.J., Cappuccio, F.P. et al. 2007. A prospective study of change in sleep duration; associations with mortality in the Whitehall II cohort. *Sleep* 30(12): 1659–66.

Fobian, A.D., Elliott, L. and Louie, T.A. 2018. Systematic review of sleep, hypertension, and cardiovascular risk in children and adolescents. *Current Hypertension Reports* 20(5): 42. doi:10.1007/s11906-018-0841-7.

Frank, S., Gonzalez, K., Lee-Ang, L. et al. 2017. Diet and sleep physiology: Public health and clinical implications. *Frontiers in Neurology* 8: 393.

Gleeson, M. and Higgins, A. 2009. Touch in mental health nursing: An exploratory study of nurses' views and perceptions. *Journal of Psychiatric and Mental Health Nursing* 16: 382–9.

Harris, R., Sims, S., Levenson, R. et al. 2017. What aspects of intentional rounding work in hospital wards, for whom and in what circumstances? A realist evaluation protocol. *British Medical Journal Open* 7: e014776. doi:10.1136/bmjopen-2016–014776.

Hartescu, L. and Morgan, K. 2018. Regular physical activity and insomnia: An international perspective. *Journal of Sleep Research* 28(2): 127–45.

Hawley, M.P. 2000. Nurse comforting strategies: Perceptions of emergency department patients. *Clinical Nursing Research* 9: 441–59.

Hessel, JA. 2009. Presence in nursing practice: a concept analysis. *Holistic Nursing Practice* 23(5): 276–81.

Huang, I., Short, M., Bartel, K. et al. 2020. The roles of repetitive negative thinking and perfectionism in explaining the relationship between sleep onset difficulties and depressed mood in adolescents. *Paediatric and Adolescent Sleep Health* 6(2): 166–71.

Husack, A. and Blair, M. 2020. Chronic pain and sleep disturbances: A pragmatic review of their relationships, comorbidities, and treatments. *Pain Medicine* 21(6): 1142–52.

Iber, C., Ancoli-Israel, S., Chesson, A. et al. 2007. *The AASM Manual for the Scoring of Sleep and Associated Events: Rules, Terminology and Technical Specifications*. Westchester, NY: American Academy of Sleep Medicine.

Jagan, S., Park, T. and Papathanassoglou, E. 2019. Effects of massage on outcomes of adult intensive care unit patients: A systematic review. *Nursing in Critical Care* 24(6): 414–29.

Kings College, London. 2012. *Intentional Rounding: What Is the Evidence? Policy.* London: KCL.

Kolcaba, K.Y. 1995. Comfort as process and product, merged in holistic art. *Journal of Holistic Nursing* 13: 117–31.

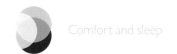
Kolcaba, K.Y. 2003. *Comfort Theory and Practice: A Vision for Holistic Health Care and Research.* New York: Springer.

Kornhaber, R. Walsh, K. Duff, J. Walker, K. 2016. Enhancing adult therapeutic interpersonal relationships in the acute health care setting: an integrative review. *Journal of Multidisciplinary Healthcare* 9: 537–46.

Lastella, M., Rigney, G., Browne, M. and Sargent, C. 2020. Electronic device use in bed reduces sleep duration and quality in adults. *Sleep Biological Rhythms* 18: 121–9.

Mcdonald, L. 2009. *Florence Nightingale: The Nightingale School: Volume 12 of Collected Works of Florence Nightingale.* Ontario: Wilfrid Laurier University Press, p. 108.

McFarlane, M., Rajapakse, S. and Loughran, S. 2019. What Prevents sleeping on an acute medical ward – An actigraphy and qualitative sleep study. *Journal of National Sleep Foundation* 5: 666–9.

McHill, A. and Wright, K. 2017. Role of sleep and circadian disruption on energy expenditure and in metabolic predisposition to human obesity and metabolic disease. *Obesity Reviews* 18(1): 15–24.

Mondanaro, J.F., Homel, P., Lonner, B. et al. 2017. music therapy increases comfort and reduces pain in patients recovering from spine surgery. *American Journal of Orthopaedics* 46(1): 13–22.

Morse, J.M. and Proctor, A. 1998. Maintaining patient endurance: The comfort work of trauma nurses. *Clinical Nursing Research* 7: 250–74.

Mottram, A. 2009. Therapeutic relationships in day surgery: A grounded theory study. *Journal of Clinical Nursing* 18: 2830–7.

Nasca, T. and Goldberg, R. 2017. American Association of Sleep Apnoea [online] the importance of sleep and understanding the stages. Available from: https://www.sleephealth.org/sleep-health/importance-of-sleep-understanding-sleep-stages/ (Accessed on 10 August 2020).

National Health Service 2018. Live well – Why lack of sleep is bad for you: Sleep and Tiredness. Available from: https://www.nhs.uk/live-well/sleep-and-tiredness/why-lack-of-sleep-is-bad-for-your-health/ (Accessed on 20 August 2020).

Pedrazza, M., Berlanda, S., Trifiletti, E. and Minuzzo, S. 2018. Variables of individual difference and the experience of touch in nursing. *Western Journal of Nursing Research* 40(11): 1614–37.

Picco, E., Santoro, R. and Garrino, L. 2010. Dealing with the patient's body in nursing: Nurses' ambiguous experience in clinical practice. *Nursing Inquiry* 17(1): 39–46.

Pinto, S., Caldeira, S., Martins, J. and Rodgers, B. 2017. Evolutionary analysis of the concept of comfort. *Holistic Nursing Practice* 31(4): 243–52.

Poulsen, MJ. and Coto, J. 2018. Nursing music protocol and postoperative pain. *Pain Management Nursing: Journal of the American Society of Pain Management Nurses* 19(2): 172–76.

Proctor, A., Morse, J.M. and Khonsari, S. 1996. Sounds of comfort in the trauma centre: How nurses talk to patients in pain. *Social Science Medicine* 42: 1669–80.

Roche-Fahy, V. and Dowling, M. 2009. Providing comfort to patients in their palliative care trajectory: Experiences of female nurses working in an acute setting. *International Journal of Palliative Nursing.* 15(3): 134–41.

Roth, T., Bhadra-Brown, P., Verne, P. and Renick, M. 2016. Characteristics of disturbed sleep in patient with fibromyalgia compared with insomnia of with pain-free volunteers. *The Clinical Journal of Pain* 32(4): 302–7.

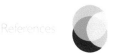

The Royal College of Nursing. 2017. Verbal communication. Available from: https://rcni.com/hosted-content/rcn/first-steps/verbal-communication (Accessed on 10 August 2020).

Royal College of Psychiatrists (RCP). 2015. Sleeping well. Available from: https://www.rcpsych.ac.uk/mental-health/problems-disorders/sleeping-well (Accessed on 10 August 2020).

Sekse, R.J.T., Hunskär, I. and Ellingsen, S. 2018. The nurse's role in palliative care: A qualitative meta-synthesis. *Journal of Clinical Nursing* 27: 21–38.

Sharine, A., Ferguson, S., Jay, M. and Vincent, G. 2020. Sleep hygiene in shift workers: A systematic literature review. *Sleep Medicine Reviews* 53: 101–36.

Sheild, S., Shiers, N. and Glanville, R. 2016. The acoustic environment of inpatient hospital wards in the United Kingdom. *The Journal of Acoustical Society of America* 140(3): 2213–2224.

Shi, L., Chen, S., Meng-Ying, M. et al. 2017. Sleep disturbances increase the risk of dementia: A systematic review and meta-analysis. *Sleep Medicine Reviews* 40: 4–16.

Speigel, K., Knutson, K., Leproult, R. et al. 2005. Sleep loss: A novel risk factor for insulin resistance and type 2 diabetes. *Journal of Applied Physiology* 99(5): 2008–19.

Stone, K., Leng, Y., Redline, S., Ancoil-Israel, S. and Yaffe, K. 2019. Objective napping, cognitive decline and cognitive impairment in older men. *Alzheimer's and Dementia* 15(8): 1039–47.

USA National Sleep Foundation. 2020. Alzheimer's disease and sleep. Available from: https://www.sleepfoundation.org/articles/alzheimers-disease-and-sleep. (Accessed on 20 August 2020).

Van Rompaey, B., Elseviers, M.M., Van Drom, W. et al. 2012. The effect of earplugs during the night on the onset of delirium and sleep perception: A randomized controlled trial in intensive care. *Critical Care* 16(R73): 1–10.

Waugh, A. and Grant, A. 2018. *The Blood: Ross and Wilson Anatomy and Physiology.* Chapter 2. Edinburgh: Elsevier, 61–80.

Wensley, C.A., Botti, M., McKillop, A. and Merry, A. 2017. Multidimensional framework of comfort for practice and quality improvement. *International Journal of Quality in Healthcare* 29(2): 151–62.

Wensley, C.A., Botti, M., McKillop, A. and Merry, A. 2020. Maximising comfort: How do patients describe the care that matters? A two-stage qualitative descriptive study to develop a quality improvement framework for comfort-related care in inpatient settings. *British Medical Journal Open* 10(5). doi:10.1136/bmjopen-2019–033336

Wilby, M.L. 2005. Cancer patients' descriptions of comforting and discomforting nursing actions. *International Journal for Human Caring* 9(4): 59–63.

Williams, A.M. and Irurita, V.F. 2006. Emotional comfort: The patient's perspective of a therapeutic context. *International Journal of Nursing Studies* 43: 405–15.

Xie, H., Kang, J. and Mills, G.H. 2009. Clinical review: The impact of noise on patients' sleep and the effectiveness of noise reduction strategies in intensive care units. *Critical Care* 13(2): 208.

Yardley, S. and Rolph, M. 2020. Death and dying during the pandemic. *British Medical Journal.* Available from: https://www.bmj.com/content/369/bmj.m1472 (Accessed on 10 February 2021).

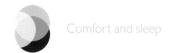

USEFUL WEBSITES

Alzheimer's Society, Alzheimer's disease. Available from: www.alzheimers.org.uk/about-dementia/types-dementia/alzheimers-disease

Alzheimer's Society. This is me. Available from: www.alzheimers.org.uk/sites/default/files/2020-03/this_is_me_1553.pdf

Diabetes UK. 2020. Diabetic neuropathy. Available from: www.diabetes.org.uk/guide-to-diabetes/complications/nerves_neuropathy.

National Health Service: Live well – Why lack of sleep is bad for you: Sleep and tiredness. Available from: www.nhs.uk/live-well/sleep-and-tiredness/why-lack-of-sleep-is-bad-for-your-health/

Royal College of Psychiatrists (RCP) Sleeping well. Available from: www.rcpsych.ac.uk/mental-health/problems-disorders/sleeping-well

The Royal College of Nursing Verbal communication. Available from: https://rcni.com/hosted-content/rcn/first-steps/verbal-communication

USA National Sleep Foundation. Alzheimer's disease and sleep. Available from: www.sleepfoundation.org/articles/alzheimers-disease-and-sleep

9 Assessing and managing pain

Lindsey Pollard and Harriet Barker

People in all healthcare settings experience pain whether it is physical, emotional, or spiritual. Evidence suggests that the proportion experiencing significant pain in an in-patient setting does not differ between medical and surgical specialities with 16.7% of people experiencing severe pain while on medical wards, and 19.9% on surgical wards (Rockett et al. 2013). Furthermore, 43% of the UK population experience chronic pain and for 14.3%, this is moderate to severe and causes significant disability (British Pain Society 2016). Managing pain and promoting function is a principal skill in daily nursing practice.

Pain impacts upon many aspects of individuals' lives including eating, drinking, moving around and sleeping.

This chapter aims to help you understand what pain is and will enable you to develop your nursing skills to effectively assess and manage pain.

This chapter includes the following topics:

- Defining pain
- Differentiating between the different types of pain
- Effective pain assessment
- Pharmacological pain management
- Non-pharmacological pain management.

Box 9.1 Recommended biology reading – pain

The following questions will help you to focus on the biology underpinning the skills used in pain management (but note pain is not only a biological experience). Use your recommended textbook to find out:

- How is pain defined?
- Is pain useful? Why?
- What are the three distinct parts of the nociceptive pathway?
- What are the differences between C-fibres and Aδ-fibres?
- Name three parts of the brain that are involved in the perception of pain.
- What can affect pain perception?
- What physiological signs may indicate that a person is in acute pain?
- How does chronic pain differ from acute pain?

DOI: 10.4324/9781003020660-9

PRACTICE SCENARIOS

The following scenarios illustrate when pain assessment and management is needed. They will be referred to throughout this chapter.

Adult

Thomas is 34 years old, married, with young children. He is a self-employed graphic designer who contracts out for work. Some time ago, Thomas was diagnosed with Crohn's disease, the impact of which has been affecting his home, work, and leisure activities. He was admitted via the enhanced recovery programme for a laparotomy, division of adhesions and formation of an **ileostomy**. Post operatively he was transferred to the high observation bay on the surgical ward. He initially had bilateral rectus sheath catheters infusing local anaesthetic alongside a morphine patient-controlled analgesic (PCA) device for pain relief. He was converted to oral analgesics after 3 days and was discharged at 6 days with pain management and stoma advice.

Learning disability

Maria is a 58-year-old woman with a moderate learning disability who has been living in a group home for the last 5 years. She has long-standing diabetes mellitus, which has been treated with insulin and has recently developed painful diabetic neuropathy. She has pain in both legs below the knees, which she finds particularly distressing when she is walking and during the night. Her sleep is disturbed by pain. She is in the care of both her GP and the diabetic team at her local hospital. Maria's mother, who is 85 years old and recently widowed, visits on a weekly basis and is concerned about Maria's distress. Her community learning disability nurse would like to understand more about how he can support Maria, her mother and the group home staff on how to manage Maria's pain.

Mental Health

Violet Davies, aged 76 years, has moderate Alzheimer's disease. She has been admitted to a care home for respite as her husband is physically and emotionally exhausted and needs a break. He has refused help in the past as he has been determined to look after his wife, but he has now agreed to take a holiday visiting friends. Violet is physically well, but she is also known to have osteoarthritis in her right hip and knee. She looks permanently worried and is agitated; she keeps repeating the same phrase over and over. Mr Davies looks shaky and tearful at the thought of leaving his wife for a week.

ASSESSING AND MANAGING PAIN IN A VARIETY OF SETTINGS

Painful diabetic neuropathy

The presence of symptoms and/or signs of peripheral nerve dysfunction in people with diabetes after the exclusion of other causes.

Box 9.2 Learning outcomes

By the end of this section, you will be able to:

1   discuss the nature of pain;
2   consider the biopsychosocial complexity of pain;
3   identify appropriate pain assessment tools for different groups;
4   demonstrate understanding of pharmacological approaches to managing pain;
5   explore non-pharmacological approaches to managing pain.

Learning outcome 1: discuss the nature of pain

ACTIVITY

Box 9.3 Activity: practice experiences

Reflect on your practice experiences. Write down a few examples of people you have met with pain and the setting in which you met them.

Alzheimer's disease

Alzheimer's disease is the most common cause of dementia, affecting around 850,000 people in the UK. The term 'dementia' describes a set of symptoms, which can include loss of memory, mood changes, and problems with communication and reasoning (Alzheimer's Society 2017).

The challenge with pain is that it is both a personal and subjective experience. Each person will have a unique experience, which makes pain difficult to assess and manage. It can influence every aspect of life as the impact is biopsychosocial.

Epidemiological studies show 15–30% of children experience pain (The Scottish Government 2018). Population estimates suggest 14.3% (with some studies showing up to 30%) of 18–25 year olds experience chronic pain. This increases as people get older with 62% of over 75 year olds experiencing chronic pain (Fayaz et al. 2016). However, it is estimated that up to 93% of older people could be experiencing pain (Schofield 2018).

Therefore, managing pain is relevant to every field of nursing.

Defining pain

ACTIVITY

Box 9.4 Activity: defining pain

Think back to a time when you have experienced pain and write down the experience. Looking at your notes, how would you define pain?

Osteoarthritis

A joint disease caused by cartilage loss in a joint. Pain and stiffness are symptoms.

Pain is a complex, personal experience that has been defined in various ways. For example, the International Association for the Study of Pain (IASP) defines pain as follows:

An unpleasant sensory and emotional experience associated with, or resembling that associated with, actual or potential tissue damage.

(IASP 2020)

Modern definitions of pain are moving on from unidimensional biological definitions of pain towards a focus on the difference between pain and nociception. Although we are aware that older commonly used definitions such as that of McCaffery (1968) who defined pain as it being 'whatever the patient says it is' still have a place in modern practice. However, solely treating the person's pain score with analgesics can lead to unintended harm. Modern pain management includes an assessment of the individual's function as well as their pain severity score. This will be discussed later within the chapter.

An individual's response to pain will vary significantly depending on their social and psychological experiences, and their individual relationship with pain. By solely assessing and managing pain as a biological process, and ignoring psycho-social aspects, their suffering is likely to persist.

However, it is worth remembering as Moskow (1987) points out:

> Pain occurring in unicorns, griffins, and jabberwockies is always imaginary pain, since these are imaginary animals; patients on the other hand are real and so they always have real pain.
>
> (Moskow 1987, p. 68)

To make sense of the concept that all pain is "real", we need to explore the different ways in which pain is perceived.

Experiencing pain

ACTIVITY

Box 9.5 Activity: experiencing pain

Access the IASP website and their most recent definition of pain. Using their six bullet points of the definition of pain, how do you think they may affect your own personal perception of pain?

Sensory signalling systems

When there is tissue damage, an inflammatory response is triggered. Various chemicals (sometimes called the 'sensitising soup') are released reducing the firing threshold of the nociceptors (or 'pain receptors'). When these pain receptors are activated, a nerve impulse or action potential travels to the dorsal horn in the spinal cord. There are two main groups of pain nerves, Aδ- or C-fibres. The Aδ-fibres are larger and myelinated and transmit impulses more quickly than the C-fibres. The Aδ-fibres conduct 'fast pain, often described as sharp pain, and the C-fibres conduct slow, aching pain'. These pains are called nociceptive (see Box 9.6).

Box 9.6 Sensory signalling – definitions and information

Action potential

The process by which neurons (cells within a nerve) alter their electrical charge so that impulses are carried down the nerve.

(Continued)

Box 9.6 (Continued)

Nerve fibres

The Aβ (beta)-fibres are larger myelinated fibres; they transmit touch, mild pressure, joint position sense and vibration. When pain occurs, signals travel up Aδ (delta)-fibres, causing a sharp sudden pain, – or C-fibres, resulting in a dull ache.

Central sensitisation and wind-up

Wind-up is a short-term reversible increase in the sensitivity of the pain nervous system. This can happen when tissues become inflamed, for example, after a burn. Central sensitisation happens when wind-up continues for a longer time – such as ongoing joint inflammation in rheumatoid arthritis. This results in longer-term changes in the pain nervous system, which may become more or less permanent and irreversible as in chronic pain. The pain nervous system is up-regulated and works in a state of 'high alert'. This lowers the threshold of what the person perceives as a painful stimulus (Institute for Chronic Pain 2017).

The first theory to explain the apparent inconsistency in pain responses to a set stimulus was suggested by Melzack and Wall in 1965 (Melzack and Wall 1996). Although now of historical interest only, this theory explained how descending nerve impulses and the effects of activating other nerve fibres (such as Aβ fine touch fibres) might increase or decrease pain perceived. The impulses from the periphery arrive at the dorsal horn of the spinal cord where they can be modified before continuing their journey to the brain. The various parts involved are referred to as the "salience matrix", which applies to all attention-grabbing stimuli, including light, sound and pain. Information from the sensory signalling system is linked with those from the emotion-related brain areas (the limbic system) and the cognition-related brain areas. These emotion- and cognition-related areas may send impulses back down the spinal cord, resulting in changes in the signal transmitted up from the periphery. The sum of these factors changes how an individual will perceive pain.

Pain can also be caused by damage to the nerves themselves, either in the periphery or centrally. This is called neuropathic pain and is relatively rare. Sometimes, people may have both nociceptive and neuropathic pain. For example, people who have undergone an amputation may experience nociceptive pain at the site of surgery in the stump, as well as peripheral and central neuropathic pain, where they feel pain in the limb that is no longer physically present; this is called phantom limb pain.

With reference to the scenarios at the start of the chapter:

- Thomas will have pain as a consequence of the surgical incision and the resultant tissue damage, activating the sensory signalling system. His pain is clearly related to his injury and is expected to subside as the healing process occurs. This is acute nociceptive pain. Thomas may also have central sensitisation from long-term pain in his bowel; this may continue post-op, resulting in visceral hyperalgesia (increased sensitivity of his bowel to painful stimuli); this pain will not respond to the local anaesthetic infusion, which only affects the nerves of skin and muscle. If he has had a lot of pain preoperatively, he may feel relieved that the surgery has been done and that he can start getting better (emotional and cognitive input that may reduce his perception of pain).

- Maria's leg pain is due to damage to the nerves by diabetes. The damaged nerves continuously send action potentials, which are perceived as painful. She may struggle to understand why she has pain; therefore, using cognitive skills to modify or reduce the pain perception can be challenging for her carers. The underlying problem causing Maria's pain is unlikely to heal, and this long-term pain is known as chronic or persistent pain. In this case, it is also neuropathic pain.

- Violet's situation is complex, with pain caused by the mechanical stimulation of osteoarthritis and changes to her brain arising from her Alzheimer's disease that appear to alter her emotional and cognitive processing. Her agitation activates the reticular activating system, a part of the brain involved in the pain pathways. These combined influences may make it difficult for her to change the pain perception (and the changes in her brain may also make it difficult for her to communicate – we will look at pain assessment for Violet later in the chapter).

- Violet's husband may be suffering from social isolation in addition to his mental and physical exhaustion. He may need comforting and active support if he is going to be able to look after his wife in the future.

Reticular activating system

A network of brain cells concerned with arousal and awareness.

Box 9.7 Activity: pain thresholds

ACTIVITY

- How often have you or friends commented that someone has a 'high (or low) pain threshold'? Think for a minute what you meant by this. Jot down your feelings about people with a low threshold and those with a high threshold.
- Now consider what you understand by the word olerance'.

In pain management, 'threshold' refers to the level at which the population at large perceives a stimulus as painful, rather than uncomfortable. In theory, we all feel pain at about the same level. Therefore, pain threshold is essentially a physiological measurement. It is common for practitioners to believe that people with cognitive impairment have a higher threshold to pain than those in the general population; however, it is argued that this may actually be the opposite (Barney et al. 2020). What makes us feel pain differently is pain 'tolerance'. This refers to the amount of pain an individual can tolerate, or put up with, at any given time. It is not affected by age, gender or culture, but rather by the thoughts and feelings we are experiencing at that point in time, and it is thus an outcome of the combination of sensory, cognitive and emotional input and processing. In struggling to communicate her pain, Maria may have a lower tolerance than Thomas whose surgery could be seen as an improvement in his condition. Pain with a negative emotional connotation is more difficult to tolerate than pain related to a positive emotional experience.

To illustrate pain tolerance, think of two individuals. One has had a formation of a colostomy as part of a curative procedure for bowel cancer. The next person has had a colostomy formed following trauma. The person who has had a curative procedure is feeling positive about their future, which has now been given back to them; the stoma is a small price to pay for their life, and they were prepared for it during clinic appointments. The person who has undergone trauma has had their life changed very quickly; they are likely to be experiencing a great deal emotionally, and are trying to process how their life will change; they would not have undergone a pre-operative work up. In these two very similar procedures, these individuals are likely to have very different levels of pain.

ACTIVITY

Box 9.8 Activity: perceptions of pain

Using the idea of cognitive and emotional input, try to map your different responses to both situations above. How might these affect your perception of the pain and the action you take?

Pain tolerance varies from one individual to the next and within an individual from one minute to the next. Some factors that increase or decrease pain perception are listed in Box 9.10.

ACTIVITY

Box 9.9 Activity: factors influencing Violet's pain perception

Look at the scenario of Violet and list the factors that may be influencing her pain perception. Note down an explanation for each factor.

- Mr Davies's emotional and physical exhaustion, his desire to support Violet at home and his tearfulness may be transmitted to Violet and increase her worry.
- The strange and potentially frightening environment may reduce Violet's sense of personal control and enhance her feelings of social isolation.
- The prolonged nature of Violet's osteoarthritis may have reduced her pain coping strategies.
- Violet's agitation will prevent her from relaxing and increase her tension.
- The lack of information about the immediate future may reduce Mr and Mrs Davies's abilities to maintain any sense of cognitive control.
- The pathophysiology of Alzheimer's disease may alter Violet's pain experience (covered further in learning outcome 3).

Knowing and understanding the factors that reduce pain perception can help guide your approach to pain management. A further concept you need to consider is pain behaviour.

Box 9.10 Examples of factors that increase or decrease our perception of pain

Increasing

- Anxiety, fear, worry, tension
- Lack of control
- Tiredness
- Prolonged or recurrent pain
- Previous poor experiences with pain

Decreasing

- Analgesic medication
- Information (if not anxious)
- Relaxation, distraction
- Control
- Touch, social interaction, reassurance
- Meditation
- Known positive outcome (e.g. childbirth)
- Previous positive experience with pain

ACTIVITY

Box 9.11 Activity: thinking about headaches

- How do you behave when you have a headache?
- How does your best friend behave?
- How do other people you know behave?

Perhaps one of the people you thought of wants attention, while others prefer to be on their own. Maybe some frown, grimace and become irritable, while others try to relax their facial expression and carry on as normal. As with non-verbal and social responses, verbal and vocal responses (e.g. shouting, moaning) also vary. These are all different pain behaviours or pain expressions.

Pain expression and pain behaviour are learned through our families and cultural beliefs are a strong determinant of pain expression and behaviour.

ACTIVITY

Box 9.12 Activity: pain behaviours

- Think of the different pain behaviours you have seen. List the ones you think Thomas, Maria and Violet might be adopting.
- Scenarios often push you into stereotyping (as do handovers). Consider the behaviours you have listed for each scenario and ask yourself why you identified those ones.
- Access Lovering's (2006) article online and make some notes about the different cultural perspectives of those involved in her study.

During this activity, keep in mind that what the person says about their pain is invariably true and is a much better indicator of pain than behaviour and physiological signs, although sometimes one has to rely on the latter, such as in Violet's case.

In summary, an appreciation of the differences between pain threshold, pain tolerance and pain behaviour will help you to understand how people's pain and their reactions to it vary. Remember, an individual's pain experience is very real to them, even if you cannot empathise with it yourself.

You may want to re-read this section to ensure that you understand the knowledge underpinning some of the practical skills that will be discussed later.

Learning outcome 2: consider the biopsychosocial complexity of pain

We have already suggested above that pain is a complex mix of physical sensation, emotions and cognitions that influence pain perception and behaviour. Both acute and chronic pains have these components.

Box 9.13 Activity: the biophyschosocial model

Many of you will be familiar with the biopsychosocial model. If you are not, you will need to look up the model before completing this activity. Thinking of someone you have recently nursed:

- What was the cause of their pain sensation?
- What were their worries and fears?
- What were their home, leisure and, if appropriate, work circumstances?
- How did all this impact upon their pain?

Thomas's biopsychosocial experience might look something like that shown in Figure 9.1.

As a self-employed graphic designer, Thomas is likely to both want and need to get back to work sooner than healthcare practitioners might advise, as well as having increased anxiety from social acceptance and body dysmorphia. This is a good example of where using a biopsychosocial model differs from the bio-medical model.

Box 9.14 Activity: knowledge and skills to improve Violet's pain management

Have a go at drawing your own diagram for Violet. Once you have done so:

- Give some thought to the knowledge and skills that you would need to improve Violet's pain management and reduce her pain perception
- Find an article that discusses biopsychosocial pain. Depending on your learning needs and stage of course, this could be an opinion article, a research paper or a video for example https://vimeo.com/86977616 by the Pain Community Centre at Cardiff University (2014).

Maria's more complex chronic pain experience is shown in Figure 9.2.

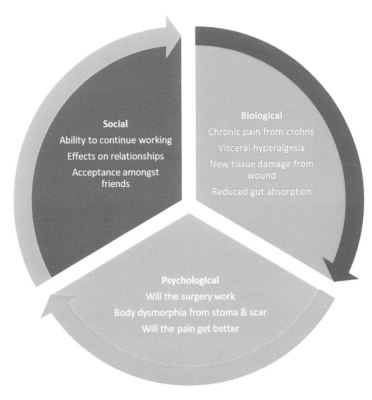

Figure 9.1: Thomas's biopsychosocial experience.

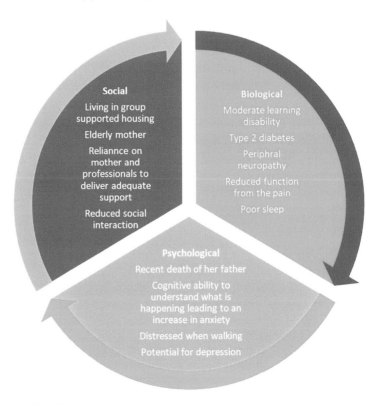

Figure 9.2: Maria's biopsychosocial experience.

Learning outcome 3: identify appropriate pain assessment tools for different groups

Pain is assessed in a variety of ways in different clinical settings. It is a key aspect of pain management; research has consistently demonstrated that accurate pain assessment is a prerequisite of effective pain management (Wood 2008). All individuals should have their pain assessed and recorded at the beginning of each episode of care and at suitable intervals thereafter.

Unidimensional pain assessment tools

Earlier in the chapter, we learned that sensory signalling and emotional and cognitive inputs are involved in the perception of pain. It makes sense then, that to assess someone's pain, we need to consider those different domains. In some settings, we prioritise the domain that we assess. For instance, in Thomas's situation on a busy acute ward, it may be appropriate to simply ask:

- Have you any pain or discomfort?' or 'Are you sore? (Not everyone will call pain "pain")'
- Where is the pain/where is it sore?'
- How bad is it when you are still? What about when you move or cough?'

These questions help identify the whereabouts (location) and intensity of the person's pain.

For a clinician to assess the intensity of a person's pain, unidimensional rating scales have been devised to help with the assessment. Commonly, nurses and doctors ask: 'On a scale of zero to ten, with zero being no pain and ten being the worst pain you can *imagine*, where is your pain?' Using the word imagine is a key flaw with this tool. If I asked your class to all draw a scene out of your imagination, you will all draw a very different scene, this is because our imaginations are all very individual; this in turn devalues the assessment. Also, by using our imagination, people are at risk of rating their situation to other, potentially more painful situations "the pain in my broken leg is very severe nurse, but I'm sure it would be much worse if I'd been attacked with a machete, therefore, maybe a 4?". What we know is that severe pain will lead to significant distress, and a reduction in function; therefore, requires treatment irrespective of the origin of the pathology. Figure 9.3 is an example of this type of numerical rating scale (NRS).

Other types of scales are the visual analogue scale (VAS) (Figure 9.4) and verbal (categorical) rating scale (VRS) (Figure 9.5). All these scales have varying risk of failure; however, the VRS has been shown to have a slightly increased efficacy due to its simplicity (Ballantyne et al. 2019). Many acute hospitals use a numerical rating score of 0–3, which links closely to the verbal descriptors none, mild, moderate and

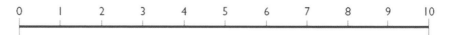

Figure 9.3: A numerical analogue scale (NRS).

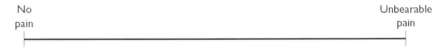

No
pain

Unbearable
pain

Figure 9.4: Visual analogue scale (VAS).

Pain intensity

None	0
Mild	1
Moderate	2
Severe	3

Figure 9.5: Verbal (categorical) rating scale (VRS).

severe within the VRS. In turn, these levels of pain intensity alongside functional assessment tools can be linked to pharmacological strategies (see the next section).

These tools were originally devised following the American Pain Association reclassifying pain as the 'fifth vital sign'; however, the extensive use of unidimensional pain scales has not resulted in improved pain scores, and outcomes for the person but ironically has led to causing harm, and the current opioid crisis within the US (Levy et al. 2019). Below we will discuss functional pain assessment tools.

Assessment of pain in people with dementia is complex but can be achieved using simple pain assessment tools such as the ones already covered, as well as tools that look at behavioural cues (Dowding et al. 2016). People with dementia may not use the non-verbal cues or behaviours we might recognise in others. The Abbey Pain Scale is an example of a tool for assessing pain in older people with severe cognitive impairment (Abbey et al. 2004). Other tools recommended for pain assessment in people with cognitive impairment include the Pain in Advanced Dementia (PAINAD) and Doloplus-2 scales (Schofield 2018). Using a validated pain scale together with discussion with Mr Davies would facilitate an accurate assessment of whether Violet is experiencing pain. This should be done alongside an assessment of her function, can she still carry out the activities she would normally do, e.g. washing and dressing, getting up and walking, socialising.

The most important aspect of assessing pain in people with dementia who are not able to express their own pain, is to ask family, friends, carers or anyone who know the person well "how do they express pain?" or "How do you know if they are in pain?". Often pain coincides with a change of behaviour. The "See Change, Think

Pain" campaign focuses on this and although behaviour change can be due to several factors, pain needs to be considered (NAPP 2014).

Agitation, which is one of Violet's symptoms, may be a sign that she is in pain, equally, it may be a reaction to her being parted from her husband and in a strange environment. The challenge for nurses is to try and identify if Violet is in pain and then manage it appropriately.

> ### Box 9.15 Activity: approaching Violet to assess her pain
>
> Make some notes on how you would approach Violet to assess her pain, taking into account ways of communicating with people who have Alzheimer's disease and how you could explain the chosen scale to her and her husband.

ACTIVITY

Pain assessment has also been identified as a major issue with people with learning disabilities as they can struggle to communicate their pain effectively. A study by Stone-Pearn (2002), which continues to be cited by various authors, including Beacroft and Dodd (2010), suggests that people with learning difficulties tend to be nonspecific about the duration of their pain and use external body locations and unusual terms in describing it. There are a number of pain assessment tools available including the FLACC Scale (1997), which was developed for pain assessment with children, and which has been found to be reliable and valid for children with severe learning difficulties. An example of the FLACC pain scale can be found at on the Health.gov.au website.

A fascinating service development by Kingston and Bailey (2009) describes the development of a protocol for assessing and managing pain with adults with learning difficulties. The protocol includes a 'pain story' template that enables individuals and their family to talk about their pain in a systematic and reflective manner. A visual pain diary and pictorial body chart were also trialled, amended and implemented. Maria's community learning disability nurse might be encouraged to contact the Portsmouth team who undertook this work to discuss their ideas and request a copy of the protocol.

Learning disability nurses and those working with adults with cognitive difficulties, such as those Violet experiences, should be aware of and be able to detect subtle behavioural changes that might indicate the presence of pain and distress. They need to be cautious about attributing behavioural change to cognitive impairments (McKay and Clarke 2012). In Maria's case, the focus on family involvement and liaison across the multidisciplinary team will help practitioners determine the underlying causes of behavioural change.

Body charts or verbal questions about pain location can also be useful in acute pain assessment, particularly when used with a categorical or numerical scale to provide insight into the areas that are the most painful. It is important to be aware that just because someone is complaining of pain in one area does not mean that they do not have pain elsewhere. In postoperative settings, it is not unusual for nurses to give opioids in response to a complaint of pain, when the problem is a post-intubation sore throat or long-standing back pain, rather than incisional pain. Thomas may also have discomfort or pain resulting from his cannula and/or catheter. Many people with chronic pain also have multiple pain foci.

Multidimensional pain assessment

Tools for multidimensional pain assessment are useful for people with complex needs and those experiencing chronic pain. One of the best-known tools is the short-form McGill Pain Questionnaire (SF-MPQ) (Melzack 1987). Using descriptor words, it enables practitioners to identify the nature and quality of pain; however, it is long and needs to be used by skilled practitioners so it would be unlikely to use it in an acute setting.

Another example of a multidimensional tool is the Disability Distress Assessment Tool or DisDAT (©2005 Northgate & Prudhoe NHS Trust and St Oswald's Hospice), which ends with the poignant words 'Distress may be hidden, but it is never silent'. This tool measures distress, rather than pain specifically, but it might be a useful tool for the community learning disability nurse to complete with Maria and her mother to gain an in-depth understanding of the way in which Maria is currently, or might in the future, express her distress. The findings can then be used to inform analgesic and non-pharmacological management.

Violet's team might want to consider the PAINAD scale or the Doloplus-2, which are both recommended for use in people with cognitive impairment (Schofield 2018). Both scales show reliability and validity for this group. The Abbey Pain Scale is still very commonly used throughout the UK; however, it has not been evaluated recently (Schofield 2018).

Functional pain assessment

The introduction of "Pain as the 5th vital sign" was intended to improve acute pain but unfortunately has led to an unhelpful emphasis on making people "pain free" and an excessive use of opioids (Levy 2018; PAINS 2017). Although the opposite was intended, in reality, it reduced pain assessment to just being about intensity and recording a number on a chart. Rather than measuring pain intensity alone, which encourages the expectation that a zero pain score is the aim, staff should ensure the person is not suffering and then manage pain to improve their ability to function. Focusing on whether a person can maintain normal activity e.g. eat, drink, sleep, reposition, walk and cough (if appropriate) without being limited by excessive pain is a better way to assess the effectiveness of an analgesic strategy. Emerging evidence shows that the use of functional pain assessment tools provides a valid way to measure pain (Halm et al. 2019) (Table 9.1).

Table 9.1: The functional activity score (FAS)[a]

A – No limitation able to undertake the activity without limitation due to pain (pain intensity is typically zero to three)
B – Mild to moderate limitation able to undertake the activity but experiences moderate to severe pain (pain intensity score typically 4–10)
C – Severe limitation unable to complete the activity due to pain, or pain treatment-related adverse effects, independent of pain intensity scores

Schug et al. (2020)

[a] Measures limitation of function due to pain compared with normal activity.

When assessing Thomas' pain using a functional pain assessment tool, alongside assessing pain intensity, will ensure that his pain is not limiting activity and will help staff titrate analgesia (Tong et al. 2018). This in turn may reduce the risks he may face from immobility, lack of sleep, not eating or drinking adequately, while ensuring as he recovers he gets appropriate analgesia (Levy 2018).

This pain scale might be useful for Maria, as it is an observational tool and Maria's mum might be able to keep a record of how Maria has been able to function to discuss with her healthcare providers.

Psychological and coping strategies assessment

We have discussed how a person's psychological state can have an impact on their pain perception; there are many tools available to assess the psychological components of pain and the ways in which people cope with their pain. These measurements are generally administered by pain experts and tend to be used in people with chronic pain. They include anxiety and depression scales, such as the PHQ-9 which can be found at www.patient.co.uk, coping strategy questionnaires, and impact of pain on function and physical activity profiles. One that tries to capture the wide impact that pain can have is the brief pain inventory, which is a self-assessment of pain: intensity, impact on daily function, location, duration and what medication is being used. Available from: https://static.medicine.iupui.edu/divisions/rheu/content/physicians/BRIEF_PAIN_INVENTORY.pdf (Accessed on 9 June 2021).

Box 9.16 Activity: brief pain inventory

ACTIVITY

Look up the brief pain inventory and thinking about someone you have cared for, decide whether it would have given you useful information to manage their pain.

Depending on your experience of pain, you may or may not have been aware of some of the strategies you use when in pain. We will consider how you might support the person's own strategies later in the chapter.

In summary, there are a variety of approaches to pain assessment. Each has its place with different client groups and different dimensions of pain. Whatever the approach, the response should be recorded so that it can be compared with the pain experience following an intervention. In acute pain settings, recordings should be made at rest and upon movement. As deep breathing, leg movements and mobilisation are important to postoperative recovery and the prevention of complications; it is imperative that pain does not prevent movement and rehabilitation. In chronic and palliative pain, post-intervention comparisons are likely to be more wide ranging.

Box 9.17 Activity: pain assessment tools in your locality

ACTIVITY

Investigate what pain assessment tools are used in your locality for different client groups.

Learning outcome 4: demonstrate understanding of pharmacological approaches to managing pain

Analgesic

A drug for relieving pain ('painkiller').

Analgesia

Another word for pain relief.

Knowledge of pharmacology and analgesic management may help enhance analgesia, which in turn can decrease anxiety, increase functional activity, improve mood and promote comfort and sleep.

Key principles in promoting analgesia include:

* assessing pain at the beginning of each episode of care and at appropriate intervals thereafter;
* giving analgesics before or as soon as acute pain begins;
* giving sufficient and regular analgesics to ensure comfort and function;
* assessing pain relief and side effects;
* balancing medication approaches with non-pharmacological strategies;
* aiming for a realistic outcome for pain management – not promising complete relief from the pain.

Box 9.18 Activity: letting pain take control

Why should you never let pain take control?

ACTIVITY

You may have come up with a number of ideas, such as that it is inhumane, places the person at risk of physical and emotional complications and increases the likelihood of hospital admissions for those living in the community or residential homes.

Pharmacological management of pain is a team effort, involving the person with pain, their family, the doctor, pharmacist, nurse, physiotherapist and others. Nurses should:

* listen and demonstrate compassion;
* record pain assessments, believing what they say about their pain;
* manage and evaluate pain competently and confidently;
* work with relevant members of the multidisciplinary team towards effective pain control;
* ensure that their knowledge is sufficient to achieve comfort and function;
* work to educate the individual and their families. The Royal College of Anaesthetists, Faculty of Pain Management (2018) have a variety of information leaflets, these can be used. See: https://www.fpm.ac.uk/about-pain-medicine-patients-relatives/patient-information-leaflets.

Individuals should be encouraged to request pain relief and take sufficient regular and as required (PRN) medication to enable them to carry out appropriate activities, readjusting dosages if necessary.

Concerns may include:

Insufficient or no regular analgesia.

Wrong analgesic for the type of pain the person is experiencing.

Fears of stopping the pain medication – a pseudo-addiction.

And more rarely but to be considered, if the person is developing a tolerance or dependency to the medication especially if it is an opioid or gabapentinoid.

Box 9.19 Activity: medicines used in your locality

Make a list of medicines used in your locality for pain relief.

Opioids

Drugs that bind with opioid receptors in the central and peripheral nervous systems to reduce the frequency of pain signals.

Opioids have been used for many years to manage pain; however, our understanding of the impact of long-term use has only recently started to be explored. Opioids have a valid place in managing acute pain and pain at the end of life but there is little evidence for their use in chronic or persistent pain.

Box 9.20 Key messages about opioids

Key messages about opioids

1 Opioids are very good analgesics for acute pain and for pain at the end of life but there is little evidence that they are helpful for long-term pain.

2 A small proportion of people may obtain good pain relief with opioids in the long-term if the dose can be kept low and especially if their use is intermittent (however, it is difficult to identify these people at the point of opioid initiation).

3 The risk of harm increases substantially at doses above an oral morphine equivalent of 120 mg/day, but there is no increased benefit: tapering or stopping high-dose opioids needs careful planning and collaboration.

4 If the person has pain that remains severe despite opioid treatment, it means they are not working and should be stopped, even if no other treatment is available.

5 Chronic pain is very complex and if the person has refractory and disabling symptoms, particularly if they are on high opioid doses, a very detailed assessment of the many emotional influences on their pain experience is essential.

Opioids Aware: Faculty of Pain Medicine of the Royal College of Anaesthetists (2018).

The best guide to their use, prescribing, opioid equivalences and risks can be found at https://www.fpm.ac.uk/opioids-aware

Nurses must be aware of how they can have a role in improving the safety and reducing harm with opioids. This should include understanding the differences between tolerance, dependence and addiction to opioids.

Nurses must also ensure that they understand side effects associated with opioids and safe dosing for each person. Doses for an opioid-naïve individual will differ from someone who is opioid dependent (Table 9.2).

Table 9.2: Commonly used analgesics

Drug	Location on ladder	Administration	Side effects
Paracetamol	Simple analgesic; helpful for mild pain, but effect often underestimated; potentiates (enhances) the effect of weak and strong opioids	Adult: One/two 500 mg tablets every 4 h; maximum 8 per day (4 g), unless otherwise directed	Rare; potentially fatal liver damage following overdose
Codeine	Weak opioid; helpful for moderate pain if person responsive	Adult: 30–60 mg every 4 h; maximum 240 mg per day	Constipation; initial drowsiness or dizziness not unusual; at least 8% of the population are unable to metabolise codeine Avoid in older adults as has many active metabolites and is eliminated by the kidneys
Tramadol	Opioid; helpful for moderate pain	Adult: 50–100 mg every 4–6 h; maximum 400 mg per day	Constipation; initial drowsiness or dizziness not unusual
Morphine Oxycodone Fentanyl Tapentadol	Strong opioid	Adult: varies; discuss dose examples with qualified MDT	Most commonly nausea, vomiting; may also experience light-headedness, confusion, pruritus, constipation, respiratory depression

Drugs for neuropathic pain

Neuropathic pain is defined as pain deriving from a disease or lesion to the somatosensory pathways in both the central and peripheral nervous systems (Magrinelli et al. 2013). Assessment and treatment can be complicated and should be completed by an appropriately trained professional. See Figure 9.6 for a recent assessment guideline for diagnosing neuropathic pain.

In recent years, anti-convulsant drugs used to treat neuropathic pain have become substances of abuse. Between the years 2012 and 2016, there was a significant increase in deaths in England and Wales relating to pregabalin and gabapentin of 2775% and 738%, respectively (Office of National Statistics [ONS] 2019); subsequently, these substances have now become schedule 3 controlled drugs with further emphasis on avoiding inappropriate prescribing (Lacobucci 2017). Although gabapentinoids are still licensed in the management of neuropathic pain, other, less addictive and abused medicines such as amitriptyline- and duloxetine-type medications are as, or potentially more effective for managing neuropathic pain. Once commenced, all of these drugs can take up to 6 weeks to have a full effect, and will require good compliance, therefore, quality counselling should be carried out between the prescriber and the individual at the time of commencing, alongside regular reviews.

Capsaicin creams and patches are used for focal neuropathic pain, including post-shingles pain and painful diabetic neuropathy; however, they can only be prescribed under the direct supervision of a hospital consultant (NICE 2013). Capsaicin, which is the active ingredient in chilli peppers, works as a counter irritant interfering at peripheral nerve endings with substance P, a neurotransmitter involved in pain processing. Lidocaine plasters are also licensed for use in the post-shingles pain

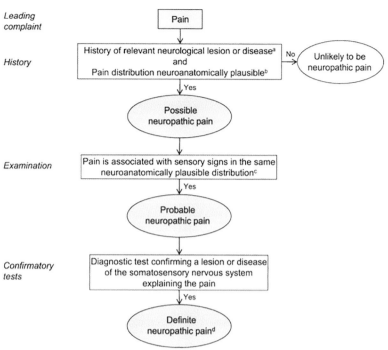

Figure 9.6: Assessment guideline for diagnosing neuropathic pain.
Finnerup et al. (2016).

causing allodynia (skin pain to non-painful stimuli). Lidocaine works by blocking sodium at the periphery and thus preventing the electrical nerve impulse from building up. Both of these should be assessed within 2–4 weeks of commencing to assess effect and if they are of no benefit, then they should be stopped.

Box 9.21 Examples of drugs used in neuropathic pain management

- Antidepressants – Amitriptyline, Nortriptyline, Duloxetine, Venlafaxine
- Anticonvulsants – Gabapentin, Pregabalin, Carbamazepine
- Local anaesthetic – Lidocaine plasters
- Rubefacients – Capsaicin

Box 9.22 Activity: applying NICE guidelines to pharmacological management of Maria's diabetic neuropathy

ACTIVITY

Visit the NICE website and look at guideline 173: 'Neuropathic pain in adults: pharmacological management in non-specialist settings' (2013), https://www.nice.org.uk/guidance/cg173

How would you manage Maria's painful diabetic neuropathy pharmacologically?

Drugs for inflammatory pain

Non-steroidal anti-inflammatory drugs (NSAIDs) reduce inflammation and are effective for mild to moderate pain. They are available in oral, transdermal, rectal (PR) and topical preparations. They are commonly used postoperatively in combination with other analgesics and are also the drug of choice in conditions such as arthritis and some other chronic pain conditions.

NSAIDs impact on multiple systems in the body as they inhibit prostaglandin synthesis.

Box 9.23 Activity: side effects/adverse effects of NSAIDs

ACTIVITY

Look up the potential side effects/adverse effects of NSAIDs and group them into body systems. Which groups of people would you avoid giving this group of drugs to and why?

If a NSAID is indicated, then the lowest effective dose for the shortest duration should be given (NICE 2020b). Nurses need to be conscious that a history of asthma, gastritis, ulcers, kidney problems, myocardial infarction and stroke may exclude an individual from using NSAIDs and be observant for side effects.

Violet has osteoarthritis in her right hip and knee; this can cause pain on movement and gradually worsen towards the end of the day. NSAIDs, such as Naproxen, could be effective in combatting her pain, allowing her to mobilise more easily and perhaps decrease her agitation. However, due to her age, they could cause more problems than they resolve. A risk-benefit assessment would be needed and ongoing monitoring for adverse effects. A topical NSAID might be considered first to decrease the risk of adverse effects.

For more information, see: https://www.nice.org.uk/advice/ktt13/chapter/evidence-context

Box 9.24 Activity: medications to help Maria and Violet

ACTIVITY

Make a list of the different medications you think might help Maria and Violet. Look up these drugs and understand their effects, side effects, doses and how long they should be given prior to review. You might find this NHS site useful when thinking of Maria- www.nhs.uk/conditions/Peripheral-neuropathy/

Other routes for administering analgesia

There are a variety of other routes for administering pain relief over and above oral and transdermal routes. Some of these are explained below.

Patient-controlled analgesia is an approach to pain management in which the individual controls the dose and frequency of analgesics up to a predetermined limit.

When practitioners refer to PCA, they generally mean the intravenous system that delivers opioids, such as morphine, oxycodone or fentanyl when a demand button is pressed. These systems are most commonly used in surgical settings and their management is covered by local protocols that include the administration of oxygen to minimise respiratory depression.

Epidurals are another route for administration, involving the infusion of a local anaesthetic, with or without an opioid, through a fine catheter into the epidural space (Middleton 2006). Historically, epidurals were seen as the 'Gold Standard' of postoperative acute pain management; however, in recent years this theory has been argued. Only people with significant cardiovascular and pulmonary risks benefit from receiving epidural analgesia over other, and less dangerous, regional techniques (Rawal 2012).

Regional analgesia is when local anaesthetics are injected into either a muscle plane (between muscles), or into a nerve plexus to block pain signalling of the peripheral nerve within the area that it is injected. Regional analgesia can be delivered as a single injection that lasts up to 12 h, or via an infusion that generally continues for up to 72 h. These are normally delivered alongside regular oral analgesics, and or a PCA. They are considered to have significantly less risk than epidurals (Wilkinson et al. 2014).

> ## Box 9.25 Activity: local protocols for PCA, regional analgesia and epidural
>
> Look up your local protocols for PCA, regional analgesia and epidural. List the recordings that must be made by nurses and state why.

ACTIVITY

Entonox is a 50:50 mixture of nitrous oxide and oxygen delivered through a handheld mask or mouthpiece. If the person becomes drowsy, because of the drug, their hand and therefore the delivery set will fall away. As such, Entonox is another form of PCA. It should not be used by people with Vitamin B12 deficiency and caution should be applied to those at risk of deficiency (Schug et al. 2020). It is effective for mild to moderate, short-lasting pain and is used by paramedics, in emergency care, for procedural pain and during labour. There is no absolute contraindication for the use of Entonox in the first 16 weeks of pregnancy (BOC 2016)

Syringe drivers should be considered when oral or transdermal routes are no longer feasible for those approaching end of life. Syringe drivers involve a fine needle being inserted just under the skin of the abdomen or arm, attached to tubing, which, in turn is attached to the pump. The drugs used, which are dependent on the individual person's needs, are made up to a 24 h dose and delivered via the syringe driver so that the individual receives a continuous dose. Other medications such as anti-emetics can also be added. (See also Chapter 15).

Epidural space

The space between the spinal canal and dura mater.

Box 9.26 Activity: resources for end of life care for people with dementia

Access the following sites and look at the resources available for end of life care for people with dementia:

- www.alzheimers.org.uk/get-support/help-dementia-care/end-life-care
- My future wishes Advance Care Planning (ACP) for people with dementia in all care settings (NHS England 2018) https://www.england.nhs.uk/publication/my-future-wishes-advance-care-planning-acp-for-people-with-dementia-in-all-care-settings

And end of life care for people with a learning disability:

- Delivering high-quality end of life care for people who have a learning disability https://www.england.nhs.uk/publication/delivering-high-quality-end-of-life-care-for-people-who-have-a-learning-disability/

British Institute of Learning Disabilities https://www.bild.org.uk/resource/my-pain-profile/

Write some notes on the ideas you have for managing pain with people who have dementia or learning disabilities and are coming to the end of their lives. How might you involve their families?

Resources

Many resources are available to help nurses develop their pharmacological knowledge. These include standard pharmacological and pain management texts, specialist texts such as those by Schug et al. (2020), websites such as the British National Formulary (BNF) site (www.bnf.com), pharmaceutical literature, journal articles and nursing, medical and pharmacist colleagues. Understanding how a drug affects the human body (pharmacodynamics) and how the body can affect the drug (pharmacokinetics) can be a rewarding addition to a nurse's knowledge base and practice.

Learning outcome 5: explore non-pharmacological approaches to managing pain

While pain-relieving medications can modify the pain processing systems to reduce pain intensity and distress, they should not be the only approach in managing the biopsychosocial complexity of pain. The current opioid crisis has led to there being a further emphasis on the non-pharmacological treatment options for chronic pain, as well as new and exploring techniques in acute pain management. However, many of these strategies have significantly differing outcomes in studies, and further research is required for efficacy of these treatments.

Heat and cold are useful non-pharmacological pain-relieving strategies. Heat can be comforting, improving blood flow and relaxing muscles (Malanga et al. 2015). It should not be used for acute pain as it can increase swelling. In these instances, ice might be used, although neither should be applied directly over wounds as they can interfere with healing. There are also cautions expressed over the use of heat for cancer pain as tumour growth is a possibility and in body areas where sensation is altered, such as with painful diabetic neuropathy.

Both methods are frequently used in managing musculoskeletal pain despite the evidence base being limited (Malanga et al. 2015). Neither one is shown to be superior to the other, so if used, should be tolerated by the person and if perceived by them to provide benefit.

Heat can be applied using covered hot water bottles, wheat bags, heat pads, disposable single use wraps and creams and via warm baths and showers. Cold tends to be applied for 5–10 min 3–4 times daily using ice packs, cold packs and cold gels. With both approaches, care should always be taken to ensure the skin is protected against burns or cold-induced injuries.

Information and education are important to increase understanding and reduce anxiety. Studies indicate that it can also reduce postoperative and cancer pain, with the most recent meta-analysis suggesting that educational interventions in the management of cancer pain may be more effective than medication management (Bennett et al. 2009)

In chronic pain, management resources such as the Pain Toolkit are available to aid self-management. A recent survey found that of the 12 strategies, individuals found the most useful to be activity pacing, acceptance of the long-term nature of the pain condition, being patient with oneself, stretching and exercising and learning to prioritise and plan (Sanderson and Cole 2011).

Box 9.27 Activity: self-management strategies

- Go to the Pain Toolkit website at and read about the different self-management strategies. Available from: www.paintoolkit.org/ (Accessed on 9 June 2021).
  - Could Maria and Violet benefit from any of these approaches and, if so, how might they be put into practice in residential and group settings?
  - Could Violet's husband be able to make use of any of the approaches with Violet at home?
  - How do these strategies help to counteract the biopsychosocial experience of pain?
- Next, have a look at the following link to the NHS Website https://www.nhs.uk/conditions/enhanced-recovery/
  - What information might Thomas benefit from preoperatively?
  - How might this help him manage any pain and distress postoperatively?
  - How does this fit with his biopsychosocial experience of pain outlined earlier in this chapter?

Exercise It may seem counterintuitive to move when someone has chronic pain, but the evidence indicates that exercise is beneficial in improving quality of life, physical function, and fatigue in people with fibromyalgia (Bidonde et al. 2019).

The Draft NICE Guidelines (2020a) for Chronic Pain: Assessment and Management is suggesting that clinicians utilise social prescribing and exercise goals when treating this group. Regular exercise types used include walking, t'ai-chi, pilates and swimming.

TENS (transcutaneous electrical nerve stimulations) is a form of electrotherapy that is used in both acute and chronic pain management. A small battery-powered device delivers an electric current via adhesively attached electrodes, with the aim of blocking the pain messages to the brain and, in low-frequency TENS, of producing the body's natural painkillers: endorphins. The latter can produce analgesia for 5 min to 18 h post-stimulation. Breaks between treatments are advised to reduce habituation in long-term use (Wright 2012). TENS is not recommended as a sole treatment but should rather be used in combination with other pharmacological and non-pharmacological strategies (Table 9.3).

Evidence about how helpful TENS is remains variable due to the different settings and frequencies that can be used, making comparison of studies difficult (Schug et al. 2020). A Cochrane review looking at TENS in chronic pain (Gibson et al. 2019)

Habituation

This is where the nervous system becomes accustomed to the stimulation resulting in reduced pain relief.

Table 9.3: Examples of supporting individuals to use their own pain-relieving strategies

Identify the strategies the person uses	Understand how the strategy works	Work with the person to enable them to use their strategy in the clinical setting
Distraction	Focusing on something other than pain Useful for brief periods Can increase perception of self-control and reduce pain intensity	May include watching TV, reading, listening to music, visits from family and friends. For example: if they says they watch television help them to the day room
Relaxation	Directs attention away from pain Useful for mild to moderate pain Can reduce muscle tension, distress, anxiety and fatigue	Find out the person's technique and support them with it if asked Ensure periods of relative peace and quiet to enable them to use the strategy. Teach short and long techniques
Imagery	Using imagination to create mental pictures: directs attention away from pain by imaging sights, sounds, odours, taste and touch (e.g. a garden on a warm summer's day). Can alter pain experience	Find out the person's preferred image and talk them through it if asked. Ensure periods of relative peace and quiet to enable them to use the strategy
Warmth	Promotes relaxation and comfort, reduces muscle tension	Hot water bottles cannot be used in hospital settings for safety reasons Wheat packs, heat pads and wraps, warm water, baths and showers are alternatives
Cold	May help reduce inflammatory pain Should not be used over wounds, as cold will decrease healing rate	Provide cold flannels, water, ice or cold packs and gels. Even better, in the clinical area, show the person/family where to access them
Positioning	Eases stiffness and enhances comfort	Help the person to adopt the most comfortable position, using own special pillows or cushions Encourage changes of position

could not give a definitive opinion as to whether TENS is useful or not. It would be worth a trial if pain remains challenging or analgesics are causing side effects. TENS is usually used in conjunction with other pain-relieving methods. A referral via a person's GP to a chronic pain clinic would be a good start.

For Violet, TENS might be worth trialling but a risk assessment should be done to ensure that she is able to tolerate it and not get entangled in the wires that could be a frightening experience.

In acute pain, the Cochrane review (Johnson et al. 2015) concluded that despite the limited evidence, it was worth trialling TENS for acute pain, as it is safe, self-administered and easily available in pharmacies or online.

There are a number of contraindications and cautions to the use of TENS, which are outlined in this NHS guide: www.nhs.uk/conditions/transcutaneous-electrical-nerve-stimulation-tens/

Relaxation (mindfulness) is a form of pain management that aims to reduce the physical and mental tension that enhances pain and pain perception. There are a variety of techniques such as breathing, imagery and meditation, among others; many of which are now available as apps on smart phone devices. A systematic review by Hilton et al. (2017) found evidence that mindfulness improved chronic pain, depression and improved quality of life. McClintock et al. (2019) showed that brief mindfulness interventions may have some benefit in managing both acute and chronic pain, though were best when taught by a trained practitioner. As with many non-pharmacological research studies, many of the primary studies were methodologically weak. Relaxation is often thought to be quite personal with some individuals preferring one method over another; it maybe that this also influences the studies.

ACTIVITY

Box 9.28 Activity: stress, anxiety, depression and pain

Visit NHS Choices at http://www.nhs.uk/Conditions/stress-anxiety-depression/Pages/ways-relieve-stress.aspx (Accessed on 20 November 2020). Although this page is about stress, anxiety and depression, the relaxation techniques described can also be used for pain.

There are many other non-pharmacological approaches, some of which you are likely to come across during your nursing studies. Not all strategies are appropriate for all people, in all situations. Those with neuropathic pain may actively avoid massage and touch because of altered sensation. In summary:

ACTIVITY

Box 9.29 Activity: factors influencing Violet's pain

Look again at the list of factors that may be influencing Violet's pain perception. What strategies might be used to counter these?

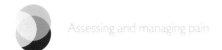

You might have thought of:

- supporting Mr Davies in his role of being a carer, for example, by referring him to the resources of the Carers Trust, https://carers.org/. You might want to go onto the site yourself and type 'pain' into the search box to see what you come up with. Alternatively, you could direct Mr Davies to a site specifically for carers of people with dementia such as https://www.alzheimers.org.uk/get-support/help-dementia-care
- ensuring that Violet has familiar objects around her
- using a mix of pharmacological and non-pharmacological pain and comfort measures to help her relax, reducing muscle tension, agitation and pain
- increasing cognitive control by providing information about the techniques you are using in an understandable format, perhaps using pictures as well as verbal explanations.

For most people, the most effective approach to pain management is to listen to what the person and their families say about his/her pain and its effect on their home, leisure and work activities; to work with the multidisciplinary team, individual and his/her family to combine pharmacological and non-pharmacological strategies, and to monitor the effectiveness of pain relief with all involved.

 Box 9.30 Children and young people: practice points – pain management

Effective pain assessment and management are essential for infants and children. There are pain assessment charts specifically developed for use with children so, if working with children, ensure that you seek out guidance about using your organisation's pain assessment tool for children. Many of the pain management techniques discussed in this section are used for children too, including distraction, relaxation and guided imagery as well as analgesics, but all will need to be administered appropriately depending on the child's age and development stage, with analgesics prescribed according to weight.

For further information, see:

Twycross, A. and Saul, B. 2017. Assessment and management of pain in children and young people. In: Price, J. and McAlinden, O. (eds.) *Essentials of Nursing Children and Young People*, 2nd edn. London: Sage, Chapter 3, 36–54.

Seeman, C. 2013. Caring for children and young people in the medical setting. In: Thurston, C. (ed.) *Essential Nursing Care for Children and Young People Theory, Policy and Practice*. Oxon: Routledge, 151–4.

Box 9.31 Pregnancy and birth: practice points – pain management

Drugs can have harmful effects on the embryo or fetus at any time during pregnancy and in the postnatal period. This includes over-the-counter medicines.

- During the first trimester (first 12 weeks), drugs can produce congenital malformations.
- During the second and third trimester, drugs can affect the growth and functional development of the fetus.
- Drugs given towards the end of pregnancy or during labour can have adverse effects on the labour or on the neonate at birth.
- For many drugs, there is insufficient information about the levels of the drug in breastmilk and as such care is needed when prescribing in breastfeeding.
- Pregnant mothers may rely on non-pharmacological pain relief such as keeping active, warm baths, relaxation techniques, deep breathing and back massages, to assuage their discomfort.
- Always seek expert advice.

Further guidance:

British National Formulary. Available from: https://bnf.nice.org.uk/ (Accessed on 5 May 2021).

Breastfeeding and Medicines. Available from: https://www.nhs.uk/conditions/baby/breastfeeding-and-bottle-feeding/breastfeeding-and-lifestyle/medicines/ (Accessed on 5 May 2021).

Pain relief in labour. Available from: https://www.nhs.uk/pregnancy/labour-and-birth/what-happens/pain-relief-in-labour/ (Accessed on 8 May 2021).

Summary

- Pain is a subjective, multidimensional experience, unique to each individual.
- Nurses need to differentiate between the terms 'pain threshold', 'pain tolerance' and 'pain behaviour'.
- Effective pain assessment is the key to successful pain management, and pain assessment tools can facilitate communication about pain.
- Pain management comprises both pharmacological and non-pharmacological approaches.

CHAPTER SUMMARY

Throughout this book, practical nursing skills are contextualised within a philosophy of caring. This final chapter has focused on some fundamental aspects of nursing: assessing and managing pain and has emphasised a caring approach, including compassion, competence and effective communication. Nurses have an important role in promoting comfort, a role recognised by Florence Nightingale who wrote in 1854:

The benefits which this Institution [hospital] ought to afford to the sick are perhaps best seen when we are enabled to give comfort in the time of danger and to lessen the agony of death.

(Quoted in Verney 1970)

Pain management is a huge topic with a developing theoretical base, and this chapter's material aimed to provide a firm basis from which to build your nursing practice. Pain management requires nurses to integrate a range of skills, with an appropriate attitude and a sound underpinning knowledge base.

ACKNOWLEDGEMENT

The authors thank Dr Mark Rockett for his vital assistance and commentary on the pain section.

REFERENCES

Abbey, J., Piller, N., DeBellis, A. et al. 2004. The Abbey pain scale: A 1-minute numerical indicator for people with end-stage dementia. *International Journal of Palliative Nursing* 10(1): 6–13.

Alzheimer's Society. 2017. What is Alzheimer's disease? Available from: https://www.alzheimers.org.uk/sites/default/files/2018-10/400%20What%20is%20dementia_0.pdf (Accessed on 1 October 2020).

Ballantyne, J.C., Fishman, S.M. and Rathmell, J.P. 2019. *Bonica's Management of Pain*, 5th edn. Philadelphia, PA: Wolters Kluwer.

Barney, C., Andersen, R., Defrin, R. et al. 2020. Challenges in pain assessment and management among individuals with intellectual and developmental disabilities. *Pain Reports*. 5(4): 821. (Accessed on 22 November 2020).

Beacroft, M. and Dodd, K. 2010. 'I feel pain' – audit of communication skills and understanding of pain and health needs with people with learning disabilities. *British Journal of Learning Disabilities* 39: 139–47.

Bennett, M.I., Bagnall, A.M. and Closs, S.J. 2009. How effective are patient-based educational interventions in the management of cancer pain? Systematic review and meta-analysis. *Pain* 143(3): 192–9.

Bidonde, J., Busch, A.J., Schachter, C.L. et al. 2019. Mixed exercise training for adults with fibromyalgia. *Cochrane Database of Systematic Reviews* 5. Art. No.: CD013340. doi: 10.1002/14651858.CD013340.

BOC Healthcare. 2016. *ENTONOX®: Essential Safety Information*. Guildford: BOC Healthcare.

British Pain Society. 2016. *The Silent Epidemic: Chronic Pain in the UK*. Available from: https://www.britishpainsociety.org/mediacentre/news/the-silent-epidemic-chronic-pain-in-the-uk/ (Accessed on 01 November2020).

Dowding, D., Lichtner, V., Allcock, N., Briggs, M., James, J., Keady, J., Lasrado, R., Sampson, E.L., Swarbrick, C. and Closs, S.J. 2016. Using sense-making theory to aid understanding of the recognition, assessment and management of pain in patients with dementia in acute hospital settings. *International Journal of Nursing Studies* 53: 152–62.

Fayaz, A., Croft, P., Langford, R.M., Donaldson, L.J., Jones, G.T. 2016. Prevalence of chronic pain in the UK: A systematic review and meta-analysis of population studies. *BMJ Open* 6(6). Available from: Prevalence of chronic pain in the UK: A systematic review and meta-analysis of population studies | BMJ Open (Accessed on 23 November 2020).

Finnerup, N., Haroutounian, S., Kamerman, P. et al. 2016. Neuropathic pain: An updated grading system for research and clinical practice. *Pain* 157(8): 1599–606. (Accessed on 22 November 2020).

FLACC Behavioral Pain Assessment Scale. 1997. Available from: https://wps.prenhall.com/wps/media/objects/3103/3178396/tools/flacc.pdf (Accessed on 10 June 2021).

Gibson, W., Wand, B.M., Meads, C. Catley, M.J. and O'Connell, N.E. 2019. Transcutaneous electrical nerve stimulation (TENS) for chronic pain – an overview of Cochrane Reviews. Cochrane database of systematic reviews. Available from: https://researchonline.nd.edu.au/cgi/viewcontent.cgi?article=1157&context=physiotherapy_article (Accessed on 10 June 2021).

Halm, M., Bailey, C., St.Pierre, J. et al. 2019. Pilot evaluation of a functional pain assessment scale. *Clinical Nurse Specialist* 33(1): 12–21.

Hilton, L., Hempel, S., Ewing, B A. et al. 2017. Mindfulness meditation for chronic pain: Systematic review and meta-analysis. *Annals of Behavioural Medicine* 51(2): 199–213.

Institute for Chronic Pain. 2017. What is central sensitization? Available from: https://www.instituteforchronicpain.org/understanding-chronic-pain/what-is-chronic-pain/central-sensitization. (Accessed on 17 February 2021).

International Association for the Study of Pain. 2020 *IASP Announces Revised Definition of Pain*. Available from: https://www.iasp-pain.org/PublicationsNews/NewsDetail.aspx?ItemNumber=10475 (Accessed on 17 February 2021).

Johnson, M.I., Paley, C.A., Howe, T.E. and Sluka, K.A. 2015. Transcutaneous electrical nerve stimulation for acute pain. Cochrane Database of systematic reviews. Available from: https://pubmed.ncbi.nlm.nih.gov/26075732/ (Accessed on 10 June 2021).

Kingston, K. and Bailey, C. 2009. Assessing the pain of people with learning disability. *British Journal of Nursing* 18(7): 420–3.

Lacobucci, G. 2017. UK government to reclassify pregabalin and gabapentin after rise in deaths. *British Medical Journal* 358: j4441.

Levy, N,. Sturgess, J. and Mills, P. 2018. Pain as the "fifth vital sign" and dependence on the "Numerical pain scale" is being abandoned in the US: Why? *British Journal of Anaesthesia* 120(3): 435–8.

Levy, N., Mills, P. and Rockett, M. 2019. Post-surgical pain management: Time for a paradigm shift. *British Journal of Anaesthesia* 123(2): 186–8.

Lovering, S. 2006. Cultural attitudes and beliefs about pain. *Journal of Transcultural Nursing* 17(4): 389–95.

Magrinelli, F., Zanette, G. and Tamburin, S. 2013. Neuropathic pain: Diagnosis and treatment. *Practical Neurology* 13: 292–307.

Malanga, G.A., Yan, N. and Stark, J. 2015. Mechanisms and efficiency of heat and cold therapies for musculoskeletal injury. *Post Graduate Medicine* 127(1): 57–65.

McCaffery, M. 1968. *Nursing Practice Theories Related to Cognition, Bodily Pain, and Man-Environment Interactions*. Los Angeles: University of California at Los Angeles Students' Store.

McClintock, S., McCarrick, S., Garland, E. et al. 2019. Brief mindful-based interventions for acute and chronic pain: A systematic review. *JACM* 25(3): 265–78.

McKay, M. and Clarke, S. 2012. Pain assessment tools for the child with severe learning disability. *Nursing Children and Young People* 24(2): 14–25.

Melzack, R. 1987. The short-form McGill pain questionnaire. *Pain* 30(2): 191–7.

Melzack, R. and Wall, P. 1996. *Challenge of Pain*. Harmondsworth: Penguin.

Middleton, C. 2006. *Epidural Analgesia in Acute Pain Management*. Chichester: John Wiley.

Moskow, S.B. 1987. *Human Hand and Other Ailments*. Boston, MA: Little, Brown.

NAPP Pharmaceuticals Ltd. 2014. Pain in people with dementia: A silent tragedy. Available from: https://www.scie-socialcareonline.org.uk/pain-in-people-with-dementia-a-silent-tragedy/r/a11G0000005Xy4BIAS (Accessed on 10 June 2021).

National Health Service. 2018. My future wishes: Advanced Care Planning (ACP) for people with dementia in all care settings. Available from: my-future-wishes-advance-care-planning-for-people-with-dementia.pdf (england.nhs.uk). (Accessed on 17 February 2021).

National Health Service. 2019. *Enhanced Recovery*. Available from: https://www.nhs.uk/conditions/enhanced-recovery/ (Accessed on 19 November 2020).

National Institute for Clinical Excellence. 2013. Neuropathic pain in adults: Pharmacological management in non-specialist settings (cg173). Available from: https://www.nice.org.uk/guidance/cg173 (Accessed on 9 June 2021).

National Institute of Clinical Excellence. 2020a. Chronic pain: assessment and management [D] Evidence review for social interventions. Available from: https://www.nice.org.uk/guidance/ng193/documents/evidence-review-4 (Accessed on 10 June 2021).

National Institute of Clinical Excellence. 2020b. NSAIDs – prescribing issues. Available from: NSAIDs – prescribing issues | Health topics A to Z | CKS | NICE (Accessed on 17 February 2021).

Office of National Statistics. 2019. Deaths related to drug poisoning in England and Wales: 2016 registrations. Available from: https://www.ons.gov.uk/peoplepopulationandcommunity/birthsdeathsandmarriages/deaths/bulletins/deathsrelatedtodrugpoisoninginenglandandwales/2019registrations (Accessed on 10 June 2021).

PAINS Project. 2017. Policy and educational brief: An important view on pain as a 5th vital sign. Available from: http://www.practicalbioethics.org/files/pains/PAINS-policy-brief-8.pdf (Accessed on 9 June 2021).

Rawal, N. 2012. Epidural technique for postoperative pain: Gold standard no more? *Regional Anesthesia & Pain Medicine* 37: 310–17.

Royal College of Anaesthetists: Faculty of Pain Management. 2018. *Patient Information Leaflets*. Available from: https://www.fpm.ac.uk/about-pain-medicine-patients-relatives/patient-information-leaflets (Accessed on 22 November 2020).

Rockett, M.P., Simpson, G., Crossley, R. and Blowey, S. 2013. Characteristics of pain in hospitalized medical patients, surgical patients, and outpatients attending a pain management centre. *British Journal of Anaesthesia* 110: 1017–23.

Sanderson, T. and Cole, F. 2011. *An Audit of the Value of the Pain Toolkit in Facilitating Self-Care: The Patient's Perspective*. Poster Presentation. Bath Pain Management Programmes Conference, Bath.

Schofield, P. 2018. The Assessment of Pain in Older People: UK National Guidelines. *Age and Aging* 47: 1–22.

Schug, S., Scott, D., Mott, J., Palmer, G., Halliwell, R. and Alcock, M. (eds.). 2020. *Acute Pain Management: Scientific Evidence*, 5th edn. Available from: Acute-Pain-Management-Scientific-Evidence-5th-edition (anzca.edu.au) (Accessed on 17 February 2021).

Stone Pearn, H. 2002. An exploratory study to investigate how people with learning disabilities understand and describe pain. (Thesis) Available from: https://openresearch.surrey.ac.uk/esploro/outputs/doctoral/A-Portfolio-of-Study-Practice-and/99513876302346 (Accessed on 4 November 2021)

The Scottish Government. 2018. *Management of Chronic Pain in Children and Young People: A National Clinical Guideline*. Edinburgh: The Scottish Government. Available from: https://www.gov.scot/publications/management-chronic-pain-children-young-people/ (Accessed on 11 June 2021).

Tong, Y.G., Konstantatos, A.H., Cheng, Y. and Chai, L. 2018. Improving pain management through addition of the functional activity score. *Australian Journal of Advanced Nursing* 35(4): 52–60.

Twycross, A. and Saul, B. 2017. Assessment and management of pain in children and young people. In: Price, J. and McAlinden, O. (eds.) *Essentials of Nursing Children and Young People*, 2nd edn. London: Sage, 36–54.

Verney, H. 1970. *Florence Nightingale at Harley Street: Her Reports to the Governors of Her Nursing Home 1853–4*. London: J.M. Dent.

Wood, S. 2008. Assessment of pain. Available from: http://www.nursingtimes.net/nursing-practice-clinical-research/assessment-of-pain/1861174.article (Accessed on 23 November 2020).

Wilkinson, K.M., Krige, A., Brearley, S.G. et al. 2014. Thoracic epidural analgesia versus rectus sheath catheters for open midline incisions in major abdominal surgery within an enhanced recovery programme (TERSC): Study protocol for a randomised controlled trial. *Trials* 15: 400.

Wright, A. 2012. Exploring the evidence for using TENS to relieve pain. *Nursing Times* 108(11): 20–3.

USEFUL WEBSITES

Alzheimer's Society. This is me. Available from: www.alzheimers.org.uk/sites/default/files/2020-03/this_is_me_1553.pdf

Breathing exercises for stress. Available from: www.nhs.uk/mental-health/self-help/guides-tools-and-activities/breathing-exercises-for-stress/

Chronic Non-Malignant Pain: Biopsychosocial Model. Available from: https://vimeo.com/86977616

Enhanced Recovery. Available from: www.nhs.uk/conditions/enhanced-recovery/

The Pain Toolkit. Available from: www.paintoolkit.org/

See Change Think Pain. Available from: https://dementiaroadmap.info/wp-content/uploads/See-Change-Think-Pain-Napp-Report.pdf

TENS (transcutaneous electrical nerve stimulation). Available from: www.nhs.uk/conditions/transcutaneous-electrical-nerve-stimulation-tens/

Medicines management

Kirsty Andrews and Martina O'Brien

In most healthcare settings, nurses administer medicines or supervise their administration. To administer and supervise medicines safely, nurses require a breadth of knowledge, including pharmacology and legal and policy issues. They also need to know how to administer medicines via a variety of routes and how to perform medicine dose calculations. Nurses must have the skills to work in partnership with individuals in their care and their colleagues. To administer medicines safely requires considerable experience and practice and therefore, students should take every opportunity to develop their knowledge and skills during their nursing programme. The Nursing and Midwifery Council's (NMC 2018a) Future nurse: standards of proficiency for registered nurses and standards of proficiency for nursing associates (NMC 2018b) for best practice, safe and effective evidence-based medicines administration and optimisation are addressed in this chapter's content.

This chapter includes the following topics:

- legal and professional issues in medicine administration including methods of prescribing
- safety, storage and general principles of medicine administration
- administering oral medication
- applying topical medication
- administering medication by injection routes
- administering inhaled and nebulised medication
- administering enteral medication
- intravenous fluid and blood administration
- calculating medicine and intravenous fluid administration doses
- preventing and managing anaphylaxis.

Box 10.1 Recommended pharmacology reading

It is important to have an understanding of the pharmacology of medicines, which includes how medicines work in the body (pharmacodynamics) and how medicines are absorbed into the body, distributed to body tissues, metabolised and excreted from the body (pharmacokinetics). There are pharmacology

(Continued)

DOI: 10.4324/9781003020660-10

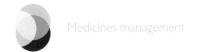

Box 10.1 (Continued)

books available that are applied to nursing and healthcare practice, and you may find these helpful. Examples are:

- Adams, M.P., Holland, L.N. and Urban, C.Q. 2020. *Pharmacology for Nurses; A Pathophysiologic Approach*, 6th edn. London: Pearson.
- McCuiston, L.E., Vuljoin-DiMaggio, K., Winton, M.B. and Yeager, J.J. 2018. *Pharmacology: A Patient Centered Nursing Process Approach*, 9th edn. St. Louis: Elsevier.
- McFadden, R. 2019. *Introducing Pharmacology for Nursing and Healthcare*, 3rd edn. Abingdon: Routledge.

Heparin

An anticoagulant that works by prolonging the anticoagulation time.

Diuretics

Medicines that cause increased excretion of urine by the kidneys.

Fucidin

A topical antibiotic cream used for treatment of a wide variety of infected skin conditions.

Anticonvulsant medication

Medicines used to treat or control seizures particularly in those with epilepsy.

Multicompartment Compliance Aids or Monitored Dosage Systems (MDS)

An aid to support medication compliance. A pre-prepared box of medication with identified doses for each day. Nomad or Dosette is another similar system.

PRACTICE SCENARIOS

The following practice scenarios illustrate situations where medicines are being administered via several different routes and where nurses require knowledge of these drugs' actions and side effects, as well as how to store and administer them safely. These scenarios are referred to throughout the chapter.

Adult

Mercy Makumbe is 72 years old. She has recently had a below-knee amputation of her leg, has a long history of cardiovascular disease and has now been transferred to her local community hospital, where she is currently receiving subcutaneous (SC) heparin, as well as oral morphine solution for pain. For years, she has taken diuretics and other medication for her cardiac problems, and she is concerned about having to take regular strong pain-relieving medicines too. She has a known penicillin allergy. She has also been prescribed fucidin cream for a small infected area behind one ear. A recent urinalysis showed blood in her urine.

Learning disability

Carol Lee is a 57-year-old woman who has a mild learning disability and has been diagnosed as having symptoms of early-onset **dementia**. She lives with another person with a learning disability, and both are supported by a sleep-in support worker. Over the past year, Carol has experienced two seizure-like episodes and has been prescribed anticonvulsant medication. She wishes to maintain her independence and self-medicate. The community learning disability nurse is working with her and her support worker to enable her to manage this. They are using a multicompartment compliance aid (MCA) known as a Dosette box system and pictures as prompts. They are also helping her to record any side effects.

Mental health

Malcolm Barber is 49 years old and has a history of schizophrenia. His main carer is his wife. His condition was stabilised on oral medication, until he experienced side effects of weight gain and akathesia (an inability to sit still). Because of these side effects, he stopped taking the medication, began to neglect himself and developed symptoms of psychosis. This deterioration led to his admission to an acute mental health unit as a voluntary patient. On admission, he was given a test dose of a depot, which is a slow-release injection of an antipsychotic drug. This treatment led to an improvement in his mental state, with minimal side effects. The plan is for him to continue with these injections administered twice-monthly by his community mental health nurse. Malcolm also has mild asthma and has a salbutamol inhaler that he uses occasionally.

LEGAL AND PROFESSIONAL ISSUES IN MEDICINE ADMINISTRATION

Nurses must adhere to many legal and professional issues relating to safe medicine administration.

Box 10.2 Learning outcomes

By the end of this section, you will be able to:

1. identify key aspects of legislation, policies and professional issues governing medicine administration;
2. discuss important professional issues for nurses who are administering medicines;
3. discuss the importance of working in partnership;
4. understand prescribing methods and how they are used in practice.

Learning outcome 1: Identify key aspects of legislation, policies and professional issues governing medicine administration

Box 10.3 Activity: rules about medicine administration

ACTIVITY

Who do you think might provide rules about medicine administration? Discuss this issue with one of your colleagues. Consider abuse of drugs and related regulations. What have you seen about drug safety in the media?

All major issues related to managing the prescribing and safety of medicines are regulated by government legislation. Nurses and all healthcare professionals are advised to follow professional guidance distributed by the Royal Pharmaceutical Society (RPS) on the safe and secure handling of medicines (RPS 2018) and joint professional guidance issued by the RPS and the Royal College of Nursing (RCN) on the administration of medicines in healthcare settings (RPS and RCN 2019).

Government legislation covers the abuse of drugs, labelling of medicines and sale of medicines over the counter and in pharmacies and supermarkets. Two important Acts of Parliament, the Misuse of Drugs Act 1971 and the Medicines Act 1968, provide public protection in these and related matters and infringement of these acts

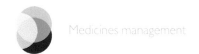

is a criminal offence. There are other related acts and reports too. The main acts are as follows:

- *The Misuse of Drugs Act 1971* lists and classifies controlled drugs (CDs). It details special controls for the manufacture, supply and possession of CDs.
- The *Misuse of Drugs Regulations 2001* identifies five schedules for CDs and specifies requirements for their import, export, manufacture, supply, possession, prescribing and record keeping.
- The *Medicines Act 1968* controls the manufacture, importation, exportation, labelling, sale and distribution of all medicines and established a compulsory licensing system (known as a marketing authorisation) for all medicines before they can be used.
- The *Mental Capacity Act 2005* defines and advises on an individual's capacity to understand treatment, including medicine administration. It also covers the role of professionals in protecting such individuals.
- The *Health Act 2006* requires the appointment of an accountable officer for each healthcare organisation who is responsible for the safe use and management of CDs.
- The *Psychoactive Substances Act 2016* restricts the production, sale or supply of psychoactive substances (referred to as legal highs).

Categories of medicines defined in the Medicines Act 1968

- **Prescription-only medicines** (POMs). POMs can be obtained only on prescription from any registered independent prescriber. In hospitals, almost all medicines are POMs. Each individual has a medicines administration record (MAR) (usually electronic) where the medicines to be administered are detailed. If you have any medicines prescribed by your general practitioner (GP), in many cases you will see POM printed on the packet.
- **Pharmacy-only medicines (P).** These medicines can be sold only in the presence of a pharmacist, but they do not require a prescription. The pharmacist may ask the customer questions relating to their symptoms to ascertain that the medicine they are requesting is appropriate. These medicines are identified by the letter 'P' on the packaging.
- **General sale list (GSL).** These are a restricted list of medicines that can be freely sold through almost any outlet, for example, garages and supermarkets. Although there are no general restrictions on their sale, as with any medicine, there is potential to misuse them. The Medicines and Healthcare products Regulatory Agency (MHRA) provides guidance for some medicines. For example, paracetamol may only be sold in packets of 16 tablets/capsules as a GSL (The Medicines (Sale or Supply) (Miscellaneous Provisions) Amendment No. 2, 1997).

Box 10.4 Activity: three categories of medicines

ACTIVITY

Can you think of an example for each of the above-mentioned three categories of medicines?

Suggested examples are antibiotics (POM), cough mixtures (P) and aspirin (GSL). Note that the category into which a medicine is placed can change because of safety concerns. For example, diclofenac was a P but is now a POM medicine because of a small increased risk of cardiovascular effects requiring individuals to undergo a medical assessment to determine their suitability to take diclofenac (MHRA 2015).

Controlled drugs

> **Box 10.5 Activity: need for drug controls**
>
> CDs were mentioned briefly above. Why would a drug need to be controlled in some special way? What might make a drug particularly dangerous if people could access it easily?

A CD is addictive, because of the dependency that could result. Medicines such as morphine or any other medicines of the opiate family can cause addiction, with all its consequences, if taken for non-therapeutic reasons. These medicines are therefore dangerous, and their sale is controlled because of their addictiveness. They are controlled by the legislation detailed above. Since the Shipman Inquiry, their control has been further tightened, including electronic prescribing in primary healthcare settings (Department of Health [DH] 2007). The move to implementing electronic prescribing in all acute healthcare settings has been slower with the expectation that all healthcare providers will implement such systems by 2024 (NHS 2019). Mercy, like many others, may be anxious about taking morphine because of this view of potentially addictive drugs.

The Misuse of Drugs Act 1971 and the Misuse of Drugs Regulations 2001 identify five categories of CDs, with category 1 being those drugs requiring the most control because of their serious addictive qualities and category 5 drugs requiring the least control. It also underlines that CDs must be kept in a separate locked cupboard with no other medicines in them and supplied with a key that is different from any other key in that setting. It does not stipulate the need for a locked cupboard within a locked cupboard, although this practice is common in acute healthcare settings for additional safe storage. In addition, a light is situated on the outside of the cupboard to alert staff when the cupboard is open or has not been locked. The cupboard must adhere to the specifications of the Misuse of Drugs (Safe custody) regulations 1975 and meet British Standards BS2881:1989 security level 1 (Care Quality Commission [CQC] 2019). In people's homes, too, drugs must be kept very securely and advice regarding storage options should be made available (National Institute for Health and Care Excellence [NICE] 2016). The level of safety has to be negotiated with the person concerned, because it is within their property. Carol's nurse will have to consider this negotiation and either carry out a risk assessment or work with the support staff to complete a risk assessment.

CDs can be ordered only by a registered nurse. They must be administered by a registered nurse with a second checker, who fits the local medicines management

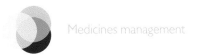
policy criteria for a checker. Criteria may vary in community settings and where people are self-medicating. You should check these details in every setting you work in and try to access the appropriate medicines management policy (RPS 2018). Checking administration of CDs requires an understanding of the gravity of the issue, as detailed above. Thus, student nurses may be able to check these medicines, but in some areas such checks may not be permitted. Do check your hospital or Trust medicines management policy in conjunction with your university medicines management policy to ascertain whether you are allowed to act as a second checker.

Checking during administration involves the whole procedure from preparing the medicine, each checker individually calculating the dose, administration of the medicine and disposal of any remaining medicine and equipment (NMC 2018a). Therefore, if you were the second checker when Mercy receives her morphine, you would have to accompany the registered nurse throughout the procedure.

CD registers must include details of stock and medicines administered and must be signed by both persons providing such detail. They should be kept for at least 2 years from the date of the last entry (Misuse of Drugs Regulations 2001).

Box 10.6 Activity: organisations involved in medicine regulation

What other organisations may be involved in medicine regulation?

You should have included professional bodies and employers.

Professional bodies

Professional bodies involved in medicine regulation in the United Kingdom (UK) include the British Medical Association (BMA), the RPS and the General Pharmaceutical Council (GPC). The NMC, while it does not offer advice on clinical guidance in relation to medicines, stipulates procedural competencies that Registered Nurses and Registered Nursing Associates must achieve for managing and administering medicines safely (NMC 2018a, 2018b).

It is also important that you know the expectations and limitations of your colleague's roles and responsibilities in medicines administration.

Box 10.7 Activity: NMCs standards of proficiency for registered nurses and nursing associates

Access and familiarise yourself with the NMC's standards of proficiency for registered nurses and nursing associates in relation to medicines administration and optimisation. Identify the similarities and differences in the competencies between what a registered nurse and a registered nursing associate should achieve.

You should have identified the competencies each role is expected to achieve on registration with the NMC. Similarities include:

- undertaking accurate drug calculations
- administering medicines via oral, topical, inhalation, intramuscular, subcutaneous and enteral routes
- professional accountability to ensure the safe administration of medicines
- recognition and responding appropriately to adverse or abnormal reactions to medications

Differences include:

- only registered nurses can administer via the intradermal and intravenous routes
- only registered nurses can prescribe or administer medications via a Patient Group Direction

Patient Group Direction

A Patient Group Direction (PGD) is a legal framework allowing certain healthcare professionals to supply and administer medicines to groups who fit certain criteria, laid down in a previously agreed PGD. There does not need to be an individual prescription.

Employers

Employers produce medicine policies. Independent care providers will each have their own medicine administration policies, which Carol's community nurse must comply with. Similarly, Malcolm's Mental Health Trust will have a policy about the person's mental capacity to understand and adhere to prescribed treatments.

Staff must work to the regulations set out in their particular employer's policy. These policies contain useful information. They refer to the student role and other issues too.

Learning outcome 2: discuss important professional issues for nurses who are administering medicines

Professional issues of particular relevance are personal accountability, knowledge, honesty and ethical practice.

Personal accountability

When administering medicines, a registered nurse takes personal accountability for his or her actions, as with all interventions carried out by registered nurses (NMC 2018c). Therefore, if you as a student give out medication under supervision, the registered nurse is accountable for what you do, as well as their own actions. There are no legal frameworks governing who can actually administer medicines, although local policies will stipulate how medicines should be administered. The RPS and RCN (2019) state that the person administering medication (e.g. Carol's sleep-in support worker) should be someone who is appropriately trained, has been assessed as competent and is able to meet relevant professional and regulatory standards and guidance.

Box 10.8 Activity: accountability for Carol's medication arrangements

Who do you think would take accountability for Carol's medication arrangements?

Accountability may vary according to local policy and arrangements. Carol's support worker is likely to have operational responsibility for supervising her self-medication, understanding medication use and side effects and reporting to the community nurse or senior support worker. NICE (2017) recommends that where MCAs or MDS are used, the pharmacists should provide a description of the appearance of each medicine. The community learning disability nurse is likely to be accountable for educating Carol and the support worker about her medication in the community, using picture prompts. She also has overall responsibility as the registered nurse for ensuring processes are carried out properly, according to Carol's level of capacity (Mental Capacity Act 2005), in view of her dementia.

Although students are not professionally accountable, you should consider these issues in preparation for becoming a registered nurse or registered nursing associate (NMC 2018c).

Knowledge of medicines

Nurses need a working understanding of medicines administered, therapeutic dosages and side effects (Dougherty et al. 2015) and must exercise professional judgement at all times (RPS, RCN 2019). As a student, you need basic knowledge of the medicines you are involved in administering, and you should continue to develop your knowledge throughout your preregistration programme and after registration. New medicines are constantly being developed, and knowledge about existing medicines is expanding.

Box 10.9 Activity: side effects of medicines

ACTIVITY

Review the scenarios. Are there any particular issues about side effects of medicines? Why should nurses know about side effects of the medicines they administer? Where can you find out about these side effects?

The side effects from Malcolm's oral medication were so unpleasant that he stopped taking these medicines, leading to a recurrence of his mental health symptoms. A urinalysis showed blood in Mercy's urine (haematuria). Nurses caring for her should be aware that this could be a side effect of her prescribed heparin, which is an anticoagulant. Morphine has various unpleasant side effects, including constipation, so these might cause Mercy's reluctance to take them. People like Carol with learning disabilities may be hypersensitive to medication. Staff such as Carol's support worker should be extra vigilant for any unusual effects when medication is prescribed.

There is a compendium called the British national formulary (BNF), which provides up-to-date information about all aspects of medicines, including side effects. This book should be available in all clinical settings, but it can also be accessed at www.bnf.org or downloaded as an app for you to use on a portable electronic device This compendium would help you understand why Malcolm's medication has been changed and would also assist in Mercy's case; she is taking various medicines together, so you need to know about their interactions.

Honesty about possible errors

If you suspect a medicine administration error, always report it immediately to the nurse in charge. Similarly, if you do not agree with a dosage or any other aspect of a prescription, always have the courage to speak up. Errors cannot be retracted, and the individual is the one who ultimately suffers. An atmosphere of openness and honesty is positively encouraged and expected in this respect at all times as registered nurses and nursing associates have a professional duty of candour (NMC 2018c).

Ethical practice and covert administration of medicines

The NMC Code (NMC 2018c) expects all of its registrants to be trustworthy and practice in an ethical manner. Covert administration of medicines is when medicines are administered in a disguised format; often hidden in food or drink (CQC 2020) and without the knowledge or consent of the person receiving them (NICE 2015).

Box 10.10 Activity: consequences for individuals who receive medicines covertly

Consider the possible consequences for individuals who receive medicines covertly.

You may have considered the following:

- Crushing or mixing certain medicines with food can alter their pharmacological properties and affect how they work;
- Some medicines, if mixed with food, can cause adverse reactions;
- If someone discovers they have been given medicines disguised in food or drink, this can lead to mistrust;
- This practice can violate the principle of autonomy and does not respect individual wishes in respect of their treatment and care.

If a person refuses their medicines, covert administration should only ever be considered in exceptional circumstances and in accordance with the principles of the Mental Capacity Act 2005. It is always best practice to discuss with them the reasons why they do not want to take their medicines. You should ask the prescriber to review their medicines to see if they are necessary.

Working with those in your care to understand their reasons for refusing to take their medicines, respecting their decision to take or not take their medicines is a good example of partnership working.

Learning outcome 3: discuss the importance of working in partnership

The RCN (2020) states that for effective medicines management, the person should be seen as the main focus with care targeted to that individual. It is also a professional requirement to work in partnership with people to ensure effective delivery of care (NMC 2018c).

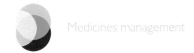

NICE (2019a) discuss shared decision-making amongst healthcare professionals and individuals who work together to make informed choices about medicines based on clinical evidence and individual preference. Working in partnership necessitates good communication and an acknowledgement of the person's views about their condition and its treatments (NICE 2019a). There may be situations where the person decides to stop or not take their medication. This situation can be difficult for healthcare professionals to accept, after all, they want the best treatment and care for those in their care. However, providing that the individual has capacity to make decisions, based on the principles of the Mental Capacity Act (2005) and you have provided the necessary information to aid in making an informed choice over their treatment, then you will need to accept and respect their right not to take the medicine (NICE 2019a).

The terms *adherence* and *concordance* are also concepts relevant to medicine management. The European Patients Forum (EPF 2015) identifies that adherence can be considered as the extent to which the person's behaviour aligns with the agreed recommendations from the prescriber, whereas concordance focuses on the interaction and relationship between the individual and the prescriber, and the extent to which the medicines prescribed represent a shared decision. Guidelines are also offered by NICE (2019a) to support the involvement in decision-making about the individual's medicines and adherence.

Box 10.11 Activity: healthcare professionals working in partnership

Reread the scenarios. What signs are there that healthcare professionals are working in partnership with Mercy, Malcolm and Carol, in relation to their medicines?

ACTIVITY

There is no obvious indication of partnership working with Mercy from the scenario provided; in particular, it does not appear that pain management methods were discussed with her and an agreement reached as she apparently remains concerned about taking opiates. Mercy should be encouraged to discuss her values and beliefs about her medicines. There should be recognition that the beliefs and preferences of each individual are paramount (EPF 2015). With Carol, partnership working seems more evident as the community learning disability nurse is working with her and her support worker. In Malcolm's scenario, a lack of partnership working could have underpinned his decision to stop taking his oral antipsychotic medication, when he experienced side effects, rather than an alternative treatment plan being developed with him. Hopefully, this time, the acute mental health unit staff have worked in partnership with Malcolm in relation to his depot injections, so that medication adherence is more likely.

Learning outcome 4: understand prescribing methods and how they are used in practice

There are a number of different ways in which people can receive their medicines by a range of non-medical healthcare professionals. The NMC (2018a) requires all registered nurses and registered nursing associates (2018b) to have knowledge of the different ways in which prescriptions can be generated and how they should be administered.

Supplementary prescribing

Supplementary prescribing involves a voluntary partnership between an independent prescriber such as doctor or a dentist and a supplementary prescriber such as a nurse (Graham-Clark et al. 2019). The supplementary prescriber is able to prescribe and review medicines once the independent prescriber has made an initial diagnosis. They can only prescribe for conditions and medicines listed on an individual agreed clinical management plan (Graham-Clarke et al. 2019).

Non-medical prescribing

Traditionally, medicines were prescribed only by doctors or dentists. Non-medical prescribing responsibilities have been assigned to a variety of registered healthcare professionals including nurses, pharmacists, physiotherapists, podiatrists, therapeutic radiographers, optometrists and paramedics (Nuttall and Rutt-Howard 2019).

More recently, the NMC has updated its guidance and under the future nurse proficiencies, newly qualified nurses will have a higher level of proficiency in skills such as pharmacology, assessment, diagnostics, planning and managing care and leadership. There is an expectation that at the point of registration they will be equipped with underpinning knowledge and be able to demonstrate the ability to progress to the completion of a prescribing qualification following registration (NMC 2018a) This type of prescribing is called **non-medical prescribing** and was introduced into the UK to enhance person-centred care by enabling healthcare professionals to extend their roles (Graham- Clark et al. 2019) Once on the register, nurses can undertake an NMC approved prescribing programme that meets the outcomes of the RPS's competency framework for all prescribers (NMC 2018d; RPS 2016).

Patient group directions

While student nurses cannot initiate PGDs, not even under the direct supervision of a registered nurse, you should understand what PGDs entail. Registered nursing associates are also not allowed to administer PGDs (Health Education England [HEE] 2017). In certain circumstances, healthcare professionals can administer prescription-only drugs without a prescription, using a PGD (MHRA 2017). This is a legal framework allowing certain healthcare professionals to supply and administer medicines to groups of people who fit certain criteria, laid down in a previously agreed PGD. Their use is limited to certain conditions where it will benefit the person in terms of speed and continuity of care (because they do not need to wait to see a doctor) without compromising individual safety. They are very useful for supplying or administering medicines such as vaccines, analgesics, antibiotics and emergency contraception. A prescription is not required, but there are strict considerations that must be adhered to when supplying or administering medicines under a PGD. For example, certain travel vaccines can be administered to groups of people who fit certain criteria – people who are medically fit, blood pressure within normal limits or no known allergies. The medicine does not need to be prescribed by a doctor or a non-medical prescriber, but it can be given by someone trained in the use of PGDs and related pharmacology, for a particular group. PGDs are often used in areas where there is not always a doctor, such as clinics or some emergency settings. Covid-19 vaccines such as the Pfizer/BioNTech and the AstraZeneca are usually administered by a PGD. Take a look at Public Health England's (PHE) website to see what information is required to be able to safely administer these vaccines via a PGD (PHE 2021a, 2021b).

PGDs are not suitable for those whose care needs are more complex. In these situations, individuals would need to see the prescriber for a thorough assessment and a prescription based on the outcome of this assessment.

Box 10.12 Activity: safety in PGDs

ACTIVITY

Consider what would be needed for safety in PGDs.

You may have thought of the following:

- A clear framework that identifies who can be given the medicine, and in what circumstances.
- Extra training for professionals in pharmacology, understanding the group.
- Ongoing effective monitoring of processes and personal competency.

Box 10.13 Activity: RPS prescribing competency framework

ACTIVITY

Read the RPS Prescribing Competency Framework and identify the competencies that a prescriber should be able to demonstrate.

You should have listed ten competencies and identified how the prescriber should demonstrate that they meet each competency.

 Box 10.14 Pregnancy and birth: practice points – medicine administration

The Human Medicines Regulation 2012, amended in 2016 consolidated many of the pre-existing pieces of legislation relating to medicines management. Within this, there is specific guidance on Midwives Exemptions, which means that at the point of registration, midwives are able to supply and administer on their own initiative, a range of permitted drugs within the regulations above. These may be GSL, pharmacy and prescription-only medicines. The ultimate aim is to ensure timely, safe and effective care of women and their babies and to respond appropriately in an emergency. It is also important to remember that some over the counter and prescribed medicines may be harmful during pregnancy or breastfeeding and as such guidance on prescribing and administering is available in the BNF.

British National Formulary and Guidance. Available from: https://bnf.nice.org.uk/ (Accessed on 12 May 2021).

Nursing and Midwifery Council. 2017, updated 2021. Practising as a Midwife in the UK. Available from: https://www.nmc.org.uk/globalassets/sitedocuments/nmc-publications/practising-as-a-midwife-in-the-uk.pdf (Accessed on 12 May 2021).

Summary

- Medicine administration by students must be under the direct supervision of a registered nurse.
- Medicine administration must comply with legal and professional requirements. Therefore, nurses must be familiar with the relevant legislation and professional guidance and work within their employers' policies.
- Nurses must take responsibility for developing their knowledge about the medicines they are administering, recognising their personal accountability in relation to medicine administration.
- Nurses and other professionals must work in partnership for effective medicine management.
- Appropriately trained nurses can initiate medicine administration using PGDs and non-medical prescribing.

SAFETY, STORAGE AND GENERAL PRINCIPLES OF MEDICINE ADMINISTRATION

Box 10.15 Learning outcomes

By the end of this section, you will be able to:

1. discuss issues concerning the safety and storage of medicines;
2. understand the general principles of medicine administration, including recording of administration.

Learning outcome 1: Discuss issues concerning the safety and storage of medicines

The RPS (2018) has produced a framework for the safe and secure handling of medicines, and includes advice relating to the safe storage of medicines outside of pharmacies or pharmacy departments.

Box 10.16 Activity: safety procedures

ACTIVITY

When you are next in practice, ask a practitioner what these safety procedures are and check them with the points below.

Safe storage

To assure the quality of medicines, manufacturers advise on appropriate storage and environmental conditions. Healthcare providers are responsible for keeping the medicines in the conditions specified.

Storage will vary depending on the setting. In a hospital, there will be a locked cupboard or immobilised medicine trolley; these must conform to the British Standard for Medicines Storage (BS2881). In a person's home, it could be the kitchen table. If children reside in the home, medicines including lotions and cleaning agents must be stored in a locked or safe place. As previously stated, there should be separate locked cupboards for CDs (RPS 2018).

In some inpatient settings, such as where Mercy is an inpatient, patients may have their own locked receptacles known as PODs (Patients' Own Drugs), where they can access their medication themselves. Continuous assessment of the person's competency to self-medicate must be performed and appropriate documentation completed.

Human factors need to be taken into consideration when storing medicines. Store medicines that have similar sounding names, or similar packaging, away from each other to minimise the risk of error (MHRA 2018).

A cool place

Medicines can be chemically unstable and may even be manufactured with a stabiliser included in the chemical compound. They generally become more unstable if warm; hence a cool dark place, away from direct sunlight, is most suitable for storage. This is why medicines are usually stored in dark bottles. Some medicines must be stored in a refrigerator, for example insulin. Separate locked drug fridges should be used with a visible temperature gauge on the outside; the temperature is regulated between 2°C and 8°C and must be monitored, recorded and reset each day (RPS 2018).

Stock rotation

Medicines should be kept in chronological order, with new items put to the back, and the older ones used first. Where the expiry date is given as a month and year, the medicine can be used until the last day of that month.

Labelling of medicines

Most UK medicines have an approved (non-proprietary) name and a brand (proprietary) name. The approved name is the chemical name and is used by all prescribers. The brand name may be different, depending on the company who produced it. All prescriptions should display the approved name (Medicines Act 1968).

European law now requires use of the recommended International Non-proprietary Name (rINN) for medicines. Most British-approved names (BANs) are the same as the rINNs, but a few BANs have had to be altered and are listed in the BNF. For example, frusemide, a commonly prescribed diuretic, is now known as furosemide.

Medicine containers are labelled with a number specific to a batch of medicines produced at the same time. For this reason, medicines should never be transferred from one container to another.

Holding drugs keys

Keys should always be held by a registered nurse, preferably the nurse in charge. Students should never hold the drug keys.

Learning outcome 2: understand the general principles of medicine administration, including recording of administration

Medicine administration must be under direct supervision of a registered nurse until you qualify as a registered nurse or nursing associate; even then your employer may require you to undergo assessments to ensure you are competent in all aspects of medicines management before allowing you to administer independently.

Medications will be prescribed on a MAR chart; either paper or electronic. The Academy of Medical Royal Colleges (2016) recommends that these records are standardised. It is essential to check the individual before, during and after administering medicines, monitoring for adverse effects. Checks that may be required include weighing them, blood monitoring for those who are taking insulin or anticoagulants and taking observations for people who have hypertension, atrial fibrillation and heart failure.

There are a number of variations on how many rights to consider when administering medicines. This section will discuss six rights (commonly referred to as 'the 6 R's') that must be taken into account when administering medicines. This is to ensure that the *right* person receives the *right* medicine and *right* dose via the *right* route at the *right* time ensuring that the *right* documentation procedure is used to record medicines administered or not (NICE 2015).

Right person

How do you know that this is the correct person for the medicine? For hospital inpatients in acute hospitals, identity bands are recommended (NHS Improvement 2018) with the standardisation of their design and the information on them to improve safety (NHS Improvement 2018). However, the person may not have a name band, for example in outpatient settings, when someone is newly admitted, or long-term residents in settings for older people or people with a learning disability (like Carol). You will need to ask the person to tell you their name and date of birth, where possible as well.

You must also gain informed consent from the individual prior to administering their medicines. You will encounter situations where it may be difficult to obtain informed consent. For example, does Carol understand what the medicine is for and agree to it being given? Only in rare circumstances does consent not need to be given – for example, if the medicine is considered essential (e.g. life-saving) and the person is unconscious.

The Mental Capacity Act (2005) states that, when working with potentially incapacitated people, the healthcare professional must assess their individual capacity at that moment when making decisions on their behalf regarding their care, which includes medicine administration. An individual's capacity can fluctuate, and a capacity assessment can recognise this and may require consideration at each administration.

In some instances, it is necessary to organise a meeting to discuss what medication is in the person's best interests. If Carol's dementia increased and she eventually lacked capacity to make decisions about her medication in the community, the community learning disability nurse would coordinate such a meeting, ensuring the relevant people are invited (e.g. Carol's GP, a family member or advocate). It is the person asking the question (in this case, does Carol understand what the medicine is for and agree to it being given?) who completes the capacity assessment. If Carol required medication in an inpatient setting, then the nurse would have to consider assessment of her capacity at that point, identifying in her care plan the best interest decision on administration. (Chapter 3 has more details about the Mental Capacity Act and also see: www.gov.uk/government/publications/mental-capacity-act-code-of-practice).

People who are detained under Section 3 of the Mental Health Act 1983 may be administered medicines to treat their mental health condition without consent, even if they have declined this treatment, for up to 3 months. However, it is only the medication required for their mental health condition, as specified on their section papers, which can be given without consent. A clear explanation about the medicine and rationale for its prescription is essential. The explanation should take into account the level of understanding and developmental stage, as in Carol's case using picture prompts.

Right medicine

It is vital to have a good understanding of all medicines that you are administering. You must ensure that it is suitable for the person's condition and that it is not contraindicated because of any other medicines they are taking or treatments they are undergoing. The name of the medicine must be written clearly, avoiding abbreviations. Care should be taken to match the name of the prescribed medicine against that on the medicine packaging. Any allergies should be noted and clearly visible on the MAR and in their individual records. Rather than a separate wrist band to indicate an allergy, some trusts may use red wrist bands with identification details to alert nurses that the person has a known risk. For example, Mercy is allergic to penicillin. An allergic reaction to a medicine could produce a serious local or systemic reaction – anaphylaxis. Anaphylaxis is a potentially life-threatening condition.

Right dose

Nurses must decide or advise how much of a medicine to administer if the prescription gives a varied dose (e.g. 5–10 mg), thus exercising professional judgement. The nurse should consider whether the dose seems correct for the person and if it falls within the normal dose range for that particular medicine. Some medicines are used for different conditions and will fall outside the normal dose range. The preparation of the medicine may also determine its dose (Carter 2019). If the dose involves a complex calculation, two nurses will be required, both nurses would need to work out the calculation separately and then compare their answers.

Right route

It is important to administer the medicine by the correct route. Doing so will ensure that the medicine is utilised appropriately within the body. Consideration also needs to be given to the preparation of the medicine; e.g. a tablet cannot be prescribed for intravenous administration.

Right time

Medicines must be administered at the correct time. Malcolm and his wife need to understand the importance of him receiving his depot injection on exactly the correct day. Some medicines should be taken with food if they need an acid medium in which to be metabolised, whereas others (e.g. the antibiotic flucloxacillin) should be taken on an empty stomach because an acid medium would break the medicine down before it can be absorbed in its useful form. Mercy is taking diuretics, which are usually prescribed in the morning to prevent a diuresis late in the day or at night. She needs to understand that it is preferable to take morphine at regular intervals, instead of waiting until the pain is already severe.

Right documentation

It is vital that all medicines administered are recorded on the individual MAR as soon as it is taken.

Box 10.17 Activity: consequences of failing to record if a person has taken their medicine

ACTIVITY

What could the consequences be of failing to record if a person has taken their medicine?

You may have realised that the nurse who is next to administer their medicines will be faced with the dilemma of whether to administer the medicine or not. If they decide to administer the drug, based on the assumption that it has not been given, the person may receive an additional dose.

You should note that 'dispensing' a medicine is not the same as administering it. It is therefore not appropriate to sign that you have given a medicine if you have simply just dispensed it into a medicine pot. The registered nurse must follow the correct procedure for their organisation in terms of how this is recorded. Any medicine refused or intentionally withheld must also be clearly recorded. A single signature is permitted for administration of any GSL, POM or P medicines (although local policies may require two signatories). Students must ensure that they always administer medicines under direct supervision of a registered nurse, countersigned by that individual. In respect of CDs, a second signatory is recommended, although when drawing up local policies, appreciation to administering CDs by lone workers in settings such as people's own homes must be taken into consideration. The second signatory is usually another registered healthcare professional, such as a nurse, doctor or pharmacist. Any alteration to a prescription must be signed and dated by the doctor.

Verbal orders

In an emergency, verbal messages may be taken over the phone by a registered nurse. However, the prescriber must update the MAR within 24 hours (RPS/RCN, 2019). Students should *not* become involved in verbal messages.

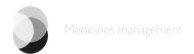

Abbreviations

The BNF states that, while generally directions on prescriptions should be written in English without abbreviations, it is recognised that some Latin abbreviations are used.

ACTIVITY

Box 10.18 Activity: BNF abbreviations

The BNF recognises all the following abbreviations. Do you know what they mean? Answers are at the end of the chapter.

b.d., o.d., o.m., o.n., q.d.s., t.d.s., stat, e/c, i/m, m/r, mL, p.r.n.

 Box 10.19 Children and young people: practice points – medicine administration

Nurses administering prescribed medicine to children must ensure that the dose is correct for the individual child's weight. Calculation of children's medicine doses is more complex than for adults because the doses are calculated according to either the child's weight (mg/kg) or body surface area (mg/m^2), although body weight is more common in practice. When nurses administer medicines to children, they must take into account the child's developmental stage and find out how the child usually takes medicines (e.g. from a spoon) and continue familiar processes.

Administration of medicines to children is specifically addressed in:

Brady, M. and Moore, L. 2018. Medication management: Administration and compliance. In: Price, J. and McAlinden, O. (eds.) *Essentials of Nursing Children and Young People*, 2nd edn. London: Sage, 55–65.

Summary

- Nurses need to be familiar with legislation and local policies concerning medicine storage and be aware of issues that could affect safe storage.
- It is crucial that medicines are stored safely, whether in a hospital or in the community, and in appropriate conditions, thus maintaining their effectiveness.
- There are a number of key safety principles that apply to medicine administration by any route to any individual, and it is very important to adhere to these, to uphold these safety principles.

ADMINISTERING ORAL MEDICATION

Box 10.20 Learning outcomes

By the end of this section, you will be able to:

1. identify the different types of oral medication available;
2. discuss how to administer oral medication safely.

Learning outcome 1: identify the different types of oral medication available

> **Box 10.21 Activity: types of oral medication**
>
> What types of oral medication have you seen?

- **Tablets**. These come in various shapes, sizes, colours and types. They often contain additives to prevent disintegration in the gastrointestinal tract. An enteric coating is used if the drug is a gastric irritant. Some tablets are formulated to control the rate of release; these preparations are referred to as 'sustained-release', 'controlled-release' and 'modified release' (Dougherty et al. 2015).
- **Capsules**. These are oval-shaped, with a coat of hard gelatin. They are useful for bitter drugs, and for unpleasant liquid like chlormethiazole. Capsules should not be opened as they are made to be swallowed whole.
- **Elixirs and syrups**. These flavoured and sweetened liquids are particularly useful for children and many are sugar-free.
- **Emulsions**. These are a mixture of two liquids. They need to be shaken well to mix the contents.
- **Linctus**. This is a sweet syrupy preparation, for example, cough linctus.

There are two other forms of medicines, which, although taken into the mouth, are not swallowed:

- **Sublingual medication**. These are produced as sprays or tablets and are absorbed through the mucosa under the tongue. As the sublingual area is very vascular, absorption and effect of the drug occur rapidly.
- **Buccal medication**. These medicines are usually produced as tablets and are put on to the gum under the lip. Again, the effect of the drug is rapid.

Learning outcome 2: discuss how to administer oral medication safely

Before administering any medicine, you should know:

- what the medicine is;
- how it works;
- the normal dosage;
- any known side effects;
- any extra precautions you should tell the person.

We are now going to look at how you would administer oral medication. Hand hygiene and gaining the person's consent must always be the first consideration. You should identify the appropriate bottle or packet of medicine that corresponds to the prescription. Check all the prescription details with the medicine label, the expiry date and any special instructions. Think about the person's positioning before

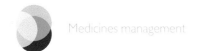

administering, as sitting up well (if not contraindicated) makes swallowing easier and safer.

Liquids

For people with swallowing difficulties, most oral medicines prescribed will be in liquid form. Many suspensions are sold with a double-ended spoon, which can measure 2.5 and 5 mL volumes, but 5 mL special oral medicine syringes can be obtained from chemists.

First shake the bottle for even distribution, then hold the bottle with the label uppermost, so that the medicine cannot flow over the label and deface it. Now carefully pour into a measuring pot, preferably place at eye level on a flat surface to measure the amount dispensed for accuracy (see Figure 10.1).

If the dose is 1 mL or less, use a 1 mL syringe and aspirate it directly from the bottle or via a quill. It may be useful to use a syringe for withdrawing larger quantities too, as they are more accurate than medicine pots. This would be appropriate for measuring Mercy's morphine. The BNF (2020) recommends that, for any oral medication prescribed in doses other than multiples of 5 mL, an oral syringe should be used. Oral syringes have a different appearance from usual syringes, and they should be used for all oral liquid medication, to reduce risk of mistakes (Health Safety Investigation

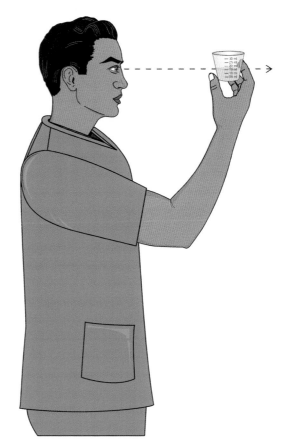

Figure 10.1: Diagram of medicine pot being looked at from eye level.

Branch [HSIB] 2019). They are often coloured, well labelled and have a different connection, preventing them from being attached to intravenous cannulae.

Tablets

If the tablets are in a bottle, tip the correct amount into the lid and then tip into a medicine pot or spoon. Many tablets are supplied in blister packs, so that they can be individually sealed and then pushed out through a foil backing into a medicine pot without being touched (Dougherty et al. 2015).

> ### Box 10.22 Activity: difficulty swallowing tablets
>
> Consider the following scenario. An individual has difficulty swallowing her tablets. A colleague suggests to you that the tablets could be crushed and given to them in food. How might you respond and why?

Crushing tablets is **not recommended** as:

- Crushing tablets could alter the medicine's therapeutic action, making it ineffective or causing adverse effects. For example, slow-release tablets that are crushed will no longer be released in the way intended. Crushing enteric-coated tablets (e.g. prednisolone) would remove the protective coating and could cause tissue damage. Particles of crushed tablets might be inhaled.
- Crushing tablets has legal consequences as it changes the product's licence (marketing authorisation) – if an adverse action resulted, then the person crushing the tablet will be responsible. Crushing must only occur if underwritten by a pharmacist who has determined that the medicine will not be compromised by crushing and that crushing is in the person's best interests.

Putting medicines in food is also not recommended as:

- It can be difficult to know how much of the tablets have been taken, when given in food.
- The food might affect the medicine's actions.
- The person may not realise they are taking medication if it is given in food or drink.

So, what should you do? Having explained to your colleague that you cannot crush tablets to be put in food for the above reasons, you should discuss the situation with the pharmacist. Most medicines are available in liquid form or there may be another alternative such as the topical route.

Administering the medicine

Next consider how to administer the medicine. Can the person self-administer or do you need to administer it on a spoon? Is the medicine best put into the mouth from a syringe? For prevention of cross-infection, never touch medication with your hand. Always provide adequate fluids, about 50 mL for an adult, to ensure medication has been swallowed, and offer a choice of fluid. Ensure that the person has swallowed all

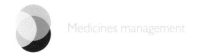
the medication before documenting. They may pocket tablets, spit them out when you have gone or be unable to totally clear them from the mouth.

In both community and hospital settings, unwanted medicines should be returned to the pharmacy. Medicines should never be disposed of in a waste bin where someone else could have access to them.

Box 10.23 Activity: medicines policy and guidance for disposal of medicines

Look in your local medicines policy and find out the guidance for disposal of medicines.

Note: Nurses and nursing associates need to evaluate whether the medication has been effective and whether side effects have occurred, as in Mercy's case, and document this.

Summary

- Both preparation and administration of oral medicines should be performed systematically, ensuring that policy is adhered to, promoting safety and prevention of cross-infection.
- Careful assessment should ensure that the oral medicine administration is performed in an acceptable and appropriate manner for each individual, taking into account factors such as swallowing ability.

APPLYING TOPICAL MEDICATION

The topical route consists of medicine administration via the epidermis (outer layer of the skin) and external mucous membranes, therefore including administration into eyes and ears.

Box 10.24 Learning outcomes

By the end of this section, you will be able to:

1. understand the indications and preparations used for the topical route;
2. show awareness of how topical medication is administered.

Learning outcome 1: understand the indications and preparations used for the topical route

Box 10.25 Activity: why has a topical antibiotic cream been prescribed for Mercy?

Mercy is prescribed fucidin cream for the small infected area behind her ear. Why might a topical antibiotic cream have been prescribed for her?

The topical route permits local rather than systemic absorption of the medicine and reduces its side effects on the body. In Mercy's case, it would have been considered appropriate as the lesion is small and superficial.

Medications are increasingly available in topical form. Common examples are patches applied to the skin being used for pain relief (fentanyl) or angina (glyceryl trinitrate). Many topical medications are designed to give a 24-hour slow release of the drug and therefore continuous action. Topical preparations also include drops into eyes and ears, where absorption occurs through the mucous membranes.

Topical preparations

- **Pastes.** These contain a large amount of powder and a little water in their composition and are therefore fairly stiff and may be difficult to spread. Lids must be carefully secured to prevent drying when exposed to the air.
- **Creams.** These are easier to spread and less prone to solidification as they are emulsions – either oil dispersed in water (e.g. aqueous cream) or water dispersed in oil.
- **Ointments.** These may be water- or oil-based, are semi-solid and are usually available in a tube. They are more occlusive and therefore better for dry lesions. Creams and ointments should be applied exactly as prescribed; for example, steroid creams are always applied very sparingly.
- **Patches.** Medication in this form is sealed in a small patch, with a peel-off sheet, which exposes the adherent part to be placed on the skin. You must follow the instructions for where it should be placed, but most are applied to the abdomen or chest, in a relatively hairless region if possible. The site is alternated each time the patch is changed, usually every 24 hours. The skin needs to be sufficiently permeable to allow absorption, so areas with good vascularity, like the trunk, are preferable. Always remove old patches before applying a new one (MHRA 2018).
- **Drops.** Drops are presented in solution in either single-use containers called minims, or in a larger bottle with a pipette-type end or dropper. Care must be taken to ensure that they are used for one person only, that the expiry time once opened is observed, usually 28 days, and that they are refrigerated if indicated.
- **Sprays.** These are produced in containers under pressure and enable a fine spray to be directed on to the area requiring it, for example nasally.

Learning outcome 2: show awareness of how topical medication is administered

Applying medication to eyes, ears and nose

Eyedrops and eye ointments should be applied with the face horizontal, the person preferably lying flat. Looking up reduces the blink reflex, as well as making it easier to apply the drops or ointment into the correct place.

Slowly squeeze the bulb when applying drops and drop vertically, from as near to the person as possible, without touching the eye. Always put the drop inside the lower lid (see Figure 10.2) (Shaw 2014). Ensure the eye is kept shut for 60 s after application, and always instil drops before an ointment (Shaw 2014), if both are being used, as the ointment leaves a film over the eye, preventing the drops being absorbed. As with drops, eye ointment should be applied to the inside of the lower lid. The eye should be held closed afterwards for a short time, where possible, enabling the ointment to settle. Vision may be blurred afterwards for a while. Excess medication should be wiped away with a clean tissue. Eyedrops can sting and some leave an after-taste at the back of the throat (Figure 10.3).

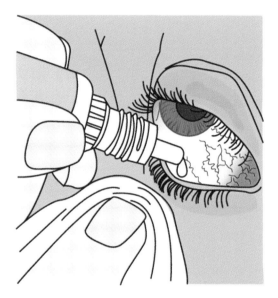

Figure 10.2: Administration of eyedrops.

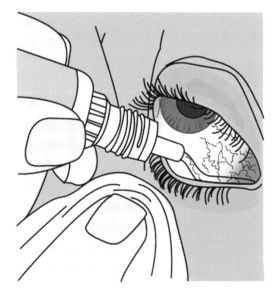

Figure 10.3: Administration of eye ointment.

If eye medication is being applied to both eyes, use separate products for each eye, ensuring bottles and tubes are labelled R and L. Apply to the least affected eye first, to reduce the risk of spreading the infection. If more than one medication is being used, leave at least 3–5 min between applications.

For application into ears, lying with the ear to be treated uppermost is most effective. For nasal sprays, the person should be upright. Nasal medication should be administered 20 min before food so that the nasal passages are clear, which makes eating easier. Ensure the person has blown their nose or cleared their mouth or throat before administration and follow closely any special instructions accompanying the spray.

Applying topical medication to the skin

Gloves should be worn when applying ointment or cream to the skin if someone other than the individual is applying the medication. This is partly to prevent cross-infection from you to them and vice versa, but also to prevent absorbing any of the medication applied into your own skin.

Where possible, encourage people to apply topical medication themselves to promote independence and reduce the risk of cross-infection. In Mercy's case, it might be difficult with the sore area being behind her ear. All stages of the skill will need to be taught, with handwashing explained carefully so that the medicine is not inadvertently transferred to other parts of the body. Creams and ointments should be gently massaged in the direction of the hair flow. Steroid creams thin the skin, so apply them sparingly.

Following application, they should remain still for several minutes and the type of covering to be applied, if any, must be considered. People may require advice about clothing and instructions about possible staining. Remember to always evaluate the effectiveness of the treatment and report and document progress or deterioration to the doctor or nurse in charge.

Box 10.26 Children and young people: practice points – topical medicines

Children can be susceptible to several skin conditions, which will require topical medication. Atopic eczema is particularly common and is a chronic, dry and itchy condition, necessitating emollient application.

For detailed information about administering topical medicines to children, see

Bruce, E.A. 2012. Administration of medicines. In: Macqueen, S., Bruce, E.A. and Gibson, F. (eds.) *The Great Ormond Street Hospital Manual of Children's Nursing Practices.* Chichester: Wiley-Blackwell, 357–95.

Keeton, D. 2010. Skin Health Care (A) Normal skin conditions and managing common skin conditions. In: Glasper, A., Aylott, M. and Battrick, C. (eds.) *Developing Practical Skills for Nursing Children and Young People.* London: Hodder Arnold, 312–23.

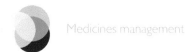

Summary

- Topical medicines are prepared in several formats and have many advantages such as direct action on the affected area and slow absorption through the skin.
- Specific instructions should be followed carefully.
- Measures to prevent cross-infection when administering topical medication are particularly important.

ADMINISTERING MEDICATION BY INJECTION ROUTES

Nurses in most settings give injections, but intramuscular (IM) injections are being used less often nowadays, so you should make the most of any opportunity to gain this experience.

Box 10.27 Learning outcomes

By the end of this section, you will be able to:

1. understand the rationale for using the injection route;
2. outline the principles of, and issues relating to, administering medicine by injection;
3. discuss health and safety issues, especially for nurses, when giving injections;
4. identify key principles of practice for administering intramuscular and sub-cutaneous injections.

Learning outcome 1: understand the rationale for using the injection route

---

Box 10.28 Activity: injection routes

ACTIVITY

What injection routes have you seen used? Why do you think these routes were chosen?

You may have seen injections into muscle (**intramuscular**), into the fat layer under the skin (**subcutaneous**), into veins through a cannula (**intravenous**), or under the skin (**intradermal**). Injections can also be given into joints, into the epidural space or directly into the heart. Students can only give intramuscular and subcutaneous injections and this must be under direct supervision of a registered nurse. Injections must always be given by the person who has drawn them up – this includes you as a student.

The intradermal route is used mainly for local anaesthetic prior to invasive procedures. Registered nurses in some specialities undergo preparation to give intradermal injections.

Rationale for injections

There are a number of situations in which an injection will be used rather than other routes for medicine administration:

* when speed of effect is required – medicines are more rapidly absorbed into the circulation when they avoid the gastrointestinal tract completely;
* when people are 'nil by mouth';
* when the drug is destroyed by digestive enzymes in the gut – for example, insulin;
* when long-term release of a drug is required – for example, depot injections for mental health clients, as in Malcolm's case.

Key features of the intramuscular route

* The effects are more rapid than the subcutaneous route because of the good blood supply to skeletal muscles, so it takes approximately 10 min for the effect to begin (Perry and Potter 2014).
* Absorption can last for 2–5 weeks if desired, using oil-based, slow-release preparations, as in Malcolm's scenario.

Key features of the subcutaneous route

* A large variety of sites are available as any subcutaneous tissue can be used (Gradel et al. 2018).
* The speed of action is slower than with the IM route because of the poorer blood supply. The medication administered therefore has a longer duration.
* The person's ability to absorb needs to be considered. If peripheral circulation is poor, the drug may stay in the subcutaneous region and not be absorbed.

Learning outcome 2: outline the principles of, and issues relating to, administering medicine by injection

Remember, all safety procedures for the oral route apply to injections too.

Box 10.29 Activity: considering issues in relation to IM and SC injections

ACTIVITY

Consider the following issues in relation to IM and SC injections. What have you seen in practice regarding: skin cleaning, injection sites, syringe and needle selection? Compare what you have observed with the points made below.

Skin cleaning

There are a number of varying views with some studies suggesting that social cleanliness is sufficient (Dougherty et al. 2015; Ogston-Tuck 2014; PHE 2020). Skin cleaning prior to injections for those who are immunocompromised and thus susceptible to infection continues to be recommended.

The Green Book (PHE 2020) advises that skin cleansing is unnecessary in socially clean individuals and only visibly dirty skin be cleaned with soap and water, although some still recommend cleansing prior to administering intramuscular injections

(Dougherty et al. 2015). If spirit swabs are used, the site must be left to dry for 30 s as vaccines can be inactivated by alcohol. Alcohol swabs are always contraindicated when subcutaneous insulin and heparin are administered, as alcohol interferes with the medicines' action and hardens the skin. Individual skin assessment is important especially in the older person or if they are immunocompromised and it is important to follow local policy (Shepherd 2018a).

Injection sites

The site used is influenced by such factors as age, medication to be injected and general client condition. Figure 10.4 shows skin, subcutaneous and muscle layers, and needle insertion. The healthcare professional must use their clinical judgement to select an appropriate site and consider the inherent risks (Shepherd 2018a).

Intramuscular sites

Intramuscular sites are shown in Figure 10.5. In adults, up to 4–5 mL can be given into most sites, but only 1–2 mL in *deltoid* muscle.

The *gluteus maximus* muscle has the slowest uptake of medication, whereas the *deltoid* has the fastest (Shepherd 2018a). The deltoid is excellent for small volumes as the site area is small and minimal undressing is required and is used for administering vaccinations. The site selected depends on the age of the person and also the needle size (Shepherd 2018a). The antero-lateral aspect of the thigh, the *vastus lateralis*, is easy to access, has few major blood vessels in the area and is suitable for all age groups. The *ventrogluteal* site is free of penetrating blood vessels and nerves and contains a large muscle mass.

If the gluteus maximus muscle in the buttock is used, it is important to quarter the buttock first and then administer in the upper outer quarter, thus avoiding the **sciatic nerve**. Any other quarter could cause nerve injury. When injecting intramuscularly, spreading the skin 2–3 cm sideways (see Figure 10.6) to provide a Z-track reduces the chance of leakage and pain (Shepherd 2018a). This method will be advantageous when giving Malcolm his injection, as depot injections can cause discomfort.

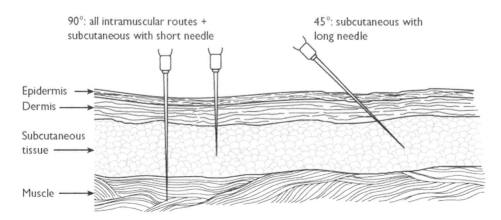

90°: all intramuscular routes +
subcutaneous with short needle

45°: subcutaneous with
long needle

Epidermis

Dermis

Subcutaneous
tissue

Muscle

Figure 10.4: Subcutaneous (SC) and intramuscular injections: diagram showing skin, SC and muscle layers and needle insertion.

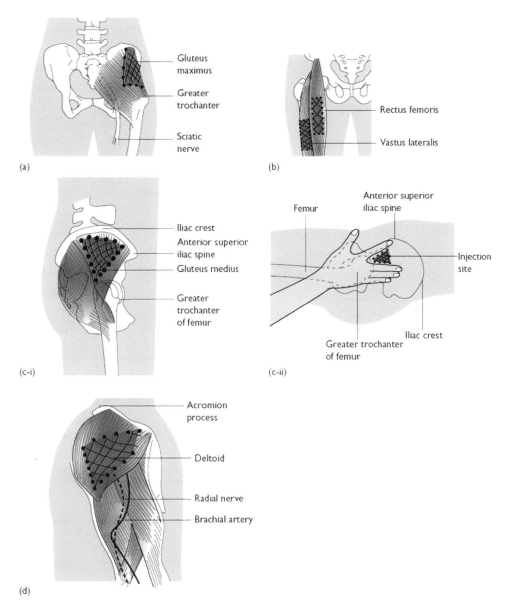

Figure 10.5: Intramuscular injection sites: (a) gluteus maximus site (upper outer quadrant of buttock); (b) quadriceps sites – vastus lateralis (outer middle third of thigh), rectus femoris (anterior middle third of thigh); (c-i) ventrogluteal site (hip); (c-ii) locating the ventrogluteal site; (d) deltoid site (upper arm).

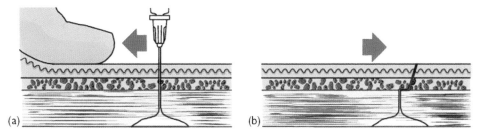

Figure 10.6: The Z-track technique: (a) skin spread to the left on administration of intramuscular medication; (b) skin released afterwards, showing formation of Z-track as a result.

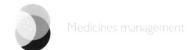

Subcutaneous sites

Subcutaneous sites are numerous, but the main ones are shown in Figure 10.7. When administering by this route, ensure a skin fold is gently pinched to free the adipose tissue from the underlying muscle (Shepherd 2018b).

Syringe and needle selection

Syringes are selected according to the volume to be given. Volumes of 1 mL and under must be given in a 1 mL syringe, because of the smaller units of graduation, usually 0.1 mL. Some drugs require a special syringe. For example, insulin needs a syringe that is marked in units, which is how insulin is prescribed. Insulin syringes incorporate a needle as well. Some injections (e.g. low-molecular-weight heparin) are pre-prepared and these also have a needle attached.

Otherwise, needles are selected according to the route and sometimes according to the body adipose of the person. For example, for an intramuscular injection, if there is a large amount of adipose, a longer needle will be required to ensure the drug enters the muscle. Nurses sometimes underestimate the required needle length by trying to be kind but using too short a needle means that the drug does not enter the muscle (Shepherd 2018a).

Needles are colour-coded according to their gauge (G); the higher the gauge, the narrower the lumen of the needle. The standard UK sizes are:

- **green**: 21G and 38 mm (1½ in) length
- **blue**: 23G and 25 mm (1 in) length
- **orange**: 25G and 10 mm (^{38} in.), 16 mm (5⁄8 in.) or 25 mm (1 in.) length.

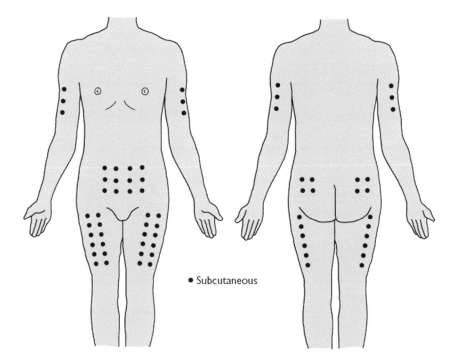

Figure 10.7: Subcutaneous sites for injection.

In general, green needles (21G) are used for adult IM injections, so the nurse should use a green needle for Malcolm's depot injection. Orange needles are used for SC injections, although the most commonly given SC injections have a short thin needle already attached to the syringe (for insulin or low-molecular-weight heparin). When drawing up liquids, the aseptic non-touch technique should be used (ANTT 2015). It is important to use a needle with a built-in filter when drawing up from a glass ampoule syringe to minimise the risk of particles of glass being withdrawn (Carraretto et al. 2011).

Learning outcome 3: discuss health and safety issues, especially for nurses, when giving injections

Box 10.30 Activity: hazards when administering injections

What hazards might nurses encounter when administering injections?

Drug contamination

There can be a danger of **contact dermatitis**, particularly if there is frequent exposure to a certain drug. For example, a nurse preparing a penicillin solution for injection could contaminate their hands with the drug. Repeated contact can cause skin sensitisation and so gloves should be worn.

Needlestick injury

The Health and Safety Executive (2013) accepts that recapping a needle is safe if you use a one-handed technique and this technique is only recommended when transporting the drug to prevent contamination.

Needlestick injuries can still occur (particularly when sharps boxes are overloaded), so what should you do if this happens?

- Remove the needle from your skin quickly.
- Encourage the wound to bleed by applying *indirect* pressure.
- Place the injured area under cold running water.
- Cover with a dressing or plaster if required.
- Complete an incident form.

The Occupational Health Department policy will advise you about further action. You should also follow your university policy regarding managing and reporting sharps injuries.

Legislation requiring safety syringes or equivalents was introduced in the UK (EU Council Directive 2010/32/EU) to prevent needlestick injuries. Safety syringes or resheathed needles have a built-in safety mechanism to reduce the risk of needlestick injuries. On some models, a sheath is placed over the needle, whereas in others, the needle retracts into the barrel.

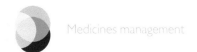

Learning outcome 4: identify key principles of practice for administering intramuscular and subcutaneous injections

The steps to take when giving an intramuscular or subcutaneous injection are set out below:

1. Ensure that the injection is *due* to be given, is written up correctly, and that consent has been given.
2. Perform hand hygiene and put on disposable gloves.
3. Assemble equipment: cleaned reusable injection tray or equivalent, appropriate syringe and needle, alcohol swab (if local policy), medication and diluent if required.
4. Check details of the medication, then draw it up either directly from the vial or, if powder, by mixing according to the manufacturer's instructions.
  * Always use the exact volume and diluent recommended to provide the most therapeutic concentration. Holding the syringe at eye level ensures you get the exact volume.
  * Remember to check the vial for cracks, precipitation or cloudiness.
  * Clean the rubber septum on vials with an alcohol wipe and allow to dry for 30 s. Inject an equal volume of air to that of the volume being withdrawn, to make withdrawal easier.
5. Recheck the person's details and medication, consent and name band. Your approach to the person is very important in developing rapport and reducing anxiety about the injection.
6. Position the person comfortably, supporting the limbs if necessary. Depot injections like Malcolm's can be very uncomfortable.
7. Identify the site. Take into account the volume to be administered and convenience to the person when choosing the site. You should also rotate sites if repeated injections are being given.
8. Check that the skin is socially clean and clean the skin if required to do so according to local policy.
9. For IM injections, spread the skin in a Z-track fashion to prevent seepage (see Figure 10.6). For SC injections, bunch the skin to release the subcutaneous tissue from the muscle. Hold the needle at approximately 90 degrees for all IM and most SC injections (as for insulin or low-molecular-weight heparin) (Shepherd 2018a, 2018b). Having first warned the person, gently insert two-thirds of the needle into the skin.
10. With IM injections, pull back on the plunger. If blood appears in the syringe, support the skin, withdraw the needle and discard the medication. This is because the needle must have entered a capillary and the route would then be intravenous rather than intramuscular. Repeat the above process. If no blood appears, administer the injection slowly (especially when giving a depot as with Malcolm). Use the recommended rate if one is given, or at 1 mL per 10 s.
11. Observe the person carefully throughout the procedure, providing reassurance as necessary.

12. Wait 10s before removing the needle (Ogston-Tuck 2014). Quickly withdraw the needle, supporting the skin with the swab and apply gentle pressure over the site. Do not rub the skin as you will cause local irritation and may alter the drug absorption rate.

13. Ensure the person is comfortable. Check for reaction, either systemic or local. All nurses should be aware of signs of anaphylaxis, a severe allergic reaction. Some drugs are known to be more likely to cause a severe allergic reaction.

14. Dispose of equipment according to local policy.

15. Document on the MAR and in the person's notes or wherever is required.

16. Return about 15 min later to check the effectiveness of the drug. The site itself should be checked 2–4 hours after administration.

Box 10.31 IM site choices

What would be the IM sites of choice for:

a a fully dressed woman who is prescribed an IM tetanus injection (0.5 mL); and

b someone lying on their back in bed, who has abdominal pain that is worse on movement, and is prescribed an IM injection of 100 mg of pethidine (2 mL) and 10 mg of metoclopramide (2 mL)?

ACTIVITY

For case a, the obvious site would be the *deltoid*, because this muscle can take an injection of 1–2 mL and is less intrusive for this woman, who need only roll her sleeve up. You will remember from earlier that this muscle is the preferred site for vaccinations. In case b, the volume for injection is too great for the *deltoid*. Because this man has pain on movement, it would be better to inject into his thigh (*vastus lateralis*) or the *ventrogluteal* site so that he does not have to move.

Main problems associated with injections
Pain

Pain may be unavoidable but can be reduced by using distraction techniques. Applying a local anaesthetic cream (EMLA) will reduce the pain but can be impractical to use before vaccinations. However, it may be useful for those with a needle phobia. Keeping the skin taut helps to reduce pain because it stretches the small nerves and reduces sensitivity. With an IM injection, try to encourage the person to relax by choosing a comfortable position for them, because injecting into a tense muscle will be more painful (Dougherty et al. 2015).

Tissue damage

Damage can be caused by the drug being administered. This can be avoided by ensuring correct dilution according to the manufacturer's instructions, and by using the appropriate technique; for example, always use the Z-track technique for depot injections like Malcolm's. Bruising may sometimes be unavoidable especially when giving subcutaneous anticoagulants. The nurses administering Mercy's injections

EMLA cream

EMLA (eutectic mixture of local anaesthetics) contains local anaesthetic and when applied to the skin enables an intravenous cannula to be inserted or blood to be taken (venepuncture) without causing pain. It is used extensively with children but can also be used for adults with needle phobia. At least 45 min must be allowed after application to produce adequate analgesia.

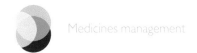

should rotate the site to prevent local damage. You should never inject into an already bruised area.

Infection

Using an aseptic technique in the preparation and administration of an injection and ensuring that skin is socially clean, should reduce the risk of infection.

Hypersensitivity

It is important to obtain a clear allergy history before giving a medicine for the first time. Observe the person carefully during administration and after, especially during the first few doses. Because of the first-pass effect, the action and therefore reaction to the drug will be faster than when it is given orally.

Staining of the skin

This may occur with pigmented drugs like iron. Using the Z-track method should leave intact tissue above the injected material in an indirect line, thereby preventing leakage to the surface tissue.

Summary

- Students can give IM and SC injections under supervision. It is advisable to take opportunities to observe and then practise injection administration so that skill and confidence develop.
- It is important to understand the sites, equipment and hazards involved in IM and SC injections and to be aware of how complications can be avoided.

ADMINISTERING INHALED AND NEBULISED MEDICATION

The inhaled route permits medication to go directly to where it is needed in the mucous membranes of the bronchioles, providing an effective method of absorption. Examples of drugs commonly inhaled are bronchodilators and steroids.

The nebulised route is the passage of medication directly to the bronchioles, as with inhalers, but by vapourising the particles in a stream of air or oxygen. Nebulised particles are much smaller in diameter than inhaled particles (British Thoracic Society/Scottish Intercollegiate Guidelines Network [BTS/SIGN] 2019). Medication for nebulisers is normally supplied in solution in single-use plastic sealed containers called **nebules**. As with inhalers, the most common drugs given by nebuliser are bronchodilators and steroids (NICE 2019b).

Box 10.32 Learning outcomes

By the end of this section, you will be able to:

1. understand why inhalers are used and how they can be used effectively;
2. demonstrate knowledge of various types of inhaler;
3. identify indications for nebulised rather than inhaled therapy;
4. administer nebulised therapy safely and effectively.

Learning outcome 1: explain why inhalers are used and how they can be used effectively

Box 10.33 Activity: inhalers

For what reasons, and by whom, have you seen inhalers used?

Chronic obstructive pulmonary disease

Chronic obstructive pulmonary disease is a chronic respiratory disease, including conditions such as emphysema, chronic bronchitis and chronic asthma.

Allergen

Allergen is a foreign substance that initiates an allergic response.

You have probably seen inhalers used by both children and adults. Asthma is probably the commonest reason for inhaler use. Inhalers are used in chronic obstructive pulmonary disease (COPD). Inhalers may be used as maintenance therapy (called **preventers**), as well as in emergency situations where acute breathlessness occurs (called **relievers**) (Asthma UK 2019; NICE 2019b). Malcolm's inhaler is therefore a reliever. Inhalers can be used as prophylactic (preventative) treatment, for example, before coming into contact with animal fur, grass, pollen, etc., which may be allergens to people with asthma, or before taking strenuous activity where extra oxygen is needed. If steroid inhalers are being used, they need to be taken after bronchodilators.

Box 10.34 Activity: instructions for using an inhaler

Instructions for using an inhaler are listed in Box 10.35. Think about how you would actually explain this to somebody.

To ensure concordance and maximum benefit, consider the individual's ability to understand instructions. Demonstration is a useful teaching strategy. Common errors have been found to be failure to shake the device, having a poor lip seal, poor coordination of actuation and inhalation, and absence of breath holding and not waiting between puffs. Frequent re-assessments and re-education are needed as correct technique usually deteriorates over time.

Did you know?
- An inhaler and spacer, used correctly, can be just as effective as nebulisers.
- You can get an inhaler aid device from pharmacists, which fits over the traditional inhaler, so that a squeezing rather than pushing-down action can be used.

Measuring the effectiveness of inhalers

Peak flow measurements can be helpful in monitoring effects of inhaled medication. Observation of respiration, including difficulty, rate and sound are important indicators of whether the medication has been effective. You can also ask the person how they are feeling and observe their colour, mental state and how well they are able to talk.

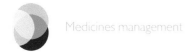

Box 10.35 Instructions for inhaler use

The person should be sitting or preferably standing, to maximise lung expansion, with their head slightly tilted to give them a clear airway. They should clear the respiratory tract by coughing if necessary, and then inhale and exhale deeply before commencing.

- Check inhaler details (medication and dose) and prescription.
- Remove the cap and shake the inhaler.
- Place the mouthpiece into mouth and at the start of a slow deep inspiration, press the canister down, and continue to inhale deeply.
- Remove the inhaler from mouth and hold breath for 10 s, or as long as possible.
- Wait several seconds before repeating for a second time if prescribed (note that most people are prescribed two puffs at a time).
- Record administration on the prescription chart.
- Wash and dry mouthpiece twice weekly.

Learning outcome 2: demonstrate knowledge of various types of inhaler

Box 10.36 Activity: types of devices currently in use

Think back to inhalers that you have seen and identify different types of devices currently in use.

The most commonly used is the pressurised metered-dose inhaler (pMDI), which contains liquid medication under pressure. This is released in the form of a mist when the inhaler is used. Other examples you might have remembered include the diskhaler and the rotohaler. With a diskhaler, the inhaled particles are contained within a disc, and with a rotohaler, the particles are enclosed in a capsule. The disc or capsule is then inserted into the inhaler to deliver a metered amount and activated by inspiration. Individual preference regarding device is crucial, so a good assessment is very important. Autohalers and the Easi-breathe are alternative types, which are both breath-activated, removing the need for good coordination, but the range of drugs is restricted in these devices. Another device you have probably seen is a spacer (see Figure 10.8).

Spacers

Spacers, sometimes referred to as a holding device, can be large (e.g. the Volumatic), or small (e.g. the Aerochamber). They are often more effective than any other hand-held inhaler (BTS/SIGN 2019) and preferred by many people. The spacer holds the medication that has been released, allowing time for the drug to be inhaled through a mouthpiece by activating a one-way valve. By filling the chamber with inhaled particles of drug, the person can then breathe these in at their own rate, usually two breaths per inhaled dose, and the particles are less likely to be lost into the atmosphere.

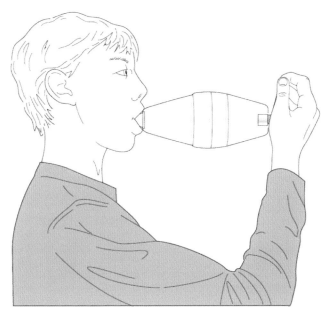

Figure 10.8: The volumatic inhaler.

Learning outcome 3: identify indications for nebulised rather than inhaled therapy

Box 10.37 Activity: advantages of nebulised therapy

Can you identify the advantages of nebulised therapy over inhaled therapy?

The nebulised route enables bronchodilators to be transported more effectively than inhalers to the bronchioles because the oxygen or air in which it is converted into a vapour reduces the size of the particles, preventing them from sticking to the oral mucosa, and therefore being lost to the respiratory tract. The smaller particles can also travel more easily into the respiratory tract.

Nebulisers are useful for people who cannot manage to hold and coordinate a metered-dose inhaler. Nebulised medication can be delivered without a high degree of cooperation, for example by a mask, or holding a nebuliser mouthpiece between the lips and breathing normally.

Learning outcome 4: administer nebulised therapy safely and effectively

Box 10.38 Activity: special instructions to someone receiving nebulised therapy

Are there any special instructions you would need to give someone receiving nebulised therapy?

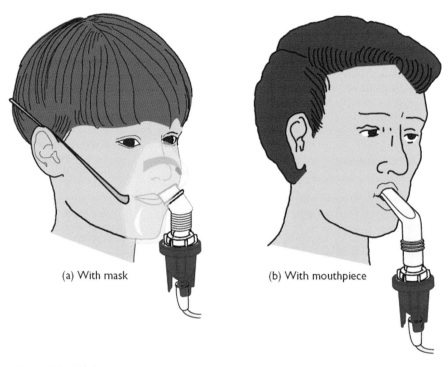

Figure 10.9: Nebuliser equipment; either a mask or mouthpiece can be used with the nebuliser.

The following points are all important:

- Sitting upright to ensure an optimum position for ventilation.
- Safety measures if oxygen is being used.
- The need to explain the noise of the nebuliser and the sensation within the mouth.

Box 10.39 Activity: considerations before administering a nebuliser

Before administering a nebuliser, what questions would you need to ask yourself?

Does the peak flow need to be measured first?

This measurement would serve as a baseline for comparison afterwards. (Chapter 14 has information about peak flow measurement.)

Should the person use a mouthpiece or a mask?

Mouthpieces are used where the person is physically and cognitively able to cooperate with holding it in the mouth. They should sit with their chest in a vertical position to ensure good ventilation, and mouth breathe to gain maximum effect. Someone who is very breathless may find this too difficult and prefer to use a mask. However, masks can be distressing to some people.

If using a cylinder (either air or oxygen) or piped oxygen/air, what flow rate would be set on the flow meter?

The flow rate must at least 6 L per minute (BTS/SIGN 2019); otherwise, the particles will not be reduced to the appropriate size for inhalation.

Should the nebuliser be administered via air or oxygen?

Some people with chronic respiratory disease continually have a high level of carbon dioxide in their blood, and their breathing is only stimulated by lack of oxygen. Nebulisers for these individuals should therefore be administered via air (Rickards 2021). If ongoing nebulisers are required at home, portable air compressor machines are much more convenient than oxygen cylinders. They extract air from the atmosphere and are available on prescription.

For people who are hypoxaemic, with acute severe asthma, should receive oxygen-driven nebulisers to help them maintain oxygen levels between 94% and 98% (BTS/SIGN, 2019; O'Driscoll et al. 2017).

What instructions would I need to give to the person?

The person will need to understand that the mouthpiece or mask must be kept in place and that nebulisation only occurs on inhalation, so it is important to inhale well. There is no need to remove to exhale. The nebuliser unit must be kept vertical throughout administration and continued until all the liquid disappears from the unit, usually within 10 min.

> **Box 10.40 Activity: considerations after administering a nebuliser**
>
> After administering a nebuliser, what questions might you ask yourself?

ACTIVITY

What should be done with the equipment?

You need to check the manufacturer's instructions as to whether the equipment is 'single-use only' or 'single-patient use'. If it is 'single-patient use', you should clean the mouthpiece or mask in warm tap water at least once daily, dry well and keep covered in a clean place. Tubing should not be washed as it cannot be dried properly.

How can I evaluate the nebuliser's effectiveness?

You can observe whether the person is still breathless, whether their colour has improved, and whether peak flow readings have increased (assess this prior to the nebuliser and post nebuliser). You should also consider whether there are any apparent side effects. Nebulised therapy can produce unpleasant side effects.

Adverse side effects of nebulised medicines can include giddiness, tremor, palpitations, wheeziness and irritable coughing. These may be related to the drugs and then dosage may need adjustment. It is also important that the nebules are not too cold as this would cause bronchoconstriction. Mouth infections (e.g. candidiasis) may occur after prolonged use of steroid-inhaled drugs, so rinsing the mouth after use is beneficial in this case. If a nebulised steroid is being administered, delivery via a mask

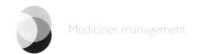

may cause irritation to the eyes and skin. Ipratropium bromide, a quite commonly prescribed bronchodilator, can also be irritating to the eyes when given via a mask, so washing the face afterwards may help.

> ### Box 10.41 Children and young people: practice points – inhalers and nebulisers
>
> Children under 5 years who need inhaler administration will need to use a spacer and facemask because they will not be able to make a good seal around a mouthpiece or coordinate their inhalation with the inhaler's use. Inhalers are more effective when the child is relaxed rather than distressed, which affects respiratory patterns. Children over 5 years should be able to use a mouthpiece. Consideration of age, motor skills and understanding needs to be considered with each individual child for the appropriate technique. For a detailed review of inhaler and nebuliser administration to children, see
>
> Fanning, L. 2018. Inhaled drug administration. In: *Children and Young People's Nursing Skills at a Glance*. Gormley-Fleming, E. and Martin, D. (eds.) Chichester: Wiley, 48–49.

Summary

- Inhaled medication is frequently prescribed, particularly for people with COPD disease and asthma.
- Inhaled medication is taken both prophylactically and as an emergency measure.
- Inhalers act directly on the respiratory tract, so doses can be lower than when medication is taken systemically.
- Inhaler technique must be effective so that the correct dose of medication is inhaled.
- Nebulised therapy is widely used, particularly for people with acute respiratory disease.
- Appropriate decisions must be made as to whether to administer a nebuliser with a mask or a mouthpiece, and via air or oxygen.
- Nurses should be aware of side effects and how these side effects can be prevented or reduced.

ADMINISTRATION OF MEDICINES VIA ENTERAL ROUTE

As a student you will come across people who are unable to take medication orally. It is common practice to administer medication via nasogastric (NG) or percutaneous endoscopic gastrostomy (PEG).

Box 10.42 Learning outcomes

By the end of this section, you will be able to:

1 identify the main problems that may be encountered when administering medicines via the enteral route;
2 administer medications via a NG tube or PEG.

Learning outcome 1: identify the main problems that may be encountered when administering medicines via the enteral route

Box 10.43 Problems when administering medicines via the enteral route

What problems do you think you might encounter when administering medicines via the enteral route?
  You might have identified:

* interaction of drugs
* liability
* medicine preparation

The timing of medication can interfere with the absorption and effect of the medication. It is important that when administering medicines, you are aware of the potential interactions as well as the required time-gap between medication and feed. Never add medicines to enteral feed containers. Each medicine must be given individually and medicines must not be crushed unless there are no alternative preparations and only if advised by the pharmacist (Shepherd 2020). There should be a flush of 10 ml of water between each medicine administered (British Association for Parenteral and Enteral Nutrition [BAPEN] 2017). Medicines that should not be crushed include enteric-coated (EC), modified/slow-release (MR, SR, LA, LX), cytotoxic medications, sublingual, buccal, melt or chewable preparations and proton-pump inhibitors. A soluble or liquid formulation should be given when administering medicines via NG or PEG. About 30 mL of fresh water (tap or sterile) should be used to flush the tube prior to administering the drug (Thompson 2017).

Learning outcome 2: how to administer medications via a NG tube or PEG

Ensure that you follow your local policy when administering drugs via NG tube or PEG. You will need to check the position of the enteral tube (NHS Improvement 2016).

Before administering medicines, you will need to stop the feed being administered. When drawing up water for flushing, use a 50/60 mL purple enteral syringe. Be aware when flushing that this water forms part of the overall fluid intake so care should be taken for those on fluid restrictions. You can use one of two methods to

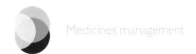

administer medicines using a gravity method where the plunger is removed or by slowly depressing the plunger. Always flush between drugs.

Summary

- Checking the position of an enteral tube before drug administration is essential.
- Drugs should be given separately.
- Stop the feed prior to administering the medication.
- Use a purple enteral syringe.

INTRAVENOUS FLUID AND BLOOD ADMINISTRATION

Student nurses, healthcare assistants and nursing associates are not allowed to administer intravenous fluids or blood. This means you cannot connect up a bag of infusion fluid, or alter the flow rate, as both actions mean you are administering the intravenous fluid. However, you may well be caring for people receiving infusions, so you need to know how to care for them safely and general precautions and signs to look for if the infusion is causing problems.

ACTIVITY

Box 10.44 Learning outcomes

By the end of this section, you will be able to:

1 understand the main indications for administration of intravenous fluids and medicines;
2 know how to care for a person with an infusion or transfusion;
3 recognise some common problems and safety issues surrounding intravenous fluid and blood administration and understand your role.

Learning outcome 1: understand the main indications for administration of intravenous fluids and medicines

Intravenous infusions can be given peripherally into a vein (Dougherty et al. 2015) or centrally into the right atrium.

Box 10.45 Activity: intravenous administration

ACTIVITY

Why do you think fluids and medicines are administered intravenously?

You might have identified that intravenous administration is used to:

- provide large volumes of fluid, blood or other nutritional supplements;
- provide fluids when other routes are not appropriate, as with those who are nil by mouth;
- provide a route for certain drugs (e.g. chemotherapy, drugs destroyed by the gut).

Whole blood is now rarely given to because there are alternative products that can be used that are less difficult and costly to collect but are just as effective. So, packed cells, plasma and platelets are given where there is a specific need (e.g. a person with low platelets after chemotherapy), but if the individual has lost blood and is still medically stable, intravenous fluids may provide sufficient replacement while their body manufactures more blood cells.

Learning outcome 2: know how to care for a person with an infusion or a transfusion

Cannulae should be sited in the non-dominant arm where possible (Dougherty et al. 2015), avoiding the antecubital fossa unless necessary. Ensure that the drip stand is lightweight and has wheels that run smoothly to preserve independence for those who are mobile. Ensure that clothing worn is loose, and that tubing is fed through sleeves to provide maximum normality. This would have helped maintain some of Mercy's independence following surgery.

Learning outcome 3: recognise some common problems and safety issues surrounding intravenous fluid and blood administration, and understand your role

Box 10.46 Activity: problems relating to intravenous and blood transfusion

What problems and safety issues are you aware of relating to intravenous and blood transfusion?

Key problems relate to infection risk and systemic reactions.

Infection risk

One of the main risks of infusions is infection, particularly at the site of cannula insertion (RCN 2016).

Systemic reactions and care

Some people may have more central or systemic reactions to infusion management, so you need to observe for these and report them to a registered nurse. Reactions include breathlessness, which could indicate either an over-infusion of fluid (i.e. a bag that has been administered too quickly, causing cardiac failure) or an allergic reaction to an infusion fluid (e.g. blood or a drug). Postoperatively, while receiving intravenous infusions, Mercy should have been observed carefully for breathlessness because of her previous cardiac history. Also, watch and report alarms sounding on pumps and any untoward discomfort, including rashes (Robinson et al. 2017), which could be a sign of an allergic reaction. It is important to follow national and local policy and guidance regarding infection prevention, e.g. cannula change.

Ensure that you document observations or care provided and report any changes. Many individuals with infusions will have their intake and output monitored on a fluid balance chart, so then ensure all oral input and all forms of output, including vomit, are measured.

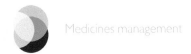
Safety issues regarding blood transfusions

Blood cells are fragile, so bags need careful handling, and some such as platelets are therefore never put through a pump which would crush them further. They are all infused through filtered giving sets, and blood products must also be used within 30 min of removal from the designated blood fridges they are kept in, otherwise the cells start to become damaged (Robinson et al. 2017).

The main problem with blood products is that they carry different antigens on their cell surfaces, which are described by the different blood groups (A, B, AB and O) and by the Rhesus factor. This means that, if the person's blood is not matched or they are not given the correct blood group (incompatibility), they will quickly become ill with a haemolytic reaction and could die if not treated fast (Serious Hazards of Transfusion [SHOT] 2020).

ACTIVITY

Box 10.47 Activity: observations when administering blood

You may have observed the process involved in administering blood. When do you think the main errors in the process are likely to occur?

You may not have been aware that these occur when the blood is collected from the designated blood fridge and also when the bedside checks are done immediately before administering the blood (Robinson et al. 2017). It is important that personal identity details are checked properly before administering blood products.

The person's temperature, pulse and blood pressure must be taken before administration and 15 min after the start of each component transfusion (Robinson et al. 2017). You must report any rise in temperature, pulse or drop in blood pressure immediately to a registered nurse. You must monitor for shivering, breathlessness, loin pain, rashes and fever, as these are all signs of reaction. If you see any of these signs, tell the nurse in charge immediately who will stop the transfusion, and call the senior member of the team. Close observation and further treatment is needed and if anaphylaxis occurs, then resuscitation may be needed.

Box 10.48 Children and young people: practice points – Intravenous therapy

For further information about intravenous fluid therapy and blood transfusion, see

Seeman, C. 2013. Caring for children and young people in the medical setting. In: Thurston, C. (ed.) *Essential Nursing Care for Children and Young People. Theory. Policy and Practice.* Oxon: Routledge, 149–71.

Hennen, S. J. 2012. Administration of blood components and products. In: Macqueen, S., Bruce, E.A. and Gibson, F. (eds.) *The Great Ormond Street Hospital Manual of Children's Nursing Practices.* Chichester: Wiley-Blackwell, 74–86.

Summary

● Students, nursing associates and healthcare assistants are not permitted to administer intravenous fluids, blood or drugs but often care for people with infusions or transfusions in progress.
● Good intravenous care requires holistic care.
● There are important safety aspects related to intravenous fluid administration and blood transfusion; students must be able to recognise problems and report these promptly.

CALCULATING MEDICINE AND INTRAVENOUS FLUID ADMINISTRATION DOSES

Nurses often worry about their ability to calculate medicine doses. Therefore, if you have a problem with basic maths, access numeracy support sessions in your university. There are also many online maths packages available to practice your numeracy skills. BBC Skillswise offers useful packages to help you to learn or refresh essential mathematical principles. These packages can be found at http://www. bbc.co.uk/teach/skillswise/maths/zfdymfr. If your university has a subscription for Clinicalskills.net, there you will find a useful section on basic mathematical principles and medicines calculations. Clinicalskills.net can be accessed via your university e-learning portal or via www.clinicalskills.net.

Tip: Try to be involved in doing calculations in the clinical setting whenever possible. Many nurses find this easier than doing calculations from a book or in the classroom.

For further explanations and more practice exercises, there are many books specifically focusing on this topic. An example is *Drugs Calculations for Nurses: A Step-by-Step Approach*, 4th edn. (Lapham 2015).

Box 10.49 Learning outcomes

By the end of this section, you will be able to:

1 appreciate the need for effective numeracy skills in practice;
2 perform calculations using decimal numbers;
3 understand units of weight and volume and their equivalences;
4 apply a variety of formulae to calculate medicine doses;
5 use formulae to calculate intravenous administration rates and volumes for pumps and administration sets.

Learning outcome 1: appreciate the need for effective numeracy skills in practice

Box 10.50 Activity: calculations going wrong

ACTIVITY

Consider what the outcome of occasionally getting a calculation slightly wrong would be. Can you ever be justified in giving a person an inaccurate dose?

The answer must always be no. You have to be 100% accurate all the time. Even a small discrepancy means the person will not receive the prescribed dose, which could be harmful. It is also a requirement that to qualify as a registered nurse or nursing associate, you must demonstrate proficiency with your calculations for a range of medicines (NMC 2018a, 2018b). As part of your course, you must pass at 100% a numeracy assessment related to nursing proficiencies and calculation of medicines (NMC 2018e, 2018f).

Debate exists about the use of calculators for working out medicine doses. They can increase accuracy and are useful for complex calculations. However, there may be occasions when a calculator is unavailable or not working. There is also the risk that a calculator will be used without an understanding of what the numbers being entered into it mean (Lapham 2015). It is also only as good as its operator; hence, if the wrong numbers, or for some calculations, the wrong order of sequence, are put in by mistake, the answer will be incorrect. Also, if you are totally unable to work without a calculator, you cannot estimate easily what the right answer will be and therefore have no way of checking that the calculator answer is about right. Having a 'sense of number' is crucial when dealing with calculations (Lapham 2015).

It is therefore sensible to be able to calculate medicine doses manually and by calculator, to prevent any chance of error.

Learning outcome 2: perform calculations using decimal numbers

Decimals or decimal fractions are often used in calculating medicine doses where less than a whole number is involved. Whole numbers and fractions of a whole number are separated by a decimal point. Numbers to the left of the decimal point are whole numbers and will always be at least 1 or greater than 1. Numbers to the right of the decimal point are fractions of a whole number and are expressed in measurements of tenths, hundredths, thousandths and so on. Each number in a decimal is 10 times larger than the number to its immediate right. In other words, each number represents a different numerical value depending on where it is positioned in relation to the decimal point.

When dealing with whole numbers only, the decimal point is omitted but when dealing with decimal fractions that involve numbers less than 1, it is necessary to place a '0' to the left of the decimal point so as not to mistake a fraction of a number with a whole number. For example, .567 should be written as 0.567.

Rounding off decimal numbers
When using decimal numbers in calculations, sometimes answers will result in many numbers after the decimal point; this is often impractical to manage and it is not always necessary to use all of these numbers since their value may be negligible. With such calculations, it is necessary to round up or round down the answer, usually to the second or third decimal place. Number digits below five are usually rounded down and digits above five are rounded up. Caution should be exercised as some drug doses are so small that to round them off may adversely affect the dose a person received and could result in the person being under- or overdosed.

Calculation exercise 1

Round off the following decimal numbers (answers are at the end of the chapter):

a. 3.666 to 1 decimal place
b. 423.12 to 1 decimal place
c. 1001.6772 to 2 decimal places
d. 964.9814 to 3 decimal places
e. 6.6666666 to 2 decimal places

Most calculations will divide into relatively easy numbers because nurses have to be able to give that portion of the drug without dividing into complicated amounts. For example, a dose of 3/8th of a tablet or 0.0065 mL of a liquid would be unrealistic to administer and unsafe. A sensible rule to follow is if your calculation requires you to administer a fraction of a tablet or a very small amount of a liquid, it is worthwhile rechecking your calculation; equally, if your calculation results in a large number of tablets or liquid to administer please recheck. You should also recheck the dose prescribed as this may be wrong!

To add and subtract decimals

The same mathematical principles of addition and subtraction apply when using decimal numbers as when using whole numbers. The only additional action to consider is ensuring that the decimal point is inserted into the correct place in your answer.

Calculation exercise 2

Calculate the following (answers are at the end of the chapter):

a. $154 + 36.21$
b. $98.4 + 106.2$
c. $456.789 - 45.67$
d. $200 - 145.98$
e. $5723.9 + 47.8 - 4056.438$

To multiply and divide decimals

When dealing with calculations that require you to multiply or divide decimals, it is usually easier to convert the decimals to whole numbers. This conversion will involve multiplying and dividing by units of 10. Since decimals represent fractions in tenths, this representation makes these processes very easy.

- To multiply by 10, move the decimal point one place to the right. For example, $0.05 \times 10 = 0.5$; $5.8 \times 10 = 58$.
- If you want to multiply by a different unit of 10 (e.g. 1000), move the decimal point to the right by the number of 0's – in the case of 1000, three places, in the case of 100, two places. For example, $0.06 \times 1000 = 60$; $5.23 \times 1000 = 5230$; $0.67 \times 100 = 67$.
- If there are no more figures to move the point over, add 0 to fill the spaces. For example, $5.8 \times 100 = 580$.

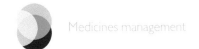

When multiplying using two decimal numbers, it is not necessary to multiply each decimal number by the same amount (i.e. 10, 100, 1000). Only multiply enough to reach a whole number. For example, to calculate 0.05 × 1.3, do the following:

0.05 × 100 = 5
1.3 × 10 = 13
5 × 13 = 65

At this stage, your answer now needs to reflect its correct value; therefore, the decimal point needs to be placed in the correct position. To do this, count how many digits there were to the right of the decimal point in both the numbers used in your calculation and place the decimal point with this number of digits to its right. Since 0.05 has two digits and 1.3 has one digit, this totals three digits to the right of the decimal point. Therefore, the answer to this calculation is 0.065.

- To divide by 10, or multiples of, do the reverse. For example, 63 ÷ 100 = 0.063; 25 ÷ 1000 = 0.025.

Division of a decimal by a whole number is a relatively straightforward process. The same principles of dividing whole numbers apply with the additional step of ensuring that the decimal point is correctly placed. The decimal point in the answer is positioned directly above the number being divided. For example, to calculate 8.6 ÷ 2

$$\frac{4.3}{2)8.6}$$

Division of a decimal number by another decimal number requires the number you are dividing by to be converted into a whole number first. It is therefore necessary to multiply the dividing number by 10, 100, 1000, and so on to reach a whole number. It is also essential to multiply the number being divided by the same amount to ensure the numerical value in the answer is correct. For example, to calculate 10.55 ÷ 0.5.

Multiply the dividing number 0.5 × 10 to give a whole number of 5.
Multiply the number being divided 10.55 × 10 to give 105.5.
Then, carry out the calculation as follows:

$$\frac{21.1}{5)105.5}$$

Calculation exercise 3

Calculate the following. Where necessary, round off your answers to two decimal places (answers are at the end of the chapter).

a. 2.5 × 3.06
b. 678.98 × 3
c. 78 ÷ 3.2
d. 0.032 ÷ 0.6
e. 156.1 ÷ 9.87

Learning outcome 3: understand units of weight and volume and their equivalences

Medicine doses are expressed in units of weight (e.g. grams, micrograms) or volume (e.g. litres, millilitres). It is essential to use the same units throughout a medicine calculation – you cannot work with both micrograms and milligrams, or millilitres and litres. Therefore, you need to convert the medicine doses in the calculation into the same units. It does not matter which unit you change them into. There is a simple rule for conversion, which is the rule of thousands: everything that needs converting is achieved by either dividing or multiplying by a thousand. In Table 10.1, you can see the most common units of weight and volume and their abbreviations. Each unit has been multiplied by 1000 to give its equivalent unit of weight or volume.

With a few exceptions, these are the units used in medicine prescriptions. So, to convert 5 milligrams (mg) into micrograms (mcg), you need to multiply by 1000 (equals 5000 micrograms). To convert the other way, you need to divide by 1000. For example, 50 micrograms to milligrams equals 0.05 mg. Therefore, to convert to a larger unit, you need to divide the figure, so there will be less numerical digits. To convert to a smaller unit, you need to multiply, so there will be more numerical digits. Nanograms and micromoles are rarely used in medicine doses for adults; however, they are used for children's doses. When dealing with plurals in a dose abbreviation, the 's' is not included (write 8 mg and not 8 mgs). Also, when writing litres or millilitres, you may see the letter 'L' in both abbreviations written as a capital letter 'L' rather than in lowercase, that is, 'l'.

Note: Recommended practice is to write micrograms and nanograms in full, rather than their abbreviated terms (BNF 2020), to prevent such abbreviations being misread, which could result in the person receiving the wrong dose of a medicine.

Calculation exercise 4

Convert the following to their equivalent units (answers are at the end of the chapter) (Table 10.2):

a. 2000 mg = __ g (d) 3 mg = __ microgram
b. 2 L = __ mL (e) 3500 mL = __ L
c. 50 mg = __ g

Table 10.1: Performing calculations using decimal numbers

The number 1234.567 is made up of the following values:							
Whole numbers				Decimal point	Decimal fractions		
Thousands	Hundreds	Tens	Units		Tenths	Hundredths	Thousandths
1	2	3	4		5	6	7

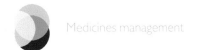

Table 10.2: Common units of weight and volume and their abbreviations

Unit	Abbreviation	Multiply by 1000	Equivalent	Abbreviation
1 kilogram	kg	× 1000	1000 grams	g
1 gram	g	× 1000	1000 milligrams	mg
1 milligram	mg	× 1000	1000 micrograms	mcg
1 microgram	mcg	× 1000	1000 nanograms	ng
1 litre	l or L	× 1000	1000 millilitres	ml or mL
1 mole	mol	× 1000	1000 millimoles	Mmol
1 millimole	mmol	× 1000	1000 micromoles	Mcmol

Learning outcome 4: apply a variety of formulae to calculate medicine doses

Tablets and capsules

The formula to use for these calculations is as follows:

$$\frac{\text{What you want}}{\text{What you've got}} \quad \text{or} \quad \frac{\text{Dose prescribe}}{\text{Stock dose}}$$

This means that the prescribed dosage needs to be divided by the stock dose that is available.

For example, 80 mg of furosemide (a diuretic) is needed for Mercy, and the stock dose is 40 mg tablets. Thus, to follow the formula:

Dose prescribed = 80 mg

Stock dose = 40 mg

$$\frac{80}{40} = 2 \text{ tablets.}$$

Liquids

The formula to use for these calculations is as follows:

$$\frac{\text{Dose prescribed}}{\text{Stock dose}} \times \text{the volume of the stock dose}$$

A useful mnemonic to remember this formula is NHS:

N – What you Need (i.e. dose prescribed)
H – What you Have (i.e. stock dose)
S – The Solution (i.e. stock volume)

$$\frac{N}{H} \times S$$

Now try exercise 5.

Calculation exercise 5

How much would you dispense for the following (answers are at the end of the chapter)?

a. 200 mg of trimethoprim required; stock dose is 100 mg tablet
b. 100 mg of chlorpromazine required; stock dose is 25 mg tablet
c. 10 mg of diazepam elixir required; stock dose is 5 mg per 5 mL
d. 1.2 g of augmentin required; stock dose is 600 mg tablet
e. 240 mg of paracetamol elixir required; stock dose is 120 mg per 5 mL

Doses based on body weight

Sometimes doses of medicines are calculated according to how much the person weighs. Their weight must always be recorded in kilograms (kg) to enable you to apply the correct calculation formula to check that the correct dose has been prescribed and to work out how much of the medicine needs to be administered. Common medicines include heparin and gentamicin, which are prescribed in this way. The medicine dose will be prescribed in milligrams/micrograms/nanograms per kilogram of body weight.

To calculate the correct dose simply multiply the prescribed dose by the person's body weight in kilograms. For example, an individual is prescribed 2 mg of a medicine per kilogram of their body weight; this is commonly written as 2 mg/kg. They weigh 64 kg. To calculate how much should be prescribed:

$$64 \times 2 = 128$$

The person should be prescribed 128 mg of the medicine.

It is important to note that if the medicine is prescribed in divided doses, then it is necessary to divide the total amount by the number of doses. In the example above, if they were to be given this medicine twice daily, then divide 128 mg by 2. Therefore, $128 \div 2 = 64$ mg. Therefore, the individual would receive 64 mg per dose.

Calculation exercise 6

How much would you give (answers are at the end of the chapter)?

a. Furosemide 0.5 mg/kg. The person weighs 60 kg.
b. Heparin 250 units/kg. The person weighs 88 kg.
c. Tinzaparin sodium 175 units/kg. The person weighs 74 kg.
d. Gentamicin 3 mg/kg. The person weighs 65 kg.
e. Heparin 250 units/kg every 12 hours. The person weighs 55 kg. How many units of heparin should be administered in a 24-hour period?

Learning outcome 5: use formulae to calculate intravenous administration rates and volumes for pumps and giving sets

Intravenous infusions are often used for fluid replacement therapy, to administer electrolytes such as sodium and potassium, as a medium for administering medicines and to deliver blood products. This section will enable you to understand how to calculate drip rates (an amount per unit of time) to ensure that the person receives the correct volume in a prescribed period of time.

Pump rates

Look at a pump and see how fluid rates are measured. They are all in millilitres (mL) per hour. Per means divided by, so you need to divide the total volume prescribed by the number of hours it has been prescribed over and that will give you the pump rate.

Example:

Prescribed: 1 litre (1000 mL) of normal saline over 8 hours:

$$\frac{\text{Total volume in mL}}{\text{Time in hours}} \quad \frac{1000}{8} = 125 \text{ mL per hour}$$

Like calculators, its accuracy in its rate of delivery will depend on the correct information inputted by the administering nurse.

Calculation exercise 7

How many millilitres per hour should be administered (answers are at the end of the chapter)?

a. 500 mL of normal saline in 6 hours

b. 1 litre of dextrose in 10 hours

c. 50 mL of normal saline in 2 hours

Manual administration sets

Depending on the type of administration or giving set used (the device used to deliver the infusion), the drop factor will vary.

A standard giving set for administering a crystalloid (such as normal saline) will hold 20 drops in 1 mL and for infusion of a colloid (such as blood or blood products) will hold 15 drops per mL. Other giving sets such as a microdrop giving set (or burette) can hold 60 drops in 1 mL. It is therefore necessary to use the correct giving set for fluids being administered and to know their drop factor to ensure the correct numbers are used in the calculation.

The formula to use when calculating how many drops per minute should be infused is

$$\frac{\text{Total volume (mL)} \times \text{drop factor}}{\text{Time (minutes)}}$$

Example:

To calculate how many drops per minute should be infused when delivering 1 litre of fluids in 6 hours, with a drop factor of 20 drops per mL:

$$\frac{1000 \times 20}{360} = 55.5 \text{ drops per minute}$$

Since it is not possible to count half a drop, the answer should be rounded off to 56 drops per minute.

Calculation exercise 8

Calculate these rates in drops per minute, all with a drop factor of 20 drops per mL. Answers are at the end of the chapter.

a. 500 mL in 4 hours
b. 1 litre in 10 hours
c. 1000 mL in 12 hours

Summary

- All nurses must be able to calculate medicine doses accurately, so a basic understanding of fractions and decimals is needed.
- There are formulae that can be used when a calculation is required, and it is important to develop skill in their application.
- Students do not carry out medicine calculations unsupervised. However, it is advisable to start working on this skill at an early stage, in preparation for registration, because students may be asked to be second checkers for a calculation at some stage during the preregistration programme.

PREVENTING AND MANAGING ANAPHYLAXIS

Anaphylaxis is a severe, life-threatening allergic reaction (NICE 2020) that requires rapid recognition and treatment (Resuscitation Council (UK) 2021). The allergen (the substance causing the reaction) may be a drug, so it is important that when medicines are being administered (especially straight into a vein), nurses observe the person closely. It often occurs after the second dose rather than the first, when the body has already become sensitised to the drug. Such allergic reactions may also be caused by plaster, tape, dressings and food.

Useful reading: The Resuscitation Council (UK) (2021) details guidelines on the emergency treatment of anaphylactic reactions (available from www.resus.org.uk). NICE (2020) provides guidelines for assessment and referral following a suspected anaphylactic episode.

Box 10.51 Learning outcomes

By the end of this section, you will be able to:

1. identify how to prevent anaphylaxis;
2. know how to recognise and manage anaphylaxis.

Learning outcome 1: identify how to prevent anaphylaxis

When you assess a new admission, always ask about any allergies they may have. These allergies must be documented clearly in their records and on the MAR and checked before any medicine is given. Mercy is an example of someone with a known allergy

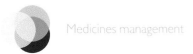

to penicillin, and this should be recorded and checked so that there is no possibility that penicillin is administered to her.

Knowing how to recognise anaphylaxis and when it is most likely to occur will help you respond promptly and effectively.

Learning outcome 2: know how to recognise and manage anaphylaxis

Recognition is often difficult because the symptoms can vary so much. With drugs, the speed of onset is usually linked to the route; for example, if intravenous, it will be much quicker (10 min) than if oral (several hours). The severity of symptoms is associated with how quickly they appear (Perry 2019). The body's reaction to an allergen is to produce histamine in large quantities, which can induce severe bronchospasm and swelling of the bronchioles and face.

It should be noted that while severe allergic reactions may display some of the signs of anaphylaxis, they do not include life-threatening airway, breathing or circulatory symptoms. Allergic reactions are treated differently to anaphylaxis.

ACTIVITY

Box 10.52 Activity: recognising and managing anaphylaxis

List how you would recognise and manage anaphylaxis. Box 10.53 outlines what you need to consider.

Box 10.53 Recognising and managing anaphylaxis (adapted from Resuscitation Council (UK) 2021)

Recognition of symptoms

- Early call for help
- Airway problems – swelling, stridor
- Breathing problems – shortness of breath, wheeze, cyanosis
- Circulation – shock, blood pressure drop, pulse raised, consciousness reduced
- Disability – neurological status – confusion, agitation, loss of consciousness
- Exposure – skin colour: flushing, facial swelling, etc.

Management

Positioning – *airway/breathing problems:* sit-up; *low blood pressure:* lie down and raise legs where possible; *unconscious:* recovery position.

- Remove triggering source where possible, e.g. stop infusion of medication.
- Give high-concentration oxygen.
- Get intramuscular adrenaline/epinephrine ready or get person to self-administer their Epi-pen.
- Be prepared to resuscitate.

Hydrocortisone and chlorphenarimine may be given as second-line drugs.

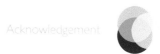

> ### Box 10.54 Children and young people: practice points – anaphylaxis
>
> The Resuscitation Council (UK) advise that treatment of anaphylaxis for adults and children is mainly the same but provides different drug doses for children <6 months, 6 months–6 years, 6–12 years and >12 years, and fluid regimes differ from adults. Anaphylaxis is more likely to be caused by food in children than it is in adults. Some children in anaphylaxis may present with signs and symptoms very similar to severe asthma. For full details and algorithm, see http://www.resus.org.uk/pages/reaction.pdf.
>
> Also see:
>
> Durack, T. 2012. Allergy and anaphylaxis. In: Macqueen, S., Bruce, E.A. and Gibson, F. (eds.) The Great Ormond Street Hospital Manual of Children's Nursing Practices. Chichester: Wiley-Blackwell, 38–51.

Summary

- Everyone must be asked about allergies and the information recorded.
- Anaphylaxis can be rapidly fatal, so be sure you know how to recognise it.
- The body may react more severely to a second dose of a drug where the antibodies remember the allergen.
- Adrenaline is the main medicine used to correct anaphylaxis but be prepared to resuscitate too. Medical help will be needed.

CHAPTER SUMMARY

This chapter has explained the importance of having a basic understanding of the laws concerning medicine administration and of ensuring that local drugs policies are adhered to in practice. You should now be able to understand the need for a working knowledge of the medicines you are giving and be able to calculate doses accurately. The chapter has stressed the importance of safe practice with regard to medicine administration and the student role and should have helped you to understand the reasons for different routes of administration and key principles for safe and evidence-based practice. It should have prepared you to administer medicines safely in a variety of clinical settings.

ACKNOWLEDGEMENT

With thanks to Veronica Corben for her contributions to previous editions of this chapter.

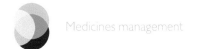

ANSWERS TO EXERCISES

Drug calculation exercises

Exercise 1

  a. 3.7

  b. 423.1

  c. 1001.68

  d. 964.981

  e. 6.67

Exercise 2

  a. 190.21

  b. 204.6

  c. 411.119

  d. 54.02

  e. 1715.262

Exercise 3

  a. 7.65

  b. 2036.94

  c. 24.38

  d. 0.05

  e. 15.82

Exercise 4

  a. 2 g

  b. 2000 mL

  c. 0.05 g

  d. 3000 mcg

  e. 3.5 L

Exercise 5

  a. 2 tablets

  b. 4 tablets

  c. 10 mL

  d. 2 tablets

  e. 10 mL

Exercise 6

  a. 30 mg

  b. 22,000 units

  c. 12,950 units

  d. 195 mg

  e. 27,500 units

Exercise 7

  a. 83 mL per hour

  b. 100 mL per hour

  c. 25 mL per hour

Exercise 8

  a. 42 drops per minute

  b. 33 drops per minute

  c. 28 drops per minute

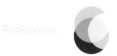

ABBREVIATIONS

b.d. = twice daily;	o.d. = daily;
o.m. = every morning;	o.n. = every night;
q.d.s = to be taken 4 times daily;	t.d.s. = to be taken 3 times daily;
stat = immediately;	e/c or EC = enteric-coated;
i/m = intramuscular;	m/r = modified release;
mL = millilitre;	p.r.n = when required.

Source: www.bnf.org.

REFERENCES

Academy of Medical Royal Colleges. 2016. *Standards for the Design of Hospital In-patient Prescription Charts.* London: AMRC. https://www.aomrc.org.uk/wpcontent/uploads/2016/05/Standards_design_hospital_prescription_charts_0411.pdf.

Aseptic Non-Touch Technique. 2015. The ANTT clinical practice framework; 4. Available from: https://www.antt.org/antt-practice-framework.html (Accessed on 9 June 2021).

Asthma UK. 2019. *Home Page.* Available from: www.asthma.org.uk.

BAPEN. 2017. *Medications. Administering Medicines via Enteral Feeding Tubes.* Available from: https://www.bapen.org.uk/nutrition-support/enteral-nutrition/medications

BBC. 2020. Skillswise: Maths for adults. Available from: https://www.bbc.co.uk/teach/skillswise/maths/zfdymfr (Accessed on 14 May 2021).

British National Formulary (BNF). 2020. *Prescriptionwriting.* Available from: https://bnf.nice.org.uk/guidance/prescription-writing.html (Accessed on 9 June 2021).

British Thoracic Society/Scottish Intercollegiate Guidelines Network (BTS/SIGN). 2019. *British Guidelines on the Management of Asthma.* London and Edinburgh: BTS/SIGN. Available from: https://www.brit-thoracic.org.uk/quality-improvement/guidelines/asthma/.

Care Quality Commission (CQC). 2019. *Storing Controlled Drugs in Care Homes.* Available from: https://www.cqc.org.uk/guidance-providers/adult-social-care/storing-controlled-drugs-care homes.

Care Quality Commission (CQC). 2020. *Covert Administration of Medicines.* Available from: https://www.cqc.org.uk/guidance-providers/adult-social-care/covert-administration-medicines.

Carraretto, A. R., Curi, E. F., de Almeida, C. E. and Abatti, R. E. 2011. Glass ampoules: Risks and benefits. *Revista Brasileira di Anestesiologia* 61(4): doi: 10.1016/S0034-7094(11)70059-9.

Carter, A. 2019. Medication Administration: Why it's important to take drugs the right way Healthline. Available from: https://www.healthline.com/health/administration-of-medication#dosage-and-timing (Accessed on 9 June 2021).

Department of Health (DH). 2007. *Learning from Tragedy, Keeping Patients Safe: Overview of the Government's Action Programme in Response to the Recommendations of the Shipman Enquiry.* London: DH. Available from: https://www.gov.uk/government/uploads/system/uploads/attachment_data/file/228886/7014.pdf. (Accessed on 10 June 2021).

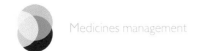

Dougherty, L., Lister, S. and West-Oram, A. 2015. *The Royal Marsden Manual of Clinical Nursing Procedures*, 9th edn. East Sussex: John Wiley.

European Patients Forum (EPF). 2015. *Adherence and Concordance: EPF Position Paper.* Available from: https://www.eu-patient.eu/globalassets/policy/adherence-compliance-concordance/adherence-paper-final-rev_external.pdf. (Accessed on 10 June 2021).

Gradel, A.KJ., Porsgaard, T. Likkesfeldt, J. et al. 2018. Factors affecting the absorption of subcutaneously administered insulin: Effect on variability. *Journal of Diabetes Research.* doi: 10.1155/2018/1205121

Graham-Clarke, E., Rushton, A., Noblet, T. and Marriott, J. 2019. Non-medical prescribing in the United Kingdom National Health Service: A systematic policy review. *PLoS One* 14(7). doi: 10.1371/journal.pone.0214630

Health Act. 2006. London: HMSO.

Health and Safety Executive (HSE). 2013. *Health and Safety (Sharp Instruments in Healthcare) Regulations 2013.* London: HSE.

Health Education England (HEE). 2017. *Advisory Guidance Administration of Medicines by Nursing Associates.* London: HEE.

Healthcare Safety Investigation Branch (HSIB). 2019. *Inadvertent Administration of an Oral Liquid Medicine into a Vein.* Farnborough: HSIB. Available from: https://www.hsib.org.uk/documents/98/hsib_summary_report_inadvertent_administration_oral_liquid_medicine_vein.pdf (Accessed on 9 June 2021).

Lapham, R. 2015. *Drugs Calculations for Nurses: A Step-by Step Approach*, 4th edn. London: Taylor and Francis Group.

Medicines Act. 1968. London: HMSO.

Medicines and Healthcare products Regulatory Agency (MHRA). 2015. *Oral Diclofenac Presentations with Legal Status 'P'- Reclassified to POM.* London: MHRA.

Medicines and Healthcare products Regulatory Agency (MHRA). 2017. Patient group directions: Who can use them. Available from: https://www.gov.uk/government/publications/patient-group-directions-pgds/patient-group-directions-who-can-use-them (Accessed on 9 June 2021).

Medicines and Healthcare Products Regulatory Agency (MHRA). 2018. *Drug-name Confusion: Reminder to be Vigilant for Potential Errors.* London: MHRA. https://www.gov.uk/drug-safety-update/drug-name-confusion-reminder-to-be-vigilant-for-potential-errors

The Medicines (Sale or Supply) (Miscellaneous Provisions) Amendment no.2 regulations. 1997. Available from: https://www.legislation.gov.uk/uksi/1997/2045/regulation/2/made (Accessed on 9 June 2021).

Mental Capacity Act. 2005. London: HMSO.

Mental Health Act. 1983. London. HMSO.

Misuse of Drugs Act. 1971. London: HMSO.

Misuse of Drugs Regulations. 2001. London: HMSO.

National Institute for Health and Care Excellence (NICE). 2015. *Medicines Management in Care Homes.* Quality Standard QS85. Available from: https://www.nice.org.uk/guidance/qs85/chapter/quality-statement-6-covert-medicines-administration (Accessed on 10 June 2021).

National Institute for Health and Care Excellence (NICE). 2016. *Controlled Drugs: Safe Use and Management.* NICE Guideline NG46. Available from: http://www.nice.org.uk/guidance/ng46/chapter/recommendations. (Accessed on 9 June 2021).

National Institute for Health and Care Excellence (NICE). 2017. *Managing Medicines for Adults Receiving Social Care in the Community.* NICE Guideline NG67. Available from: https://www.nice.org.uk/guidance/NG67/chapter/Recommendations#ordering-and-supplyingmedicines. (Accessed on 10 June 2021).

National Institute for Health and Care Excellence (NICE). 2019a. Shared decision making. Key therapeutic topic KTT23. Available from: https://www.nice.org.uk/advice/ktt23/chapter/Key-points. (Accessed on 10 June 2021).

National Institute for Health and Clinical Excellence (NICE). 2019b. *Chronic Obstructive Pulmonary Disease in Over 16s: Diagnosis and Management.* London: NICE. Available from: https://www.nice.org.uk/guidance/NG115. (Accessed on 9 June 2021).

National Institute for Health and Clinical Excellence (NICE). 2020. *Anaphylaxis: Assessment to Confirm an Anaphylactic Episode and the Decision to Refer after Emergency Treatment for a Suspected Anaphylactic Episode.* Clinical Guidelines 134. London: NICE. https://www.nice.org.uk/guidance/cg134/evidence/anaphylaxis-full-guidance-pdf-184946941.

NHS Improvement. 2016. *Resource Set: Initial Placement Checks for Nasogastric and Orogastric Tubes.* Available from: http://rightbiometrics.com/wp-content/uploads/2018/04/Resource_set_-_Initial_placement_checks_for_NG_tubes_1.pdf (Accessed on 9 June 2021).

NHS Improvement. 2018. *Recommendations from National Patient Safety Agency Alerts That Remain Relevant to the Never Events List 2018.* Available from: https://www.england.nhs.uk/wp-content/uploads/2020/11/Recommendations-from-NPSA-alerts-that-remain-relevant-to-NEs-FINAL.pdf (Accessed on 9 June 2021).

NHS. 2019. *The NHS Long Term Plan.* Available from: https://www.longtermplan.nhs.uk/wp-content/uploads/2019/08/nhs-long-term-plan-version-1.2.pdf (Accessed on 9 June 2021).

Nursing and Midwifery Council (NMC). 2018a. *Future Nurse: Standards of Proficiency for Registered Nurses.* London: NMC.

Nursing and Midwifery Council (NMC). 2018b. *Standards of Proficiency for Nursing Associates.* London: NMC.

Nursing and Midwifery Council (NMC). 2018c. *The Code: Professional Standards of Practice and Behaviour for Nurses, Midwives and Nursing Associates.* London: NMC.

Nursing and Midwifery Council (NMC). 2018d. *Realising Professionalism: Standards for Education and Training; Part 3: Standards for Prescribing Programmes.* Available from: https://www.nmc.org.uk/globalassets/sitedocuments/education-standards/programme-standards-prescribing.pdf (Accessed on 9 June 2021).

Nursing and Midwifery Council (NMC). 2018e. *Realising Professionalism: Standards for Education and Training: Part 3: Standards for Pre-registration Nursing Programmes.* Available from: https://www.nmc.org.uk/globalassets/sitedocuments/education-standards/programme-standards-nursing.pdf (Accessed on 10 June 2021).

Nursing and Midwifery Council (NMC). 2018f. *Realising Professionalism: Standards for Education and Training: Part 3: Standards for Pre-registration Nursing Associate Programmes.* Available from: https://www.nmc.org.uk/globalassets/sitedocuments/education-standards/print-friendly-education-framework.pdf (Accessed on 10 June 2021).

Nuttall, D. and Rutt-Howard, J. 2019. *The Textbook of Non-medical Prescribing*, 3rd edn. Chichester: John Wiley and Sons Ltd.

O'Driscoll, B.R., Howard, L.S., Earis, J. et al., on behalf of the British Thoracic Society. 2017. BTS guideline for oxygen use in adults in healthcare and emergency settings. *Thorax* 72(Suppl. 1): ii1–ii90. PMID: 28507176. doi: 10.1136/thoraxjnl-2016-209729

Ogston-Tuck S. 2014. Intramuscular injection technique: An evidence-based approach. *Nursing Standard* 29(4): 52–9. PMID: 25249123. doi: 10.7748/ns.29.4.52.e9183

Perry, A. and Potter, P. 2014. *Clinical Nursing Skills and Techniques*, 8th edn. St Louis: Elsevier Mosby.

Perry, M. 2019. Assessing and managing anaphylaxis in primary care. *Independent Nurse*. Available from: https://www.independentnurse.co.uk/clinical-article/assessing-and-managing-anaphylaxis-in-primary-care/221141/ (Accessed on 10 June 2021).

Psychoactive Substances Act. 2016. London: HMSO.

Public Health England (PHE). 2020. *The Green Book*. Available from: https://www.gov.uk/government/collections/immunisation-against-infectious-disease-the-green-book#the-green-book. (Accessed on 10 June 2021).

Public Health England (PHE). 2021a. *Patient Group Direction for COVID-19 Vaccine Astra-Zeneca (ChAdOx1-S [Recombinant])*. Available from: https://www.england.nhs.uk/coronavirus/wp-content/uploads/sites/52/2021/01/C1012-patient-group-direction-for-covid-19-vaccine-astra-zeneca-ChAdOx1-S-6-jan-2021.pdf (Accessed on 9 June 2021).

Public Health England (PHE). 2021b. *Patient Group Direction for COVID-19 mRNA Vaccine BNT162b2 (Pfizer/BioNTech)*. Available from: https://www.england.nhs.uk/coronavirus/publication/patient-group-direction-for-covid-19-mrna-vaccine-bnt162b2-pfizer-biontech/ (Accessed on 9 June 2021).

Resuscitation Council (UK). 2021. *Emergency Treatment of Anaphylactic Reactions: Guidelines for Healthcare Providers*. Available from: https://www.resus.org.uk/library/additional-guidance/guidance-anaphylaxis/emergency-treatment (Accessed on 9 June 2021).

Rickards, E. 2021. Pulmonary administration medicines 2: Dry powder inhalers and nebulisers. *Nursing Times* 117(2): 45–7.

Robinson, S., Harris, A., Atkinson, S. et al. 2017. The administration of blood components: A British Society for haematology guideline. *Transfusion Medicine*. doi:10.1111/tme.12481. https://onlinelibrary.wiley.com/doi/epdf/10.1111/tme.12481

Royal College of Nursing (RCN). 2016. *Standards for Infusion Therapy*, 4th edn. London: RCN.

Royal College of Nursing (RCN). 2020. *Medicines Management: An Overview for Nursing*. London: RCN.

Royal Pharmaceutical Society (RPS). 2016. *A Competency Framework for All Prescribers*. Available from: https://www.rpharms.com/resources/frameworks/prescribers-competency-framework (Accessed on 10 June 2021).

Royal Pharmaceutical Society (RPS). 2018. *The Safe and Secure Handling of Medicines*. Available from: https://www.rpharms.com/recognition/setting-professional-standards/safe-and-secure-handling-of-medicines (Accessed on 10 June 2021).

Royal Pharmaceutical Society and Royal College of Nursing (RPS, RCN). 2019. *Professional Guidance on the Administration of Medicines in Healthcare Settings*. Available from: https://www.pslhub.org/learn/patient-safety-in-health-and-care/medication/medication-administration/professional-guidance-on-the-administration-of-medicines-in-healthcare-settings-january-2019-r639/ (Accessed on 9 June 2021).

Serious Hazards of Transfusion (SHOT). 2020. *Annual Shot Report 2019. Haemolytic Transfusion Reactions*. Available from: https://www.shotuk.org/wp-content/uploads/myimages/18.-Haemolytic-Transfusion-Reactions-HTR-v2.pdf (Accessed on 10 June 2021).

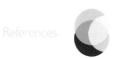

Shaw, M. 2014. How to administer eye drops and ointment. *Nursing Times* 110(40): 16–18.

Shepherd, E. 2018a. Injection technique 1: Administering drugs via the intramuscular route. *Nursing Times* 114(8): 23–5.

Shepherd, E. 2018b. Injection technique 2: Administering drugs via the subcutaneous route. *Nursing Times* 114(9): 55–7.

Shepherd, M. 2020. Medicine Administration 1: Understanding routes of administration. *Nursing Times* 116(6): 42–4.

Thompson, R. 2017. Troubleshooting PEG feeding tubes in the community setting. *Journal of Community Nursing* 31(2): 61–6.

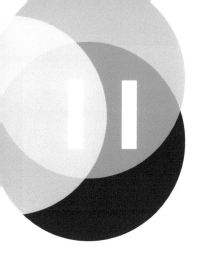

Caring for people with impaired mobility

Rowena Slope and Katherine Hopkinson

The World Health Organization (WHO) defines physical activity as 'bodily movement produced by skeletal muscles that require energy expenditure' (WHO 2020a). A healthy human body is capable of thousands of body movements every day in the course of carrying out Activities of Daily Living (Roper et al. 2000). Any restriction on mobility can have profound physical, psychological and social impacts on an individual, especially if the loss of mobility is sudden and profound. The human body is designed to move, and people with mobility restrictions are vulnerable to further deterioration of their physical and psychological health. Nurses from all specialist areas including child, mental health and learning disability, will encounter individuals with restricted mobility throughout their career and across different healthcare settings. Therefore, nurses should have a comprehensive understanding of the vulnerabilities that people with mobility problems are susceptible to, and ensure that they are up to date with the latest evidence based on correct moving and handling techniques. This is to protect the person, their colleagues and themselves from unnecessary harm. Individual assessments and care plans should be developed in collaboration with individuals with restricted mobility, which promote independence, contain realistic goals, and reduce the risk of further deterioration. Nurses must work with people in partnership and 'respond to their preferences and concerns' (NMC 2018).

This chapter includes the following topics:

- Pressure ulcer risk assessments
- Pressure ulcer prevention
- Prevention of other complications of immobility
- Key principles of moving and handling people
- Assisting with mobilisation and preventing falls

RECOMMENDED BIOLOGY READING

The questions below will help you understand the biology underpinning this chapter's skills. Use your recommended textbook to find answers.

- What body systems are involved in movement and posture? (Do not forget cellular requirements for oxygen and nutrients, and the transportation systems that deliver these and remove waste products).

DOI: 10.4324/9781003020660-11

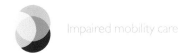
- What are the functions of our muscles and bones?
- What are joints and what are the different types of joints in the human body?
- Are all joints moveable and which types of movement are they capable of?
- How does immobility affect the following body systems: musculoskeletal system, respiratory system, gastrointestinal system, integumentary system?
- How does the integumentary system protect the body and what happens if it is compromised?
- How does immobility affect metabolic rate and energy balance?
- What is the psychological impact of reduced mobility?

PRACTICE SCENARIOS

The following scenarios illustrate situations where nurses need to assist with and promote mobility, and implement measures to prevent complications of impaired mobility.

Adult

Diane Beck is a 50-year-old woman with **multiple sclerosis** who lives at home with her husband and two teenage children. She has difficulty walking. She has tingling and burning pains and spasms in her legs, so she uses walking sticks or a wheelchair. She has a **suprapubic catheter** for her bladder problems.

Learning disability

Marion Pearce is a 42-year-old woman with a severe learning disability who lives in a community home. Due to accompanying physical disabilities, she uses a wheelchair for mobilising. She is underweight and incontinent of urine and faeces; her skin tends to be dry. Joint deformities make it very difficult to position her comfortably in the wheelchair. She has a poor appetite and is unable to eat independently or manage her own hygiene needs. Marion's health facilitator is her keyworker who liaises closely with the community nurse for learning disabilities. Marion's **Health Action Plan** includes input from many different health professionals including the general practitioner, the occupational therapist and the physiotherapist. She has also been assessed by the speech and language therapist.

Mental health

John Barnes, aged 52 years, is a client on an acute mental health admission ward. He has severe depression and also has a history of limited mobility and chronic pain after an accident 10 years ago. He needs a walking frame for support but unfortunately fell on the ward recently and sustained a fractured wrist, which is now in a plaster cast.

Pressure ulcer risk assessment

One of the greatest risks to immobile individuals is the potential to develop pressure ulcers, also known as a pressure injury, pressure sore or decubitus ulcers. In 2016, the

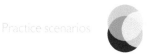

National Pressure Injury Advisory Panel (NPIAP) updated its definition, and staging, of pressure injuries as follows:

> A pressure injury is localized damage to the skin and underlying soft tissue usually over a bony prominence or related to a medical or other device. The injury can present as intact skin or an open ulcer and may be painful. The injury occurs as a result of intense and/or prolonged pressure or pressure in combination with shear. The tolerance of soft tissue for pressure and shear may also be affected by microclimate, nutrition, perfusion, co-morbidities and condition of the soft tissue.
>
> (NPIAP 2016, p. 1)

The NHS and the European Pressure Ulcer Advisory Panel (EPUAP) continue to use the term 'pressure ulcer' so this terminology will be used in this chapter (NHS Improvement 2018; EPUAP 2015). Pressure ulcers usually occur over the bony prominences in individuals who are restricted to a bed or chair due to an illness or have reduced mobility (NICE 2015a). Anyone can develop a pressure ulcer but those most at risk are the very young and the very old, and those people with cognitive impairments, nutritional deficiency, reduced sensation, restricted mobility and inadequate tissue perfusion (Alderden et al. 2017; NICE 2015a; Coleman et al. 2013). The National Health Service (NHS) recognises pressure ulcers as being a significant risk to individual safety and must be reported as a Serious Incident through the Strategic Executive Information System (StEIS) (NHS Improvement 2018). The Essence of Care (Department of Health 2010) has identified benchmarks of best practice for pressure ulcer screening, risk assessment and prevention. This section will examine the importance of risk assessment in relation to preventing pressure ulcers.

Box 11.1 Learning outcomes

By the end of this section, you will be able to:

1 Explain how pressure ulcers are formed and the areas of the body that are most at risk;
2 Discuss why some people are more likely to develop pressure ulcers;
3 Use a pressure ulcer risk calculator to identify people at risk of pressure ulcers;
4 Discuss the importance of accurate documentation of pressure ulcer risk assessment.

Learning outcome 1: explain how pressure ulcers are formed and the areas of the body most at risk

Box 11.2 Activity: identifying a pressure ulcer

ACTIVITY

Hold a clear plastic tumbler or glass in your hand using your fingertips. Press with your fingers and notice how your fingertips have become very pale. Now release the pressure and look at your fingertips: they will have a red flush.

The red flush, called reactive hyperaemia, is one of the first signs of pressure damage that occurs if skin and other tissues are compressed between bone and another surface. When this happens, the blood supply to the capillary bed is compromised leading to reduced flow of oxygen and other vital nutrients, and failure to remove products of cell metabolism (Peate and Glencross 2015). If the circulation is quickly restored, then there will be a sudden increase in blood flow to the area, called reactive hyperaemia, as the build-up of metabolites acts on the arteriole sphincters. However, if the circulation is not restored quickly enough, then cell death and necrosis will occur.

Pressure ulcers, like any wound, can become infected and therefore nurses must reduce the possibility of infection by adhering to infection-control policies including wearing personal protective equipment and adhering to the WHO's five moments of hand hygiene (before touching a person; before clean/aseptic procedures; after body fluid exposure/risk; after touching a person; and after touching a person's surroundings) (WHO 2020b). Signs of infection include exudate and an offensive smell emanating from the wound, erythema around the wound, pyrexia and pain (Sepsis Alliance 2020). It is important to undertake holistic assessments including regular monitoring of vital signs (respiration, oxygen saturation, systolic blood pressure, pulse rate, consciousness, blood sugar and temperature) of individuals in acute hospital settings using the National Early Warning Score (NEWS2) (RCP 2017). The Sepsis 6 should be initiated for people who show signs and symptoms associated with infection.

Sepsis 6

Sepsis is a dysregulated reaction by the body to an infection that can cause shock, organ failure and death. The Sepsis 6 protocol is as follows: (1) administer oxygen; (2) take blood cultures; (3) administer intravenous antibiotics; (4) administer intravenous fluids; (5) check serial lactates; (6) measure urine output (The UK Sepsis Trust 2018).

Box 11.3 Activity: pressure ulcer risk

ACTIVITY

What areas of the body are most at risk of developing pressure ulcers? Which of these sites are risk areas for the people in the scenarios at the start of the chapter?

Pressure ulcers can occur anywhere on the body. Pressure ulcers can be caused by the weight of the body or persistent contact with a medical device, or shearing and friction forces associated with poor manual handling. The most vulnerable areas of skin are around bony prominences, especially if they are in contact with hard surfaces such as an operating table or standard hospital mattress. People nursed in the supine position may develop pressure ulcers on the back of the heels and ankles; the area around the buttocks (ischial tuberosity), the elbows and shoulder blades, and the occiput (back of the head) (EPUAP 2015). Individuals nursed in the prone position are vulnerable to pressure ulcers on the toes, knees, hips, elbows and ribs (EPUAP 2015). Stephen-Haynes and Maries (2020) recommend the use of specialist equipment, silicone padding, careful positioning, and close attention to skin care for people nursed in the prone position. Wheelchair-bound individuals are at risk of developing pressure sores on their buttocks, spine, elbows, heels, back of the knees, palms and genitals (Stephens and Bartley 2018). Comprehensive assessments and care plans should be carried out for wheelchair users and their carers, which include equipment, positioning, cushions, and environment (Stephens and Bartley 2018). Medical devices and associated lines and tubes may cause pressure injuries wherever they are in contact with the skin (NPIAP 2020).

Box 11.4 Signs of early pressure ulcer development

- Non-blanching redness of a localised area usually over a bony prominence.
- Darkly pigmented skin may not have visible blanching. Its colour may differ from the surrounding area.
- The area may be painful, firm, soft, warmer or cooler compared with adjacent tissues.

Source: European Pressure Ulcer Advisory Panel, National Pressure Injury Advisory Panel and Pan Pacific Pressure Injury Alliance. 2019. Pressure and Treatment of Pressure Ulcers: Quick Reference Guide. Available from: http://www.internationalguideline.com/static/pdfs/Quick_Reference_Guide-10Mar2019.pdf (Accessed on 08 November 2020)

Box 11.5 Pressure ulcer categories

Assessment of pressure injuries

Pressure injuries are classified by the EPUAP (2015) according to the depth of injury and tissues involved:

Category 1: Non-blanchable erythema of intact skin

An area of erythema surrounds the affected area that does not blanch (whiten) when pressed, in darker pigmented skin, erythema may not be obvious but skin will be of a different colour.

Category 2: Partial thickness skin loss

There will be a break in continuity in the skin, which may involve several layers of skin with a shallow open ulcer present.

Category 3: Full thickness skin loss

The pressure ulcer now extends through all layers of the epidermis and dermis. Subcutaneous fat may be visible.

Category 4: Full thickness loss of skin and tissue

This is the most serious type of ulcer that may involve fat, muscle and bone.

Source: European Pressure Ulcer Advisory Panel (EPUAP) 2015. Pressure Ulcers: Just the Facts! Available from: www.epuap.org/wp-content/uploads/2015/09/EPUAP_Factsheet_A4.blue_.pdf (Accessed on 22 November 2020).

Inspection of vulnerable areas

Careful inspection should be undertaken at regular intervals of individuals who are at risk of developing a pressure ulcer by an appropriately trained healthcare professional. Special attention should be paid to bony prominences in areas of pressure, placement of medical devices, and any reports of pain or discomfort from

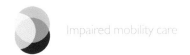

the person. Any changes in skin colour, heat, firmness or moisture should be carefully noted. If erythema or discoloration is observed, then finger pressure should be applied to identify non-blanching areas (NICE 2015a). If non-blanching areas are located, then preventative action according to NICE guidelines should be initiated and skin assessments must be repeated every 2 h (NICE 2015a). See Box 11.4 for signs of pressure ulcers and Box 11.5 for categories of pressure ulcers.

Learning outcome 2: discuss why some people are more likely to develop pressure ulcers

Box 11.6 Activity: pressure ulcer development

If you can, lie down on a hard floor in the supine and then prone position. Now see how long you can lie there without moving and which areas of the body become painful first.

How long did you manage in each position: 5 min, 10 min or longer? What made you move? You probably found that your pressure areas became uncomfortable and eventually you had to move position. Listed below are important intrinsic (individual related) risk factors and extrinsic risk factors for pressure ulcers. Remember, the more risk factors a person has, the more likely they are to develop a pressure ulcer.

Limited mobility

Immobility is the most important factor in the development of pressure ulcers. A reduction in mobility may be the result of a traumatic injury, weakness due to disease or poor diet, stroke or medical interventions such as surgery. People with limited mobility have an increased risk of developing pressure ulcers (NICE 2015a).

Stroke

A stroke occurs when the blood supply to the brain is disrupted by a blockage or rupture of an artery. If the blood supply is not quickly restored, then brain cells start to die due to lack of oxygen and other vital nutrients. According to NICE (2019), there are 100,000 strokes each year in the UK resulting in 38,000 deaths. Strokes represent a medical emergency and symptoms often present as unilateral facial droop, weakness or numbness in the upper limbs, and slurred speech.

Sensory loss

People who have reduced sensation and are unable to feel are at great risk of pressure ulcers. The body's defence against pressure is to shift weight frequently, whether asleep or awake, in response to sensory stimulation. This may be the result of damage to the nervous system such as diabetic neuropathy, affecting the lower limbs or spinal cord damage.

Diabetic neuropathy

Diabetes (mellitus) is caused by deficient insulin release, leading to inability of the body cells to use carbohydrates, and an elevated blood glucose. Elevated blood glucose

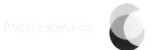

is linked to the development of diabetic neuropathy, whereby nerves supplying the hands and feet become damaged, resulting in a loss of sensation.

Previous or current pressure ulcer

It is important to undertake a head-to-toe assessment of the individual, especially elderly and frail individuals who may have been transferred from other care providers on admission to check for any signs of pressure ulcers. The persons, their family members and carers may be able to provide valuable information about whether they have previously developed pressure ulcers. Any evidence of previous or current pressure ulcers should be carefully documented in the risk assessment and a care plan initiated as well as appropriate safeguarding responses.

Nutritional deficiency

Underweight individuals with poor nutritional intake are vulnerable to pressure ulcers because they lack protective layers of subcutaneous fat around the bony prominences. Lack of adequate nutritional intake may interfere with maintenance of body systems essential for health including circulation and wound healing. Nutritional deficient individuals may also be dehydrated leading to poor tissue perfusion. Individuals going towards the end of their life such as those suffering from cancer or HIV may suffer from cachexia leading to muscle wastage. Individuals who have a high **body mass index (BMI)** can be nutritionally deficient if they are consuming the wrong types of food and the additional weight on bony prominences can contribute to pressure ulcer formation.

Cachexia

Cachexia is an involuntary loss of weight involving musculoskeletal muscle as well as fat. It is a complex, multifactorial and progressive condition often associated with long-term illnesses such as cancer or HIV.

Inability to reposition

People who are unable to position themselves are at risk of developing pressure ulcers. There might be different reasons for this, and thorough assessments should be conducted to assist individuals to reposition when they need to. Pain often prevents people from repositioning themselves, particularly at night, and pain should be managed effectively with referrals to pain specialists and thought given to the timing of analgesia administration. Someone with mental health conditions such as depression may lack the ability to reposition and require prompting.

Cognitive impairment

Cognitive impairment is defined as a deficit in at least one cognitive domain (WHO 2017). These domains include sensation and perception; motor skills and construction; attention and concentration; memory; executive functioning; processing speed; and language/verbal skills (Harvey 2019). The most common causes of cognitive impairment are dementia as well as development disorders, head injuries and substance misuse. Around 50 million people around the world suffer from a form of dementia, and of these, around 60–70% of people are diagnosed with Alzheimer's (WHO 2020c). People with Alzheimer's are vulnerable to pressure ulcers because they may have communication problems and suffer from agitation or restlessness, leading to the display of repetitive movements (Alzheimer's Society 2020). Someone with dementia including Alzheimer's is likely to have other age-related risk factors.

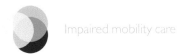

Other important risk factors

The integumentary system undergoes age-related changes causing the skin to become thinner and wound healing to slow down (Lee 2020). The skin provides an important barrier to infection, protects deeper structures from friction and other forces, plays a role in the synthesis of vitamin D and regulates temperature. The skin also acts as a moisture barrier and prevents excessive moisture loss. Age-related changes mean that the body is less able to protect itself from the effects of pressure and infection.

Medicines can be implicated in increasing the risks of the individual developing pressure ulcers. Vasopressors administered to individuals to increase contractility of the heart may lead to reduced perfusion and oxygenation of the skin. Sedative drugs, both prescribed and recreational, may render the person unable to respond to stimuli such as pressure or pain. People who have had surgery have increased risk of pressure ulcers as they are unable to react to stimuli and their mobility is restricted. People who receive nerve blocks such as an epidural analgesia for labour will have reduced sensation, are at risk of developing pressure ulcers and will need support with repositioning.

Extrinsic factors

Extrinsic factors are non-individual dependent and are the result of actions by external factors such as handling by care providers and/or interaction with the environment. This would include pressure from medical devices and furniture, the effects of shearing from sliding down a bed and friction caused by rubbing against the skin. These forces may cause traumatic damage or occlusion of the capillaries supplying the skin with oxygen and other vital nutrients and prevent the removal of waste products. The skin of incontinent individuals may be compromised by altered pH and represent a source of infection, and promotion of continence is a priority.

Box 11.7 Activity: extrinsic and intrinsic factors

Think about factors other than reduced sensation and mobility that may make people susceptible to pressure ulcers. Try to think of some extrinsic factors and some other intrinsic factors, then consult the NICE guidance in Box.11.8.

Box. 11.8 Factors contributing to pressure ulcer formation (NICE 2015a)

The following factors are risk factors for adults, neonates, children and young people according to NICE (2015a)

- significantly limited mobility (for example, people with a spinal cord injury)
- significant loss of sensation
- a previous or current pressure ulcer
- nutritional deficiency
- the inability to reposition themselves
- significant cognitive impairment

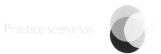

Learning outcome 3: use a pressure ulcer risk calculator to identify people at risk of pressure ulcers

The NICE (2015a) quality standard (QS89) on pressure ulcers in hospital and nursing homes recommends the use of clinical judgement and validated risk-assessment tools. Examples of these validated tools for adult individuals include the Waterlow scale, the Norton risk-assessment scale, the Braden scale, and the Braden Q scale for paediatrics (NICE 2015a). A systematic review by Moore and Patton (2019) for the Cochrane library found over 40 pressure ulcer tools in use and concluded that it might not be possible to have one pressure ulcer tool to cover all, given the diversity of individual factors and clinical care settings.

Box 11.9 Activity: ulcer risk calculators

Have you seen any pressure ulcer risk calculators used in the practice setting? If so, which ones have you seen?

Here is a selection of some that you may have seen:

The Norton score

The Norton risk-assessment score was published by Norton et al. in 1962. This score identified five separate risk factors: physical condition, mental condition, activity, mobility and incontinence. Each factor is scored from 1–4 and then totalled; the lower the score, the higher the risk of contracting a pressure ulcer. For example, a person who was in very poor physical condition, in a coma, unable to move, immobile and doubly incontinent would be given a score of 5 and deemed high risk.

The Braden Score and Braden Q Score

The Braden Score was developed by Braden and Bergstrom in 1987 for use in the adult population. It uses a similar scoring system to the Norton Scale with each factor graded 1–4 and a lower score indicates high vulnerability to pressure ulcers. The Braden Score includes factors associated with sensory perception, moisture, activity, mobility, nutrition, friction and shear. The authors considered intrinsic and extrinsic factors and focused on intensity of pressure and length of contact time, as well as tissue resilience (Braden and Bergstrom 1987). Quigley and Curley (1996) took inspiration from the Braden Score and used it to develop a paediatric version for use in a children's hospital in Boston, USA. This included a recommendation for separate algorithms for prevention of pressure ulcers and staging and managing pressure ulcers (Quigley and Curley 1996).

The Waterlow Score

The Waterlow risk-assessment card was developed for the general adult population and identifies three degrees of risk status: at risk, high risk and very high risk. The tool provides guidelines on nursing care, preventative aids and equipment, wound

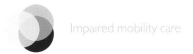

assessment and dressings (Waterlow 2005). It is widely used in the UK, sometimes in adapted forms. The developer of the tool emphasises the use of professional judgement when assessing the risk of individuals and the importance of recognising different care environments. The Waterlow risk-assessment tool is available as a poster and downloadable app from www.judy-waterlow.co.uk.

Box 11.10 Activity: Waterlow scale/pressure ulcer risk-assessment tool

Use either the Waterlow scale or the pressure ulcer risk-assessment tool used in your practice setting to assess the people in the scenarios for pressure ulcer risk.
Ask a colleague to undertake the same exercise and compare your answers. Did you both arrive at the same score for each person?

Learning outcome 4: discuss the importance of accurate documentation of pressure ulcer risk assessment.

Box 11.11 Activity: recording information

Consider why it is important to record information relating to pressure ulcer risk in nursing documentation.

The NMC code (2018) outlines the standards and behaviours expected of nurses and midwives. The section on Practising Safely states that nurses must 'keep clear and accurate records relevant to your practice' which includes assessing risk and measures undertaken to mitigate these risks (2018, p.11). According to the Royal College of Nursing (RCN), a care plan is a written document based on a template, developed with the person or for a person, and may be simple, single goal-orientated or complex (RCN 2016). The care plan is the principal means of communication between the nurses caring for an individual and the other members of a multidisciplinary team.

According to NICE (2015a) Quality Standards, individuals must have a pressure ulcer risk assessment undertaken within 6 h of admission to a care home or hospital setting, using a validated tool (such as Waterlow, Braden or Norton). Individuals including adults, young people, children, infants and neonates identified as being at risk of a pressure ulcer should have this carefully documented and an individualised care plan activated (NICE 2014a). People who have multiple risk factors for pressure ulcers and/or have a past medical history of pressure ulcers or an existing ulcer should be assessed as high risk (NICE 2014a). Even if a person is initially assessed as low risk, they should be reassessed if their clinical situation changes such as undergoing surgery (NICE 2014a). The Essence of Care (DH 2010) best practice indicator states that the plan of care should be continuously evaluated and revised to meet individual needs. If there is concern that pressure ulcers have been caused by poor practice, then this should be carefully documented according to the Safeguarding Adults Protocol: Pressure Ulcers and the Interface with a Safeguarding Enquiry (2018) in relation to Section 42 of The Care Act.

Pressure ulcers cause pain, discomfort, disablement and disfigurement and are potentially fatal for people. It is estimated that pressure ulcers cost the NHS between £1.4 and £2.1 billion per year according to the Department of Health and Social Care (2018, p.11). They are a source of complaint from individuals and relatives and may result in litigation. In 2017/2018, the NHS paid out over £20.8 million in compensation in relation to pressure ulcer care (Stephenson 2019).

PRESSURE ULCER PREVENTION

Many pressure ulcers are preventable if the correct procedures are followed and there is a growing evidence base of how to prevent them; indeed, they are a key measure of nursing care (Department of Health and Social Care 2018). Pressure ulcer prevention involves timely and effective assessment, comprehensive care plans for those at risk or high risk, effective pain management, adequate nutrition, promotion of continence and skin care, appropriate individual handling and repositioning and use of pressure-relieving devices.

Box 11.12 Learning outcomes

By the end of this session, you will be able to:

1. Explain why pressure ulcer prevention is an important aspect of the nurse's role;
2. Discuss ways of preventing pressure ulcers in people at risk.

Learning outcome 1: explain why pressure ulcer prevention is an important aspect of the nurses' role

---

Box 11.13 Activity: pressure ulcer prevention

ACTIVITY

Why is it important that pressure ulcer prevention is implemented for people identified at risk of pressure ulcers?

You may have thought of some or all of the following points:

- Pressure ulcers can have serious physical effects. They can lead to local infection, and this may develop into osteomyelitis (infection of the bone), representing a grade IV pressure ulcer, which occurs in approximately one-third of cases (Bodavula et al. 2015). These types of pressure ulcers commonly develop around the sacrum, femoral heads and the ischial bones, but osteomyelitis may be difficult to detect especially in people with neurological compromise (Bodavula et al. 2015). Individuals who develop severe pressure ulcers may require amputation of affected limb, may have their hospital stay extended, and can die of complications

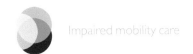

(NHS Stop the Pressure 2018). The scar tissue resulting from pressure ulcers predisposes the person to further pressure ulcers owing to the reduced tissue strength.

- Pressure ulcers can have serious psychological effects on the person. These psychological effects can be caused by discharge, odour, pain and altered body image. Discharge and the need to change dressings regularly, may reduce social opportunities while females in particular may be affected by a perceived loss of femininity (Charalambous et al. 2018). Pain, discharge and altered body image can lead to reduced mobility, confidence and independence.

- Pressure ulcers are a financial drain on the NHS with an estimated cost in the UK of £3.8 million every day (NHS Improvement 2018). The government has introduced improvements to pressure ulcer reporting via the NHS Safety Thermometer, and Serious Incidents to improve data on pressure ulcers (NHS Improvement 2018). NHS Improvement (2018) has also developed a national Stop the Pressure to disseminate recommendations to local NHS trusts on how to prevent pressure ulcers.

There are therefore many reasons why pressure ulcers must be prevented. Prevention of pressure ulcers has always been a nursing role – Florence Nightingale believed that good nursing care could prevent pressure ulcers. However, there should be a multidisciplinary team approach, with support from tissue viability nurses, physiotherapists, dietitians and doctors (Samuriwo 2012); a view also supported by The Essence of Care (DH 2010). Nevertheless, as nurses assess, plan, implement and evaluate care to meet all aspects of a person's needs, they are in a key position to minimise pressure ulcers.

Learning outcome 2: discuss ways of preventing pressure ulcers in people at risk.

Pressure ulcer prevention can take several forms. It includes maintaining and improving tissue tolerance to pressure; protection against pressure, shear and friction forces; and education of staff, individuals and carers. NHS Improvement (2017) identified five key elements in the SSKIN care bundle: surface, skin inspection, keep people moving, incontinence/moisture and nutrition/hydration.

Care bundle

A care bundle is a set of evidence-based interventions, which, used together, improve the person's outcomes.

ACTIVITY

Box 11.14 Activity: methods of pressure ulcer prevention
List some methods of pressure ulcer prevention that you have observed in practice. Consider which might be suitable for individuals in the scenario.

Surface

The surface area on which the person is in contact requires careful thought especially if they are at risk of pressure ulcers. A wide range of pressure-relieving devices have been developed to assist in protecting skin against pressure damage. The Essence of

Care benchmark for best practice recommends the use of pressure redistributing support surfaces to prevent and manage pressure ulcers (DH 2010). Specialist beds, mattresses and cushions can help relieve pressure areas by supporting vulnerable areas of the body such as the heels and sacrum and redistributing pressure more evenly (McInnes et al. 2015). Remember, it is important to check the manufacturers guidelines and check equipment regularly to ensure it is designed for the purpose intended and is in good working order.

Seat cushions

Marion and Diane spend a lot of time in their wheelchairs and need appropriate wheelchair cushions that will relieve pressure. Wheelchair cushions should fit the seat and the user; be at the right height; be stable, promote symmetrical posture and positioning and be comfortable. The EPUAP (2019) recommends that a pressure redistributing cushion should be used for wheelchair users who are at high risk of developing a pressure ulcer. Infants, children and young people should be offered frequent wheelchair assessments as well as pressure redistribution and relief systems (NICE 2014a). The seat and cushion should be carefully selected to ensure that it is compatible with the size, weight, form, posture, lifestyle factors and mobility of the individual (EPUAP 2019). If a person has developed a pressure ulcer on the sacrum/coccyx or ischia, then sitting should be minimised to 3 times a day for no more than 60 min at a time and specialist advice sought (EPUAP 2019).

Mattresses

A standard foam mattress will not be a suitable surface for Marion and may not be appropriate for Diane or John either. A systematic review for the Cochrane library recommended the use of higher specification foam mattresses instead of standard hospital mattresses to redistribute pressure and support vulnerable areas of the body as well as medical grade sheepskin (McInnes et al. 2015).

When choosing a surface, other criteria need to be considered too. Individual acceptability is very important. If the equipment is uncomfortable, increases pain or disturbs sleep, then its use must be reconsidered. Another vital consideration is effects on mobility. The goal is to increase mobility, so using a support system that reduces mobility is inappropriate. Alternating pressure systems can make it difficult for a person to get into or out of bed due to increased bed height and lack of a firm mattress edge.

Medical devices

Medical devices are believed to cause around 30% of all pressure-related injuries (Black et al. 2010). A systematic review and meta-analysis conducted by Jackson et al. (2019) found that tubing, splints, cervical collars, intravenous catheters and respiratory aids were most commonly associated with pressure damage. Oedematous individuals are particularly at risk of skin break down and pressure ulcer damage (NPIAP 2020). The oedema places additional pressure on the blood vessels that compromise oxygen, nutrient and waste transportation. The NPIAP (2020) have produced best practice guidance on preventing pressure injuries from medical devices. This involves choosing the appropriate size of medical device for the person, cushioning vulnerable areas,

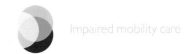

rotating and repositioning devices, daily inspections, staff education, not situating devices under the individual or damaged skin and carefully noting oedematous areas (NPIAP 2020).

Skin inspection

Comprehensive skin inspections should be undertaken as early as possible after admission or transfer, during risk assessments, whenever risk of pressure ulcer increases and before discharge (EPUAP 2019). Where possible, individuals should be asked whether they are experiencing any pain or discomfort and skin integrity should be carefully assessed in these areas as well as areas vulnerable to pressure such as bony prominences and medical devices (NICE 2014a). These inspections should look for evidence of blanchable and non-blanchable erythema, oedema, temperature and moisture levels (EPUAP 2019). Changes in colour and skin consistency should be noted also, and appropriate dressings used for wounds (NHS Modernisation 2017). Remember to carefully document any changes and use a body map to mark the location of any wounds or areas of concern.

Scanner devices

In people with darkly pigmented skin, it can be more difficult for nurses to identify non-blanching erythema. Devises such as the Sem Scanner may play a useful role in detecting pressure ulcers as it measures sub-epidermal moisture levels. These are hand-held wireless devices that scan pressure areas and provide a reading based on moisture content of the skin to a depth of around 4 mm according to the manufacturer (Provizio Sem-Scanner 2020). However, NICE (2020) have stated that although this product has potential, further randomised controlled trials are needed to demonstrate its efficacy.

Keep individuals moving

The human body is designed to move. Encouraging and assisting people to move is an important aspect of pressure ulcer prevention and management. Individuals at risk of pressure ulcers should move position at least every 2 h and independence with activities such as getting up, dressed and washed should be encouraged (NHS Improvement 2017). Nurses must ensure that they follow manual handling regulations when repositioning a person and use specialist equipment that reduce friction and shear (EPUAP 2019). Individuals should be repositioned so that weight is off loaded from bony prominences and pressure is redistributed, and reminder strategies should be employed to ensure people are repositioned frequently (EPUAP 2019).

Incontinence/moisture

There is an association between moisture and pressure ulcers. The normal pH of the skin is between 4.0 and 5.5, but the breakdown of urea in urine produces ammonia, which will increase skin pH. Frequent washing with soap can change skin pH from acidic to alkaline-causing dryness and cracking and can remove natural lipids that help to create a protective barrier. Superabsorbent incontinence pads help to keep skin dry, and faecal incontinence must be dealt with promptly. SSKIN emphasises the importance of barrier creams to prevent moisture reaching the skin, the use of continence wipes to help maintain personal hygiene, and emollients to stop skin from drying out (NHS Improvement 2017). Chapter 13 deals with this topic in more detail.

Nutrition

Nutritional status should be assessed using a screening tool such as the Malnutrition Universal Screening Tool (MUST) (British Association for Parenteral and Enteral Nutrition 2020). This tool calculates the risk of malnutrition using BMI, effects of disease and percentage weight loss of the previous 6 months. A score of two or more requires a referral to a dietician. Some people's dietary intake may need to be supplemented, particularly to increase vitamin and trace elements, as nutrition is important for maintaining skin integrity and healing. Consider referring the person with high and low BMIs as both are at risk of pressure ulcers. Underweight individuals have fewer nutritional reserves, less cushioning around bony areas such as the spine and may have thinner skin which is at risk of abrasions while people with a high BMI are less mobile, with deep folds of skin and are at risk of tissue necrosis (NHS Improvement 2017).

Pain control

Another important consideration in addition to SSKIN is pain management. Uncontrolled pain prevents people from moving, so adequate pain control is essential. Diane has tingling and burning pains in her legs, and John has chronic pain from his previous injury and acute pain from his newly fractured wrist. Marion may not be able to report pain sensations, but those who know her well may report changes in her presentation and non-verbal communication that would indicate discomfort. Nurses caring for them, in conjunction with the multidisciplinary team, must implement appropriate pain management strategies and promote their comfort. The EPUAP (2019) recommends the use of topical opioid analgesics and administration of regular pain relief to reduce pain caused by pressure ulcers. You can read about pain management strategies in Chapter 9.

ACTIVITY

Box 11.15 Activity: methods of pressure ulcer prevention you have observed in practice

List some methods of pressure ulcer prevention that you have observed in practice. Consider which might be suitable for the people in the scenarios.

Interface pressure

Interface pressure is a measurement of the amount of pressure applied to the skin. It is often used to describe properties of pressure-relieving devices such as cushions or mattresses and may be included in manufacturer's descriptions.

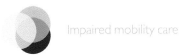

Box 11.16 Activity: local resources

In your clinical setting find out about;

- any local guidelines for pressure ulcer prevention
- whether there are locally based tissue viability specialist nurses and how they can be contacted for advice
- how pressure-relieving equipment is ordered locally

 Box 11.17 Children and young people practice points – pressure ulcer prevention

NICE (2014a) includes guidelines for preventing pressure ulcers in children as well as adults and published quality standards for both in 2015.

Anthony, D. 2017. What do we know about paediatric pressure ulcer risk assessment? Available from: www.wounds-uk.com/journals/issue/51/article-details/what-do-we-know-about-paediatric-pressure-ulcer-risk-assessment

For further reading, see

Macqueen, S., Bruce, E.A. and Gibson, F. 2012. Personal hygiene and pressure ulcer prevention. In: *The Great Ormond Street Hospital Manual of Children's Nursing Practices.* Chichester: Wiley-Blackwell. 167–220.

Summary

- Pressure ulcers can have serious consequences. They are a significant cause of pain, deformity, disability and embarrassment, and can lead to delayed discharge, infection and death.
- Appropriate assessment tools should be used to identify individuals at risk of pressure ulcers; those assessed as low risk must be reassessed again if their nursing and medical needs change.
- A care plan must be documented for those identified as being at risk of pressure ulcers, and effective measures must be taken to present pressure ulcer formation.
- Appropriate preventive measures for people at risk of pressure ulcers must be planned and carefully documented. These measures should include appropriate pressure-relieving devices, regular skin inspections, encouraging people to move, effective management of incontinence and excessive moisture, and adequate nutrition and hydration.
- Individuals/carers should be involved in decision-making processes about pressure ulcer prevention.

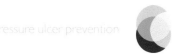

Prevention of other complications of immobility

Pressure ulcers are a significant potential problem for people with impaired mobility, but there are many other possible complications.

Box 11.18 Learning outcomes

By the end of this section, you will be able to:

1 Identify physical and psychosocial problems arising from impaired mobility;
2 Explain ways in which nurses can prevent complications of immobility.

Learning outcome 1: identify physical and psychosocial problems arising from impaired mobility

---

Box 11.19 Activity: reduced mobility

Think of people you have cared for whose mobility was reduced for some reason. They may have been confined to bed or were dependent on a wheelchair, or physical or psychological problems may have made walking difficult. What problems did their limited mobility cause them?

Compare your answers with the list of problems in Box 11.20. You may observe that immobility affects many bodily functions, as well as having psychosocial effects; this list highlights the multidimensional nature of immobility.

Box 11.20 Physical and psychosocial problems caused by reduced mobility

- Cardiovascular – deep vein thrombosis, orthostatic hypotension
- Respiratory – pneumonia, pulmonary embolism
- Gastrointestinal – loss of appetite, constipation, faecal impaction
- Urinary – renal calculi, urinary tract infection, incontinence
- Musculoskeletal – osteoporosis, muscle wasting, contractures
- Psychosocial – loss of self-esteem, depression, frustration, boredom, isolation

Adapted from: Crawford and Harris (2016).

Circulatory and respiratory problems

There are many circulatory and respiratory problems that can occur; some are discussed below.

Deep vein thrombosis (DVT): Normally, movement of the legs contracts the muscles, which press on the veins and cause them to empty. Legs that are not mobile cannot maintain this pumping action, so the venous blood pools, causing a blood clot (DVT). The blood clot or part of it may break off and travel to the lungs, causing a pulmonary embolism, which may be fatal (Waldron and Moll 2014). There are many risk factors for DVT, but increased age, obesity, active cancer, pregnancy and the puerperium, surgery, acute medical illness and fractures (particularly with plaster immobilisation of the lower limb) carry a particularly high risk (Di Nisio et al. 2016). NICE (2018a) gives further guidance on high-risk categories, but also reminds that risk should be assessed in all those admitted to hospital.

Orthostatic hypotension (when blood pressure falls on moving to an upright position) can quickly develop in people confined to bed or chair. Marion, for example, may feel faint and dizzy when she is transferred from bed to wheelchair. The act of lying down shifts 11% of the blood volume away from the legs, with most going to the chest. Normally, about 30% of circulating blood volume is in the thoracic cavity. When moving to an upright position, the effect of gravity causes a volume drop of about one-third, reducing venous return to the heart and consequently reducing blood pressure. This reduction triggers physiological responses to return the blood pressure to normal. In cases where the person has been confined to bed, these response mechanisms may be hindered by reduced blood volume from increased diuresis, reduced venous return and cardiac deconditioning reducing the effectiveness of the heart's function as a pump (Lainer et al. 2011).

Decreased cardiac output and reduced tissue perfusion related to immobility can cause venous leg ulcers, particularly if there is associated poor calf muscle function or venous incompetence (Day 2015). Leg ulcers will limit a person's mobility as standing and walking may cause pain. Wound dressings, swollen legs, leakage and the need to wear large shoes compromise mobility too and potentially increase the risk of falls (Humphreys et al. 2016).

Impaired mobility can cause *reduced ventilation of the lungs* and *reduced stimulation for coughing*, leading to a build-up of secretions in the bronchi and bronchioles, which can become infected. If the person is on bed rest, the normal lung clearing functions of the mucociliary escalator, cough reflex and drainage are compromised by the supine position increasing the risk of infection (Vollman 2010). Marion could be at risk of chest infections. Individuals with paralysis of their abdominal and intercostal muscles, for example, people with spinal cord injury, will have reduced lung ventilation affecting their ability to cough, putting them at risk of a chest infection.

Gastrointestinal problems

Impaired mobility can predispose to constipation as exercise stimulates digestion and the movement of the gastrointestinal system (Weaver 2005) and can also affect diet and fluid intake, further increasing the risk. Immobility may also cause weakening of the abdominal wall muscles, making straining and therefore defecation difficult (Kyle 2006). Immobility can impair appetite, and people with reduced mobility may find it difficult to pour out their own drinks or eat independently.

Urinary problems

Usually when toileting in the upright position, gravity assists with the position of urine in the bladder and when lying in bed, people can find it hard to empty or completely empty their bladder (Knight et al. 2019a). Reduced mobility can cause urinary stasis, which in turn can cause urinary tract infection or renal calculi (stones) and individuals with spinal cord injury are particularly at risk of developing upper urinary tract stones (Ramsey and McIlhenny 2011). People who are immobile rely on staff to take them to the toilet or provide bedpans, urinals or commodes. Impaired mobility may also cause difficulties removing or adjusting clothing, which could be an issue for all the people in this chapter's scenarios. Some people can experience incontinence due to inability to get to the toilet quickly because of impaired mobility. Having to be dependent on staff to assist with elimination can threaten dignity. Chapter 6 discusses how to assist people with going to the toilet, in a way that promotes safety and dignity.

Musculoskeletal problems

Disuse of muscles leads to atrophy and loss of muscle mass and strength. It is estimated that 12% of muscle strength can be lost each week with atrophy occurring after only 72 h of immobility, and after one week of bedrest up to 40% of muscle strength is lost (Knight et al. 2019b). The lack of muscle activity causes degenerative changes involving the release of calcium from the bones (osteoporosis), with loss of bone density. A study of 10 healthy men found that deconditioning of the muscles and bone loss occurred after 5 weeks of bedrest and was not fully reversed after 4 weeks of active weight-bearing, which highlights the importance of exercise and early mobilisation (Berg et al. 2007).

If joints remain in one position for too long, the connective-tissue collagen fibres around the joint shorten, straighten and become tightly packed. This can occur after less than 1 day and if allowed to progress, the muscles, tendons, ligaments and joint capsule become involved causing a stiff joint that is limited in its use and range of movement – this combined process causes a contracture (Knight et al. 2019b). Joints particularly at risk are the shoulders, elbows, wrists, neck, fingers, hips, knees, ankles and toes. For people with paralysed limbs, a range of positions should be adopted to discourage the development of abnormal tone and contractures (Kneafsey 2007), but Marion already has some joint deformities, and this is likely to be irreversible now. Diane has spasm in her legs, which leads to a restricted range of joint movement due to muscle shortening or contractures, and attention will need to be paid to prevent this from progressing further. Upper limb contractures reduce the ability to carry out activities of living such as showering, dressing and feeding, while lower limb contractures affect walking and increase the risk of falls, thus restricting mobility further (Clavet et al. 2008).

Immobility causes a drop in calcium levels and bone mass and density loss due to lack of skeletal loading; this is termed 'disuse osteoporosis' (Knight et al. 2019c). This causes the bones to become fragile and more prone to fracturing.

People with learning disabilities have a high risk of developing osteoporosis, and the prevalence of fractures is higher than that in the general population. This prevalence may be partly due to medication taken for epilepsy, and instability causing

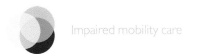

falls. There are also several other factors that contribute to this high risk, such as poor nutrition due to food spillage and low vitamin D levels due to lack of exposure to sunlight (Srikanth et al. 2011), which may apply to Marion.

Psychosocial problems

Loss of mobility can cause people to experience loss of self-esteem. Self-esteem and self-concept are made up of a person's body image, achievement, social functioning and self-identification. Knight et al. (2019c) suggest that loss of mobility affects three aspects of self:

- The achieving self – if they are unable to pursue their work or hobbies
- The social self – interactions with friends and family
- The private self – loss of independence and reliance on others

Mobility problems can also contribute to depression and social isolation. John has had impaired mobility resulting from his accident for some time, and this could have contributed to his depression. Bed rest can also lead to a decline in cognitive functions (Marusic et al. 2019) and people who live on their own or who have low social participation are more likely to experience functional disability (Nilsson et al. 2011). Diane may be frustrated that her mobility problems limit her ability to actively participate in activities with her family. Marion, would be at a similar risk but she'd have less ability to communicate/ understand any mobility issues.

Learning outcome 2: explain ways in which nurses can prevent complications of immobility

Roper et al. (2000) suggest that when planning care, the objective is to:

- prevent identified potential problems from becoming actual problems;
- solve actual problems;
- where possible, alleviate problems that cannot be solved;
- prevent reoccurrence of problems that have been resolved;
- help the person to cope positively with those problems that cannot be alleviated or solved.

Box 11.21 Activity: problems related to impaired mobility

ACTIVITY

We have identified many potential and actual problems related to impaired mobility in our three individuals. Consider the nursing interventions that could be implemented to prevent or solve these problems.

A few points that you may have considered are discussed below.

Deep vein thrombosis/pulmonary embolus

Observations for signs and symptoms of DVT (painful, swollen calf) and of pulmonary embolus (chest pain, cough) are all part of ongoing nursing assessment. NICE (2018a) provides detailed guidelines for venous thromboembolism (VTE) prevention and advice for all individuals: dehydration should be prevented, and mobility should be encouraged. Nurses, in liaison with physiotherapists, can help people with passive and active exercises of the legs. These activities help to break the cycle of immobility and increase circulation (Van Wicklin et al. 2006).

Graduated compression stockings, intermittent pneumatic compression pumps and venous foot pumps are other preventive measures; these devices enhance venous return and blood flow. When using these devices, it is essential that the correct size is chosen and that they are applied correctly and are removed only for a short time each day (Gee 2019). Anticoagulants such as heparin and/or oral anticoagulants may be prescribed for those at high risk; the NICE (2018a) guidelines for reducing the risk of VTE in people who are admitted to hospital recommend that after following risk assessment for VTE, and an assessment of bleeding risk, a decision about pharmacological prophylaxis must be made, balancing the risk of clotting with risk of bleeding.

Orthostatic hypotension

For Marion, orthostatic hypotension can be alleviated by gradually sitting her up in bed before she transfers into her chair. Marion's carers should be aware of the signs and symptoms of orthostatic hypotension as Marion may not be able to verbally communicate if she feels dizzy. It is also important to explain to Marion what is happening to reduce any anxiety relating to these symptoms.

Chest infection

Frequent repositioning and encouragement to do deep breathing exercises can help to prevent chest infection. The person can also be encouraged to cough to clear secretions and prevent them pooling in the lungs. Chapter 14 has a section on observation of sputum, which includes tips on how to encourage expectoration of sputum.

Loss of appetite and constipation

An adequate fluid and diet intake should be provided, taking individual preferences into account and ensuring that sufficient fibre is included. A persons' food and drinks should be positioned so that they can reach them. An individual with hemiplegia needs be provided with a non-slip mat to prevent the plate moving, a plate guard to help keep the food on the plate, and an appropriate cup for drinking from. John's dominant arm is in plaster, making it difficult to cut up his food, so he may need help. People with profound learning and multiple physical disabilities, like Marion, may have difficulty with eating and drinking; carers should aim to enhance the quality of their mealtime experience. Chapter 5 has more detail about these issues.

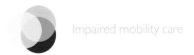
Urinary tract infection and incontinence

People who are at risk of urinary tract infection should be observed for signs such as cloudy, foul-smelling urine. Chapter 6 has a section on urinalysis and explains how urinary tract infection might be suspected and when a specimen of urine should be sent for microscopy, culture and sensitivity. Marion would require continence aids, but consideration must be given to body image, comfort and skin care and as to how continence can be promoted, rather than only contained. People with impaired mobility (e.g. after a stroke) should be positioned within a short walking distance from the toilet when they start to mobilise. People who are confused may need guidance with orientating to where the toilet is located. Diane will need to learn how to manage a suprapubic catheter as blockage, leakage and infection can be a problem. Chapter 6 explores these issues and will help you to develop your skills to assist people who need help with elimination.

Muscle wasting and contractures

As muscle contraction increases, joint movement becomes further limited, which is an issue for Marion and Diane. People with profound learning disabilities who are immobile are particularly at risk of developing deformities. Diane's spasms can be helped by careful positioning. Pillows or wedges positioned under the legs to put them in flexion can reduce extensor and adductor spasm (Pellatt 2007). Splints may be prescribed, and physiotherapy and occupational therapy play an important role in preventing contractures.

Botulinum toxin can be used to reduce muscle tone and increase the range of movements in a joint. It can be targeted to individual muscles (Gibbon 2002). Antispasmodic drugs such as baclofen can be used to reduce spasm. However, some spasm can help maintain blood circulation and aid transfers and walking, by acting as a splint to limbs, so treatment of spasticity should be selected carefully and regularly reviewed to maintain function (Thompson et al. 2005).

Loss of self-esteem, frustration, boredom and isolation

As discussed in Chapter 1, how nurses carry out care may affect how people feel about themselves. A caring and empathetic approach from nurses can assist in reducing the psychosocial effects of impaired mobility. Chapter 2 looks at the approach of nurses when carrying out practical skills and emphasises self-awareness. Family and friends have an important role in providing support too.

Box 11.22 Pregnancy and birth: practice points – VTE risk and prevention

Although most are active and mobile, some pregnant or recently delivered mothers may have impaired mobility due to prolonged epidural anaesthesia, caesarean birth or coexisting debilitation, for example, pelvic girdle pain (PGP) or spinal injury. A significant risk for these mothers is VTE. If these factors are compounded by additional risks such as obesity, high maternal age, excessive blood loss/blood transfusion, multiple pregnancy or pre-eclampsia, then the risk increases significantly. All pregnant mothers, even those who have had a recent miscarriage or ectopic pregnancy should be risk assessed and have ongoing risk assessments as to whether they require VTE prophylaxis. This usually consists of avoidance of dehydration, mobilisation, antiembolic stockings) and pharmacological management (NICE 2018a).

Not all mothers will require all of these and there is some helpful guidance by the Royal College of Obstetricians and Gynaecologist in the green top guideline 37a. Available from: www.rcog.org.uk/en/guidelines-research-services/guidelines/gtg37a/

For further reading about PGP, see www.pelvicpartnership.org.uk

Summary

- People who have reduced mobility are at risk of several physical and psychosocial complications.
- Nurses have an important role in identifying potential complications and implementing preventive care.

Key principles of moving and handling

During the course of their treatment and care, many individuals may require assistance with moving themselves; whether this is required and how much help they need may change over time. For example, Diane does not currently need help with moving, but if her condition deteriorates, this situation may change. While the focus in this chapter is on the safety, comfort and dignity of the person, it is also important that carers are protected from harm. All moving and handling including individual handling practice is governed by both legislation and NHS trust policies. To ensure the safety of both the person and of themselves and their colleagues, the principles of safe handling must be learned by all nurses. Smith's (2011) Guide to the Handling of People is a very useful resource for safe handling of individuals and should be available in your organisation.

Box 11.23 Learning outcomes

By the end of this section, you will be able to:

1. Conduct a moving and handling risk assessment.
2. Identify barriers to mobilising/assisting to move a person.
3. Identify appropriate equipment for a specific individual's needs.
4. Discuss the importance of communication when handling a person.
5. Explain the legal implications of handling an individual.

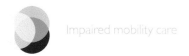
Learning outcome 1: conduct a moving and handling risk assessment

Box 11.24 Activity: moving and handling assessment tools

Find out about the moving and handling assessment tools in use in your clinical area.

When you are in a practice setting, you will see moving and handling assessment tools being used for carrying out and documenting a systematic assessment. They can vary between organisations but are likely to include sections relating to task, individual capability, load and environment (as outlined in the Manual Handling Operations Regulations 1992) along with the equipment used. This is sometimes referred to by the acronym TILEE (or ELITE). Some considerations for each of these elements are outlined below:

Task. What exactly is the activity to be carried out? What needs to be moved from where to where? Does it really need to be done? Is there an alternative? How many people are needed to carry out the task? What elements of the activity does the person need help with?

Individual capability. This is about you and the others carrying out the task. Registered nurses are responsible for their own health (NMC 2018) and need to assess their own ability in terms of physical fitness and whether they have the required knowledge and skills. You need to ensure you have attended suitable and sufficient training before carrying out individual handling tasks. Other things that need to be considered are whether the handler is wearing suitable clothing, whether any special strength is required and whether they have a pre-existing injury.

Environment. Is there enough room for you, the individual, other staff members as well as any equipment used, to work in and to maintain a safe posture? Is the area free from obstacles? Is the flooring in good condition? Slippery floors are a danger for people like Diane and John who have difficulty walking or who are unsteady on their feet. Is the floor suitable for the equipment being used? For example, carpets can stop a hoist from moving smoothly. Are there noise levels which would impede members of team hearing the instructions?

Equipment. What is required, how and when should it be used and is it available? Has it been appropriately checked? Is the equipment acceptable to the person?

   If people cannot move themselves independently, then equipment is likely to be required. You will be able to practise using different equipment and techniques in your moving and handling practical training sessions. The Moving and Handling of People; An Illustrated Guide (Ruszala 2010) is a pictorial guide to equipment and techniques, but it is not a substitute for having the opportunity to practise using the equipment in a safe environment. Equipment will be discussed further in Learning Outcome 3.

Load. The load in this case is the individual. How much can people do by themselves? Do they have the ability to co-operate?

When the load is a person, there are many factors that will need to be considered; these may affect them as a load and their ability to mobilise/ participate in the moving and handling task.

A person who is generally fit and has no communication problems, with support and training, may eventually be able to transfer from bed to wheelchair using a lateral transfer board. Marion, although not particularly heavy, is unable to move and therefore needs a hoist to move her out of bed. Those who know Marion well will be able to identify risks such as sudden unexpected movement or specific aids required.

If a person is in pain, they will be reluctant or unable to help, so pain relief is vital before the move is carried out and proper handling techniques will help to reduce pain.

Learning outcome 2: identify barriers to mobilising/assisting to move a person

Box 11.25 Activity: barriers to mobilisation

What factors about a person may pose a risk when moving and handling them or present a barrier to mobilisation? Think particularly about the people in the scenarios.

Some possible answers are given below but there are many more you may have included in your answer.

Pain: this could be from their medical condition or after surgery. Pain or fear of pain can prevent someone from mobilising, and this is an important issue for John. Therefore, pain must be assessed and controlled (Kneafsey 2007). Read more about pain assessment and control in Chapter 9.

Medical condition: many conditions can impact on balance, posture and strength; examples include multiple sclerosis and Parkinson's disease. In such cases, it is important that any associated medication is administered regularly, ensuring it is given before mobilisation is attempted.

Fatigue: this can be a common symptom of some medical conditions, including multiple sclerosis (Swann 2006) or could occur following surgery or illness. The person may experience an overwhelming feeling of exhaustion in response to minor exertion. Diane is able to walk with sticks sometimes but needs a wheelchair when she becomes severely fatigued.

Mental health: many mental health conditions and behaviours could affect mobilisation. A lack of motivation or reduced cognitive function, perhaps where people have depression or dementia, may lead to reluctance to mobilise (Swann 2006). It may take longer to assist these individuals with a moving and handling task, and some may present with challenging behaviour. John's depression could therefore present a further barrier to his mobilisation.

Foot problems: this can include ingrowing toenails, corns and bunions. Foot problems can impede mobility (Soliman and Brogan 2014); additionally, many foot problems can make it difficult to wear normal shoes, but unsuitable footwear also makes mobilising difficult and dangerous (Woodrow et al. 2005).

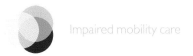

Falls/Fear of falling: if a person is worried about falling and/or is prone to falls, then this may lead to them becoming reluctant to mobilise. A full falls risk assessment (see later in the chapter) needs to be completed and interventions implemented to reduce the risk. When a person, like John, has already had one fall causing a significant injury, fear of another fall and a lack of confidence in mobilising are understandable.

Muscle tone: both increased and decreased tone can affect the person's ability to mobilise. High muscle tone, often a result of certain medical conditions including multiple sclerosis, can prevent a full range of movement (Swann 2006). This will impact on the moving, handling and positioning for both Diane and Marion.

Weight: a person who is significantly overweight (often referred to as bariatric or plus size) may require specialist equipment for all aspects of care and more carers to assist with moving and handling tasks. This client group is discussed further later in the chapter.

Getting dressed: a national campaign #endPJparalysis worked on the principle that getting people out of bed, dressed and moving would promote recovery and length of stay (Somerville et al. 2020). This will in turn reduce the risk of loss of muscle strength during their stay and improve privacy and dignity (Mckew 2017).

Learning outcome 3: identify appropriate equipment for individual needs

Box 11.26 Activity: equipment commonly used in your clinical area

What handling equipment is commonly in use in your clinical area?

If you are working in a clinical area that has very dependent individuals, you may have a wide range of equipment available. Hignett (2003) suggests that the minimum equipment list for a clinical environment where handling activities occur on a regular basis includes hoists, stand aids, sliding sheets, lateral transfer boards, walking belts and height-adjustable beds. Even within these broad categories, equipment manufacturers and usage can vary so be sure to familiarise yourself with the equipment used within your practice area, ask if you are not sure and do not use equipment you are not familiar with and have not been trained to use.

Nurses will need to use a hoist to move Marion from a height-adjustable bed to wheelchair and back. They will also need to use a sliding sheet to move her around in bed. You may be working in an area where people are mostly independent – such as an acute mental health unit – but staff must have access to equipment if it becomes necessary and staff must keep their skills up to date. For example, if John falls and is unable to get himself up from the floor, a hoist will be needed. Some people will have equipment designed for their particular needs and this must be sourced for safe practice.

In children and young people's nursing, the same principles apply even though the "load" (the individual) may be smaller. Poor posture can give rise to musculoskeletal pain, so it is important to ensure you are working at a suitable height and adopt approaches that minimise the high-risk manoeuvres such as twisting, stooping and repetition (Health and Safety Executive 2020). You should ensure you familiarise yourself with the local risk-assessment tool/procedures in place. For further information about moving and handling risk assessments for children, please see the article by Johnstone and Owen (2017).

Learning outcome 4: discuss the importance of communication when handling a person

Box 11.27 Activity: handling manoeuvres

Why is it important to communicate with your colleagues and people involved in handling manoeuvres?

When moving and handling, both the person and the carers are working as a team. It is imperative that a single person leads and coordinates the activity. All participants, including the individual, need to know exactly what to expect and what their role is (Green 2012). The team leader must communicate the command to the team, check that everyone is ready and give the command clearly (e.g. '*Ready … Steady … Move*') so that the manoeuvre is smooth and coordinated.

Learning outcome 5: explain the legal implications of handling an individual

Box 11.28 Activity: legal implications

Identify some possible legal implications of handling a person.

The focus of this chapter is on the care of the people in relation to their immobility; however, it must be acknowledged that there are multiple pieces of legislation related to moving and handling that focus on the health and safety of the carers carrying out the moving and handling procedure, for example the Health and Safety at Work Act 1974 and Manual Handling Operations Regulations 1992. These are summarised clearly by Tofts and Arnold (2012).

The law relating to protecting the person include common law that imposes a duty of care on health and social care staff to take reasonable steps to avoid acts or omissions that are likely to cause foreseeable harm (Sturman and Varnham 2019) as well as elements of the Human Rights Act (1998), including article 3, prohibition of torture, for example hoisting someone against their will.

Poor moving and handling practice has implications for the persons safety. Moving someone in bed without using appropriate equipment can cause a risk of tearing or causing friction burns to persons' skin (Thompson and Jevon 2009). The 'drag lift' (whereby nurses hook their arms under the person's armpits and drag them up the bed, or on to their feet from sitting) can cause bruising, fractures or dislocation of shoulders; this can be considered as abuse with associated legal consequences (Pellatt 2005).

Box 11.29 Children and young people practice points: moving and handling

Key principles of assessment, use of correct techniques and selection of appropriate equipment should be applied when moving and handling children across the age range just as it would for adults. There are paediatric sizes and child-friendly versions of the equipment available, for example, hoist slings and slide sheets.

The National Back Exchange publication Manual Handling of Children (Alexander and Johnson 2011) focuses on the physical handling of children in the community; however, the practical guidance can be used to guide the approach used in hospital and facilitate continuity of care from home to hospital and back again.

Summary

- A risk assessment must be carried out before any moving and handling activity takes place to protect both the individual and the carers.
- It is important that appropriate handling equipment is available for individuals where it is required.
- Handling requires teamwork that includes the person being moved.
- Using inappropriate handling techniques compromises safety and can have legal consequences.
- Nurses should be aware of barriers to mobilisation so that they can be addressed.

Moving, turning and positioning individuals

Assisting with mobility is an important role of nurses in many settings and involves overcoming barriers and working closely with the multidisciplinary team, particularly physiotherapists and occupational therapists.

Box 11.30 Learning outcomes

By the end of this section, you will be able to:

1 Identify a range of movements that a person may need assistance with;
2 Discuss how people can be assisted to complete these moves;
3 Identify barriers to mobilisation.

There are a range of moving and handling tasks you may need to consider for the individual. Each one needs to be assessed to ascertain whether your person can complete this independently or whether they need assistance – and then to establish the most appropriate technique and/or equipment for the individual.

The multidisciplinary approach helps to ensure high quality, personalised care. For example, the orthotist can supply walking sticks for Diane, and callipers, adapted shoes or knee braces, may overcome some of the barriers to mobility. Physiotherapists will assess people for mobility aids such as crutches, or walking frames, both standard or wheeled for people who cannot lift a standard frame, and the use of gutter frames to help people with arthritis.

Learning outcome 1: identify a range of movements a person may needs assistance with

Box 11.31 Activity: movements in daily life

Make a list of the movements a person might need to make in the course of a normal day.

ACTIVITY

A basic range of tasks might include:

- Moving within the bed
- Lying to lying
- Lying to sitting
- Sitting to standing
- Walking
- Standing transfer
- Sitting transfer.

Learning outcome 2: discuss how people can be assisted with mobilisation

Box 11.32 Activity: assisting with mobilisation

Focus on the practice scenarios and identify strategies and equipment that might assist with mobilisation.

ACTIVITY

Each section below outlines a range of ways you could approach assisting a person to accomplish each task. You must consult the patient's moving and handling risk assessment before attempting any moving and handling procedure. Where equipment is identified, remember to always check the safe working load (SWL) and that the equipment is in good working condition. These descriptions are to give an indication of the range of methods available and are not a substitute for attending practical moving and handling training.

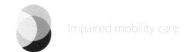

Moving within the bed

Independent: The person can be given equipment to help them move themselves within the bed. This could include a bed ladder, hand blocks and slide sheets, which, when under the individual, allow them to glide up the bed. This level may be sufficient for Diane, to allow her to maintain her independence where possible.

Rolling an individual: This is a fundamental moving and handling task that is required for many of the other techniques in this section, as well as for basic hygiene, pressure areas checks and changing of the bed sheets.

Guided: Ask the person to turn their head towards you, ensure the arm closest to you is away from the body, ask them to reach the other arm towards you, bending their far knee and pushing with the foot and reach towards you on the command *Ready, Steady, Roll*.

Assisted: As above but stand facing the individual in a walk stance (one foot in front of the other). Place a hand on their shoulder and hip but do not grip hold of them. On the command *Ready, Steady, Roll*, transfer your weight backwards as the person attempts to push with their foot and reach with their hand as above.

Dependent: You will need at least two carers. Start in the same position as above as far as the individual can manage. This time the carer on the far side will place their hands on the person's hip and shoulder as well. On the command *Ready, Steady, Roll* the carer on the far side will push, while the carer on the near side pulls using weight transfer from one foot to the other to provide the power behind the move. Marion will need at least two carers to help her roll, possibly more due to her joint deformities and frailness.

Slide sheets: The rolling techniques above can be used to place slide sheets under the individual. Slide sheets are made from low friction material used in two layers so one surface moves smoothly and easily on the other. Once the slide sheets are under the person, they can then be used to move the individual in a variety of ways, most usually to reposition them up the bed. During your practical moving and handling session, you will be shown a variety of ways to insert, use and remove slide sheets.

Lying to lying: A lying to lying transfer would be used for example when moving a person from a bed onto a trolley, for example, if Marion needed to attend theatre or for an X-ray. Using the rolling technique described above a transfer sheet is inserted underneath the individual, at the same time placing a full length lateral transfer board partially under them (make sure their head is on the board). The trolley is brought up alongside the bed on the same side as the transfer board allowing it to act as a bridge between the bed and the trolley. The carers on the bed side place their hands on the person ready to push and the carers on the trolley side grasp the transfer sheet handles assuming a walk stance. On the command *Ready, Steady, Slide*, the carers transfer the individual by the bed side, carers pushing and the trolley slide carers transferring their weight from their front legs to the back legs to slide the person towards them. This may take more than one manoeuvre.

Lying to sitting: In many healthcare settings, the use of electric profiling beds is now widespread. A key feature is that they electronically raise and lower the headrest, making many moving and handling procedures much safer and easier for both person and staff. Sitting a person up in bed can now be achieved using the electric profiling bed, and Diane and John could use the controls to reposition themselves.

Where there is no electric profiling bed available, or where a person is being encouraged to become independent in the task perhaps; ready for discharge home, other approaches can be considered.

These techniques require the individual to have sitting balance and to be able to participate in the activity.

Guided activity: John may be able to achieve this himself – consideration should be given to selecting which side he gets out of bed based on his fractured wrist; he could be guided by taking him through the steps required. Think about how you get out of bed yourself and ask him to do the same. Get him to roll onto his side in the bed bringing both legs out over the edge of the bed. As he swings his legs down, he pushes himself from the bed. Manual assistance can be given from one or two carers if required.

Assisted activity: using a bed ladder – a piece of equipment that is anchored to the bottom of the bed and the person pulls themselves up by grabbing one handle after another until they are in a sitting position.

Dependent individual: if the person cannot participate and there is no electric bed available, then the safest alternative is to use a hoist and sling to sit the person up in bed.

Sitting to standing (ready to walk)

Guided activity: Encourage the individual to assume a ready to stand position – place their feet one in front of the other and lean forward slightly (nose over toes). Their hands should be on the arms of the chair ready to push up. Recommend they rock themselves backwards and forwards to gain momentum and then push themselves into a standing position.

Assisted activity: one or two carers, with or without handling belt (a device applied around the person's waist with handles for carers to hold onto, see Figure 11.1). The carer(s) take on a walk stance at the side of the person, reach across the individual's back and hold the handle on the far side of the person or resting their hands on the individual's opposite hip. The carers' free hand then rests at the front of the person's shoulder. As in the guided activity, encourage or assist the person into position ready for standing. Explain what will happen next and co-ordinate the move, by giving the command *Ready, Steady, Stand* rocking on the words ready and steady and standing with the person on stand. There may be times when Diane needs this level of assistance even though she may normally achieve it independently.

Dependent individual: not applicable

Walking: Once the person is up on their feet using one of the previous techniques, give them enough time to stabilise their balance before continuing. If using a walking frame, place this in front of them now.

Prompt the individual to look forward (and not at their feet). If not using a frame, to make them feel secure, you can keep your hand on their shoulder or support at the elbow or hand; if supporting with the hand, ensure that your thumb is NOT interlinked with that of the individual.

Stand beside them, facing forward so you both move the same way; this is where a handling belt around the person's waist can give you something to hold. If on your own, consider which side of the person to stand on. For example, if someone has a slight weakness on the left side, you stand at their left side in a walk stance, with your right hand holding the belt around their waist, and their left hand placed on your left hand (Figure 11.1). You can now maintain this hold to give the person confidence to walk.

A very important aspect is not to hurry the person, maintaining a slow steady pace. It is important that you have assessed how long the person is able to stand, how far they can walk and if these abilities fluctuate (Chadwick 2010). Consider use of a chair or wheelchair behind them in case they need to sit down, especially with Diane who is known to need one on occasions.

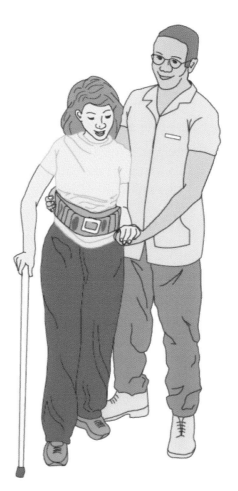

Figure 11.1: Helping a person walk.

Standing transfer: Where the individual cannot take some steps once standing, the techniques above cannot be used and, as long as the person can maintain a standing position, a standing transfer may be suitable.

Assisted activity higher ability: using a standing turner device. These devices have a footplate and a long handle. As well as sitting balance and the ability to follow instructions clearly, the person must have good arm and leg strength to use this equipment as, once their feet are on the footplate, they reach up to the handle and pull themselves into a standing position. The carer can then turn the device on the spot so that the person can sit down in a second location (e.g., from bed to chair). There are some specialised versions of this device that can also be used to transport the individual a short distance.

Assisted activity lower ability: using a standing hoist (active hoist). For this transfer, the person needs some weight-bearing ability and some ability to co-operate with instructions. The standing sling is applied to the individual ensuring it is in good condition, it fits, and it is comfortable. The person's feet are assisted onto the foot platform and their knees bent so that the shins are in contact with the pads; apply the brakes. The sling is attached to the hoist and checked. The carer raises the hoist up until the person is high enough for the transfer to be completed. Remove the brakes, turn the standing hoist to the new location, leave the brakes off and lower the person onto the new surface. If Diane's mobility deteriorates further, this may become a more suitable option for her.

Sitting Transfer: Where a person cannot stand as described in the sections above, to move for example from the bed to the chair, there are alternative approaches.

Guided/assisted/independent activity: using a transfer board (sometimes called a banana board). Transfer boards enable people with upper body balance stability to transfer independently or with minimal assistance from one seated position to another (Chadwick 2010). This board is often curved and is placed between the two surfaces (for example, the bed and the chair). The individual slides along the board bridging the gap between the two surfaces. This can be assisted with by a carer and possibly a handling belt if required.

Dependent individual: where the person does not have the ability to use the transfer board, then it is likely they will need hoisting with a full body hoist (passive hoist). This technique can be used with a fully dependent individual such as Marion. You must be familiar with the specific type of hoist and sling. Different manufacturers have different attachment styles (loop and clip), and it is imperative that the sling is correctly sized and fitted for the individual as well as being compatible with the hoist used. Hoists must be checked under Lifting Operations and Lifting Equipment Regulations (LOLER 1998) to ensure they are fit for use.

Once the sling has been correctly applied to the individual, it is then attached to the hoist. Leaving the brakes off, raise the boom of the hoist to the level where the task can be safely completed and then carefully turn the hoist around to the new surface and gently lower the person onto the new surface.

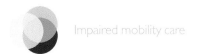

In all cases you should only use equipment you have been trained to use, following the recommendations in the moving and handling assessment.

Summary

- There are lots of moving and handling tasks that individuals may need assistance with.
- Moving and handling risk assessments are necessary before carrying out these tasks.
- Nurses work as a key member of the multidisciplinary team in managing and facilitating mobilisation.
- Nurses should have an understanding of a range of equipment and techniques to meet the variety of individual needs.
- Nurse must attend suitable practical moving and handling training before attempting moving and handling tasks to protect both the individual and themselves.

PREVENTING FALLS

Box 11.33 Learning outcomes

By the end of this section, you will be able to:

1 Consider a range of risk factors for falls;
2 Examine ways of preventing falls.

Falls in older people cost the NHS 2.3 billion a year (NICE 2013). However, people in other age groups like Diane and John are at risk of falls as well. In-hospital falls are the most reported safety incident, numbering at least 235,000 a year, with many more going unreported and 3,000 of these falls result in a hip fracture or brain injury (NHS England & NHS Improvement 2019). It is unsurprising therefore that there are ongoing initiatives to reduce these figures. The effects of falls extend beyond cost and the pain and distress of the physical injury, as a subsequent lack of confidence and development of a fear of falling has the potential to limit an individual's mobility and therefore their independence, resulting in functional decline and dependency further increasing their risk of falling (McCarter-Bayer et al. 2005) and increasing the chance of them being unable to return home.

Learning outcome 1: consider a range of risk factors for falls

There are more than 400 risk factors that are associated with falls (NICE 2015b) and the risk increases further where more risks are present.

The WHO (2007) identified that fall risk factors can be grouped into four main categories:

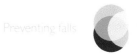

- **Biological**: can include anything relating to the body, from age and gender through to changes due to ageing or co-morbidity associated with chronic illnesses. These usually cannot be changed.
- **Behavioural**: includes risk associated with our actions, emotions or choices and are potentially modifiable.
- **Environmental**: relates to the interplay of the person's physical conditions with the surrounding environment, such as hazards in the home, the outside world or within the hospital.
- **Socioeconomic**: involves the influence of social conditions and the economic status of individuals on the likelihood of falling.

ACTIVITY

Box 11.34 Activity: people who have fallen

Think of people you have looked after who have fallen. Make a list of the reasons why they fell and then group these risk factors into groups based on the categories above.
Your list might have included the following:

Biological

- **Vision:** Visual impairment is when a person's vision is too poor to carry out everyday tasks and is a major risk factor for falls (Windsor and Dix 2017). Poor vision can be due to age-related deterioration or other visual problems (Lyons 2005). Cataracts, glaucoma, diabetic retinopathy, hemianopia and macular degeneration could all increase a person's risk of falling by altering their perception of the environment. People may trip over objects in the dark, trip on carpets or uneven floors or miss stairs and fall.
- **Cognitive impairment:** For example, dementia can cause cognitive impairment, memory loss and confusion, all of which may contribute to the danger of falling (Chaâbane 2007). We will explore dementia and mobility later in the chapter.
- **Balance and gait:** Poor mobility with age-related changes in gait, posture and balance. Neurological diseases cause motor and sensory impairment; for example, Parkinson's disease causes people to stoop, lean forward and develop a short-stepped, shuffling gait. Multiple sclerosis causes gait problems due to spasm, and motor and sensory changes, and this will impact on Diane's risk levels. Diabetic neuropathy may cause decreased sensation in legs and feet. Stroke affects mobility and balance (Lyons 2005).
- **Loss of muscle strength and flexibility**. Loss of muscle strength and flexibility can cause difficulty in holding handrails or getting out of chairs and walking (Kneafsey 2007).
- **Changes in the inner ear.** Inner-ear changes can affect a person's sense of balance and an ear infection could increase the risk of falling (Nazarko 2015).
- **Problems with bladder and bowels**. Falls can result from lack of bladder or bowel control, such as with urge incontinence (McCarter-Bayer et al. 2005).

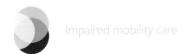

Behavioural

- **Psychosocial factors:** Fear of falling is a real anxiety and can result in physical symptoms such as nausea (While 2020a). Fear increases with age and is more common in women; a previous fall is not necessary to trigger this fear (Halvarsson et al. 2011).
- **Medication:** Medications and alcohol can cause dizziness, hypotension, blurred vision, weakness, poor balance and drowsiness (Jasniewski 2006). John's medication for his depression could have these effects. Diuretics and laxatives increase the number of trips to the toilet, often in a hurry. Taking more than four different medicines, particularly sedating or blood pressure lowering medicines, is a predisposing factor in falls (Anderson 2008).
- **Footwear:** Suitable supportive footwear with a large surface-area contact can reduce fall risk (Swann 2014) as well as ensuring that shoes or slippers are correctly fitting. Fall risk also increases when walking barefoot (Borland et al. 2013).

Environmental

- **Mobility aids:** Mobility aids are used to decrease the risk of falls; however, they are often left out of persons' reach, resulting in people being unable to mobilise or at increased risk of falling (Bolwell et al. 2016).
- **Unsafe home/hospital environment:** examples of hazards include obstacles on the floor, wet floors, poor lighting, broken call bells, all of which could increase the risk of falling (Nazarko 2012).

Socioeconomic

- Older people with lower economic status, especially those who are female, live alone or in rural areas face an increased risk of falls (WHO 2007).

Learning outcome 2: examine ways of preventing falls

Older people are more likely to fall (NICE 2018b) and rather than use risk prediction tools (which have been found to be inaccurate). NICE 2013 gave a recommendation that any person aged 65 or over, where there has been a fall or a history of falls, should have a multifactorial risk assessment completed (this guideline is under review in 2020). The guideline also states that people aged 50–64 admitted to hospital and considered to be at higher risk of falling because of an underlying condition are also covered by the recommendations. This multifactorial assessment should include a discussion about falls history, checks on gait, balance, mobility and muscle weakness, assessment of osteoporosis risk, perceived functional ability and fear of falling, eyesight check, neurological and cognitive functioning examinations, discussion about continence and home hazards, cardiovascular examination and a review of medication.

All nurses should understand risk factors for falls and be aware of the falls service within their area and how referrals are made.

Box 11.35 Activity: how falls can be prevented

Think of how falls can be prevented for people who are identified as being at risk.

Commissioning for Quality and Innovation (CQUINs) require trusts to demonstrate improvement in a specified area of care, and in 2019, a Preventing Hospital Falls CQUIN was introduced to encourage trusts to focus their improvement efforts on the delivery of three high-impact actions for falls prevention in hospital (NHS England and NHS Improvement 2019). These were:

- **Lying and standing blood pressure**, as a drop in blood pressure on standing (orthostatic hypotension) is a common occurrence in acutely unwell hospitalised individuals and is a risk factor for falls (Windsor et al. 2016).
- **No hypnotics or antipsychotics or anxiolytics** given during stay OR rationale for giving hypnotics or antipsychotics or anxiolytics documented, as falls are associated with polypharmacy and psychotropic drug use.
- **Mobility assessment documented within 24 h** of admission to the inpatient unit identifying if walking aid required or not, and walking aid provided within 24 h of admission if required, as a lack of suitable mobility aid increases the risk of falling.

Additionally, the following interventions can be effective in preventing falls:

- Call bell within reach
- Suitable footwear
- Muscle strengthening, gait and balance training and exercise (Halvarsson et al. 2011)
- Home hazard assessment and modifications such as handles and rails to a person's home (While 2020b)
- Review and possible withdrawal of medications where appropriate (Anderson 2008)
- Cardiac pacing where appropriate (NICE 2013)
- Full eye examination and ensure wearing glasses appropriately (Windsor and Dix 2017)
- Continence management (Anderson 2008)
- Hip protectors may be provided to prevent hip fractures in older people who have a high risk of falling; research evidence to support this function is equivocal (Parker et al. 2006).

There is some evidence to suggest that Tai Chi exercises may help to prevent falls by improving balance and improve muscle and cardiorespiratory strength and fitness (Halvarsson et al. 2011).

For detailed guidance on preventing falls, including falls in hospital, see NICE (2013).

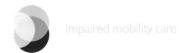

Summary

- Nurses should be aware of the risk factors for falls and ensure a multifactorial risk assessment is completed where appropriate.
- Nurses should be aware of key interventions to prevent falls and ensure they are implemented.
- Nurses should be aware of how to access the fall prevention service for their organisation.

Moving and handling of specific client groups

> **Box 11.36 Learning outcomes**
>
> By the end of this section, you will be able to:
>
> 1 Consider the specific needs of a person with dementia when assisting with moving and handling tasks;
> 2 Identify strategies to assist when moving and handling people who are bariatric (plus size).

Learning outcome 1: consider the specific needs of a person with dementia when assisting with moving and handling tasks

The number of people diagnosed and living with dementia-related illnesses in increasing and there are currently around 850,000 people in the UK with dementia (Alzheimer's Society 2017).

Dementia is an umbrella term for a range of conditions affecting the brain and the different types can affect people in different ways and therefore the approach to supporting them with their mobility. Common symptoms include difficulty in communicating, memory loss, lack of orientation to time and place, visual difficulties, mood changes and mobility issues. This section identifies some key points to consider when assessing and assisting a person with dementia for mobility activities.

Often people with dementia demonstrate 'challenging behaviour', that is behaviour that makes it difficult to provide safe care; this needs to be acknowledged and assessed as part of the moving and handling risk assessment prior to assisting with mobility. The potential for unmet needs such as pain, anxiety, hunger, thirst and the need for the toilet should be considered and addressed before commencing mobilisation as it may affect their behaviour and co-operation.

Promoting mobility in people with dementia has physiological, psychological and social benefits (Jootun and Pryde 2013), but restoring or minimising loss of mobility in people with dementia is challenging. Logsdon et al. (2005) suggest an activity programme that uses both behavioural and exercise strategies. These strategies are enjoyable and help to improve physical and emotional health.

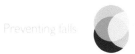

Varnham (2011) and Sturman and Varnham (2019) identify some general tips for practical manual handling tasks with the person with dementia:

Visual cues – approach from the front so they are not startled, make good eye contact and smile as you approach; standing to the side will keep their line of vision clear and maintain safety from grabbing. Use gestures to show how you want them to move and place mobility aids so that the person can see them.

Verbal cues – keep your face level with theirs; using their preferred name clearly state what you are going to do and what you expect them to do; keep each step simple and use a calm and reassuring tone.

Touch cues – ensure you have their consent to use touch, touch can cue the direction of movement, guide the person with your own body movements. Touch and hand massage may reduce agitated behaviour.

Sound cues – this can be used to attract their attention and show the direction of movement, for example, patting on the bed surface to direct them.

Equipment and environment – reduce background noise, have enough space and remove obstacles, and ensure adequate lighting.

People with dementia: walking and moving about

Box 11.37 Activity: dementia care

ACTIVITY

Reflect on situations where you have been caring for a person with dementia in hospital. Were there any issues related to their moving about the ward? If so, how have you dealt with these?

Alzheimer's Society (2009) identified that nurses experienced difficulties regarding people with dementia walking and moving about in a hospital setting, for example, trying to leave the ward. Alzheimer's Society (2019) has since developed some guidance for carers to help the person to walk safely as well as suggesting reasons for them walking, some of which are summarised below in Box 11.38.

As an example, in a study of students' experiences of caring for people with dementia in hospital, a student nurse explained how a man with dementia who was a former naval captain, kept packing his bags and attempting to leave the ward to 'go to sea' (Baillie et al. 2012, p. 23). The student engaged him in conversation about the navy:

He started telling me about all the ports and places he'd been what he had done during his service.

The student found that he then calmly walked with her back to his bed to continue the conversation.

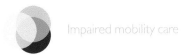

Box 11.38 Moving and walking about for people with dementia

- People with dementia can experience problems with orientation, which are increased in unfamiliar environments such as hospital wards.
- Try to understand why the person wishes to walk about so that you can find ways of meeting their needs. It is essential to help people with dementia maintain their independence and dignity.
- Some people with dementia find it comforting to walk, so try to accommodate this comfort. Find out from the family or carers what support or supervision they usually need.
- People often walk about if they are bored, so ensure the person has enough things to do. Involve the person in suitable activities on the ward, which will give a sense of purpose and self-worth.
- Help the person find their way about the ward, for example, ensure they know where the toilet is and ask if they need to go there.
- People often walk when in pain to try to ease discomfort. If the person cannot communicate, they are in pain, investigate further.
- If a person is feeling agitated or anxious, they may want to walk about. Try to encourage the person to tell you about their anxieties and reassure them.
- Short-term memory loss can lead a person with dementia to start moving for a specific purpose but then forget where they were going, and find themselves lost, which is very distressing.
- They may set out to search for someone or something related to their past. Encourage them to talk about this and show them that you take their feelings seriously. Try to avoid correcting things that the person may say. It is important to focus on what the person feels rather than the factual accuracy of what they say.
- People with dementia often become confused about time. They may wake in the middle of the night and get dressed, ready for the next day. Try putting a clock, where they can see it, which shows the date, time, a.m. and p.m.
- The person with dementia may walk because they feel they need to carry out a certain activity, which may be one they carried out in the past, for example, going to work. This action may be because they are feeling unfulfilled, so try to find them an activity that gives them a sense of purpose.
- If the person is determined to leave, try not to confront them, as this could be upsetting. Instead, accompany them a little way and then divert their attention so that you both return.

Adapted with permission from original information produced by Alzheimer's Society alzheimers.org.uk

Learning outcome 2: identify strategies to assist when moving and handling individuals who are bariatric (plus size)

About 64.2% of adults in England were overweight or obese in 2019, with similar figures for Scotland, Wales and Northern Ireland (Baker 2021). The term bariatric is used to describe the field of medicine that focuses on the causes, prevention, treatment and management of obesity, and while the term obesity has been used for people with a BMI of 30+, it is individuals who have a BMI of 35+ who are eligible for bariatric surgery (NICE 2014b). The term plus size was introduced in a key publication by Muir and Rush (2013) as a term that the client group preferred and is intended to shift away from the medical model, that 'bariatric' focused on, to consider their holistic needs.

Challenges can present when providing care and equipment for this client group. Attention must be given to the provision of suitable equipment that both has a sufficient SWL and physical dimensions to cater to the person's body shape, and further problems can be caused by issues of space within building design. It is important that staff caring for plus size individuals have an appropriate attitude to obesity (Sturman-Floyd 2013) and treat all people with dignity (NMC 2018). Body shape and weight distribution have been categorised into five distinct categories, with different moving and handling and positioning considerations:

Box 11.39 Body shape (somatotypes)

Apple-shaped (android) – the weight is predominant around the waist area
- the adipose tissue can cause limited bending at the waist

Pear-shaped (gynoid) – the weight is concentrated in the hips and thighs
- if the adipose tissue is predominantly on the inside of the thighs, it will be hard for the person to roll/be rolled

Proportional – carries their weight in proportion to their height

Anasarca – severe generalised oedema
- reduced ability to flex limbs or at the waist and will be at high risk of skin tears from assisted moving

Bulbous gluteal – excessive buttock tissue, creating protruding posterior shelf
- will affect their sitting and lying posture

(adapted from Muir and Rush 2013 and Sturman-Floyd 2013)

Revisiting the TILEE risk assessment for this client group, consideration should be given to specific factors including:

Task: increased exertion and force, holding parts of the body for prolonged periods and possibly at a distance from the body

Individual: there is the potential for a higher risk of injury to carers who support bariatric individuals (Hignett et al. 2007); carers need to have had appropriate training and there needs to be enough staff for the risk assessed task

Load (person): need to know an accurate weight, as well as the adipose distribution factors identified earlier, and an appreciation of tolerance of certain positions

Environment: sufficient room for the number of carers and equipment, width of doorways and safe working load of the floor all need to be considered

Equipment: needs to have a suitable and sufficient SWL and needs to be available without undue delay

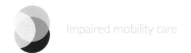

Summary

- Nurse should understand the specific needs of people with dementia and how to address this in moving and handling tasks.
- Nurses should understand how to access appropriate equipment to meet the care needs of bariatric individuals.
- Nurses should maintain a non-judgemental, caring and understanding approach when dealing with all client groups.

REFERENCES

Alderden, J., Rondinelli, J., Pepper, G., Cummins, M. and Whitney, J. 2017. Risk factors for pressure injuries among critical care patients: A systematic review. *International Journal of Nursing Studies* 71: 97–114.

Alexander, P. and Johnson, C. 2011. *Manual Handling of Children.* Towcester: National Back Exchange.

Alzheimer's Society. 2009. *Counting the Cost: Caring for People with Dementia on Acute Hospital Wards.* London: Alzheimer's Society.

Alzheimer's Society. 2017. What is dementia? Factsheet 400LP. Available from: https://www.alzheimers.org.uk/sites/default/files/2018-10/400%20What%20is%20dementia_0.pdf (Accessed on 31 January 2021).

Alzheimer's Society. 2019. Walking about. Factsheet 501LP. Available from: https://www.alzheimers.org.uk/sites/default/files/2019-05/501lp-walking-about-190521.pdf (Accessed on 31 January 2021).

Alzheimer's Society. 2020. Pressure ulcers and bed sores. Available from: https://www.alzheimers.org.uk/get-support/daily-living/pressure-ulcers (Accessed on 9 November 2020).

Anderson, K.E. 2008. Falls in the elderly. *Journal of Royal College of Physicians of Edinburgh.* 38(1): 38–43.

Baillie, L., Merritt, J. and Cox, J. 2012. Caring for older people with dementia in hospital: Part II: Strategies. *Nursing Older People* 24(9): 22–6.

Baker, C. 2021. *Obesity Statistics. House of Commons Briefing Paper no. 3336.* London: House of Commons Library. Available from: https://researchbriefings.files.parliament.uk/documents/SN03336/SN03336.pdf (Accessed on 31 January 2021).

Berg, H., Eiken, O., Miklavic, L. et al. 2007. Hip, thigh and calf muscle atrophy and bone loss after 5-week bedrest inactivity. *European Journal of Applied Physiology* 99(3): 283–9.

Black, J.M., Cuddigan, J.E., Walko, M.A. Didier, A.L., Lander, M.J. and Kelpe, M.R. 2010. Medical device related pressure ulcers in hospitalized patients. *International Wound Journal* 7: 358–65.

Bodavula, P., Liang, S.Y., Wu, J. et al. 2015. Pressure ulcer-related pelvic osteomyelitits: A neglected disease? *Open Forum Infectious Diseases* 2(3): ofv112 doi: 10.1093/ofid/ofv112

Bolwell, C., Hughes, C. and Wyrko, Z. 2016. Can I reach my walking aid? Assessment on three acute medical wards within a tertiary hospital setting. *Age and Ageing* 45: i1–i9.

Borland, A., Hollins Martin, C. and Locke, J. 2013. Nurses' understandings of suitable footwear for older people. *International Journal of Health Care Quality Assurance* 26(7): 653–65.

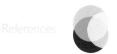

Braden, B. and Bergstrom, N. 1987. A conceptual schema for the study of the etiology of pressure sores. *Rehabilitation Nursing* 12: 8–12.

British Association for Parenteral and Enteral Nutrition. 2020. The 'MUST' toolkit. Available from: https://www.bapen.org.uk/screening-and-must/must/must-toolkit/the-must-itself (Accessed on 18 November 2020).

Chaâbane, F. 2007. Falls prevention for older people with dementia. *Nursing Standard* 2(6): 50–5.

Chadwick, M. 2010. Providing excellent service for those with mobility impairment. *Nursing and Residential Care* 12(6): 278–82.

Charalambous, C. Vassilopoulos, A., Koulouri, A. et al. 2018. The impact of stress on pressure ulcer wound healing process and on the psychophysiological environment of the individual suffering from them. *Medical Archives Journal of the Academy of Medical Sciences in Bosnia Herzegovina* 72(5): 362–6. doi: 10.5455/medarh.2018.72.362-366

Clavet, H., Hébert, P.C., Fergusson, D. et al. 2008. Joint contracture following prolonged stay in the intensive care unit. *Canadian Medical Association Journal* 178(6): 691–7.

Coleman, S., Gorecki, C., Nelson, E.A. et al. 2013. Patient risk factors for pressure ulcer development: systematic review. *International Journal of Nursing Studies* 50(7): 974–1003.

Crawford, A. and Harris, H. 2016. Caring for adults with impaired mobility. *Nursing* 46(12): 36–41.

Day, J. 2015. Diagnosing and managing venous leg ulcers in patients in the community. *Community Wound Care* 20(Sup 12): S22–30.

Department of Health. 2010. *Essence of Care: Benchmarks for Prevention and Management of Pressure ulcers*. Norwich: The Stationary Office.

Department of Health and Social Care. 2018. Safeguarding adults protocol: Pressure ulcers and the interface with a safeguarding enquiry. Available from: https://assets.publishing.service.gov.uk/government/uploads/system/uploads/attachment_data/file/756243/safeguarding-adults-protocol-pressure-ulcers.pdf (Accessed on 18 November 2020).

Di Nisio, M., van Es, N. and Büller, H.R. 2016. Deep vein thrombosis and pulmonary embolism. *The Lancet* 388(10063): 3060–73.

European Pressure Ulcer Advisory Panel (EPUAP) 2015. Pressure ulcers: Just the facts! Available from: https://www.epuap.org/wp-content/uploads/2015/09/EPUAP_Factsheet_A4.blue_.pdf (Accessed on 22 November 2020).

European Pressure Ulcer Advisory Panel, National Pressure Injury Advisory Panel and Pan Pacific Pressure Injury Alliance. 2019. Pressure and treatment of pressure ulcers: Quick reference guide. Available from: http://www.internationalguideline.com/static/pdfs/Quick_Reference_Guide-10Mar2019.pdf (Accessed on 08 November 2020)

Gee, E. 2019. How to apply antiembolism stockings to prevent venous thromboembolism. *Nursing Times* 115(4): 24–6.

Gibbon, B. 2002. Rehabilitation following stroke. *Nursing Standard* 16(29): 47–52, 54–5.

Green, D. 2012. Moving and positioning individuals. *Nursing and Residential Care* 14(10): 506–9.

Halvarsson, A., Olsson, E., Farén, E. et al. 2011. Effects of new, individually adjusted, progressive balance group training for elderly people with fear of falling and tend to fall: A randomised control trial. *Clinical Rehabilitation* 25(11): 1021–31.

Harvey, P.D. 2019. Domains of cognition and their assessment. *Dialogues in Clinical Neuroscience* 21(3): 227–37. doi: 10.31887/DCNS.2019.21.3/pharvey

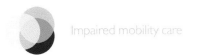
Health and Safety Executive. 2020. *Manual Handling at Work. A Brief Guide.* Available from: https://www.hse.gov.uk/pubns/indg143.pdf (Accessed on 31 January 2021).

Hignett, S. 2003. Systematic review of patient handling activities in lying, sitting and standing positions. *Journal of Advanced Nursing* 41(6): 545–52.

Hignett, S., Chipchase, S., Tetley, A. and Griffiths, P. 2007. Risk assessment and process planning for bariatric patient handling pathways. Available from: https://www.hse.gov.uk/research/rrpdf/rr573.pdf (Accessed on 31 January 2021).

Human Rights Act. 1998. C42. Available from: https://www.legislation.gov.uk/ukpga/1998/42/data.pdf (Accessed on 31 January 2021).

Humphreys, C., Moffatt, C. and Hood, V. 2016. Risk of falling for people with venous leg ulcers: A literature review. *Community Wound Care* 21: S34–8.

Jackson, D., Sarki, A.M., Betteridge, R. and Brooke, J. 2019. Medical device-related pressure ulcers: A systematic review and meta-analysis. *International Journal of Nursing Studies.* Apr 92: 109–20. doi: 10.1016/j.ijnurstu.2019.02.006

Jasniewski, J. 2006. Putting a lid on medication-related falls. *Nursing.* 36(6): 22–4.

Johnstone, J. and Owen, K. 2017. Implementation of an infant manual handling risk assessment tool. *Journal of Neonatal Nursing* 23: 290–3.

Jootun, D. and Pryde, A. 2013. Moving and handling of patients with dementia. *Journal of Nursing Education and Practice* 3(2): 126–31.

Judy-waterlow.co.uk. 2005. Pressure ulcer risk assessment and prevention. Available from: http://www.judy-waterlow.co.uk/index.htm (Accessed on 17 November 2020).

Kneafsey, R. 2007. A systematic review of nursing contributions to mobility rehabilitation: Examining the quality and content of the evidence. *Journal of Clinical Nursing* 16(11c) 325–40.

Knight, J., Nigam, Y. and Jones, A. 2019a. Effects of bedrest 4: Renal, reproductive and immune systems. *Nursing Times* 115(3): 51–4.

Knight, J., Nigam, Y. and Jones, A. 2019b. Effects of bedrest 5: The muscles, joints and mobility. *Nursing Times* 115(4): 54–7.

Knight, J., Nigam, Y. and Jones, A. 2019c. Effects of bedrest 6: Bones, skin, self-concept and self-esteem. *Nursing Times* 115(5): 58–61.

Kyle, G. 2006. Assessment and treatment of older patients with constipation. *Nursing Standard* 21(8): 41–6.

Lainer, J.B., Mote, M.B. and Clay, E.C. 2011. Evaluation and management of orthostatic hypotension. *American Family Physician* 84(5): 527–36.

Lee, A.C.W. 2020. Management of integumentary conditions in older adults. In: Avers, D. and Wong, R. (eds.) *Guccione's Geriatric Physical Therapy*, 4th edn. St Louis: Elsevier, 486–501.

Lifting Operations and Lifting Equipment Regulations. 1998. SI 1998/2307. Available from: https://www.legislation.gov.uk/uksi/1998/2307/made/data.pdf (Accessed on 31 January 2021).

Logsdon, R., McCurry, S. and Terry, L. 2005. A home health care approach to exercise for people with Alzheimer's disease. *Care Management Journals* 6(2): 90–7.

Lyons, T. 2005. Fall prevention for older adults. *Journal of Gerontological Nursing* 32(11): 9–14.

Macqueen, S., Bruce, E.A. and Gibson, F. 2012. Personal hygiene and pressure ulcer prevention. In: Macqueen, S., Bruce, E. A. and Gibson, F. (Eds). *The Great Ormond Street Hospital Manual of Children's Nursing Practices.* Chichester: Wiley-Blackwell. 167–220.

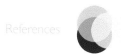

Manual Handling Operations Regulations. 1992. SI 1992/2793. Available from: https://www.legislation.gov.uk/uksi/1992/2793/made/data.pdf (Accessed on 31 January 2021).

Marusic, U., Kavcic, V., Pisot, R. and Goswami, N. 2019. The role of enhanced cognition to counteract detrimental effects of prolonged bed rest: Current evidence and perspectives. *Frontiers in Physiology* 9: 1864.

McCarter-Bayer, A., Bayer, F. and Hall, K. 2005. Preventing falls in acute care: An innovative approach. *Journal of Gerontological Nursing* 31(3): 25–33.

McInnes, E., Jammali-Blasi, A., Bell-Syer, S.E.M. et al. 2015. Support surfaces for pressure ulcer prevention. *Cochrane Database of Systematic Reviews.* https://doi.org/10.1002/14651858.CD001735.pub5

McKew, M. 2017. 'PJ paralysis' campaign gets patients up and trusts moving. *Nursing Standard* 31(40): 12–13.

Moore, Z.E.H. and Patton, D. 2019. Risk assessment tools for the prevention of pressure ulcers. *Cochrane Systematic Reviews.* Available from: https://www.cochranelibrary.com/cdsr/doi/10.1002/14651858.CD006471.pub4/full (Accessed on 11 November 2020).

Muir, M. and Rush, A. 2013. *Moving and Handling of Plus Size People – An Illustrated Guide.* Towcester: National Back Exchange.

National Health Service (NHS) England and NHS Improvement. 2019. CQUIN CCG7: *Three High Impact Actions to Prevent Hospital Falls. Advice and FAQs.* Available from: https://improvement.nhs.uk/documents/5335/Falls_CQUIN_FAQ_Final.pdf (Accessed on 31 January 2021).

National Health Services (NHS) Improvement. 2017. *Using SSKIN to Manage and Prevent Pressure Damage.* Available from: https://improvement.nhs.uk/resources/Using-SSKIN-to-manage-and-prevent-pressure-damage/ (Accessed on 1 November 2020).

National Institute for Health and Care Excellence (NICE). 2013. Clinical guideline 161, Falls: The assessment and prevention of falls in older people. Available from: https://www.nice.org.uk/guidance/cg161 (Accessed on 31 January 2021).

National Institute for Health and Care Excellence (NICE). 2014a. Pressure ulcers: Prevention and management. Available from: https://www.nice.org.uk/guidance/cg179 (Accessed on 22 November 2020).

National Institute for Health and Care Excellence (NICE). 2014b. Obesity: Identification, assessment and management. Clinical guideline CG189. Available from: https://www.nice.org.uk/guidance/cg189 (Accessed on 31 January 2021).

National Institute for Health and Care Excellence (NICE). 2015a. *Pressure Ulcers: Quality Standard (QS89).* Available from: https://www.nice.org.uk/guidance/qs89/chapter/Introduction (Accessed on 18 November 2020).

National Institute for Health and Care Excellence (NICE). 2015b Falls in older people. Quality Standard 86. Available from: https://www.nice.org.uk/guidance/qs86/resources/falls-in-older-people-pdf-2098911933637 (Accessed on 31 January 2021).

National Institute for Health and Care Excellence (NICE). 2018b. Impact: Falls and fragility fractures. Available from: https://www.nice.org.uk/media/default/about/what-we-do/into-practice/measuring-uptake/nice-impact-falls-and-fragility-fractures.pdf (Accessed on 31 January 2021).

National Institute for Health and Care Excellence (NICE). 2019. NICE Impact Stroke. Available from: https://www.nice.org.uk/Media/Default/About/what-we-do/Into-practice/measuring-uptake/NICE-Impact-stroke.pdf (Accessed on 3 November 2020).

National Institute for Health and Care Excellence (NICE). 2020. Sem Scanner 200 for preventing pressure ulcers. Available from: https://www.nice.org.uk/guidance/mtg51 (Accessed on 16 November 2020).

National Institute for Health and Clinical Excellence (NICE). 2018a. Venous thrombo-embolism in over 16s: reducing the risk of hospital-acquired deep vein thrombosis or pulmonary embolism. Clinical Guideline 89. Available from: https://www.nice.org.uk/guidance/ng89/resources/venous-thromboembolism-in-over-16s-reducing-the-risk-of-hospitalacquired-deep-vein-thrombosis-or-pulmonary-embolism-pdf-1837703092165 (Accessed on 31 January 2021).

National Pressure Injury Advisory Panel (NPIAP). 2016. NPIAP pressure injury stages. Available from: https://cdn.ymaws.com/npiap.com/resource/resmgr/online_store/npiap_pressure_injury_stages.pdf (Accessed: 08 February 2021).

National Pressure Injury Advisory Panel (NPIAP). 2020. Best practise for prevention of medical device-related pressure injuries. Available from: https://cdn.ymaws.com/npiap.com/resource/resmgr/MDPI-Poster2020.pdf (Accessed 13 November 2020).

Nazarko, L. 2012. Falls: Environmental risk factors. *British Journal of Healthcare Assistants*. 6(3): 111–15.

Nazarko, L. 2015. Modifiable risk factors for falls and minimizing the risk of harm. *Nurse Prescribing* 13(4): 2192–98.

NHS Improvement. 2017. Using SSKIN to manage and prevent pressure damage. Available from: https://improvement.nhs.uk/resources/Using-SSKIN-to-manage-and-prevent-pressure-damage/ (Accessed on 8 February 2021).

NHS Improvement. 2018. *Pressure ulcers: revised definition and measurement Summary and recommendations*. Available from: https://www.england.nhs.uk/wp-content/uploads/2021/09/NSTPP-summary-recommendations.pdf (Accessed on 8 February 2021).

NHS Modernisation. 2017. *Pressure Ulcers: Revised Definition and Measurement*. Available from: https://improvement.nhs.uk/documents/2932/NSTPP_summary__recommendations_2.pdf (Accessed on 12 November 2020).

NHS Stop the Pressure. 2018. Available from: https://nhs.stopthepressure.co.uk/professionals.html (Accessed on 16 November 2020).

Nilsson, C.J., Avlund, K. and Lund, R. 2011. Onset of mobility limitations in old age: The combined effect of socioeconomic position and social relations. *Age and Ageing* 50(5): 607–14.

Norton, D. Mclaren, R. and Exton-Smith, A. 1962. *An Investigation of Geriatric Nursing Problems in Hospital*. Edinburgh: Churchill Livingstone.

Nursing and Midwifery Council (NMC). 2018. *The Code. Professional Standards of Practice and Behaviour for Nurses, Midwives and Nursing Associates*. Available from: https://www.nmc.org.uk/globalassets/sitedocuments/nmc-publications/nmc-code.pdf (Accessed on 31 January 2021).

Parker, M.J., Gillespie, W.J. and Gillespie, L.D. 2006. Effectiveness of hip protectors for preventing hip fractures in elderly people: systematic review. *British Medical Journal* 332(7541): 571–4.

Peate, I. and Glencross, W. 2015. *Wound Care at a Glance*. New Jersey: Wiley Blckwell.

Pellatt, G. 2005. The safety and dignity of patients and nurses during patient handling. *British Journal of Nursing* 14(21): 1150–6.

Pellatt, G. 2007. Clinical skills: Bed making and patient positioning. *British Journal of Nursing* 16(5): 302–5.

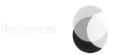

Provizio Sem Scanner. 2020. Sem Scanner FAQ. Available from: https://sem-scanner.com/product/sem-scanner-faq/ (Accessed 3 November 2020).

Quigley, S.M. and Curley, M.A.Q. 1996. Skin integrity in the pediatric population: preventing and managing pressure ulcers. *Journal for Specialists in Pediatric Nursing* April 1(1): 7–18. https://doi.org/10.1111/j.1744-6155.1996.tb00050.x

Ramsey, S. and McIlhenny, C. 2011. Evidence-based management of upper tract urolithiasis in the spinal cord-injured patient. *Spinal Cord* 49(9): 948–54.

Roper, N., Logan, W. and Tierney, A.J. 2000. *The Roper-Logan-Tierney Model of Nursing.* Edinburgh: Churchill Livingstone.

Royal College of Nursing (RCN). 2016. *Care Plans.* Available from: https://rcni.com/hosted-content/rcn/first-steps/care-plans (Accessed on 19 September 2020).

Royal College of Physicians (RCP). 2017. *National Early Warning Scores (NEWS) 2 Standardising the Assessment of Acute Illness Severity in the NHS.* Available from: https://www.rcplondon.ac.uk/projects/outputs/national-early-warning-score-news-2 (Accessed 16 November 2020).

Ruszala, S. 2010. *Moving and Handling People. An illustrated Guide.* London: Clinical Skills Ltd.

Samuriwo, R. 2012. Pressure ulcer prevention: the role of the multidisciplinary team. *British Journal of Nursing* 21(5): S20–4.

Sepsis Alliance. 2020. *Pressure Ulcers (Pressure Injuries).* Available from: https://www.sepsis.org/sepsisand/pressure-ulcers-pressure-injuries/ (Accessed on 18 November 2020).

Smith, J., ed. 2011. *The Handling of People a Systems Approach*, 6th edn. Teddington: BackCare.

Soliman, A. and Brogan, M. 2014. Foot assessment and care for older people. *Nursing Times* 110(50): 12–15.

Somerville, C., Harper, M. and O'Neill, A. 2020. Up, dressed and mobilised: Embedding end PJ paralysis on a stroke ward. *Nursing Times* 116(3): 39–41.

Srikanth, R., Cassidy, G., Joiner, C. et al. 2011. Osteoporosis in people with intellectual disabilities: A review and a brief study of risk factors for osteoporosis in a community sample of people with intellectual disabilities. *Journal of Intellectual Disability Research* 55(1): 53–62.

Stephen-Haynes, J. and Maries, M. 2020. Pressure ulcers and the prone position. *British Journal of Nursing Tissue Viability Supplement* 29(12). https://doi.org/10.12968/bjon.2020.29.12.S6

Stephens, M. and Bartley, C.A. 2018. Understanding the association between pressure ulcers and sitting in adults what does it mean for me and my careers? Seating guidelines for people, carers and health and social care professionals. *Journal of Tissue Viability* 27(1): 59–73.

Stephenson, J. 2019. NHS litigation bill for pressure ulcers soars 53% in three years. *Nursing Times.* Available from: https://www.nursingtimes.net/news/technology/nhs-litigation-bill-for-pressure-ulcers-soars-53-in-three-years-08-05-2019/ (Accessed on 13 November 2020).

Sturman, M. and Varnham, W. 2019. *Dementia Care – a Behavioural Approach to Manual Handling.* Towcester: National Back exchange.

Sturman-Floyd, M. 2013. Moving and handling: supporting bariatric residents. *Nursing and Residential Care* 15(6): 432–7.

Swann, J. 2006. Keeping mobile: Part one. *Nursing and Residential Care* 8(12): 566–8.

Swann, J. 2014. Understanding multifactorial fall risks. *Nursing and Residential Care* 16(7): 387–91.

The UK Sepsis Trust. 2018. *ED/MU Sepsis Screening & Action Tool.* Available from: https://sepsistrust.org/wp-content/uploads/2018/06/ED-adult-NICE-Final-1107.pdf (Accessed on 17 November 2020).

Thompson, A.J., Jarrett, L., Lockley, L. et al. 2005. Clinical management of spasticity. *Journal of Neurology, Neurosurgery and Psychiatry* 76(4): 459–63.

Thompson, S. and Jevon, P. 2009. Manual handling part 2 – repositioning a supine patient using a slide sheet. *Nursing Times* 105(1): 14–15.

Tofts, D. and Arnold, M. 2012. Moving and handling in the community: Update on legislation and best practice. *British Journal of Community Nursing.* 17, 2: 50–57.

Van Wicklin, S., Ward, K. and Cantrell, S. 2006. Implementing a research utilisation plan for prevention of deep vein thrombosis. *AORN Journal* 83(6): 1351–62.

Varnham, W. 2011. How to mobilise patients with dementia to a standing position. *Nursing Older People* 23(8): 31–6.

Vollman, K.M. 2010. Introduction to progressive mobility. *Critical Care Nurse* 30(2): S3–5.

Waldron, B. and Moll, S. 2014. A patient's guide to recovery after deep vein thrombosis or pulmonary embolism. *Circulation* 129(17):e477–9.

Weaver, D. 2005. Helping individuals to maintain mobility. *Nursing and Residential Care* 7(8): 343–8.

While, A.E. 2020a. Falls and older people: Understanding why people fall. *British Journal of Community Nursing* 25(4): 173–7.

While, A.E. 2020b. Falls and older people: Preventative interventions. *British Journal of Community Nursing* 25(6): 288–92.

Windsor, J., Lowry, M. and Ashelford, S. 2016. Orthostatic hypotension 1: Effect of orthostatic hypotension on falls risk. *Nursing Times* 112(43–4): 11–13.

Windsor, J. and Dix, A. 2017. A bedside tool to assess eyesight in hospital patients at risk of falls. *Nursing Times* 113(5): 22–4.

Woodrow, P., Dickson, N. and Wright, P. 2005. Foot care for non-diabetic older people. *Nursing Older People* 17(8): 31–2.

World Health Organisation (WHO). 2007. *WHO Global Report on Falls Prevention in Older Age.* Available from: https://www.who.int/ageing/publications/Falls_prevention-7March.pdf?ua=1 (Accessed on 31 January 2021)

World Health Organisation (WHO). 2020a. *Global Strategy on Diet, Physical Activity and Health.* Available at: https://www.who.int/dietphysicalactivity/pa/en/ (Accessed on 1 April 2020).

World Health Organisation (WHO). 2020b. Save lives: Clean hands. Available from: https://www.who.int/infection-prevention/campaigns/clean-hands/5moments/en/ (Accessed on 18 November 2020).

World Health Organisation (WHO). 2020c. *Dementia.* Available from: https://www.who.int/news-room/fact-sheets/detail/dementia (Accessed on 3 November 2020).

World Health Organization (WHO). 2017. *Evidence Profile: Cognitive Impairment.* Available from: https://www.who.int/ageing/health-systems/icope/evidence-centre/ICOPE-evidence-profile-cognitive.pdf?ua=1#:~:text=Cognitive%20impairment%20is%20a%20strong, criteria%20for%20dementia%20(1) (Accessed on 19 November 2020).

Infection prevention and control

Jennifer Wyeth (with acknowledgements to Patricia Folan and Lesley Baillie)

The utilisation of activities aimed at the prevention and management of infection are the responsibility of all staff working in all health and social care settings (Royal College of Nursing [RCN] 2012a). While there is a risk of cross-infection occurring in any health and social care setting, this risk is significantly greater in hospital and residential care environments. Failure of healthcare practitioners to take adequate care can result in the unintentional transfer of microorganisms from one person to another. Healthcare-associated infection (HCAI), previously referred to as hospital-acquired infection or nosocomial infection, can be defined as those infections arising as a consequence of the delivery of healthcare either in acute (hospital) or community care locations. It is estimated that 300,000 individuals a year in England acquire a healthcare-associated infection as a result of care within the National Health Service (NHS) (National Institute for Health and Clinical Excellence [NICE] 2014).

The Nursing and Midwifery Council (NMC 2018a and 2018b) published revised standards of proficiency for registered Nurses and Nursing Associates, which includes the appropriate utilisation of evidence-based infection prevention and control practices, all of which are incorporated in this chapter.

- Principles for preventing healthcare-associated infection: an introduction
- Hand hygiene
- Use of personal protective equipment, including gloves, aprons and gowns, eye protection and face masks
- Healthcare waste disposal and linen management
- Sharps disposal
- Decontamination of the healthcare environment and multiuse equipment
- Aseptic technique and management of invasive devices
- Specimen collection: key principles
- Screening for methicillin-resistant *Staphylococcus aureus* (MRSA) and other organisms (carbapenemase-producing enterobacterales (CPE) and SARS-CoV-2)
- Isolation procedures (source and protective)
- Antimicrobial Stewardship
- Physical and social distancing (New Standard Infection Prevention and Control (SIPC) precaution in response to the SARS-CoV-2 pandemic)

DOI: 10.4324/9781003020660-12

Box 12.1 Recommended biology reading

These questions will help you to focus on the biology underpinning the skills required to prevent cross-infection. Use your recommended textbook to find out the following:

- What are microorganisms? Where are they found? Are all microorganisms harmful?
- Identify some of the beneficial roles of microorganisms.
- How do microorganisms enter the body?
- How are microorganisms classified?
- What are the structure and properties of bacteria, viruses, prions, fungi, yeasts and protozoa?
- How do bacteria grow and multiply?
- What factors influence the proliferation of microorganisms?
- What is meant by the terms 'commensal', 'pathogen' and 'normal flora'?
- Distinguish between endogenous and exogenous sources of infection.
- What mechanisms does the body use to defend itself from infection? Think about non-specific defences, for example, secretions, reflexes and barriers as well as specific mechanisms. Review the structure of the skin.
- How does the body fight infections?
- What are the clinical signs of infection? What role does histamine play?
- Which cells are involved in the specific immune response? Where are they found?
- What is the difference between humoral and cell-mediated immunity?
- What are antibodies? How do they help protect us from infection?
- How do we achieve an immunological memory?
- What factors can affect an individual's immune system?

PRACTICE SCENARIOS

As discussed above, activities aimed at the prevention and control of infection form an essential part of the nurse's role in all practice settings. The following scenarios are referred to throughout the text when discussing the practical skills covered in this chapter.

Adult

Mrs Winifred Lewis, aged 87 years, was widowed many years ago and lives in warden–controlled accommodation. She has a history of **rheumatoid arthritis** and **type 2 diabetes**, and she recently fell and fractured her hip, which was operated on in the hospital. She was discharged home, under the care of the district nursing team and intermediate care, but her surgical wound deteriorated and the surrounding skin showed signs of infection. Mrs. Lewis appeared unwell and dehydrated, and she had a raised body temperature, so her general practitioner (GP) requested readmission. She is now being isolated in a single room of a surgical ward, and an intravenous infusion and intravenous antibiotics have been commenced. She has a commode in the room and can transfer with help. Blood cultures, taken on admission, showed an MRSA **bacteraemia** and a wound swab confirmed the presence of MRSA in the surgical wound.

Learning disability

James Smith is a 59-year-old man with a learning disability who lives alone in a farm cottage and works on the adjacent farm. After an accident, James has an open wound on his lower left leg that shows signs of infection. There is a large amount of exudate, which has an offensive odour. The district nurse has been visiting the farm to carry out dressings, and a wound swab has been taken. James is keen to carry on with his usual work on the farm. The district nurse is liaising with the community nurse for learning disabilities to help to teach James how to care for his leg in between dressings. This information is now included in James's **Health Action Plan**. As the district nurse runs a clinic at the local GP's surgery, James is being encouraged to attend this clinic for dressings instead of receiving visits at his home.

Mental health

Stacey is 28 years old and has been addicted to opiates for 6 years. She is living with her parents, who are very supportive. Recently, Stacey began a community-based detoxification programme with support from her local drug and alcohol team. During detoxification, Stacey experienced severe withdrawal symptoms, including very high blood pressure and vomiting. As a result, she was admitted as an emergency to the acute mental health admission unit. She arrived feeling very unwell, and soon after arrival, she vomited over her bed. She was prescribed intramuscular metoclopramide (an antiemetic) to stop her vomiting. Stacey is known to have hepatitis B.

PRINCIPLES OF PREVENTING HEALTHCARE-ASSOCIATED INFECTION: AN INTRODUCTION

Healthcare-associated infections

As defined by NICE (2011) guidance, "HCAIs cover any infection contracted: as a direct result of treatment in, or contact with, a health or social care setting, as a result of healthcare delivered outside a healthcare setting (for example, in the community), or brought in by patients, staff or visitors and transmitted to others (for example, norovirus)" (NICE 2011, p. 8).

The human body is colonised by a wide variety of microorganisms the majority of which live there harmlessly without causing any detrimental effect and, in some instances, confer some protective function by reducing the availability of sites to 'foreign' pathogenic organisms. Although these colonising bacteria (commensals) form the body's normal flora, organisms that would not normally be regarded as 'normal' flora can colonise body sites if the correct conditions occur, i.e. *Pseudomonas aeruginosa* can colonise 'wet' wounds such as chronic leg ulcers but once the wound dries up and heals, it will no longer be present.

Infection

Infection is a condition in which body tissues are damaged due to the presence of microorganisms or toxins they produce. Common signs of infection include pyrexia plus pain, heat, swelling, increased wound exudate, tenderness and redness at the site of infection.

Many different microorganisms exist but very few have the ability to cause infections in individuals. Microorganisms that have the ability to cause disease are called pathogens. When pathogens are acquired from another person, or from the environment, they are described as exogenous. The transmission of pathogens, between people and across environments, is termed cross-infection. When microorganisms from one site on the host are able to enter another site on the same person causing infection, this is called self-infection or endogenous infection.

In the fourth national prevalence survey (Health Protection Agency [HPA] 2012), the prevalence of HCAI in England was 6.4%, compared with 8.2% in 2006. A similar point prevalence survey undertaken in Scotland in 2016 identified a prevalence of HCA of 4.6% in adults and 2.7% in paediatrics in acute care (hospitals) and a further 3.2% in non-acute care. According to the fourth national survey, the six most common types of HCAI, accounting for more than 80% of all HCAIs, were respiratory tract infections (pneumonia and other respiratory infections, 22.8%); urinary tract infections (UTIs, 17.2%); surgical site infections (SSIs, 15.7%); clinical sepsis (10.5%); gastrointestinal infections (8.8%); and bloodstream infections (BSIs, 7.3%). In the paediatric population, the most common HCAIs were clinical sepsis (40.2%), respiratory tract infections (15.9%) and BSIs (15.1%). Enterobacteriaceae were the most frequently reported organisms associated with HCAIs.

Box 12.2 Learning outcomes

On completion of this section, you will be able to:

1. discuss key policies and guidance influencing infection control practices;
2. outline the composition and role of infection prevention and control teams;
3. explain the chain of infection, including the routes by which microorganisms are spread.

Learning outcome 1: discuss key policies and guidance influencing infection control practices

Concern about HCAIs in the United Kingdom (UK) has led to many government publications and other guidance documents, providing recommendations for infection prevention and control. Here are some examples:

* *The Health and Social Care Act 2008: Code of Practice for Health and Adult Social Care on the Prevention and Control of Infections and Related Guidance* (Department of Health [DH] 2015a). The Code of Practice and related guidance aim to help

health and adult social care providers to plan and implement how they prevent and control infections and specifies the criteria for compliance with Care Quality Commission (CQC) standards.

- *National Evidence-Based Guidelines for Preventing Healthcare-Associated Infections in NHS England* (Loveday et al. 2014). In these DH-commissioned evidence-based infection control guidelines (referred to as epic3), the authors recommended that SIPC precautions should be applied by all healthcare practitioners to the care of all individuals. This is a requirement of the *Health and Social Care Act 2008: Code of Practice* (DH 2015a), which states that registered providers must audit compliance to key policies and procedures for infection prevention. epic4 is currently under development and should be referred to when published.
- *Prevention and Control of Healthcare-Associated Infections in Primary and Community Care* (CG139) (NICE 2017a). These guidelines apply the standard precautions of hand decontamination, use of personal protective equipment and sharps disposal to community-based care and include guidance for preventing infections associated with long-term urinary catheters and vascular access devices.
- *The Royal College of Nursing; Essential Practice for Infection Prevention and Control RCN* 2017). This guidance document, aimed at all nursing staff, describes the essential elements of good infection prevention and control practice.

New guidance to address specific infection concerns continues to be released. For example, in 2012, the DH published Health Technical Memoranda (HTM) 04.01 technical guidance aimed at those healthcare organisations providing individual care in augmented care units, such as paediatric and adult critical care, neonatal and burns units, providing advice for healthcare providers on management of *Pseudomonas aeruginosa* in water systems (DH 2016).

In response to the rapidly increasing incidence of multi-drug resistant organisms and the impact on individuals and healthcare provider services, Public Health England (PHE) have developed national guidance for the management of one of the most significant groups of multi-drug resistant organisms, CPE (PHE 2020b).

Public Health England has also produced detailed infection prevention and control guidance in response to the SARS-CoV-2 (COVID-19) pandemic of 2020. This guidance has been constantly reviewed and updated as more information becomes available in relation to the management of this new infection (PHE 2020a, 2020c).

Central to all IP&C precautions is the need to ensure that the buildings and facilities in which healthcare is delivered are fit for purpose and conducive to enabling staff to carry out safe, effective care. Consequently, there are many documents; Health Building Notes (HBN) and HTM that describe how healthcare facilities should be built and the standards that building services need to achieve. HBN 00-09 Infection control in the built environment (DH 2013b) describes the requirements, including consultation with the Infection Prevention and Control (IPC) team, to ensure that buildings are designed and built to the correct standards and that the finished project meets the IPC needs of staff and individuals in their care.

The other UK countries' administrations also provide guidance and policy on infection control: for Scotland, refer to NHS Scotland, National Infection Prevention and Control Manual (accessible at http://www.nipcm.hps.scot.nhs.uk) for Wales, see Welsh Healthcare Associated Infection Programme (https://www.wales.nhs.uk/ourservices/directory/NationalProgrammesandServices/379) and for Northern Ireland see the Department of Health, Social Services and Public Safety (www.dhsspsni.gov.uk)

Learning outcome 2: outline the composition and role of infection prevention and control teams

As you read above, there are many sources of infection prevention and control-related policy and evidence-based guidelines, the interpretation, adoption and monitoring of which are led at a local level by an infection prevention and control team (IPCT).

ACTIVITY

Box 12.3 Activity: local IPCT

When next in the practice setting, find out who the members of the local IPCT are and where they are located. Also, find out where your local infection prevention and control policy and other IP&C guidance documents are kept and familiarise yourself with their contents.

The IPCT usually consists of one or more infection prevention and control nurses (IPCN) and an infection prevention and control doctor. Due to the ever-increasing requirements for local and national reporting requirements, teams may also have access to data and office administration staff. In some smaller organisations, the IPCT function may be provided via a service-level agreement with a third party such as the local Acute Healthcare Trust. The role of the IPCT include planning, implementing and monitoring the infection prevention and control programme. They are available to offer advice on all matters relating to infection control to staff, individuals in their care and visitors. They also provide training and education to all trust/organisational employees and are responsible for ensuring that local policy and practice guidance documents reflect new advances and /or changes to national guidelines. One of the most important roles of the IPCT is the prospective monitoring of laboratory test reports for infectious organisms and the early identification of potential outbreaks. The IPCT will advise on the isolation requirements of individuals and identifies additional actions to be taken to minimise the impacts on people and healthcare provider services associated with outbreaks and periods of increased incidence of infection.

Many community healthcare providers also employ IPCNs who work closely with their local healthcare providers and the Public Health Consultant for Communicable Disease Control (CCDC), which is responsible for monitoring and controlling the spread of infection in the community, as well as other environmental hazards. Trusts work proactively in multiagency collaborations with other local healthcare and social care providers to reduce risk from infection. Many healthcare settings also use infection control link nurses/practitioners (or champions) to act as a local IPC resource and improve awareness of and compliance with infection control practices within their clinical areas. They receive specific training to help deliver local education and training, as well as undertaking audit and surveillance activities as determined by the IPC team. There should also be close liaison between the occupational health and safety teams and the IPCT to maintain the health and safety of individuals in their care and staff alike (Wilson 2019).

An infection control committee consisting of key stakeholders from across the organisation as well as external members such as the CCDC, and representatives from patient groups and local CCGs supports the IPCT to identify key initiatives and monitor the implementation of the IPC strategy and associated action plans.

Learning outcome 3: explain the chain of infection, including the routes by which microorgnisms are spread

The chain of infection can help you to understand how to prevent spread of infection (Figure 12.1). Prevention of cross-infection is about breaking the chain of infection. Each link in the chain is discussed below.

Infectious agent

An infectious agent is a microorganism with the ability to cause disease and includes bacteria (e.g. *Clostridioides difficile* and MRSA), viruses (e.g. influenza and hepatitis B) fungi (e.g. *Candida*, which causes thrush) and protozoa (e.g. *Toxoplasma gondii*, which causes fetal death or brain damage if infection occurs in early pregnancy). To identify the specific infectious agent and determine appropriate antimicrobial therapy, specimens are collected and sent to the laboratory for microscopy, culture and sensitivity (M, C & S). For example, if a UTI is suspected, a specimen of urine should be sent to the laboratory as soon as possible to identify the presence or otherwise of an infectious organism and inform the medical team of the most appropriate antimicrobial treatment (Wilson 2019). A later section in this chapter focuses on the collection of a specimen. More advanced testing available in some laboratories includes molecular tests such as polymerase chain reaction, which is a biochemical technology used to identify the presence of an organism by detecting the specific DNA or RNA of the suspected organism in a sample. Generally, the turnaround time is quicker for a result from a specimen sent in this way (Wilson 2019).

Box 12.4 Activity: microbiology laboratory

When next in the practice setting, try to arrange to spend time in the microbiology laboratory to see what happens to samples once they arrive in the lab.

Two microorganisms that have historically caused particular concern in healthcare settings and are regularly covered in the media are MRSA and *Clostridioides difficile* (formally known as *Clostridium difficile*).

Methicillin-resistant Staphylococcus aureus

Mrs. Lewis is an example of a person who has an infection caused by MRSA, a strain of *Staphylococcus aureus* (*S. aureus*) that has become resistant to the antibiotic meticillin – hence the name 'meticillin-resistant *Staphylococcus aureus*'. All strains of MRSA are inherently resistant to flucloxacillin, with some strains being resistant to a wide range of other antibiotics, in particular penicillin and cephalosporins. *S. aureus* commonly colonises the skin, in particular, the warm, moist sites such as the axillae, groin, perineum and nose. Healthy people do not usually develop an infection, even if colonised but *S. aureus* may cause a range of infections from spots, boils and abscesses to prosthetic joint infections, pneumonia, endocarditis and sepsis (Wilson 2019). Serious staphylococcal infection usually occurs in people who are vulnerable because of underlying illness or medical interventions. Mrs. Lewis, as a frail older person with diabetes and rheumatoid arthritis, fits into this vulnerable category.

MRSA can cause a range of superficial infections of the skin as well as more severe infections such as deep wound infections, as with Mrs. Lewis. The mandatory surveillance of total hip replacement surgery identifies that 0.5% of people undergoing this type of surgery developed surgical site infection with 4.2% of these being caused by MRSA (PHE 2019a). In the fourth national prevalence survey, less than 0.1% of the survey population had an HCAI caused by MRSA (HPA 2012). Although all strains of MRSA are inherently resistant to flucloxacillin and other penicillin-based antibiotics, fortunately there have always been antibiotics with clinical activity against MRSA. These tend to be relatively expensive and usually need to be administered intravenously; however, oral antibiotics can be used in some cases to treat MRSA in community settings. The commonly used antibiotics such as vancomycin, teicoplanin and linezolid require regular monitoring of blood levels as they are highly toxic.

As MRSA is usually found on the skin, the hands of healthcare workers, that may be transiently colonised, are the most likely means of cross-infection. Staff or individuals with skin conditions such as eczema or dermatitis are likely to have significantly higher levels of bacteria on their skin. This increases the risk of shedding organisms into the environment from where they can be spread to other staff and individuals in their care. Organisms can also be carried on skin scales from an infected individual or member of staff and may contaminate uniforms, clothing and bed linen as well as residing in dust should this be allowed to accumulate.

Another important feature of *S. aureus* is its ability to produce toxins, which, in turn, can have the ability to cause significant tissue damage. One of the most significant of these are the Panton-Valentine Leukocidin (PVL) toxin-producing strains that can cause septic arthritis and necrotising pneumonia. These may also be MRSA but commonly meticillin-sensitive strains are also isolated. Due to the serious nature of these infections, specific guidance in relation to the identification and management of PVL *S. aureus* has been published (HPA 2008).

Clostridioides difficile *(formerly* Clostridium difficile*)*

In response to the significant media attention caused by large scale outbreaks of infection, national guidance was published on 2008 relating to the management of *C. difficile* infections (DH and HPA 2008). In 2013, PHE revised the section of this guidance relating to the management and treatment of *Clostridium difficile* infection to include updated recommendations for the clinical management of individuals with *C. difficile* infection (PHE 2013). *Clostridioides difficile* is a spore-forming bacterium, which is commonly found in the environment but which can colonise the gastrointestinal tract of approximately 3% of healthy adults and 66% of children. *C. difficile* infection occurs when the normal gut flora is altered, for example, after taking antibiotics, allowing the proliferation and production of two main toxins (A and B) that act on the bowel lining resulting in colitis and diarrhoea (NICE 2017b). *C. difficile* produces spores that are very resistant to normal cleaning processes and can survive in the environment for long periods of time potentially resulting in a significant reservoir for future cross-infection. In response to an increasing trend in the incidence of *C. difficile*, mandatory reporting of all cases in adults over 65 years old was implemented in 2007, since when there has been a significant reduction in the number of reported cases – a 77.9% reduction reported in 2018/19 from the base-line data collected in 2007/08 (PHE. 2019a).

Individuals most at risk of *C. difficile* infection are older people and those who have recently taken antibiotics (DH and HPA 2008, NICE 2015; therefore, Mrs. Lewis could be at risk (Figure 12.1).

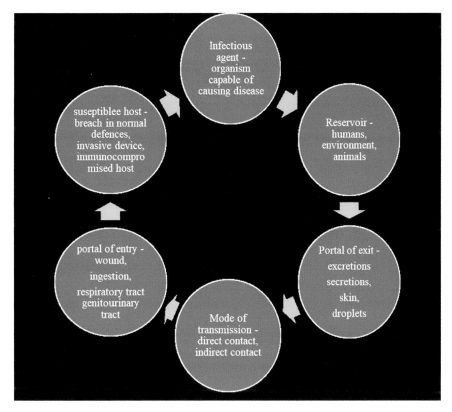

Figure 12.1: Chain of infection. (Reprinted from Sax, H., Allegranzi, B., Uçkay, I., Larson, E., Boyce, J. and Pittet, D. 2007. My five moments for hand hygiene: A user-centred design approach to understand, train, monitor and report hand hygiene. *Journal of Hospital Infection* 67(I): 9–21. With permission from Elsevier.)

Reservoir of infection

A reservoir of infection is a place within which microorganisms grow and reproduce and can include people (e.g. healthcare workers, individuals in their care), the environment, equipment and water. Mrs. Lewis's and James's wounds provide reservoirs for infection.

Portal of exit

A portal of exit provides a way for microorganisms to leave the reservoir and includes excretions (e.g. faeces from the bowel) or droplets (via the mouth or nose by sneezing or coughing). If Stacey cut herself, the cut would provide a means for the hepatitis B microorganism to leave her body via her blood.

Mode of transmission

Microorganisms can spread through many routes.

Box 12.5 Activity: pathogenic microorganisms

Read Table 12.1, which presents the routes by which pathogenic microorganisms can be transmitted or spread between people. Then reread the practice scenarios. Can you work out which transmission route would feature mostly strongly for them?

In our scenarios, it is likely that direct or indirect contact via hands of carers is going to be the principal mechanism of cross-infection. For Mrs. Lewis, infection is unlikely to be spread via the airborne route; however, both direct and indirect contact transmission are equally likely. Stacey has hepatitis B and as this virus is transmitted via blood and serum-derived fluids such as vaginal secretions, direct and indirect contact of broken skin or mucous membranes with these fluids is the principal means of transmission. As James's wound is producing a large amount of exudate, poor wound care or attention to aseptic technique could be a source of the spread of infection.

Although all routes of transmission are important, this short activity points out that the most common route of spread is via hands. The hands of healthcare workers act as one of the most likely means of transferring organisms from one source to another, leading to cross-infection. Consequently, compliance with hand hygiene policy is seen as a key performance indicator of the standard of infection prevention and control being delivered by healthcare provider services (World Health Organization [WHO] 2009). Attention to hand hygiene has the potential to break the chain of infection and is discussed in detail later in this chapter.

Portal of entry

To cause infection, microorganisms must have the means by which they can enter the body. Portals of entry include: ingestion, inhalation, inoculation, transplacental and sexual intercourse.

Table 12.1: Routes of transmission

Direct contact	**Description**
	Transmission by contact with body surfaces or fluids infected or colonised by infectious *organisms*
	Examples
	Hepatitis B could be *transmitted* by direct contact with infected blood if there is a wound or break in the skin of the recipient.
Indirect contact	**Inanimate objects (fomites)**
	Description
	Items of equipment or the environment contaminated by infectious organisms NB: Dust is composed primarily of skin scales, which may be colonised by *S. aureus* and other skin commensals
	Examples
	C. difficle transmission via soiled commodes, contact with dusty equipment
	If disturbed, small particles of dust can remain airborne for considerable periods of time and may eventually settle on wounds causing infection
	Food
	Description
	Ingestion or inhalation of food and water contaminated by infectious organisms
	Examples
	Staph aureus food poisoning following preparation of food by someone with *S. aureus* infected skin lesions, *Campylobacter* acquired following the ingestion of undercooked chicken
	Water
	Description
	Contamination of the skin and/or invasive devices following contact with contaminated water
	Examples
	– Cryptosporidium acquired following swimming in contaminated water (rivers or swimming pools)
	– Pseudomonas aeruginosa contaminated water has been identified as a source of infection in augmented care areas where individuals tend to have many invasive devices (DH 2016)
	Droplets/aerosols
	Description
	Droplets of saliva produced during talking, coughing and sneezing or contaminated water. Large droplets tend to fall rapidly to the ground and are unlikely to be inhaled; however, smaller droplet nuclei (usually derived from aerosols) can remain airborne for hours and can therefore be inhaled.
	Examples
	SARS-CoV-2 acquired from infected individuals via aerosols produced when carrying out AGP
	Legionellosis following inhalation of *Legionella* when showering
Vectors	**Description**
	Transmission by insects and animals
	Examples
	Cockroaches and ants may transfer enteric pathogens to food in food preparation areas, Malaria (protozoa) is transmitted if bitten by infected mosquitoes

Source: Adapted from Wilson 2019.

ACTIVITY

> ### Box 12.6 Activity: portals of entry
>
> Identify Mrs. Lewis's portals of entry.

Mrs. Lewis's wound (already infected) is one portal of entry, but her intravenous access site is another portal of entry. Although we have many natural defences to prevent microorganisms entering the body, individuals often have increased routes for entry because of invasive procedures (e.g. urinary catheters, vascular access devices, chest drains) and wounds. The Health Protection Scotland 2016-point prevalence survey (HPS 2017) identified that 75% of people with a Blood Stream Infection had a vascular access device (peripheral or central) in-situ within the 48 h prior to the onset of infection and 50% of individuals with a UTI had a urinary catheter present within 7 days the infection onset.

Susceptible host

Most people are vulnerable to infection because of their immunity, age, underlying disease and medical interventions.

ACTIVITY

> ### Box 12.7 Activity: factors that make people susceptible to infection
>
> Discuss with a colleague the people in the scenarios and the factors that make them susceptible to infection.

Individuals vary widely in their ability to resist infection. People are especially vulnerable to infection if they have underlying disease. Mrs. Lewis's long-term conditions of rheumatoid arthritis and diabetes and Stacey's hepatitis B render them more susceptible. Mrs. Lewis's impaired defence mechanisms could have led to her infection being more severe than in healthy people. Serious diseases, such as cancer, and associated treatments (e.g. powerful drugs including steroids and chemotherapy), affect the immune system too. Local factors, such as a poor blood supply to a wound, increase the likelihood of infection developing, and people who have diabetes, like Mrs. Lewis, can have impaired circulation. Age (especially very young or very old people) and previous exposure to infection and vaccinations, all affect levels of risk (Wilson 2019). Mrs. Lewis, as an older adult with pre-existing medical issues, is therefore more vulnerable to infection.

The presence of a wound, as in the cases of Mrs. Lewis and James, increases susceptibility to infection as the skin, which is an important bodily defence, is breached. Other reasons for susceptibility to infection include poor nutrition, which could apply to any of the people in the scenarios. You should assess individuals for underlying susceptibilities when you are in clinical practice.

Box 12.8 Children and young people practice points: infection prevention and control

Infection control precautions and control procedures are standard to all fields of nursing. For further information, specifically relating to the care of children, see

Macqueen, S., Bruce, E.A. and Gibson, F. 2012. Infection prevention and control. In: *The Great Ormond Street Hospital Manual of Children's Nursing Practices*. Chichester: Wiley-Blackwell, 240–66.

Box 12.9 Pregnancy and birth practice points: infection risks

Infection in pregnancy carries a risk to the mother, but even more to her fetus or newborn infant, who are especially vulnerable to infection, probably because of the immaturity of the immune system and other defence mechanisms. Viruses pose the greatest risk (e.g. abnormality, abortion, premature delivery) but bacterial infections, especially in the neonatal period, can be life-threatening and require prompt diagnosis and treatment. Some infections are bloodborne and cross the placental barrier; others can ascend via the vagina causing risk to the fetus or premature delivery. Any pregnant mother with gastrointestinal infection, rash, severe throat infection or offensive vaginal discharge requires isolation and immediate obstetric assessment.

For further reading, see

https://www.rcog.org.uk/en/guidelines-research-services/guidelines/gtg36/

https://www.gov.uk/guidance/group-b-streptococcal-infections

Summary

- HCAI is a major concern to governments and the general public. National infection prevention and control policies and guidelines are regularly updated and these will be incorporated into local guidelines by the IPCT for adoption and implementation by staff working for their organisation.
- It is important to keep up to date with changes to local policy and practical IPC guidance made in response to advances in the evidence relating to IP&C.
- An understanding of the chain of infection helps to explain the rationale behind infection prevention and control measures.

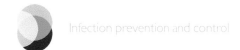

Standard infection prevention and control precautions

According to NHS England and NHS Improvement SIPC, precautions are composed of 10 elements (NHSE/NHSI 2019a);

- hand hygiene
- respiratory and cough hygiene
- personal protective equipment (PPE)
- safe management of care equipment
- safe management of the care environment
- individual placement/assessment for infection risk
- safe management of blood and body fluids
- safe management of linen
- safe disposal of waste (including sharps)
- occupational safety/managing prevention of exposure (including sharps).

In addition to the above, concerns relating to the increasing incidence of antimicrobial resistant organisms has resulted in the need to improve antimicrobial stewardship.

In this chapter, you will focus on the skills associated with standard precautions based on the principle that all blood, body fluids, secretions, excretions except sweat, non-intact skin and mucous membranes may be a source of transmissible infectious organisms. Standard IPC precautions are the essential practices that need to be used when caring for all individuals, irrespective of the known or suspected presence of infectious organisms. Standard IPC practices apply in all settings and locations where healthcare services are provided.

HAND HYGIENE

Adequate hand hygiene is the single most important practice in reducing the spread of infection during care delivery (HPS 2013). Loveday et al. (2014) identified standard principles for hand hygiene, and these principles are referred to throughout this chapter, with application to practice and this chapter's scenarios.

The term 'hand decontamination', used throughout these principles, is defined as 'the use of hand sanitiser or handwashing to reduce the number of bacteria on the hands' (NICE 2017a, p. 13). Handwashing is the key skill used for hand hygiene. Effective hand decontamination can also be achieved, in some circumstances, by using an alcohol-based hand sanitiser containing isopropyl alcohol (minimum 70% alcohol/volume).

Box 12.10 Learning outcomes

By the end of this section, you will be able to:

1 understand the importance of hand decontamination in relation to the delivery of care and the safety of both individuals in their care and nurses;
2 identify when hand decontamination is needed;
3 carry out effective hand hygiene;
4 reflect on the factors that influence compliance with hand hygiene practice.

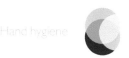

Learning outcome 1: understand the importance of hand decontamination in relation to the delivery of care and the safety of both individuals in their care and nurses

Hungarian obstetrician Ignaz Semmelweis (1815–1865) succeeded in reducing the death rate of his patients from around 1 in 8 to 1 in 79 by persuading his colleagues and medical students to wash their hands in a solution of chlorinated lime before every individual contact (WHO 2009). Since then, it has become widely recognised that the hands of those employed in healthcare settings are an important route for the transmission of infection (Loveday et al. 2014). People requiring access to healthcare services are often more vulnerable to infection for a variety of reasons; therefore, the consistent application of IPC precautions form an essential component of every healthcare interaction.

Microorganisms are important in an ecological balance on earth; some living in and on humans and other animals (normal flora) are needed to maintain health. However, as some microorganisms cause disease, how individuals interact with the environment is important. James's work environment may not be conducive to keeping his wound free from infection, especially if it was not adequately covered. As you will read in Chapter 13, 'Principles of Wound Care', traumatic wounds are nearly always contaminated, so infection poses a high risk in these situations.

It is evident that the general population requires a basic knowledge of hygiene and infection control, including handwashing to reduce their susceptibility to infection. The health promotion messages utilised by the UK Government during the COVID-19 pandemic centred on the importance of hand hygiene and environmental cleanliness as ways to avoid infection (see https://www.gov.uk/coronavirus for further information). Now that James has an infected wound, the community nurse for learning disabilities should check that he has the cognitive ability and physical dexterity to look after his wound in between dressing changes and knows when and how to carry out handwashing. The nurse should demonstrate an effective handwashing technique to James and ensure he can carry this out. She could provide pictures of the different stages in handwashing as an aide-memoire. Good handwashing can help to reduce the risk of infection being transferred to other sites in his body or prevent reinfection. James's Health Action Plan should include this information and the other care interventions associated with his leg wound, documenting the role of the different professionals involved in his care.

For some people with learning disabilities, a structured behavioural programme may be necessary to teach effective handwashing. Behavioural approaches are skilled interventions that use reinforcement, prompting and redirecting to help a person to learn new behaviour. The nurse should assess the individual's comprehension level and adapt a programme to meet the needs of the individual. Sometimes, a backward chaining technique is used, which involves teaching the final stage of the skill first, and then working consecutively backwards. Encouragement and positive reinforcement by nurses are very important.

Bacteria on hands

Resident or normal flora are those organisms that have adapted to live in stable populations within the hair follicles, sebaceous glands and dead skin scales of the epidermis and are less likely to be implicated in cross-infection due to being difficult to remove. Transient (temporary) microorganisms, however, are readily acquired on the surface of the skin following contact with bodily excretions and secretions as well as from the environment. Although these organisms tend to be short-lived due to the antibacterial properties of the skin, they are very easily transferred to the next person or object touched (Wilson 2019). The aim of hand hygiene is to remove transient bacteria to below the level likely to cause infection.

> **Box 12.11 Activity: transient microorganisms in everyday practice**
>
> Consider how you might pick up transient microorganisms on your hands during everyday nursing practice.

ACTIVITY

Some examples are

1. after the care of a person who has been incontinent;
2. when emptying urine bags and bedpans;
3. when handling the bed linen of a person who has an infection or has been incontinent;
4. when assisting a person into/out of bed;
5. when touching fomites, such as computer keyboards, persons' notes, lockers or beds;
6. when using reusable care-associated equipment such as commodes, blood pressure monitors and IV pumps;
7. when taking a person's pulse or temperature.

You can pick up microorganisms following any activity that involves direct or indirect contact with people and the care environment. Wilson et al. (2006) found that more than a third of keyboards tested in their study were contaminated with MRSA, regardless of the position of the keyboard. Hand hygiene rarely accompanied keyboard contact. Transferring bacteria from your hands to an individual can result in them becoming colonised and potentially infected. Effective hand hygiene is the single most important action that can reduce the incidence of HCAIs in all settings.

Learning outcome 2: assess when hand decontamination is needed

Loveday et al. (2014 SP6) suggest that the standard principles you should adhere to are that hands must be decontaminated:

Immediately before and after each episode of direct contact
Immediately after contact with body fluids, mucous membranes or non-intact skins

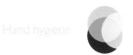

Immediately after contact with items within the immediate care environment
Immediately after the removal of gloves

Pathogens are likely to be acquired on the hands in greatest numbers when handling moist, heavily contaminated substances such as body fluids. The 'five moments of hand hygiene' (Sax et al. 2007) (Figure 12.2) have been widely adopted and describes those aspects of care irrespective of location where it is essential that hand hygiene is undertaken.

ACTIVITY

Box 12.12 Activity: five moments of hand hygiene

Consider the WHO's five moments of hand hygiene (Figure 12.2) in relation to the practice scenarios. Identify when nurses would decontaminate their hands.

Examples you could have thought of include the following:

Mrs. Lewis: before and after assisting with her personal hygiene and assisting her on and off the commode, after emptying and decontaminating the commode, after removing gloves worn to take the used linen from her bed, before and after changing her wound dressing and before and after administering intravenous medication

James: before and after changing his wound dressing.

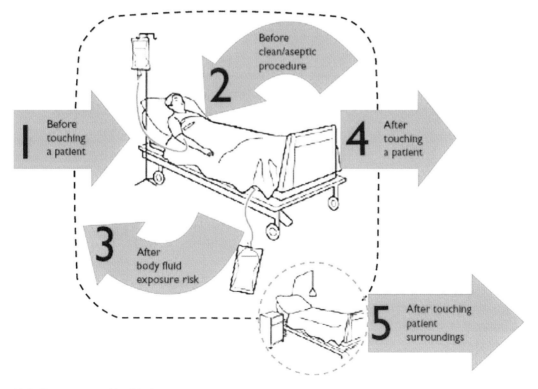

Figure 12.2: Five moments of hand hygiene.

Stacey: after dealing with her vomit and changing her bed linen, before and after giving her intramuscular injection.

Although the nurses caring for Stacey know that she has hepatitis B, in many other situations, this information is not known. Therefore, following the principles of hand decontamination and the other standard IPC precautions for each and every individual, will protect you and other people from the unwitting transmission of currently unidentified pathogens.

Public Health England (2013b) also recommends that all appropriate healthcare staff should be up to date with immunisations for vaccine preventable diseases such as hepatitis B, tuberculosis (TB), measles, mumps and rubella, influenza and chickenpox. From 2021, vaccines for SARS-CoV-2 (COVID-19) have been available to healthcare workers and the adult population of the UK.

Learning outcome 3: carry out hand hygiene effectively

Transient microorganisms are relatively easy to remove simply by washing the hands with soap and water, however, to ensure that this is an effective and reliable handwashing technique is essential.

The phrase 'Bare Below the Elbows' has been used to describe the manner in which healthcare providers should present themselves to be able to effectively carry out hand hygiene. The presence of physical barriers such as long sleeves, long, false or varnished nails, wrist jewellery and rings will inevitably result in reduced efficacy of the hand hygiene process (NHSE and NHSI 2020).

Hand hygiene products

Loveday et al. (2014) reviewed hand-cleaning preparations. They concluded that, generally, washing hands effectively with soap and water removes transient microorganisms and renders hands socially clean, which is sufficient for most care activities. Antimicrobial soap is not required for the majority of healthcare activities but should be used when there is the potential for resident flora to cause infection i.e., surgical procedures. Some antiseptics such as chlorhexidine gluconate have a residual effect, which can be beneficial where it is desirable to have sustained suppression of the growth of microorganisms. Alcohol-based hand sanitisers come in many forms; rub, gel and foam and provide an effective way to rapidly clean the hands, reducing both transient and resident flora, particularly in those locations with limited access to clean water. However, alcohol-based products are rapidly inactivated in the presence of organic matter and so should not be used on visibly soiled hands, nor are they effective against spores, so should not be used when caring for individuals with *C. difficile*. Alcohol hand rubs have been shown to increase the frequency of hand hygiene and so improve hand hygiene compliance, particularly if located at the point of care (Wilson 2019).

Effective handwashing technique involves four processes: preparation, washing, rinsing, and drying. The recommendations by Loveday et al. for these processes are summarised in Box 12.13. These processes are now discussed in more detail.

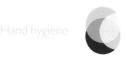

Box 12.13 Steps for an effective handwashing technique

At the start of each shift, remove all wrist and hand jewellery and cover all cuts/abrasions with waterproof dressings. Ensure nails are kept short and free from nail varnish.

Preparation

Check that you have the following: running water, soap, paper towels and a foot-operated waste bin.

- Wet hands under running water before applying liquid soap or an antimicrobial preparation.

Washing

- Rub the hands together in a methodical fashion for 10–15 s ensuring that a lather is generated and that all surfaces of the hands come into contact with the handwash solution.
- Particular attention must be paid to the tips of the fingers, the thumbs and the areas between the fingers.

Remember that your dominant hand is usually more effective and will therefore clean the non-dominant hand better unless specific effort is made to ensure that the non-dominant hand is equally effective.

Rinsing

- Hands should be rinsed thoroughly making sure to remove all soap residues.

Drying

Pat dry with good-quality paper towels ensuring that the hands are completely dry at the end of the process.

(There is some evidence that hand dryers should be avoided in clinical areas due to wide-spread contamination of the surrounding areas caused by splashing of water (Best et al. 2014).)

Preparation for handwashing

Box 12.14 Activity: preparing for handwashing

ACTIVITY

What do you think you would need to do to prepare for handwashing? Consider both facilities and yourself.

Ensure you have the necessary equipment at the sink area – liquid soap and paper hand-towels. You must have your forearms exposed and should not wear false nails (they can harbour microorganisms), wristwatches, or jewellery such as rings (excluding one plain band ring, according to local policy) and bracelets. You must keep nails short, free of nail varnish and clean. Preparation also includes covering cuts and abrasions with a waterproof dressing to prevent the risk of acquiring infections via breaks in skin integrity (NHSE and NHSI 2019a).

Washing and rinsing

Box 12.15 Activity: UV disclosing cream

Find out whether you can access UV disclosing cream from your IPCT to check how effectively you cleanse your hands using the cream as an alcohol sanitiser substitute and then how effectively you remove the cream when using your normal handwashing technique.

Figure 12.3 shows the areas most commonly missed (Ayliffe et al. 2001). How does this diagram compare with your handwashing results?

Loveday et al. (2014) stressed that all surfaces of the hands must be included during handwashing. Figure 12.4 shows an example of a technique that can help you to cover all surfaces of your hands during hand decontamination. You should finish by washing your wrists up to and just beyond where the cuff of disposable gloves would end.

Box 12.16 Activity: using UV disclosing cream

Rewash your hands using the principles in Box 12.13 and the technique in Figure 12.4 as a guide. If available, use UV disclosing cream for this activity, so you can note any improvement: did you manage to cover all areas of your hands this time? Ensure you time your handwashing with a watch and adhere to the recommended minimum of 10–15 s.

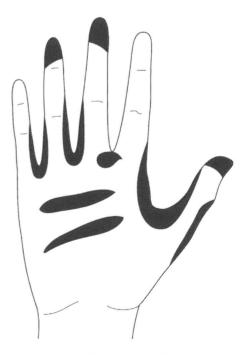

Figure 12.3: Areas commonly missed with poor handwashing. (Reproduced with permission from Ayliffe, G.A.J., Babb, J.R. and Taylor, L.J. 2001. Hospital-Acquired Infection: Principles and Prevention, 3rd edn. London: Arnold).

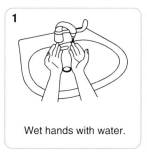
1 Wet hands with water.

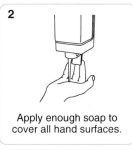
2 Apply enough soap to cover all hand surfaces.

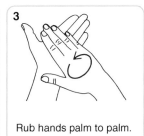
3 Rub hands palm to palm.

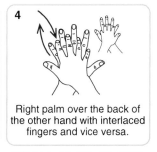
4 Right palm over the back of the other hand with interlaced fingers and vice versa.

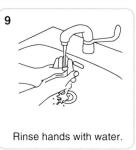
5 Palm to palm with fingers interlaced.

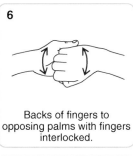
6 Backs of fingers to opposing palms with fingers interlocked.

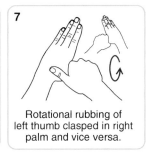
7 Rotational rubbing of left thumb clasped in right palm and vice versa.

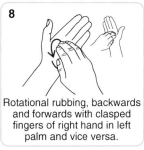
8 Rotational rubbing, backwards and forwards with clasped fingers of right hand in left palm and vice versa.

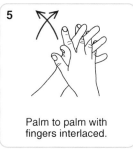
9 Rinse hands with water.

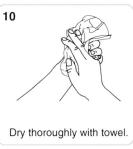
10 Dry thoroughly with towel.

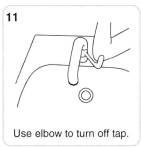
11 Use elbow to turn off tap.

12 Steps 3-8 should take at least 15 seconds.
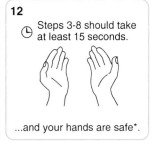
...and your hands are safe*.

Figure 12.4: Handwashing technique. (Adapted from Health Protection Scotland, NIPCM, Appendix One – Best Practice- How to handwash, http://www.nipcm.hps.scot.nhs.uk/appendices/appendix-1-best-practice-how-to-hand-wash accessed on 12 November 2020). NB. Steps 3–8 should also be used when applying alcohol-based sanitiser.

The amount of time you wash your hands is important, as the mechanical action helps to remove bacteria. As you can see, the guidelines by Loveday et al. suggest you spend a minimum of 10–15 s; when timing this action in the last activity, did it feel longer than usual? Hands should be rinsed thoroughly before patting dry with good-quality paper towels (Loveday et al. 2014). When disposing of paper towels, using 'hands-free' foot-operated pedal bins reduces the risk of recontaminating hands after washing.

Use of alcohol-based hand rubs

Alcohol-based hand rubs are quick to use and effective, although, as mentioned, they can be used only when hands are visibly clean, and they are not effective against *C. difficile* spores or fully effective against norovirus. It is also preferable that hands are washed with soap and water after glove removal (Loveday et al. 2014).

Box 12.17 Activity: principles for performing handwashing and drying when using alcohol-based hand rub

Are the principles for performing handwashing and drying that you have read about any different when using an alcohol-based hand rub? If so, how?

The principles are similar. The preparatory measures for handwashing discussed also apply to decontamination of hands with alcohol-based handrubs. Loveday et al. (2014) advise that the hand rub solution must come into contact with all surfaces of the hands, with the hands rubbed together vigorously, giving particular attention to the tips of the fingers, the thumbs and the areas between the fingers, until the solution has evaporated and the hands are dry. After several consecutive uses of alcohol-based hand rub, the hands may begin to feel 'sticky' due to the build-up of emollient and should be washed with soap and water.

Surgical hand antisepsis is the technique that needs to be undertaken prior to carrying out surgical and some invasive procedures, i.e. central venous catheter insertion and involves the use of antimicrobial soap. In some circumstances, licensed antimicrobial alcohol-based sanitisers can be utilised between surgical procedures providing the integrity of the surgeons sterile gloves has not been compromised. Prior to undertaking surgical scrubbing or rubbing the hands must be washed as per the procedure outlined in Figure 12.5. For further information on surgical scrubbing/rubbing, please refer to SIPC precautions: national hand hygiene and personal protective equipment policy (NHSE/NHSI 2019a).

Learning outcome 4: reflect on the factors that influence effective handwashing practice

There are various barriers to good hand hygiene, which affect compliance. In a large hospital-wide survey, Pittet et al. (1999) identified predictors of non-compliance with hand hygiene during routine care and found average compliance was 48%, being highest among nurses. Non-compliance was higher in intensive therapy units rather than medical wards, during procedures with a high risk for bacterial contamination, and when intensity of care was high. The results indicated that organisational factors must be considered and that hand hygiene compliance could improve if activities were targeted on certain wards, groups of staff and individual interventions. Staff champions and positive role models with an active interest in hand hygiene improvement are critical to improving compliance. Each member of the staff can exert a very powerful influence on colleagues.

The importance of hand hygiene for a person in care must not be forgotten and it is just as important for them to have ready access to hand hygiene facilities. If they are unable to access these for themselves, it is important that healthcare staff enable individuals to clean their hands, particularly after using toilet facilities and before eating and drinking, by providing them with soap and water (wet wipes) or hand sanitiser. People can also provide prompts to improve practice by reminding staff

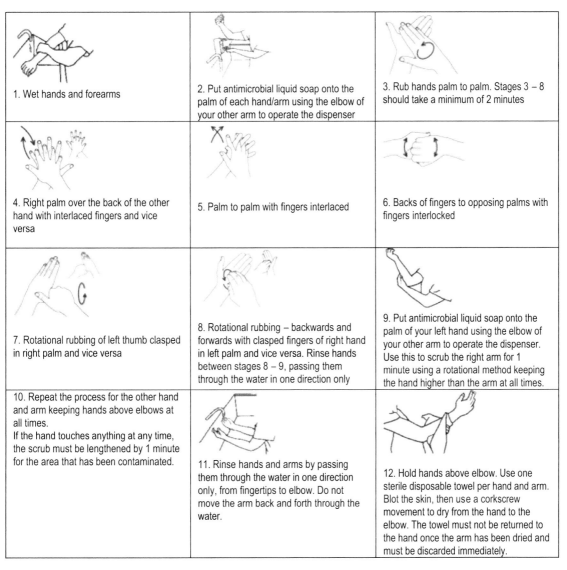

1. Wet hands and forearms	2. Put antimicrobial liquid soap onto the palm of each hand/arm using the elbow of your other arm to operate the dispenser	3. Rub hands palm to palm. Stages 3 – 8 should take a minimum of 2 minutes
4. Right palm over the back of the other hand with interlaced fingers and vice versa	5. Palm to palm with fingers interlaced	6. Backs of fingers to opposing palms with fingers interlocked
7. Rotational rubbing of left thumb clasped in right palm and vice versa	8. Rotational rubbing – backwards and forwards with clasped fingers of right hand in left palm and vice versa. Rinse hands between stages 8 – 9, passing them through the water in one direction only	9. Put antimicrobial liquid soap onto the palm of your left hand using the elbow of your other arm to operate the dispenser. Use this to scrub the right arm for 1 minute using a rotational method keeping the hand higher than the arm at all times.
10. Repeat the process for the other hand and arm keeping hands above elbows at all times. If the hand touches anything at any time, the scrub must be lengthened by 1 minute for the area that has been contaminated.	11. Rinse hands and arms by passing them through the water in one direction only, from fingertips to elbow. Do not move the arm back and forth through the water.	12. Hold hands above elbow. Use one sterile disposable towel per hand and arm. Blot the skin, then use a corkscrew movement to dry from the hand to the elbow. The towel must not be returned to the hand once the arm has been dried and must be discarded immediately.

Figure 12.5: Surgical scrub technique. (Adapted from Health Protection Scotland, NIPCM, Appendix Three – Best Practice- Surgical scrubbing, http://www.nipcm.hps.scot.nhs.uk/appendices/appendix-3-best-practice-surgical-scrubbing/, accessed on 12/11/2020).

about hand hygiene. Individuals should be encouraged to ask staff if they have cleaned their hands prior to delivering care.

The need for commitment from all levels of the organisation is necessary to support this aspect of improving compliance. The DH (2015b) requires that healthcare providers have adequate provision of handwashing facilities and antimicrobial handrub and evidence of this is obtained during external inspections such as those carried out by the CQC and the Patient-Led Assessment of the Care Environment (PLACE), which is a system for assessing the quality of the care environment.

(For more information about PLACE refer to: https://improvement.nhs.uk/resources/patient-led-assessments-care-environment-place/)

ACTIVITY

Box 12.18 Activity: factors influencing effective handwashing

What factors can you think of that might influence effective handwashing? In particular, think about when you would need to wash your hands either in the community or in a hospital setting. Referring to the scenarios will help you.

By referring to the scenarios you will probably have identified how frequently nurses need to wash their hands. Frequent handwashing can cause damage to skin, especially if antiseptic solutions are used, or if hands are not dried properly. Cracked or dry skin may harbour more bacteria and increase the risk of cross-infection. Therefore, you should apply an emollient hand cream regularly to protect skin from the drying effects of regular hand decontamination. If skin irritation or dryness persists, seek occupational health advice (Loveday et al. 2014).

Although healthcare staff are well aware of the importance of hand hygiene in reducing infections, compliance still falls below 100%. Several reasons have been identified for this including:

- Inadequate and inconveniently placed handwashing facilities;
- Lack of time due to increased workload may deter handwashing when facilities are some distance away; however, the availability of alcohol-based sanitisers at the point of care goes some way to offset this;
- Water may be too hot or too cold if there is no mixer tap present;
- Lack of knowledge or understanding of the importance of hand contamination in the transmission of infection;
- Lack of positive role models in the workplace and emphasis on handwashing by peers and managers;
- The use of gloves has been found to affect compliance with handwashing (Loveday et al. 2014).

In recent years, there have been several campaigns to improve hand hygiene, including during the Covid-19 pandemic (https://www.gov.uk/government/publications/how-to-stop-the-spread-of-coronavirus-covid-19/how-to-stop-the-spread-of-coronavirus-covid-19). For Health Protection Scotland's campaign, see http://www.nipcm.hps.scot.nhs.uk/resources/hand-hygiene-wash-your-hands-of-them/

The WHO (2009) published an extensive evidence-based review of hand hygiene for healthcare workers and recommended a multimodal hand hygiene improvement strategy, comprising system change (access to adequate facilities), education based on the WHO's five moments, evaluation and feedback, workplace reminders and creating an environment of safety. To further promote the importance of hand hygiene, WHO have also declared that May 5th should be Global Hand Hygiene Day with national and local activities being undertaken to promote hand hygiene.

ACTIVITY

> **Box 12.19 Activity: Global Hand Hygiene Day**
>
> Ask your IPC team what activities are being planned for the next Global Hand Hygiene Day and see if there is anything you can do in your clinical area to improve hand hygiene practice. Visit https://www.who.int/infection-prevention/campaigns/clean-hands/en/ for further information from WHO relating to the promotion of hand hygiene and the 'Save Lives: Clean your hands' campaign (WHO 2020b).

Summary

- Effective hand hygiene is an essential tool in preventing and controlling infection.
- Nurses need to know when and how to clean their hands as well as what product to use. For example, alcohol-based handrubs are an acceptable alternative to handwashing providing hands are not visibly soiled but not if caring for individuals with *C. difficile*.
- Handwashing must be performed correctly paying attention to preparation, washing, rinsing, and drying.
- Hands must be patted dry carefully with paper towels.
- Commitment at all levels of the organisation is needed to overcome the barriers to hand hygiene and achieve consistent hand hygiene compliance.
- Infection prevention and control champions can assist in improving compliance.
- Commitment from all levels of the organisation is needed to support aspects of improving compliance with hand hygiene.

USE OF PERSONAL PROTECTIVE EQUIPMENT, INCLUDING GLOVES, APRONS, GOWNS, FACE AND EYE PROTECTION

Loveday et al. (2014) advise that the selection of protective equipment (aprons, gowns, gloves, eye protection and face masks) should be based on an assessment of the following:

> the risk of transmission of microorganisms to the patient or to the carer and the risk of contamination of healthcare practitioners' clothing and skin by patients' blood, body fluid, secretions or excretions.

Gloves and aprons are the most commonly used items of PPE; however, masks and visors must be worn when there is a risk of blood, body fluids, secretions and excretions splashing into the face and eyes. Respiratory protective equipment (a particulate filtrate mask – FFP3 respirator) must be worn when carrying out aerosol-generating procedures for individuals with some airborne respiratory infections such as influenza and COVID-19. All members of staff who may need to wear FFP3 respirators must be fit-tested, ideally as part of departmental induction. Fit-testing is mask-specific, so staff will need to be fit-tested again if alternative respirators are provided.

ACTIVITY

Box 12.20 Activity: fit-testing

Contact your Health and Safety representative or IPC team to find out how to be fit-tested in your organisation.

Box 12.21 Learning outcomes

On completion of this section, you will be able to:

1 identify the procedures for which gloves, sterile or non-sterile, are recommended and key factors in their use.
2 discuss when plastic aprons and gowns should be worn, stating the rationale.
3 understand when to use facial protection (masks, goggles and face shields).

Learning outcome 1: identify the procedures for which gloves, sterile or non-sterile, are recommended and key factors in their use

According to epic3, gloves should be worn:

- when undertaking invasive procedures;
- for contact with sterile sites and non-intact skin or mucous membranes;
- when carrying out any all activity assessed as carrying a risk of exposure to blood or body fluids; and
- when handling sharps or contaminated devices.

(Loveday et al. 2014, SP21)

It is important not to wear gloves when not necessary as this decreases hand hygiene compliance and could increase the risk of skin irritation and sensitivity reactions. The selection of sterile or non-sterile gloves is dependent on the activity, i.e. invasive procedure and or contact with non-intact skin or mucous membranes. Refer to Figure 12.6 for PPE risk assessment.

In the next activity, you need to consider situations when sterile gloves are needed, where non-sterile gloves are satisfactory, and those situations where no gloves are needed.

Situations where sterile gloves are used

ACTIVITY

Box 12.22 Activity: use of sterile gloves

Referring to each scenario at the beginning of the chapter, write down clinical procedures and situations for which you think sterile gloves should be worn.

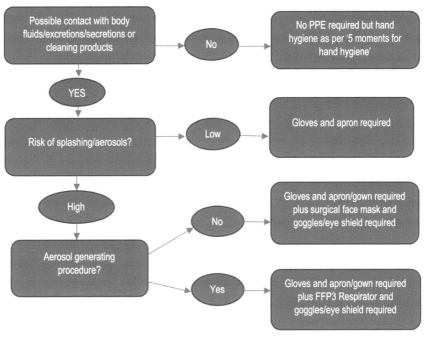

Figure 12.6: **PPE risk assessment.** (Adapted from Wilson 2019, p. 254.)

For Mrs. Lewis and James, an aseptic technique (see later section) using sterile gloves is necessary when redressing their wounds to reduce the risk of cross-infection. For Stacey, sterile gloves are not necessary from the information given in the scenarios.

Based on this activity, it can be seen that sterile gloves tend to be used when undertaking invasive procedures and when contact with non-intact skin is anticipated. An example of a procedure where sterile gloves are necessary is urinary catheterisation (for more information, see Chapter 6).

When applying sterile gloves, you must avoid contaminating the outer surface of the glove. Figure 12.7 shows the technique required.

Situations where non-sterile gloves are satisfactory

Box 12.23 Activity: non-sterile gloves

ACTIVITY

Look again at the practice scenarios and list those clinical procedures and situations when nurses and other staff should use non-sterile gloves.

As Mrs. Lewis has MRSA, non-sterile gloves should be used by all staff entering her room to carry out physical assessments and/or to deliver care; however, if no direct contact with Mrs. Lewis is anticipated, no PPE is required. Hand hygiene must be carried out as per the '5 moments for hand hygiene'. Gloves must always be worn when there is potential contact with faeces, urine or any other body fluid (Loveday et al. 2014), so non-sterile gloves must be worn when assisting Mrs. Lewis to use

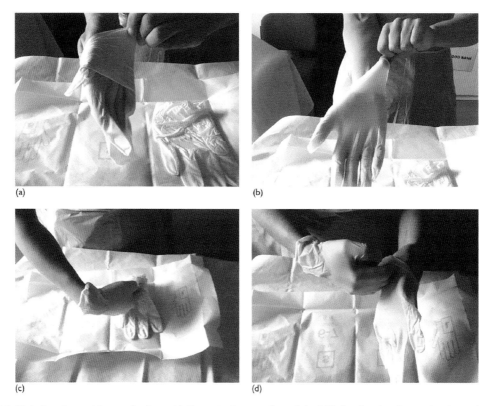

Figure 12.7: Technique for applying sterile gloves. (a) Grasp the inner surface of the folded cuff and push your hand into the glove, lining up your thumb with the thumb of the glove. (b) Pull the first glove on fully but only touch the inside of the glove to do this, so the outside remains sterile. (c) Using your gloved hand, pick up the second glove under the cuff. (d) Pull the second glove on using your other, gloved, hand to help, but it must not touch ungloved areas.

the commode and subsequently emptying and cleaning it. In addition, the domestic cleaner should be instructed to wear disposable gloves (and apron) when cleaning the room and to remove them before leaving the room. Mrs. Lewis will have her dressing changed and blood taken regularly, for which gloves should be worn (Wilson 2019).

For James, when the district nurse removes James's soiled dressing, any outer layers, such as a cotton bandage keeping the dressing in place, might be removed using non-sterile gloves, with sterile gloves preserved for the aseptic dressing procedure itself.

Considering Stacey, contact with vomit (a body fluid) requires the use of non-sterile gloves. Whether gloves would be worn for other procedures with Stacey depends on individual risk assessment and local policy. Gloves are not required for routine intradermal, intramuscular or subcutaneous injections (Wilson 2019).

Wearing gloves also protects from potential harm to nurses during preparation of specific drugs, such as antibiotics and cytotoxic materials as well as when undertaking decontamination activities. *Note:* You should adhere to local policy regarding wearing of gloves in practice.

Key factors in using gloves

All gloves can perforate and should therefore be checked for defects. Keeping fingernails short helps to avoid perforations. The standard principles by Loveday et al. (2014) include the following points:

- Gloves are single-use items and must be put on immediately before an episode of care and discarded after each care activity for which they were worn to prevent the transmission of microorganisms to other sites in that individual or to other individuals. Wilson et al. (2017) identified that on 59% of occasions, non-sterile clinical gloves were used inappropriately and that potential cross contamination occurred in 50% of care episodes. For further advice/information on the inappropriate use of gloves, please refer to the NHSE Campaign – 'the gloves are off' (NHSE 2018).

- Hands should be decontaminated after removing gloves, preferably with soap and water. The WHO (2009) highlighted that bacterial flora colonising individuals has been recovered from the hands of up to 30% of healthcare workers who wear gloves during contact, presumably via small defects in gloves or by contamination of the hands during glove removal.

- All gloves should be disposed of correctly (see the later section).

Situations where gloves are not necessary

Box 12.24 Activity: situations where gloves are not necessary

With reference to the scenarios, make a list of the procedures and situations for which gloves are usually unnecessary. Think particularly of all the individuals who may come into contact with those in need of care and try to decide whether they need to wear gloves.

Unless assisting with nursing care activities Mrs. Lewis's visitors are unlikely to have contact with body fluids; therefore, they do not need to wear gloves or an apron. However, they should be instructed to wash their hands, on arrival and before leaving the room. If Mrs. Lewis visits another department (e.g. X-ray), only those staff having direct contact will need to use gloves. As porters transferring Mrs. Lewis are unlikely to be in direct contact with her or infectious material, gloves are not needed.

Concerning James, gloves are needed only when changing wound dressings. For other aspects of his care, they are not required. Similarly, for most of Stacey's care – for example, checking her blood pressure, administering oral medication and giving psychological support – gloves are not required.

Box 12.25 Activity: gloves available to practitioners

When next in the clinical area, take note of the different types of gloves available to practitioners.

- All gloves must meet the European Standard (Loveday et al. 2014). Types of disposable gloves include natural rubber latex (NRL), vinyl and nitrile. NRL is the material of choice due to the degree of protection offered and level of dexterity.

To minimise the risk of developing latex sensitivity, NRL gloves must be low protein and powder-free. Staff who regularly use latex gloves must be monitored via occupational health for the development of latex sensitivity.

(Further information relating to latex gloves is available from the health and safety executive at https://www.hse.gov.uk/skin/employ/latex-gloves.htm).

Some staff and individuals have sensitivities to latex, so non-latex alternatives must be available, and allergies clearly documented. Nitrile gloves offer similar protection to NRL, but they may also cause sensitivities. Polythene gloves should not be used due to their permeability and tendency to damage.

The RCN publication 'Tools of the Trade' provides detailed guidance about glove use and prevention of contact dermatitis (RCN 2020).

Learning outcome 2: discuss when disposable aprons and gowns should be worn, stating the rationale

Box 12.26 Activity: plastic aprons and gowns

ACTIVITY

Make a list of occasions when you have seen plastic aprons worn and/or gowns used in clinical settings.

You may be able to relate your experiences to the advice by Loveday et al. (2014, Standard Principles 26, 27 and 28) about apron and gown use.

- Disposable plastic aprons must be worn when close contact with the person, materials or equipment may result in the contamination of clothing with pathogenic microorganisms or blood, body fluids, secretions and excretions
- Full-body gowns should be worn if there is a risk of extensive splashing of body fluids onto the skin or clothing of the healthcare practitioner (e.g. during childbirth)
- As with gloves, aprons and gowns must be worn as single-use items for one care activity and then disposed of. If used reusable gowns must be sent for laundering in a fully compliant facility

Normalisation as a concept was proposed during the 1960s by Bengt Nirje in Scandinavia and developed further by Wolfensburger in the 1970s to counter the existing practices of social exclusion and institutionalisation frequently utilised when caring for those with learning disabilities. For further information please visit:

http://www.aboutlearningdisabilities.co.uk/normalisation-learning-disabilities.html

In community/assisted living settings, there is an emphasis on social aspects of care and normalisation, so the use of plastic aprons is likely to be greatly reduced. Thinking about James, it is really important to try and 'normalise' healthcare interactions as far as possible; however, when dealing with body fluids, they are still advisable.

Learning Outcome 3: understand when to use facial protection (masks goggles/face shields)

According to Wigglesworth (2019), facial and respiratory protection should be used when there is a risk of splashing into the face and eyes as well as to protect the wearer from exposure to infectious large droplets or from inhaling infectious aerosolised droplet nuclei such as those produced when carrying out aerosol-generating procedures (AGPs). The use of surgical face masks also prevents exhaled droplets from the wearer contaminating surfaces such as surgical wounds or the environment.

Aerosol-generating procedures

This is the list of medical procedures for COVID-19 that have been reported to be aerosol-generating and are associated with an increased risk of respiratory transmission and therefore require the use of FFP3 respirators, eye protection gloves and gowns:

- tracheal intubation and extubation
- manual ventilation
- tracheotomy or tracheostomy procedures (insertion or removal)
- bronchoscopy
- dental procedures (using high-speed devices, for example, ultrasonic scalers/high-speed drills
- non-invasive ventilation (NIV); Bi-level Positive Airway Pressure Ventilation (BiPAP) and Continuous Positive Airway Pressure Ventilation (CPAP)
- high flow nasal oxygen (HFNO)
- high frequency oscillatory ventilation (HFOV)
- induction of sputum using nebulised saline
- respiratory tract suctioning
- upper ENT airway procedures that involve respiratory suctioning
- upper gastrointestinal endoscopy where open suction of the upper respiratory tract occurs
- high-speed cutting in surgery/post-mortem procedures if respiratory tract/paranasal sinuses involved (from PHE 2020c, COVID-19: infection prevention and control guidance, p 19)

Box 12.27 Activity: facial protection

Identify when facial protection might be required in your area of clinical practice.

Putting on (donning) and removal (doffing) of PPE

To minimise the potential for cross-infection, there is a specific order for the donning and doffing of PPE. When removing items of PPE, it is important not to touch the outer – potentially contaminated surfaces

Hand hygiene should be carried out prior to donning PPE. The order for donning is: apron or gown, mask (surgical mask or FFP3 respirator), eye protection and lastly gloves

Doffing should be carried out in the following order: Gloves – followed by hand hygiene, apron or gown, eye protection followed by hand hygiene and lastly mask or FFP3 respirator,

For more detailed information, please refer to the Gov.UK Coronavirus (COVID-19): personal protective equipment (PPE) hub https://www.gov.uk/government/collections/coronavirus-covid-19-personal-protective-equipment-ppe

Summary

- Selection of appropriate PPE should be based on risk assessment.
- PPE are single-use items and should be disposed of in the correct waste stream (see Table 12.2).
- PPE may need to be removed and changed several times when carrying out multiple care activities for an individual.
- The donning and doffing of PPE should be undertaken in the specified order to minimise the risk of contamination of the wearer.
- Hands must be washed immediately before donning and after doffing PPE.

HEALTHCARE WASTE DISPOSAL AND LINEN MANAGEMENT

There is a statutory duty of care that applies to all those involved in the waste management chain, including nurses. European legislation has led to changes in how waste is classified and disposed of, and new methods have been established for identifying and classifying healthcare waste (DH 2011). A revised colour-coded waste segregation and packaging system is being implemented with use of the 'List of Wastes' codes (formerly the European Waste Catalogue) (see http://www.environment-agency.gov.uk/business/topics/waste/32140.aspx)

The List of Wastes provides common terminology for describing waste throughout Europe. The DH (2011, version 2) provides detailed guidance on management of healthcare waste. For Scotland, see guidance from Health Facilities Scotland (HFS 2015).

Box 12.28 Learning outcomes

By the end of this section, you will be able to:

1. define different types of waste arising from healthcare;
2. identify how colour-coded receptacles are used for segregating different waste streams, and how waste is dealt with safely in healthcare;
3. discuss how soiled linen should be dealt with safely.

Learning outcome 1: define different types of waste arising from healthcare

Complete guidance relating to the management of waste can be found in HTM 07 01 Safe management of healthcare waste (DH 2013c) Healthcare waste is 'waste that is produced by healthcare activities, and of a type specifically related to such activities'. Different terms are used for different types of healthcare waste, according to legislation and regulations; some types are classified as hazardous and others as non-hazardous. How waste is classified affects how it is disposed of, transported and dealt with.

Clinical waste is defined in HTM 07 01 as:

a. "any waste which consists wholly or partly of human or animal tissue, blood or other body fluids, excretions, drugs or other pharmaceutical products, swabs or dressings, syringes, needles or other sharp instruments, being waste which unless rendered safe may prove hazardous to any person coming into contact with it; and

b. any other waste arising from medical, nursing, dental, veterinary, pharmaceutical or similar practice, investigation, treatment, care, teaching or research, or the collection of blood for transfusion, being waste which may cause infection to any person coming into contact with it." (DH 2013c, p. 22)

Clinical waste can be further subdivided into three groups:

1. Waste that could pose a risk of infection
2. Waste which could pose a chemical hazard
3. Pharmaceuticals and waste contaminated by pharmaceutically active (cytostatic or cytotoxic) substances.

Cytotoxic or cytostatic

A full list of medications regarded as being cytostatic or cytotoxic can be found in section 13 of HTM 0701 (DH 2013c).

Most clinical waste is classified as hazardous, however non-cytotoxic or cytostatic waste is classified as non-hazardous but may still require specific handling and disposal. but some types of medicinal waste (medicines that are not cytotoxic or cytostatic) are classified as non-hazardous, although they often possess hazardous properties and, therefore, require appropriate treatment and disposal (DH 2013c).

Mixing of infectious and non-infectious waste is prohibited in England and Wales, and segregation of infectious and non-infectious waste is considered best practice in Scotland and Northern Ireland. Waste is classified as infectious waste if (1) it arises from a person known or suspected to have an infection (whether or not the causal agent is known) and where the waste may contain the pathogen, or (2) where an infection is not known or suspected, but it is considered that there is a potential risk of infection (DH 2013c). Nurses therefore need to assess whether waste generated is likely to be infectious.

Offensive/hygiene waste is non-infectious and classified as non-hazardous, but it may cause offence due to the presence of recognisable healthcare waste items, body fluids or odour.

Box 12.29 Types of waste products

What types of wastes are the soiled wound dressings from Mrs. Lewis and James?

You should have identified that Mrs. Lewis's and James's soiled wound dressings are clinical waste as they are infectious. Both Mrs. Lewis and James are known to have infections, and their soiled wound dressings are likely to contain the pathogens.

Infectious waste is classified as hazardous. Although in these scenarios we know that Mrs. Lewis and James have infections, in other instances, nurses will need to assess the likelihood of an infection being present, as non-infectious soiled dressings can go into the non-hazardous, offensive/hygiene waste stream. Chapter 13 discusses recognition of a wound infection.

Learning outcome 2: identify how colour-coded receptacles are used for segregating different waste streams and how waste is dealt with safely in healthcare

Segregation of waste is mandatory in England and Wales so that different types of waste can be managed appropriately through incineration, treatment, recycling or landfill. To facilitate segregation, the DH (2013c) recommends the use of colour-coded receptacles, advising that a national system should be in place to achieve standardisation.

Box 12.30 Activity: colour receptacles for waste disposal

What colour receptacles have you seen used in practice for waste disposal and what type of waste are they used for?

The colours you are likely to have seen will depend on the type of healthcare settings you have worked in and the type of waste produced. The DH (2013c) recommends a colour-coded system for the different waste types, which require different management (Table 12.2). *Note:* Colour-coding for sharps bins is discussed in the next section.

Appropriate receptacles must be used. For liquid waste, the receptacle should be designed to take liquids, such as a rigid leakproof plastic drum, or a receptacle with fluid-absorbing granules. Sharps must only be placed in approved sharps bins. All other waste may be packaged in flexible bags. The bags or rigid containers must be no more than three-quarters full when they are sealed. The swan-neck method is recommended for sealing bags (HPS 2013) (Figure 12.8). The bags/containers must

Table 12.2: Colour-coding system for waste

Colour receptacle	Waste type and management
Yellow	Infectious waste that has an additional characteristic that means that it must be incinerated in a suitably licensed or permitted facility. Examples: anatomical waste, chemically contaminated samples and diagnostic kits, medicinally contaminated infectious waste; and Category A (as specified in the Carriage Regulations) pathogens (often when in culture form) as these are capable of causing permanent disability, life-threatening or fatal disease.
Orange	Infectious waste, for example, incontinence pads, stoma bags and soiled wound dressings where the individual has an infection and the causative agent is likely to be in the waste. For example, the stoma bag of a person with a gastrointestinal infection. A used wound drain would always go into this waste steam. This waste stream must not contain non-infectious waste or infectious waste with additional characteristics (chemicals, medicines, anatomical waste), which mean it must be incinerated.
Purple	Waste consisting of, or contaminated with cytotoxic and/or cytostatic products.
Yellow with black stripe	Offensive/hygiene waste, such as stoma bags, incontinence pads, catheter bags and soiled wound dressings, when they are not considered infectious. In the community, a person who is self-managing can put small amounts of these items into their domestic waste stream.
Red	Anatomical waste, which includes recognisable body parts and placenta.
Black (or clear)	Domestic waste, which is similar to waste generated at home. Domestic waste should not contain any infectious materials, sharps or medicinal products. Examples: non-recyclable packaging from single-use devices, crisp packets, polystyrene cups, flowers.

Source: Department of Health (DH). 2013. Health Technical Memorandum (HTM) 07-01: Safe management of healthcare waste.

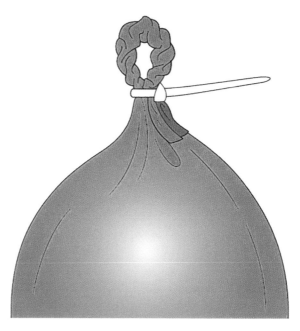

Figure 12.8: Swan-neck technique for sealing waste bags.

be labelled or tagged with their place of origin so that they can be traced back to source. All waste containers should be securely closed/sealed when ¾ full or to the fill line and stored in an area that is inaccessible to people or members of the public prior to transportation to the waste collection point and onward transport to the waste disposal plant. In the community, healthcare workers must ensure that healthcare waste awaiting collection is stored appropriately, away from children and animals.

Learning outcome 3: discuss how soiled linen should be dealt with safely

Soiled linen requires careful handling, bagging and disposal as it may be contaminated with infectious microorganisms present on the skin or body fluids.

Points to remember when changing bed linen: disposable apron (and gloves if there is visible soiling) should be worn when removing used/soiled linen and cleaning the bed, put the used linen directly into the linen skip at the bedside, never place used linen on the floor or items of furniture, do not shake the linen, do not overfill laundry bags (HPS 2013). Gloves and apron must be removed and hands washed prior to remaking the bed with clean linen. Linen bags should never be left in persons rooms and must be stored prior to collection in an area that cannot be accessed by the person or visitors.

The laundry process decontaminates linen through the mechanical process of washing, the detergent used and the temperature of the water. The process must include sufficient time for all parts of the load to be washed at an adequate temperature. Any microorganisms that remain after washing can be destroyed by tumble drying and ironing (Wilson 2019).

ACTIVITY

Box 12.31 Activity: linen categories

Can you name three different types of linen bag and the category of linen that should be placed in each? Why are the different categories needed? Which colour would be used for Mrs. Lewis's used sheets and which colour for Stacey's vomit-covered bed linen? See Table 12.3

Table 12.3: Categories of hospital linen

Category	Bag colour	Linen type	Comments
Used	White or clear	Used, soiled or foul linen	Thermally disinfected (wash at 65°C for 10 mins or 71°C for 3 mins)
Infected	Red water-soluble (alginate) bag with red outer bag	Linen from people with known/ suspected infections or as directed by the IPC team	No hand sorting, thermally disinfected
Heat labile	As per local laundry protocol	Fabric unable to tolerate thermal disinfection	40°C wash plus hypochlorite
Return to sender	As per local laundry protocol	Individuals own clothing, departmental specific items	As per local protocols

Source: Adapted from Wilson (2019, p. 269).

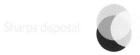

Summary

- Nurses and other healthcare workers have a duty of care to dispose of waste appropriately in order to prevent hazards to themselves, colleagues, individuals in their care and the public.
- It is important to differentiate between different categories of waste and to ensure that it is disposed of in the correct, colour-coded receptacle.
- Used linen must be disposed of correctly according to whether it is infectious or soiled only.

SHARPS DISPOSAL

Safe disposal of sharps, such as needles, blood glucose lancets, phlebotomy equipment, intravenous cannulae and catheter stylets, is important to maintain a safe environment and prevent cross-infection.

In 2013, the health and safety executive published The Health and Safety (Sharp Instruments in Healthcare) Regulations 2013 requiring employers prevent injuries and infections to healthcare workers. Employers are required to minimise the use of sharps, removing them completely where possible and, where there is no reasonable alternative, to minimise the risk of sharps injuries by utilising safety devices or needle-less systems. The regulations apply to all staff including students working in all locations where healthcare services are delivered: NHS, private and other public sector provision, such as prisons (HSE 2013). The RCN have produced detailed guidance in relation to the HSE regulations and the prevention of sharps injuries in healthcare (RCN 2013).

Box 12.32 Learning outcomes

By the end of this section, you will be able to:

1. appreciate the need and reasons for the safe disposal of sharps;
2. explain the principles for the safe use and disposal of sharps;
3. identify the actions required after sharps injury.

Learning outcome 1: appreciate the need and reasons for the safe disposal of sharps

Box 12.33 Activity: disposing of sharps safely

ACTIVITY

Identify two possible reasons for the importance of disposing of sharps safely.

The main reason for disposing of sharps safely is the physical prevention of cross-infection through sharps injuries, including needlesticks. According to epic3 guidelines the average risk of transmission of bloodborne pathogens after a single percutaneous exposure, without post-exposure prophylaxis or prior vaccination (if available), has been estimated as

* hepatitis B virus 33.3% (1 in 3);
* hepatitis C virus 3.3% (1 in 30);
* HIV 0.31% (1 in 300).

In 2011, there were 541 occupational exposures to bloodborne viruses compared to 276 in 2002 (Loveday et al. 2014).

Staff caring for Stacey know that she has hepatitis B, but this information about individuals is not always available as some individuals do not know that they have a bloodborne virus and some that do choose to withhold this information for fear of stigmatisation by family and friends.

It is because of this that all sharps should be handled with care and disposed of as if they are potentially contaminated. All healthcare workers should be vaccinated against hepatitis B. Without immunity to hepatitis B, staff who are caring for Stacey would be at risk of acquiring this virus if they sustained a needlestick injury from her used injection needle.

The safe disposal of sharps effectively removes the risk of inadvertently harming people and colleagues and prevents the fear and anxiety of the transmission of infections that naturally arises following a sharps injury.

ACTIVITY

Box 12.34 Activity: needlestick injury

Discuss with a colleague how you would feel if you sustained a needlestick injury where the individual source was suspected of having a bloodborne infection.

You might have identified fear, anxiety and panic among your emotions. It is clearly much better to prevent needlestick or other sharps injuries.

Learning outcome 2: explain the principles for the safe use and disposal of sharps

ACTIVITY

Box 12.35 Activity: disposing of sharps

Make a list of the key safety factors you think you should take into account when using and disposing of sharps.

There are many factors to take into account.

* Sharps must be disposed of by the user into a designated approved receptacle conforming to BS EN ISO 23907:2012 standards at the point of use
* Needles and syringes should not be disassembled – dispose of these as a single item

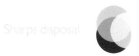

- Needles must never be resheathed, bent or broken
- Never tap or shake the sharps container to make more room
- Sharps should never be carried in the hand or passed directly to another person
- The temporary closure mechanism must be activated when sharps bins are not in use and when being carried
- Sharps bins must be correctly assembled, labelled and securely closed when ¾ full.

(Wilson 2019)

The HSE healthcare waste regulations (HSE 2013) describe the colour of lids should vary according to the nature of the contents and the risk of medicinal contamination:

- purple lid for sharps that are contaminated with cytotoxic or cytostatic medicines;
- yellow lid for sharps that are contaminated with non-cytotoxic and non-cytostatic medicines;
- orange lid for sharps not contaminated with medicines (e.g. sharps used for venepuncture).

The above applies to England and Wales. In Scotland and Northern Ireland, sharps fully discharged of medicines (non-cytotoxic and non-cytostatic) but still contaminated can, in some circumstances, be put into orange-lidded sharps receptacles.

Self-medicating community individuals (e.g. people with diabetes) should be provided with a sharps receptacle and taught to seal and label it and return it to the surgery or pharmacy for disposal when it has reached the fill line. Policies in community healthcare settings and care homes may vary, and you should ensure that you are familiar with the relevant policies for the areas that you study and work in.

Box 12.36 Activity: when a sharps receptacle is full

ACTIVITY

What should you do when a sharps receptacle is full (i.e. reached the fill line)?

You should seal a sharps receptacle according to the manufacturer's instructions, often found on the outside of the receptacle. If you observe that a sharps box is full, be proactive about sealing it. Do not leave someone else to deal with an overfilled sharps box as this is very hazardous. Never shake or tap an overfilled sharps box to try and close the lid. The entire box should be placed in a larger sharps bin which would then be sealed and an incident form completed to report this risk. Sealed receptacles should be left at identified collection points in the manner prescribed by the local policy and labelled with date and source. It is usual for facilities staff to remove the boxes and take them to a central point for transporting. The correct sealing and disposal of sharps bins are essential to protect the many people who could be injured otherwise, including porters, transport staff and waste disposal staff.

Table 12.4: Action after a sharps injury

Emergency action	*Encourage bleeding at the site by squeezing.*
	Wash the wound well with soap and running water.
	For blood splashes to eyes, mouth or into broken skin, irrigate the affected area thoroughly with plenty of running water.
	Call for assistance.
	Cover wound with waterproof dressing.
Reporting	Inform your manager immediately.
	Complete accident/incident form.
	Identify individual source if possible.
	Report to the occupational health department immediately, or if closed, attend the emergency department for further advice.
Follow-up	Make use of counselling if required.
	Attend for testing if indicated.
	Follow medical advice.

Note: You should consult and follow your local policy throughout. It is the responsibility of the member of staff involved and their manager to see that all procedures are carried out.

Learning outcome 3: identify the actions required after a sharps injury

Box 12.37 Activity: sharps injury

ACTIVITY

With a colleague, discuss what you think should be done after a sharps injury.

All healthcare employers are required to develop processes for dealing with sharps injuries. These processes include identifying the employee's responsibility to report the injury and their subsequent entitlement to be provided with counselling and testing services. However, before this stage is reached, emergency action is needed. Now check your ideas with Table 12.4.

The same policies should also be used if blood or body fluids are splashed into the eyes or mouth, or come into contact with broken skin.

Box 12.38 Activity: local clinical policy on a sharps injury

ACTIVITY

When you are next in the practice setting, seek out and read the local clinical policy on the action to be taken after a sharps injury.

Summary

- Sharps pose a potential hazard to nurses, other staff and the public.
- All nurses must follow national and local policy and handle and dispose of sharps safely to prevent the risk of sharps injuries to themselves and colleagues.
- All healthcare organisations have agreed procedures to follow in the event of a sharps injury and these procedures should be adhered to carefully.

HEALTHCARE ENVIRONMENTAL HYGIENE AND MULTIUSE EQUIPMENT

Decontamination can be defined as the chemical or physical processes required to effectively remove or destroy pathogenic organism to a level at which they are no longer present in sufficient numbers to cause harm and the item or surface is rendered safe to use. Decontamination is composed of three elements – cleaning, disinfection and sterilisation.

Cleaning

The physical removal of dirt and associated microorganisms. Cleaning does not kill infectious organisms. Cleaning must be carried out prior to disinfection and sterilisation.

Sterilisation

A process that renders an item free from microorganisms, including spores.

ACTIVITY

Disinfection

A process to reduce the number of viable microorganisms, but it may not inactivate some microbial agents (e.g. spores).

ACTIVITY

Criterion 2 of The Health and Social Care Act 2008 Code of Practice of the prevention and control of infections and related guidance (DH 2015, p. 12) requires care providers to *'Provide and maintain a clean and appropriate environment in managed premises that facilitates the prevention and control of infections'.*

Healthcare environments and equipment can easily become contaminated by pathogenic organisms found on the skin and in body fluids and excretions of infected or colonised individuals. These surfaces can then act as a potential source of harmful organisms that could be transferred directly to people or carried on the hands of healthcare workers having contact with contaminated surfaces or equipment.

Although commonly referred to as 'cleaning', the aim of these activities in relation to the healthcare environment and equipment is to 'decontaminate' the environment or equipment.

Box 12.39 Learning outcomes

On completion of this section, you will be able to:

1 discuss issues relating to healthcare environments and their cleanliness;
2 explain how and when communal equipment should be cleaned.

Learning outcome 1: discuss issues relating to healthcare environments and their cleanliness

Box 12.40 Activity: decontamination

Thinking of your current clinical area, what aspects of the environment do you think need to be decontaminated?

You probably thought of the floor; furniture, such as chairs, beds and bedside lockers; and toilets or commodes. Did you identify taps, call bells, curtains/screens, light switches, and door handles too?

The design, building and maintenance of healthcare premises all exert considerable influence on the ability to maintain a clean, safe environment. There are a number of guidelines in the form of HBN and HTM published to provide detailed advice to healthcare providers planning to build new or refurbish existing premises (DH 2013).

Box 12.41 Activity: ensuring healthcare environments are clean

Whose responsibility is it to ensure healthcare environments are clean?

You probably identified the key role that facilities staff have in ensuring that healthcare environments are kept clean, but all staff have responsibilities with respect to maintaining a clean, safe environment. The nurse in charge or senior member of staff on duty are responsible for ensuring that cleaning standards are maintained and to report faulty or damaged equipment promptly to the relevant individual/department for rectification.

Routine cleaning of non-individual contact surfaces and equipment such as telephones and keyboards can be carried out using general purpose neutral detergent (wipes or solution plus disposable cloth). Based on the premise that all people have the potential to be colonised/infected by pathogenic organisms, to make sure that reusable care-associated equipment and the person's immediate environment are safe to use, disinfection is generally required. There are a large range of disinfectant wipes and solutions available but most 'National' guidance documents recommend cleaning with detergent followed by the use of a chlorine-based disinfectant (1000 ppm available chlorine) and disposable cloths for routine disinfection (e.g. DH 2020; PHE 2020a). There are a variety of products that contain both detergent and chlorine-releasing agent, i.e. Chlor-Clean, SoChlor, which reduce the time taken to disinfect an area/item. To safely disinfect surfaces contaminated by blood, a 10,000 ppm chlorine solution is required (i.e. Haztabs, Precept, Actichlor).

Enhanced or additional 'cleaning' may be recommended by your IPC team in certain circumstances such as during outbreaks or when caring for individuals with *C. difficile* or CPE. This 'enhanced cleaning' may involve supplementary disinfection using products such as hydrogen peroxide or ultra-violet light (Wilson 2019).

All disinfectants need to be stored and used safely and come under the Control of Substances Hazardous to Health (COSHH) regulations. (For further details, refer to the health and safety executive at www.hfs.scot.nhs.uk.)

Box 12.42 Activity: COSHH

Read your organisation's decontamination guidelines to find out what products are recommended in your workplace and read the COSHH data sheets relating to these products. Note: there should be a COSHH folder in all workplaces.

After Mrs. Lewis's discharge from the side room, it will be the nursing staff's responsibility to ensure that the room, including furniture, as well as any reusable equipment such as the commode and drip stands are thoroughly decontaminated before admitting another person. This is usually a shared activity requiring liaison between nursing and facilities staff. Disposable equipment used for her care must be disposed of as infective waste.

Box 12.43 Activity: body fluid spillages

How should you deal with body fluid spillages, for example, blood, vomit or urine?

Blood and body fluid spillages pose significant cross-infection risks, so they must be dealt with immediately and appropriately – check your local policy. The following processes are recommended in Appendix 9 of the HPS National Infection Prevention and Control Manual (http://www.nipcm.hps.scot.nhs.uk/):

- Urine/faeces/vomit/sputum. Initially, soak up and remove gross contamination/spillage with paper towels. *Do not use allow chlorine-releasing agents to come into direct contact with urine as this may generate chlorine fumes*; decontaminate the area with a combined detergent/chlorine-producing solution of 1000 ppm av Cl. Leave the solution for 3 min or as per manufacturer's recommendations.

- Blood/other body fluids including cerebrospinal, peritoneal, pleural, pericardial, synovial, amniotic, semen, vaginal secretions, breast milk and other body fluids with visible blood. Apply chlorine-releasing granules to the spill or use disposable towels soaked with a solution of 10,000 ppm av Cl. Leave the solution for 3 min or as per the manufacturer's recommendations and then dispose of the waste.

Afterwards, clean the area with paper towels, warm water and detergent and then dry the area or allow to air dry. Discard all paper towels, etc. into clinical waste, remove PPE and wash hands.

Nursing staff are usually responsible for the initial removal and disinfection of the blood/body fluid spillage but subsequent cleaning could be carried out by facilities staff.

Learning outcome 2: explain how and when communal equipment should be cleaned

The HPS (2013) summarises the different types of equipment as follows:

Single-use equipment is used once and then discarded and not reused even on the same person. The packaging of these items is marked with a standardised symbol (Figure 12.9).

Single person use equipment can be reused but only on the same individual, for example, an oxygen mask.

Reusable invasive equipment is used once and then decontaminated, for example, surgical instruments returned to sterile services department for sterilisation.

Reusable non-invasive equipment (communal equipment) is reused on more than one individual after disinfection immediately after each use e.g. commodes, drip stands, hoists, blood pressure monitors

Figure 12.9: Symbol for single use only.

In general, advice would be to use single-use equipment where this is available and appropriate. For example, while it may be too expensive to provide all individuals with a single-individual-use blood pressure cuff, it may be considered appropriate for those individuals with known/suspected infections to have access to these. The use of other items such as disposable tourniquets are widely accepted as the financial cost is minimal compared with the costs associated with the risk of cross-infection and the time needed for decontamination after each use.

It is important to remember that all reusable (communal) items of equipment must be effectively decontaminated immediately after each use, before and after being stored for any length of time and prior to sending for repair or servicing. Some areas use 'I'm clean' indicator tape or labels to identify who cleaned the item and when.

Box 12.44 Activity: cleaning communal equipment

ACTIVITY

Consider each of the people in the scenarios. What communal equipment will be used in their care? How and when might you clean this equipment?

When James's wound was dressed at home, there would have been no communal equipment used in his care. At the doctor's surgery, the dressing trolley used will be in communal use. Dressing trolleys are unlikely to become contaminated during the dressing procedure, but they should be cleaned before and after use (see 'Aseptic technique'). Stacey's blood pressure monitoring equipment will be communal, although in some settings individuals are allocated their own blood pressure cuff to use until their discharge. Other equipment used is either single use (injection equipment) or washable (bed linen). Her bed and bedside locker should be decontaminated after her discharge and kept socially clean while in her use. As Mrs. Lewis has MRSA and is isolated, any equipment that is not disposable (e.g. commode, blood pressure monitoring equipment) should be designated for her use only. After discharge, the equipment must be decontaminated effectively before use by other people.

When decontaminating equipment, check any special manufacturers' instructions and local policy.

Decontamination methods for care-associated equipment should not be influenced by whether the individual is known or suspected to have an infection/colonisation All individuals are potentially colonised with infectious organisms, which will remain unknown until relevant test results reveal their presence (Wilson 2019).

Summary

- All healthcare workers have a duty to ensure that healthcare environments are clean.
- Body fluid spillages must be dealt with immediately using recommended procedures.
- All care-associated equipment must be effectively decontaminated to render it safe to use.

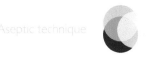

ASEPTIC TECHNIQUE

Aseptic technique describes a series of activities that are used to ensure that susceptible sites are not contaminated by microorganisms when undertaking invasive procedures, using sterile devices and carrying out wound care. The correct use of an aseptic technique ensures that non-sterile items are prevented from coming into contact with sterile or susceptible sites.

Using an aseptic no-touch technique ensures that key sterile parts of devices/equipment are protected from coming into contact with non-sterile items and or the unprotected hands of the healthcare worker. Aseptic Non-Touch Technique (ANTT™) (Rowley et al. 2010) is an example of a standardised aseptic technique for vascular access device maintenance.

> **Box 12.45 Learning outcomes**
>
> By the end of this section, you will be able to:
>
> 1 assess when aseptic technique is required;
> 2 explain how to conduct an aseptic technique, with special reference to wound dressings.

Learning outcome 1: assess when aseptic technique is required

> **Box 12.46 Activity: aseptic technique**
>
> For the items on the following list, identify whether it is true or false that an aseptic technique is required:
>
> 1 Giving food to people
> 2 Removal of sutures or clips
> 3 Inserting a urinary catheter
> 4 Taking an individual's temperature
> 5 Assisting with oral hygiene
> 6 Wound dressings

ACTIVITY

You should have identified that the answers for 2, 3 and 6 are true, as these are procedures that could introduce infection. For the three remaining procedures, 1, 4 and 5, hand hygiene is required but not aseptic technique. For oral hygiene, non-sterile gloves may be used (for more information, see Chapter 7).

Generally, aseptic technique should be used; after surgery when skin integrity has been interrupted; after trauma to skin tissue as occurred during James accident; and when undertaking invasive procedures, such as catheterisation and insertion of intravascular devices. Mrs. Lewis would require aseptic technique for her wound care and the insertion of her intravenous cannula. Any other invasive techniques that may be performed as part of her investigations and treatment such as phlebotomy would require an aseptic technique. A clean, rather than aseptic, technique is sufficient in some wound-care situations, such as with some chronic wounds (for further discussion, see Chapter 13).

Learning outcome 2: explain how to conduct an aseptic technique, with special reference to wound dressings

Because hands are not sterile, forceps were traditionally used for wound dressing, but sterile disposable gloves are used for most wound dressings now. Good gloving technique is required to prevent contamination of gloves (see the earlier section).

Preparing for aseptic technique

ACTIVITY

Box 12.47 Activity: preparing for wound dressing

Discuss with a colleague how you would prepare James to have his wound dressed.

You would need to explain the procedure to James and gain his consent and cooperation. The accident that resulted in James's wound, followed by ongoing wound dressings, could cause him anxiety, so nurses should be understanding and patient with him. The community nurse for learning disabilities could help prepare James for his dressings and will be familiar with how to communicate with him effectively. Pictures and photos may be useful to aid understanding and to chart the progress of wound healing, which may reassure James that he is getting better.

Dressings should be changed at the prescribed interval or when they are no longer able to contain the amount of exudate being produced by the wound. If exudate leaks from the wound dressing, it is no longer providing an effective microbiological barrier. Non-intact dressings can allow bacteria from the surrounding skin and other external sources to enter the wound as well as allowing organisms present in the exudate to contaminate external surfaces.

ACTIVITY

Box 12.48 Activity: preparing the environment before carrying out a wound dressing

How might you prepare the environment before carrying out a wound dressing, either in the community as for James, or in a hospital setting, as for Mrs. Lewis?

In the community, good lighting and James's comfort and privacy are key factors to consider. James has been having his dressing changed at his home near the farm, and community nurses are used to adapting practice to take account of the home environment. When James attends the local facilities for his dressings, there should be a clean treatment room and good handwashing equipment. In the hospital, privacy should be maintained. Mrs. Lewis is in a single room but for people in multiple

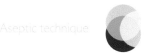

occupancy bays, privacy will usually be provided by using the curtains or, if available, a dedicated treatment room.

The dressing trolley or other surface must be clean and dry. Follow local policy regarding products used. Prior to carrying out any aseptic procedure, ensure doors and windows are closed and fans are turned off, to minimise air currents that may disturb dust.

Box 12.49 Activity: equipment required to carry out a wound dressing

ACTIVITY

Based on your experience, identify what equipment is required to carry out a wound dressing.

You will have identified that you will need a dressing pack. These packs vary in content, but they typically include sterile gloves, gauze swabs, a disposal bag, a paper towel and a container into which cleansing fluid can be poured, if required. Commercially manufactured packs often state the content on the wrapper. If there is no waste bag included, you will need to take a waste bag. You will also need to check that the gloves in the pack will fit, if not, ensure you have the correct sized sterile gloves on the trolly. You should check that the dressing pack and any other sterile items are in date and the packaging is not damaged or wet; damaged packs should not be used as the sterility of the contents cannot be guaranteed.

The choice of wound dressing depends on many factors (see Chapter 13). The wound care required for each wound, including type of dressing, frequency of dressing change and cleansing agent, should be clearly documented in the care plan. If tape is needed, it should be hypoallergenic, in good condition and clean. If needed, sterile scissors must be used to cut dressings to the required size. Some wounds may need cleansing; Chapter 13 discusses when and how to cleanse wounds. As both James and Mrs. Lewis have heavily exudating wounds due to their infections, cleansing will be necessary. A sterile solution such as normal saline may be used to clean and irrigate the wound, if indicated.

Carrying out the aseptic technique

Before starting the aseptic technique, try to ensure you will not be disturbed by telephones and so on. Box 12.50 outlines a set of guidelines that you could use to change a wound dressing by using the aseptic technique. Before starting the aseptic technique, explain to the person what you intend to do and ensure you have all the necessary items available.

Box 12.50 aims to guide you through the aseptic dressing change process, but you should follow your local policy for aseptic technique. In a person's own home, where a trolley is not available, nurses can use any suitable surface; ideally this would be a clean table. Where this is not possible, a new plastic apron should be placed on the surface.

Box 12.50 Equipment and guidelines for aseptic technique, applied to a wound dressing

Equipment

A clean dressing trolley or surface that is large enough to hold the required equipment

A sterile dressing pack with sterile gloves

Sterile cleansing solution (if cleansing required) and alcohol swab to clean its outer packaging

Wound dressing appropriate for wound, based on assessment and/or as per the person's care plan (see Chapter 13), and any additional equipment needed to apply this dressing

Hypoallergenic tape (if needed)

Sterile scissors (if needed to shape the dressing)

Clean disposable apron

Alcohol-based hand sanitiser

Waste bag if not provided in the dressing pack

Procedure

Note: Throughout the procedure, continually observe a person's condition and take into account their comfort and privacy.

- Check the individual's notes regarding wound management plan. Confirm you have the correct person and check the person's identity band.
- Explain the procedure, gain consent and cooperation.
- Wash hands and put on plastic apron.
- Prepare the environment. Clean the trolley surfaces.
- Collect equipment and place on bottom of trolley.
- Position the person and adjust clothing to expose required area.
- Loosen the dressing covering the wound (wear non-sterile gloves if necessary).
- Decontaminate hands.
- Open the outer packaging of the pack and slip the inner package onto the trolley top.
- Open the dressing pack using corners only. The sterile field should lie flat on the trolley. Avoid touching sterile inner surfaces and content (Figure 12.10). Open any additional sterile items onto the sterile field (Figure 12.11).
- Use the sterile disposal bag (if provided in the pack) over one hand to arrange the equipment (Figure 12.12).
- Remove the used dressing with your hand inside the bag, invert the bag and attach it to the side of the trolley, between you and the individual (Figure 12.13).
- If using a sachet of cleansing solution, clean the perforation area with an alcohol swab and let it dry. Tear open and pour the solution into the dressing pack's container, avoiding splashing (Figure 12.14).
- Decontaminate hands and put on sterile gloves (Figure 12.15).

(Continued)

Box 12.50 (Continued)

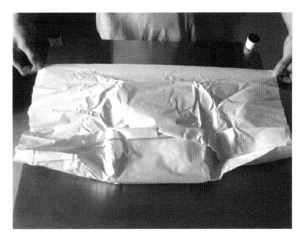

Figure 12.10: Opening a dressing pack.

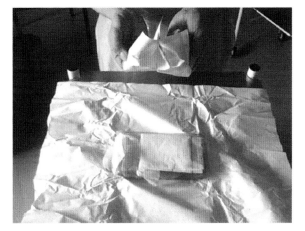

Figure 12.11: Placement of sterile items.

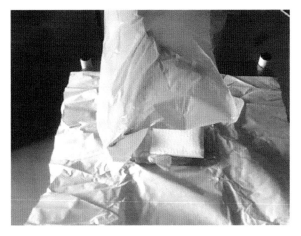

Figure 12.12: Using the sterile bag to arrange equipment.

(*Continued*)

Box 12.50 (Continued)

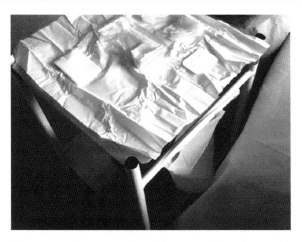

Figure 12.13: After removing dressing with sterile bag invert and attach to trolley

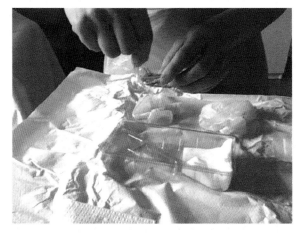

Figure 12.14: Cleansing solution.

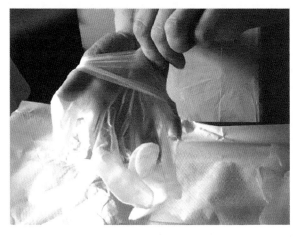

Figure 12.15: Decontamination of hands and put on sterile gloves.

(*Continued*)

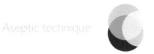

Box 12.50 (Continued)

- Place sterile towel near wound (you may need assistance to position the person so you can position the towel and/or access the wound).
- Irrigate/cleanse the wound, if required and apply new dressing according to the individual's care plan and manufacturer's instructions.
- Make the person comfortable.
- Dispose of all equipment safely. Remove and dispose of gloves and apron.
- Clean the trolley and wash hands.
- Document the care, reporting any significant findings or effects on the individual.

The important principles of aseptic technique, when applied to wound dressings, are that the open wound should not come into contact with any item that is not sterile and that any items that have been in contact with the wound must be discarded safely or decontaminated (Wilson 2019). These same principles apply to protecting the key parts involved in any other procedure requiring an aseptic technique. For example, during catheterisation (see Chapter 6), the sterile catheter, which will be inserted into the sterile urinary tract, must not be contaminated. Stacey's injection must also be carried out using an aseptic no-touch technique (see Chapter 10). Medication needs to be drawn up into the syringe aseptically and as the needle will be piercing the skin (the natural protective barrier) and entering the sterile muscle, the needle must remain sterile.

Box 12.51 Activity: opening a sterile pack

ACTIVITY

Practice opening a sterile pack and putting on the sterile gloves. If you have access to a skills laboratory and equipment, collect the equipment listed and follow the instructions in Box 12.50 to practice carrying out a wound dressing. Take particular care to ensure that you do not contaminate the sterile gloves or your sterile field.

Summary

- Aseptic technique is required to prevent cross-infection during invasive procedures.
- Effective aseptic technique requires good hand hygiene, sterile equipment and the systematic use of a non-touch technique so that sterile items/sites are not contaminated.
- Understanding the underlying principles of aseptic technique enables guidelines to be adapted safely to each individual situation.

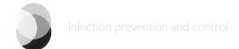
SPECIMEN COLLECTION: KEY PRINCIPLES

Laboratory tests are used to assist in the diagnosis of infection and inform the doctors of appropriate antimicrobial treatment options. It is therefore essential that clinical specimens are collected in a timely and appropriate fashion. Delays in sending samples can impact on the reliability of the result and may cause a delay in the person receiving the correct treatment. Poor collection technique or inadequate sample volumes can produce inaccurate or misleading results. Where possible, samples should be collected before commencing treatment with antibiotics or using antiseptics, as these may temporarily inhibit the growth of organisms. If antimicrobial treatment has been started, this information must be included on the specimen request form so that the microbiologist can correctly interpret the results.

A written local policy should be in place for the collection and transportation of laboratory specimens. You should be aware of this policy and its contents and be trained and competent to collect and handle specimens safely.

Box 12.52 Learning outcomes

By the end of this section, you will be able to:

1. explain the general principles relating to the collection of any specimen;
2. discuss the general principles underpinning the collection of wound swabs and pus.

Note: For urine and stool specimen collection, refer to Chapter 6. For sputum specimen collection, refer to Chapter 14.

Learning outcome 1: explain the general principles relating to the collection of any specimen

As with any procedure, you should explain the procedure to the person, gain consent and maintain privacy during the procedure.

Box 12.53 Activity: specimen collection

ACTIVITY

Have you been involved in collecting any specimens? How can you ensure that you maintain safety and accuracy?

The general principles of collecting any specimen to ensure safety and accuracy include the following:

- Carry out hand hygiene before and after the procedure.
- Wear non-sterile gloves and apron if exposure to body fluids is likely.

- Ensure that tissue and fluid samples are collected from the suspected site of the infection using an aseptic technique to avoid contamination with other organisms that may influence the result.
- If possible, it is preferable to send pus from a wound.
- Wound swabs should be taken from a representative area of the infected lesion, taking care not to touch any surrounding skin, swab the wound using a zig-zag action from the centre outward, while turning the swab over in a circular manner, and ensure it is soaked with wound exudate if present (Wilson 2019).
- Catheter urine samples need to be collected using an aseptic technique using the sampling port and must not be taken from the urine drainage bag.
- Stool samples can still be sent if the person has also passed urine. If the individual is using incontinence pads, the solid portion of the stool can be scraped off the pad; however, this should be clearly noted on the request form as the lab may reject non-liquid stool samples – Types 5–7 on the Bristol Stool Chart (PHE 2013a).
- Staff need to undertake specific training and be assessed as being clinically competent to collect blood cultures. (Refer to your organisations protocol for further information).
- Make sure specimen containers are filled to the correct volume. The laboratory may reject under/overfilled sample containers as depending on the tests requested, the sample volume may influence the final result.
- Without contaminating the outer surfaces, place the specimen in an appropriate and correctly labelled sterile container and seal it properly.
- Complete the label on the container immediately after the specimen is collected, to prevent contamination of the label, and prevent samples being mislabelled with the wrong individuals' details. Complete the specimen request form using individual's labels (where available).
- Check that all relevant information such as the indication for the test; relevant medical history and recent antimicrobial treatment is included and correct. This informs the laboratory what tests are required and ensures that the result relates to the correct person. Some individuals have multiple wounds/ specimens sent so it is really important to be able to interpret the results correctly.
- Place the sample in the zip lock part of the bag and the specimen request form in the outer pouch, taking care not to contaminate the outside of the container or the request form as this puts the laboratory staff at risk.

If specimens are not correctly labelled and match the request form, the laboratory cannot process the specimen and a further specimen will have to be obtained, thus causing unnecessary distress to the person and delaying treatment.

ACTIVITY

Box 12.54 Activity: documenting specimens

Make a list of the information that you think would be essential to document and accompany the specimen. Why is full and correct information important?

You may have identified the following:

- Person's name and location (e.g. address, ward).
- Hospital number and NHS number.
- Person's date of birth.
- Consultant's/GP's name.
- Date and time specimen collected.
- Clinical details of relevance to the specimen, for example, signs of infection and date of onset of symptoms.
- Any antibiotic therapy being taken by the person, including information about current or recent antibiotic prescriptions.
- Type of specimen and site.
- Name and telephone/bleep number of the doctor/nurse requesting the investigation – it may be necessary to telephone the result before the report is released into the computer system.

If specimens cannot be sent to a laboratory immediately, they should be stored in a dedicated specimen refrigerator at 4°C. Blood cultures, however, go in an incubator at 37°C. Cotton-wool swab sticks are used to take specimens from mucous membranes. The specimen stick is then inserted into a tube of soft agar, which preserves any microorganisms for up to 24 h. Bottles for transporting viruses need to be sent to the laboratory as soon as possible after specimen collection (Wilson 2019).

Learning outcome 2: discuss the general principles underpinning the collection of wound swabs and pus

Wilson (2019) states that infections should be diagnosed by clinical signs of infection not just following the isolation of bacteria from a specimen. As you read in the scenarios, James had a wound swab taken from his clinically infected wound.

ACTIVITY

Box 12.55 Swabbing a wound

What would prompt you to take a swab from a wound?

You would take a wound swab when the wound shows clinical signs of infection. Chapter 13 explains in detail how to recognise a wound infection, but some signs include local heat, erythema (redness), pain, pus/purulent discharge, malodour and delayed healing. If present, the collection of pus or exudate, is preferable to swabbing wounds as swabs can also pick up organisms that are just colonising the surrounding tissues. Pus can be withdrawn using a syringe and sent to the laboratory in a universal container (Ayliffe et al. 2001). If only minute amounts of pus are present, it can be collected on a swab that is put into transport medium.

When swabbing a wound, remember to follow all the principles discussed in learning outcome 1, including explaining to the individual and gaining consent. Remember that the wound may be painful, so be gentle and reassuring while taking the swab. Wound swabs or pus should be obtained after the original dressing has been removed, and dressing material traces have been removed by irrigating using saline at body temperature (Wilson 2019). Swabbing dry, crusted areas is unlikely to identify the presence of pathogenic organisms; however, if the specimen site is dry, the swab should be moistened with sterile saline before use.

Summary

- Specimens can be important diagnostic aids and should be collected in a timely fashion using recommended techniques.
- It is essential to prevent cross-infection and contamination of samples during the specimen collection process.
- Specimens should be labelled accurately and relevant clinical information included on the request form.
- Clinical signs of infection should be looked for. Collection of pus is preferable to wound swabs.

SCREENING FOR MRSA AND OTHER ORGANISMS (CPE AND SARS-COV-2)

MRSA screening is the microbiological testing of a sample taken from the potential carriage sites of a person on or before admission to hospital. It is the process by which individuals who are colonised with MRSA are identified. MRSA suppression procedures (also termed decolonisation) must then be applied, as per local protocol.

Box 12.56 Learning outcomes: MRSA

By the end of this section, you will be able to:

1. discuss when and how MRSA screening is conducted;
2. explain how MRSA suppression (decolonisation) procedures are carried out.

Learning outcome 1: discuss when and how MRSA screening is conducted

The guidelines of Coia et al. (2006) for the control and prevention of MRSA recommend an active approach to MRSA screening linked to isolation and cohorting facilities (see the next section).

Box 12.57 Activity: MRSA screening

ACTIVITY

In practice, how have you seen decisions made about MRSA screening? Are you aware of a local trust protocol on MRSA screening?

In 2014, the Department of Health published modification to the guidance relating to which individuals need to be screened for MRSA. Prior to this virtually all admissions were routinely screened for MRSA either at pre-assessment or on admission.

The purpose of screening is to identify those who are colonised/infected by MRSA with a view to ensure optimal care and antimicrobial therapy and reducing the risk of serious infection. Current guidelines currently recommend that all people admitted to high-risk specialties and those that have previously been identified to be colonised/infected by MRSA should be screened.

High-risk specialties are defined as: vascular, renal/dialysis, neurosurgery, cardiothoracic surgery, haematology/oncology/bone marrow transplant, orthopaedics/trauma and all Intensive Care/High Dependency units including Coronary Care (DH 2014).

According to Coia et al. (2006), factors that may increase the risk of MRSA colonisation include:

- Frequent admissions to healthcare facilities
- Direct transfers from other hospitals (UK or abroad)
- Residents of residential/nursing care facilities known or suspected to have a high incidence of MRSA.

Health Protection Scotland also identifies that the presence of a wound or invasive device prior to admission also increases the likelihood of being colonised with MRSA (HPS 2019).

In addition to the above groups, local risk assessment should be used to identify others where individuals may have increased risks associated with MRSA. Refer to your local MRSA screening policy to find out which groups of people need to be screened.

Based on the above, Mrs. Lewis should have been screened for MRSA when she was admitted to the orthopaedic ward after fracturing her hip and on readmission due to the pre-existing surgical wound. It is not anticipated that screening will take place in the A&E department but should be carried out within 24–48 h of admission.

People who have had emergency mental health admissions need not be screened unless they have other locally identified risk factors for MRSA (e.g. chronic wound, intravenous drug user, admitted after a surgical procedure or an admission to an acute trust). Thus, if Stacey is an intravenous drug user, the trust protocol may advise MRSA screening.

Box 12.58 Activity: MRSA screening in the practice setting

ACTIVITY

Have you observed or been involved in MRSA screening in the practice setting? If so, what sites were swabbed and how was this performed?

Which sites to swab will be part of locally agreed protocols. The NOW study identified that more that 75% of NHS providers screen the nose and groin plus others as indicated (swabs from throat, wound and invasive device sites, urine sample if catheterised) (DH 2014).

You should refer to your local policy when collecting screening specimens. Swabs used to swab drier areas, such as the nose and skin should be moistened with sterile saline or the culture medium prior to use. Ensure you follow the general principles of specimen collection described in the previous section, including the labelling of the swabs and completion of accompanying information.

The following procedures should be followed when collecting screening samples. Prior to commencing the sampling process, explain to the person what to expect and obtain verbal consent.

Nasal swab

Ask the person to blow their nose into a tissue if they have nasal discharge. Carefully open and remove the sterile swab from the packaging. Gently insert the swab 1–2 cm into the nostril next to the nasal septum and carefully rotate around the nasal mucosa for 3–5 s. Repeat for the other nostril using the same swab. Place the swab into the transport medium and secure, taking care not to contaminate it by avoiding contact with any other surfaces. Complete the label prior to leaving the person and sending to the lab.

Perineal swab

Ask the individual to loosen their clothing – assisting them if necessary. Open and remove the swab from the packaging. Taking care, rotate the swab against the perineal area (between anus and external genitalia) for 3–5 s. Place the swab back into the transport medium taking care to avoid touching other surfaces and secure. Assist the person to redress before labelling the sample container.

Throat swab

Taking care not to touch any other surfaces, open the pack and remove the swab. Carefully rotate the swab around the tonsillar area for 3–5 s. Note that this may stimulate the persons' gag reflex. Place the swab back into the transport medium and secure prior to filling in the label (HPS 2019).

Learning outcome 2: explain how MRSA suppression (decolonisation) procedures are carried out

If MRSA is identified from screening or clinical specimens, suppression procedures are commenced. The aim of suppression therapy is to reduce levels of colonisation and prevent self-infection as well as reducing the risk of cross-infection arising from the shedding of MRSA into the person's surroundings (HPS 2019).

In general, all people who have been identified as being MRSA positive should receive a 5-day course of MRSA suppression (decolonisation) therapy. If identified at pre-op assessment, the suppression therapy should be timed so that day of the surgical intervention coincides with day 5 of suppression therapy, as follows:

The use of an antibacterial shampoo and body wash daily, for 5 days. The person should moisten their skin first and then apply the solution, giving particular attention to known carriage sites such as the axilla, groin and perineum. Do not add the wash solution to the water as this affects the final concentration and may reduce the efficacy of the product. The wash lotion must be left on the skin for the required period of time as per the manufacturers advice before rinsing with clean fresh water. After washing, the person must use clean towels, sheets and clothing. The person should wash items used separately from the family's laundry, using as high a temperature as the fabric allows.

The application of an antibacterial nasal cream 3 times a day for 5 days. The person should apply a pea-sized amount to the inner surface of each nostril and should be able to taste the ointment at the back of the throat.

Box 12.59 Activity: MRSA suppression at home

What would people need to be able to carry out MRSA suppression procedures effectively at home?

People will need clear explanations about what they need to do and why it is important. They will need a prescription for the antibacterial shampoo and body wash and the nasal cream and clear instructions about how to apply these materials. They will need laundry facilities and a good supply of clean bed linen, towels and clothes. For some people, these items may not be readily available; for example, consider what facilities a person in a hostel might have.

Most people will need assistance to carry out suppression procedures as it is important that the correct contact times are achieved.

Screening for other organisms

Screening programmes also exist for some other significant organisms due to their clinical and operational impact.

Carbapenemase-producing enterobacterales (CPE)

Enterobacterales are a large family of gram-negative bacteria which includes *Escherichia coli*, *Klebsiella* spp. and *Enterobacter* spp., which usually live harmlessly in the gastrointestinal tract of humans; however, they are also some of the most common cause of urinary tract, abdominal and blood stream infections.

Carbapenems are a group of β-lactam (penicillin-like) antibiotics that include meropenem and ertapenem that are usually reserved to treat the most serious infections. Some gram-negative bacteria are naturally resistant to carbapenems, while others can produce enzymes (carbapenemase) capable of destroying carbapenem antibiotics, the genes for which tend to be located on plasmids that can be transferred from one organism to another. In this way, carbapenem resistance can be acquired (PHE 2020b).

The rapid spread of CPE will, if unchecked, inevitably result in an increased threat to public health and will potentially affect the viability of some existing treatment options, such as elective surgery, due to the increasing threat of untreatable infections.

To identify those individuals who may be colonised with CPE, all people who are admitted directly from or have been an inpatient in any hospital, either in the UK or abroad, need to be screened on admission.

Screening for CPE consists of either a rectal swab (a standard bacteriological (charcoal) swab is inserted into the rectum and gently rotated – there should be faecal matter on the swab) or a stool sample. If sending a stool sample, the indication for testing on the request form needs to clearly state 'sample for CPE screening' as most labs will reject non-diarrhoeal stools (types 5–7 on the Bristol Stool Chart). Swabs should also be sent from any wounds or skin lesions as well as a catheter urine sample if a catheter is present.

SARS-CoV-2

COVID-19 is the respiratory disease caused by infection with the SARS-CoV-2 virus, which was first identified in the city of Wuhan in China in December 2019. This infection spread rapidly, initially to Northern Italy and then to the rest of the world, resulting in a global pandemic being declared on 12 March 2020 by the World Health Organization (WHO 2020a).

Advice in relation to the management of SARS-CoV-2 has been regularly updated as more information is obtained. Due to the long incubation period for SARS-CoV-2 and the high incidence of asymptomatic infection, at the time of writing, all people admitted to hospital need to be screened on admission and, if negative, rescreened 5–7 days after admission (day of admission = day 1). Individuals would also be screened if they develop symptoms associated with COVID-19 (new continuous cough or fever or loss of/change in smell or taste) and 24–48 h prior to discharge to other healthcare provider services, including nursing/residential or domiciliary care. People booked for elective surgical procedure should be screened 48 h before their data of admission and advised to self-isolate until they come in for their procedure (DH 2020).

Testing regimens in Care Homes and Social Care settings are described in the collection of documents available at https://www.gov.uk/government/publications/coronavirus-covid-19-admission-and-care-of-people-in-care-homes; and https://www.gov.uk/government/collections/coronavirus-covid-19-social-care-guidance

Screening for SARS-CoV-2 consists of a nose and/or throat swab collected on a viral swab and placed in a vial of viral transport medium. The type of swab is dictated by the laboratory testing method being used – refer to your local protocols for the details of testing in your organisation.

Periodically, other screening programmes may be required if outbreaks are suspected. These will be implemented at the request of your IPCT or your local Health Protection Unit depending on the nature/severity of the outbreak.

Summary

- Screening is a valuable tool in the identification of people who may be colonised with MRSA and other significant organisms.
- Knowing that a person is colonised with a multi-drug resistant organism or other significant organism allows them to be given appropriate antimicrobial therapy if this is clinically indicated, as well as alerting bed managers of the need to allocate the person to a single room for source isolation purposes.
- People found to be colonised with MRSA can be prescribed suppression therapy, to be completed either before admission for people having elective surgery or after emergency admission. This reduces the risk of infection during the period when people are likely to undergo a number of invasive procedures.

ISOLATION PROCEDURES (SOURCE AND PROTECTIVE)

Isolation procedures are used in healthcare settings to prevent the spread of infection from an infected or colonised person to others.

There are two main categories of isolation precautions – 'Source' and 'Protective', the use of which are designed to prevent the transmission of infection to and/or from one person to another. Remember that the consistent use of SIPC precautions are central to all categories of isolation and must be used if there is likely to be contact with blood or body fluids.

Source isolation is used when the affected person is the potential source of pathogenic organisms, i.e. MRSA, *C. difficile*, CPE, influenza, and SARS-CoV-2. There are three categories of source isolation: contact, droplet and airborne (Wilson 2019).

Contact precautions should be used for those significant infections transmitted via direct contact with person or their environment, i.e. MRSA, CPE, and *C. difficile*.

Droplet precautions for those infections transmitted via contact with or inhalation of respiratory secretions that only remain suspended in the air for a very short time generally landing on surfaces within 1–2 m, i.e. *Neisseria meningitidis*.

Airborne infections are transmitted via the inhalation of droplet nuclei, i.e. tuberculosis and measles. Note: Aerosol-generating procedures can be an important route of transmission for some infections that would otherwise be transmitted by direct contact or droplets (e.g. SARS-CoV-2 and influenza during AGPs) (PHE 2016).

'Protective isolation' is used to protect those individuals who, by nature of their underlying medical condition or treatment, are immunosuppressed and therefore extremely vulnerable to infections. i.e. individuals with AIDS, haematology/ oncology – people undergoing chemotherapy.

Isolation precautions should be commenced as soon as the presence of an infectious organism or immunosuppression is suspected. Do not wait for laboratory results before moving individuals to a single room if the person develops symptoms associated with gastrointestinal infections such as *C. difficile* and norovirus, or respiratory viral infections such as influenza and COVID-19.

If clinical samples are being sent to the laboratory due to the presence of symptoms associated with transmissible infections, the person should remain isolated until the results are received. While it is preferable to isolate a person in single rooms sometimes, if single-room capacity is exceeded, the person can be cared for as a cohort in a clearly defined area of the ward. People should not be moved to a cohort area until the specific infection is confirmed and there are no other indications for single-room allocation, e.g. individuals with multiple infections.

For cohort nursing, the following are advised:

- Cohort nursing would be authorised by the IPC team.
- Individual movements for non-clinical reasons should be avoided if possible.
- Designated staff should be allocated to care for the cohorted individuals.
- If there is no designated isolation ward, use a clearly defined bay within a ward, ideally with doors and with access to designated washing/toilet facilities.
- In Nightingale style wards or open units such as critical care, cohorting in a clearly defined area of the unit may be used.

Box 12.60 Learning outcomes

By the end of this section, you will be able to:

1 explain when source isolation is necessary and key principles of care;
2 discuss when protective isolation is necessary and what it entails;
3 reflect on the importance of communication and be aware of whom to inform when isolation is required.

Learning outcome 1: explain when source isolation is necessary and key principles of care

---

Box 12.61 Activity: infection control measures underpinning care in isolation

ACTIVITY

Mrs. Lewis is being nursed in isolation as she has MRSA. Why is this necessary? What infection control measures would underpin her care?

When someone, like Mrs. Lewis, is identified as MRSA positive, either because they have an MRSA infection or because they have been identified through screening as being colonised, they should be isolated to reduce the risk of transmission to other people. You probably identified that infection control measures underpinning Mrs. Lewis's care include hand hygiene, PPE and correct waste disposal. However, if these measures were not implemented until lab results confirmed that Mrs. Lewis had MRSA, the risk of transmission of infection would be significant. Safe care is therefore dependent on standard precautions being used by all healthcare workers for the care of all people, and consequently, there should be minimal concerns relating to possible cross-transmission should pathogenic organisms be subsequently identified (Wilson 2019).

While it is preferable to minimise the transfer of individuals with known or suspected infections, the presence (or suspicion) of an infectious organism must not be allowed to prevent people being transferred to specialist units or accessing urgent diagnostic/treatment procedures as clinically indicated.

Prior to transferring the person, the receiving department must be informed and they should confirm that they are ready to receive the individual. People should not be left in waiting areas but should be seen immediately on arrival and return to their original clinical area as soon as it is safe for them to be moved. Individuals involved in transferring the person should also utilise relevant standard precautions.

Any other special precautions used depend on the type of infection and its specific route of transmission. Refer to Table 12.1 if you need to recap on these routes of transmission. Individuals with airborne infections (e.g. chickenpox, pulmonary tuberculosis) or those undergoing AGPs should be nursed in a well-ventilated single room with the door closed; however, if available, a negative-pressure-ventilated isolation room could be used (Wilson 2019).

The door to isolation rooms/cohort areas should be closed; however, in some instances where person safety could be compromised by closing the door, such as individuals requiring constant observation (critically unstable, falls risk, confused), the IPC team should be contacted for advice. Doors must always be closed during care or assessment activities and when undertaking decontamination procedures. Stacey, with a bloodborne infection (unless bleeding) does not need to be isolated but should be cared for using SIPC precautions in the same way as every other individual.

Box 12.62 Activity: preventing spread of infection

ACTIVITY

To prevent spread of infection to other people, what precautions should be taken if someone develops diarrhoea and vomiting? Consider both small community-based units and hospital situations.

For a community setting, you might have identified the following:

- Good personal hygiene is required, particularly handwashing before eating and after using the toilet.
- There are no specific requirements in relation to the cleaning of crockery and cutlery as bacteria and viruses are easily removed by washing in hot water and detergent, ideally in a dishwasher.
- If dishes are washed by hand, use a disposable dishcloth with clean hot water and detergent. The items should be rinsed and left to air dry, not dried with a tea towel as these are easily contaminated.
- If possible, the person should be allocated a toilet for their sole use.

• If there is a suspected outbreak of gastrointestinal illness – defined as when two or more clients or staff are affected by unexplained diarrhoea or vomiting – then further action may be needed, particularly if there are other vulnerable people within the residence (PHE 2013).

In small residential facilities, the IPCT and local Health Protection Unit need to be informed as they will be able to provide advice relating to appropriate laboratory testing and any additional outbreak measures. The other residents, and their GPs need to be informed.

If gastroenteritis occurs in an institutional setting, such as a hospital, care home or prison, affected individuals must be transferred immediately to single rooms where at all possible and the IPC team informed. Standard Infection Prevention and Control and Source Isolation precautions should already be in place but the IPC team may advise additional measures such as restricting visitors and enhanced environmental decontamination of frequently touched surfaces.

> ### Box 12.63 Activity: management of specific organisms and outbreaks
>
> All staff should know how to access their local guidelines relating to the management of specific organisms and outbreaks. Read your local guidelines for the management of viral gastroenteritis (Norovirus) and the Outbreak policy.

Neutropenia

Neutropenia is an abnormally low neutrophil count commonly associated with courses of chemotherapy. Neutrophils are the predominant white cells circulating in the blood. Having fewer of these phagocytic white blood cells significantly compromises the body's ability to fight infection.

Learning outcome 2: discuss when protective isolation is necessary and what it entails

Isolation is also used for individuals who are extremely vulnerable to infectious diseases because their immune system is compromised. Protective isolation is used to protect people from infection risks from themselves and others rather than to protect others from any risk that they pose, for example, people with neutropenia.

> ### Box 12.64 Conditions leading to a person becoming immunocompromised
>
> What conditions might lead to people being severely immunocompromised? What precautions would be necessary?

Protective isolation requires individuals to be cared for in single rooms with the strictest application of infection prevention and control precautions. Visitors and staff caring for people in protective isolation should not have any signs of infection. Ideally staff should not care for people with infections on the same shift (Wilson 2019).

Due to the extremely vulnerable nature of these individuals, the food they eat needs to be considered. Most food contains microorganisms, and while these microorganisms are not usually harmful in small numbers, they could cause infection in severely immunosuppressed individuals. Your catering department and dieticians can provide advice on appropriate food selection for people requiring protective isolation.

Invasive procedures and the use of indwelling devices are a major threat to immunosuppressed individuals; hence it is vital that the correct protocols/care bundles are utilised to ensure that these are used correctly.

Learning outcome 3: reflect on the importance of communication and be aware of whom to inform when isolation is required

Box 12.65 Activity: the decision to isolate a person

ACTIVITY

List the key people who should be informed when a decision is made to isolate a person. Try to link your answer to Mrs. Lewis's case.

You may have identified the following: Mrs. Lewis has a right to confidentiality and consequently should give permission for family and friends to be informed of the reason for her isolation. Domestic staff do not need to be told what the infectious organisms are but do need to know what precautions (in addition to standard precautions) are required if indicated. If Mrs. Lewis needs to visit other departments, they need to be aware of her MRSA status so that they can take the relevant precautions. Others who need to be informed include the IPCT, bed management and of course her GP and community nursing services who may be involved in her care following her discharge home. Further details about explanations to these key people are now discussed.

Explanations to individuals and families

Box 12.66 Activity: reducing the effects of isolation

ACTIVITY

How might Mrs. Lewis feel, being isolated in a side room?
What might nurses do to reduce the effects of isolation?

Studies of peoples' experiences of being in isolation for MRSA revealed many negative feelings, for example, anger, fear of contaminating others, fear of telling others, apathy and depression (Webber et al. 2012). Feelings of stigmatisation associated with MRSA and isolation have been expressed (Barratt et al. 2011; Webber et al. 2012). One person said, 'You don't feel like a human being' (Webber et al. 2012, p. 45). In the study by Barratt et al. (2011), some peoples' families were reluctant to visit because of fear of catching MRSA, causing the person to feel hurt and abandoned. People viewed isolation as lonely and boring, especially people in long-term care and people with few visitors (Webber et al. 2012) and being in a single room prevented socialisation with others (Barratt et al. 2011). However, some did appreciate the benefits of a single room (Barratt et al. 2011; Webber et al. 2012).

Nurses should be sensitive to the psychological implications of being labelled infectious and of being isolated.

Individuals in isolation often feel lonely, have increased levels of fear and anxiety and can become depressed due to reduced interaction with healthcare providers and other people, especially if the isolation room doors are kept closed (see Chapter 2). Nurses need to be aware of this and make an effort to reassure the individual and explain why they need to be cared for in the single room. By providing the person with clear advice and information relating to their infection, some of the negative impacts of isolation can be overcome. The infection prevention and control nurses will be happy to visit the individual (and their relatives or carers) to provide more information if you are not confident to do so. Most healthcare providers also have access to a range of information leaflets (in a range of languages) that can provide additional information to supplement verbal information (Wilson 2019).

It is important that staff and visitors know what precautions are required when caring for/entering rooms occupied by individuals with infection. To facilitate this while also maintaining confidentiality, some organisms have generic isolation signs that are displayed on the room door to remind staff of the required 'standard' precautions. The signs may be modified dependent on the need of the person for additional source or protective isolation precautions.

Visitors should be advised to speak to a member of nursing staff before entering an isolation room. Visitors may not need to wear PPE unless assisting in healthcare-related activities but should be advised to clean their hands on arrival and before leaving the isolation room. Children and vulnerable adults should be advised of any risks associated with visiting (Wilson 2019).

The fact that she has MRSA must not be allowed to delay or prevent Mrs. Lewis's access to diagnostic and rehabilitation services. In Mrs. Lewis's case, the MRSA is most likely to be transferred by direct contact with her wound, therefore, provided the dressing is intact, she can safely come out of her room to participate in physiotherapy/occupational therapy activities and so speed up her rehabilitation.

Explanations to domestic staff

The facilities supervisor and their staff working in the department should be informed of any individuals who are being isolated, however, they do not necessarily need to be informed of the causative organism. Exceptions would be when the person has infections such as measles and chickenpox as only those members of staff with confirmed immunity should enter these rooms. The cleaning of isolation rooms is usually carried out after the rest of the ward/department has been cleaned using dedicated cleaning equipment (mop, bucket, disposable cloths) should only be used to clean each isolation room. Where available, disposable mops should be used and these plus cloths and PPE should be disposed of within the room. Domestic staff need to be included in any training activities relating to the use of PPE – including fit-testing for FFP3 respirators if indicated, and need to be confident that they know how to use these items correctly (Wilson 2019).

Antimicrobial stewardship

The inappropriate use of antibiotics is fuelling the global increase in the development of antimicrobial resistance with the incidence of multi-drug resistant organisms, in turn, leading to treatment failure and increased mortality and morbidity for infected individuals. Antimicrobial stewardship is essential if the future efficacy of antimicrobial therapies is to be sustained.

Definition of 'antimicrobial stewardship'

The term 'antimicrobial stewardship' is defined as an organisational or healthcare system-wide approach to promoting and monitoring judicious use of antimicrobials to preserve their future effectiveness (NICE 2016).

Prudent prescribing of antibiotics and antimicrobial stewardship is a requirement of Criterion 9 of the 2008 Health and Social Care Act (DH 2015). In response to the increasing trends in antimicrobial resistance, the PHE toolkit 'Start smart – then focus' (DH 2015b) was produced to provide a framework that clearly describes what an effective antimicrobial stewardship programme contains. The purpose is to ensure that antimicrobial therapy is used only when clinically indicated, with the selection of antimicrobial agent and duration of therapy being prescribed in accordance with locally agreed prescribing guidelines.

Social distancing

The concept of social distancing as a means of preventing infection transmission came to prominence during the COVID-19 pandemic of 2020. The rationale for this was that the SARS-CoV-2 virus was initially thought to be predominantly transferred by droplets that will usually fall to the ground within 1–2 m. In the UK, a distance of 2 m between individuals was advised (Gov.UK 2020). Health Building Note (HBN 00-09) (DH 2013a) advised that most healthcare activities can be undertaken within a space of 3.6m wide by 3.7 m long, and so if facilities had been built to this standard, social distancing should have not been a problem. However, in many hospitals, bed spaces are considerably smaller than this, and in some cases, bed occupancy levels had been reduced to achieve 2 m separation. Various measures have been suggested in order to maintain a 2 m separation between individuals from pulling the curtains between beds, putting up additional plastic screens and/or positioning people so that the space between them is maximised. The simplest way is to ensure that individuals are separated by arranging furniture in the bed space to maximise the distance between individuals, i.e. chair, bed, locker, locker, bed and chair. The situation regarding any pandemic will be constantly changing therefore always visit government websites e.g. Gov.uk for up-to-date information.

Visits to departments

Staff in other departments and areas that the person may need to visit should be informed so that any special arrangements can be made. If possible, investigations should be carried out immediately so that the person does not wait in communal areas in contact with others (Coia et al. 2006). This information would be relevant to Mrs. Lewis if she requires a hip X-ray. Porters need not wear protective clothing, but they should be advised to wash their hands on completion of the journey (Wilson 2019). On completion of the transfer, the trolley or chair needs to be decontaminated as per your local protocol and any linen used placed in the appropriate linen bag for return to the laundry.

Summary

- Standard Infection Prevention and Control (SIPC) precautions (hand hygiene, use of PPE, decontamination, use of sharps, waste disposal, etc.) are key to the prevention of cross-infection when caring for all individuals; however, in some situations, additional source and/or protective isolation measures may be necessary.
- Source isolation requires correct use of SIPC precautions with the addition of single-room accommodation and where possible, dedicated toilet facilities and care equipment.
- For people who are severely immunocompromised, protective isolation may be required.
- When isolation is necessary, good communication with individuals, their relatives and staff is essential.
- Nurses should be aware of the psychological impact of isolation and provide support and information.

CHAPTER SUMMARY

This chapter has highlighted the problem of healthcare-associated infection and covered those aspects of care that are essential for the prevention of cross-infection. Standard infection prevention and control practices have been introduced and the practical skills required to implement these when caring for the individuals described. Having worked your way through this chapter, you should now be aware of the fundamental principles of infection prevention and control that underpin all other practical nursing interventions. This chapter is therefore referred to within many other chapters in this book.

The NMC Standards of Proficiency for Registered Nurses and Nursing Associates (NMC 2018a and 2018b) demand that nurses protect and support the health of individuals and the health of the wider community, while being personally accountable for their practice. Therefore, there is a professional as well as moral imperative to contribute towards the prevention of cross-infection, which is after all of fundamental importance to the health, safety and well-being of all in our care, nurses and other healthcare workers.

REFERENCES

Ayliffe, G.A.J., Babb, J.R. and Taylor, L.J. 2001. *Hospital-Acquired Infection: Principles and Prevention*, 3rd edn. London: Arnold.

Barratt, R., Shaban, R. and Moyle, W. 2011. Behind barriers: Patients' perceptions of source isolation for methicillin-resistant *Staphylococcus aureus* (MRSA). *Australian Journal of Advanced Nursing* 28(2): 53–9.

Best, E. L, Parnella, L.P. and Wilcox, M.H. 2014. Comparison of hand-drying methods: The potential for contamination of the environment, user, and bystander. *Journal of Hospital Infection* Dec., 88(4): 199–206.

Coia, J.E., Duckworth, G.J., Edwards, D.I. et al. 2006. Guidelines for the control and prevention of meticillin-resistant *Staphylococcus aureus* (MRSA) in healthcare facilities. *Journal of Hospital Infection* 63: S1–44. Available from: https://www.his.org.uk/media/1195/mrsa_guidelines_pdf.pdf (Accessed on 24 November 2020).

Department of Health (DH). *2008.* Health Action Planning and Health Facilitation for people with a learning disability – good practice guidance. *Available from: https://www.choiceforum.org/docs/hafa.pdf (Accessed on 24 November 2020)*

Department of Health (DH). 2011. *The Waste (England and Wales) Regulations 2011.* Available from: https://www.legislation.gov.uk/uksi/2011/988/contents/made (Accessed on 24 November 2020).

Department of Health (DH). 2012. Water sources and potential pseudomonas aeruginosa contamination of taps and water systems—advice for augmented care units. Gateway reference 17334. London: DH.

Department of Health (DH). 2013a. Prevention and control of infection in care homes – an information resource. Available from: https://assets.publishing.service.gov.uk/government/uploads/system/uploads/attachment_data/file/214929/Care-home-resource-18-February-2013.pdf (Accessed on 24 November 2020).

Department of Health (DH). 2013b. HBN 00-09 Infection control in the built environment. Available from: https://www.gov.uk/government/publications/guidance-for-infection-control-in-the-built-environment (Accessed on 24 November 2020).

Department of Health (DH). 2013c. Health technical memorandum 07-01: Safe management of healthcare waste. Available from: https://assets.publishing.service.gov.uk/government/uploads/system/uploads/attachment_data/file/167976/HTM_07-01_Final.pdf (Accessed on 24 November 2020).

Department of Health (DH). 2014. Implementation of modified admission MRSA screening guidance for NHS (2014). Available from: https://www.gov.uk/government/publications/how-to-approach-mrsa-screening (Accessed on 24 November 2020).

Department of Health (DH). 2015a. The Health and Social Care Act 2008 Code of Practice of the prevention and control of infections and related guidance. Available from: https://www.gov.uk/government/publications/the-health-and-social-care-act-2008-code-of-practice-on-the-prevention-and-control-of-infections-and-related-guidance (Accessed on 24 November 2020).

Department of Health (DH). 2015b. Antimicrobial stewardship: Start smart – then focus. Available from: https://www.gov (Accessed on 24 November 2020).

Department of Health (DH). 2016. Health Technical Memorandum 04-01: Safe water in healthcare premises: Part C – pseudomonas aeruginosa – advice for augmented care units. Available from: https://assets.publishing.service.gov.uk/government/uploads/

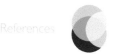

system/uploads/attachment_data/file/524884/DH_HTM_0401_PART_C_acc.pdf (Accessed on 24 November 2020).

Department of Health. 2020. COVID-19: Guidance for health professionals. Available from: https://www.gov.uk/government/collections/wuhan-novel-coronavirus (Accessed on 24 November 2020).

Department of Health and Health Protection Agency (DH and HPA). 2008. Clostridioides difficile infection: How to deal with the problem. Available from: https://www.gov.uk/government/publications/clostridium-difficile-infection-how-to-deal-with-the-problem (Accessed on 24 November 2020).

Gov.UK. COVID-19: Guidance for health professionals. Information on COVID-19, including guidance on the assessment and management of suspected UK cases. Available from: https://www.gov.uk/government/collections/wuhan-novel-coronavirus (Accessed on 24 November 2020).

Health Protection Agency (HPA). 2008. Guidance on the diagnosis and management of PVL-associated Staphylococcus aureus infections (PVL-SA) in England. Available from: https://www.gov.uk/government/publications/pvl-staphylococcus-aureus-infections-diagnosis-and-management. (Accessed on 24 November 2020).

Health Protection Agency (2012). *English National Point Prevalence Survey on Healthcare Associated Infections and Antimicrobial Use, 2011: Preliminary Data*. Health Protection Agency: London.

Health Protection Scotland (HPS). 2020. *National Infection Prevention and Control Manual. Available from:* http://www.nipcm.hps.scot.nhs.uk/ (Accessed on 25 November 2020)

Health Protection Scotland. 2017. National point prevalence survey of healthcare-associated infection and antimicrobial prescribing 2016. Available from: https://www.hps.scot.nhs.uk/web-resources-container/national-point-prevalence-survey-of-healthcare-associated-infection-and-antimicrobial-prescribing-2016 (Accessed on 25 November 2020)

Health Protection Scotland. 2019. Protocol for CRA MRSA screening national rollout in Scotland. Available from: https://hpspubsrepo.blob.core.windows.net/hps-website/nss/1899/documents/1_cra-mrsa-screening-national-rollout-in-scotland-v1.10.pdf (Accessed on 24 November 2020).

Health and Safety Executive. 2013. Health and safety (sharp instruments in healthcare) regulations 2013 guidance for employers and employees. Available from: https://www.hse.gov.uk/pubns/hsis7.pdf (Accessed on 24 November 2020).

Loveday, H.P., Wilson, J.A., Pratt, R.J. et al. 2014. Epic3: National evidence-based guidelines for preventing healthcare-associated infections. *Journal of Hospital Infection* 86 (Suppl 1): P S1–70. Available from: https://www.journalofhospitalinfection.com/article/S0195-6701(13)60012-2/fulltext (Accessed on 24 November 2020).

NHS England. 2018. *The Gloves are Off.* Available from: https://www.england.nhs.uk/atlas_case_study/the-gloves-are-off-campaign/ (Accessed on 24 November 2020).

NHS England and NHS Improvement (NHSE/NHSI).2019a. Standard infection control precautions: National hand hygiene and personal protective equipment policy, March 2019. Available from: https://improvement.nhs.uk/documents/4957/National_policy_on_hand_hygiene_and_PPE_2.pdf (Accessed on 24 November 2020).

NHS England and NHS Improvement (NHSE/NHSI). 2019b. *National Standards of Healthcare Cleanliness June, 2019.* Available from: https://docs.wixstatic.com/ugd/f70a7d_0c74562a2f1342bca8a8873af86a1b4a.pdf?index=true (Accessed on 24 November 2020)

NHS England and NHS Improvement. 2020. *Uniforms and workwear: Guidance for NHS employers*. Available from: https://www.england.nhs.uk/wp-content/uploads/2020/04/Uniforms-and-Workwear-Guidance-2-April-2020.pdf (Accessed on 24 November 2020).

NHS Scotland. 2015. Scottish Health Technical Note 3 NHS Scotland waste management guidance Part D: Guidance and example text for waste procedures. Available from: www.hfs.scot.nhs.uk (Accessed on 24 November 2020).

National Institute for Health and Clinical Excellence (NICE). 2011. Healthcare-associated infections: Prevention and control. Public health guideline [PH36] Published date: 11 November 2011. Available from: https://www.nice.org.uk/guidance/ph36. (Accessed on 24 November 2020).

National Institute for Health and Clinical Excellence (NICE). 2014. Infection prevention and control Quality standard [QS61] Published date: 17 April 2014. Available from: https://www.nice.org.uk/guidance/qs61/chapter/introduction. (Accessed on 24 November 2020)

National Institute for Health and Clinical Excellence (NICE). 2015. Clostridium difficile infection: risk with broad-spectrum antibiotics Evidence summary [ESMPB1] Published date: 17 March 2015. Available from: https://www.nice.org.uk/advice/esmpb1/chapter/Key-points-from-the-evidence (Accessed on 24 November 2020).

National Institute for Health and Clinical Excellence (NICE). 2016. Antimicrobial stewardship: Quality standard [QS121]. Available from: https://www.nice.org.uk/guidance/qs121 (Accessed on 24 November 2020)

National Institute for Health and Clinical Excellence (NICE). 2017a. Healthcare-associated infections: prevention and control in primary and community care Clinical guideline Published: 28 March 2012, Last updated Feb 2017. Available from: https://www.nice.org.uk/guidance/cg139/chapter/1-guidance (Accessed on 24 November 2020)

National Institute for Health and Clinical Excellence (NICE). 2017b. Healthcare-associated infections: prevention and control in primary and community care Clinical guideline Published: 28 March 2012, reviewed Jan 2017. Available from: www.nice.org.uk/guidance/cg139 (Accessed on 24 November 2020).

National Institute for Health and Clinical Excellence (NICE). 2017c. Preventing recurrence of Clostridium difficile infection: Bezlotoxumab Evidence summary [ES13] Published date: 06 June 2017. Available from: https://www.nice.org.uk/advice/es13/chapter/Introduction-and-current-guidance (Accessed on 24 November 2020).

Nursing and Midwifery Council (NMC). 2018a. Future nurse: Standards of proficiency for registered nurses. Available from: https://www.nmc.org.uk/globalassets/sitedocuments/standards-of-proficiency/nurses/future-nurse-proficiencies.pdf (Accessed on 24 November 2020)

Nursing and Midwifery Council (NMC). 2018b. Standards of proficiency for nursing associates. Available from: https://www.nmc.org.uk/globalassets/sitedocuments/standards-of-proficiency/nursing-associates/print-friendly-nursing-associates-proficiency-standards.pdf (Accessed on 24 November 2020)

Pittet, D., Mourouga, P., Perneger, T.V. et al. 1999. Compliance with handwashing in a teaching hospital. *Annals of Internal Medicine* 130(2): 126–30.

Public Health England. 2013. Updated guidance on the management and treatment of Clostridium difficile infection. Available from: https://assets.publishing.service.gov.uk/government/uploads/system/uploads/attachment_data/file/321891/Clostridium_difficile_management_and_treatment.pdf (Accessed on 24 November 2020).

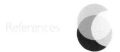

Public Health England. 2015. Start smart – then focus antimicrobial stewardship toolkit for English hospitals. Available from: https://www.gov.uk/government/publications/antimicrobial-stewardship-start-smart-then-focus (Accessed on 24 November 2020).

Public Health England. 2016, Infection control precautions to minimise transmission of acute respiratory tract infections in healthcare settings. Available from: https://assets.publishing.service.gov.uk/government/uploads/system/uploads/attachment_data/file/585584/RTI_infection_control_guidance.pdf (Accessed on 24 November 2020).

Public Health England. 2019a. Annual epidemiological commentary: Gram-negative bacteraemia, MRSA bacteraemia, MSSA bacteraemia and C. difficile infections, up to and including financial year April 2018 to March 2019 11 July 2019. Available from: https://assets.publishing.service.gov.uk/government/uploads/system/uploads/attachment_data/file/843870/Annual_epidemiological_commentary_April_2018-March_2019.pdf. (Accessed on 24 November 2020).

Public Health England. 2019b. Surveillance of surgical site infections in NHS hospitals in England, 2018/19 Dec 2019. Available from: https://assets.publishing.service.gov.uk/government/uploads/system/uploads/attachment_data/file/854182/SSI_Annual_Report_2018_19.pdf (Accessed on 24 November 2020).

Public Health England. Aug 2020a. COVID-19: Guidance for the remobilisation of services within health and care settings Infection prevention and control recommendations. Available from: https://assets.publishing.service.gov.uk/government/uploads/system/uploads/attachment_data/file/910885/COVID-19_Infection_prevention_and_control_guidance_FINAL_PDF_20082020.pdf (Accessed on 24 November 2020).

Public Health England. Sept 2020b. Framework of actions to contain carbapenemase-producing Enterobacterale. Available from: https://assets.publishing.service.gov.uk/government/uploads/system/uploads/attachment_data/file/923385/Framework_of_actions_to_contain_CPE.pdf (Accessed on 24 November 2020).

Public Health England. Oct 2020c. Guidance COVID-19 infection prevention and control guidance: aerosol generating procedures Updated 20 October 2020. Available from: https://www.gov.uk/government/publications/wuhan-novel-coronavirus-infection-prevention-and-control/covid-19-infection-prevention-and-control-guidance-aerosol-generating-procedures (Accessed on 24 November 2020).

Public Health England. Nov 2020. COVID-19: Guidance for the remobilisation of services within health and care settings Infection prevention and control recommendations Oct 2020. Available from: https://assets.publishing.service.gov.uk/government/uploads/system/uploads/attachment_data/file/910885/COVID-19_Infection_prevention_and_control_guidance_FINAL_PDF_20082020.pdf. (Accessed on 24 November 2020).

Rowley, S., Clare, S., Macqueen, S. and Molyneux, R. 2010. ANTT v2: An updated practice framework for aseptic technique. *British Journal of Nursing* (Intravenous Supplement) 19(5): S5–11.

Royal College of Nursing (RCN). 2012a. *Wipe It Out – One Chance to Get It Right: Essential Practice for Infection Prevention and Control: Guidance for Nursing Staff.* London: RCN.

Royal College of Nursing (RCN). 2013. Sharps safety RCN guidance to support the implementation of the health and safety (sharp instruments in healthcare regulations) – 2013. Available from: https://www.rcn.org.uk/professional-development/publications/pub-004135 (Accessed on 24 November 2020).

Royal College of Nursing (RCN). 2017. Essential Practice for Infection Prevention and Control. Available from: https://www.rcn.org.uk/professional-development/publications/pub-005940 (Accessed on 24 November 2020).

Royal College of Nursing (RCN). 2020. Tools of the trade guidance for health care staff on glove use and the prevention of work-related contact dermatitis. Available from: https://www.rcn.org.uk/professional-development/publications/rcn-tools-of-the-trade-covid-19-pub009109 (Accessed on 24 November 2020).

Sax, H., Allegranzi, B., Uçkay, I. et al. 2007. My five moments for hand hygiene': A user-centred design approach to understand, train, monitor and report hand hygiene. *Journal of Hospital Infection* 67(l): 9–21.

Wigglesworth, N. 2019. Infection control 5: Equipment for facial and respiratory protection. *Nursing Times* 10: 30–2.

Webber, K.L., Macpherson, S., Meagher, A. et al. 2012. The impact of strict isolation on MRSA positive patients: An action-based study undertaken in a rehabilitation center. *Rehabilitation Nursing* 37(1): 43–50.

Wilson, A., Hayman, S., Folan, P. et al. 2006. Computer keyboards and the spread of MRSA. *Journal of Hospital Infection* 62(3): 390–2.

Wilson, J. 2019. *Infection Control in Clinical Practice*, 3rd edn. London: Elsevier.

Wilson, J., Bak, A and Loveday, H.P. 2017. Applying human factors and ergonomics to the misuse of nonsterile clinical gloves in acute care, American Journal of Infection Control 45(7): 779–786.

World Health Organization (WHO). 2009. *WHO Guidelines on Hand Hygiene in Health Care*. Geneva: WHO. Available from: https://www.who.int/publications/i/item/9789241597906#:~:text=The%20WHO%20guidelines%20on%20hand%20hygiene%20in%20health, transmission%20of%20pathogenic%20microorganisms%20to%20patients%20and%20HCWs (Accessed on 24 November 2020).

World Health Organisation (WHO). 2020a. *WHO Announces COVID-19 Outbreak a Pandemic 12.03.2020*. Available from: https://www.euro.who.int/en/health-topics/health-emergencies/coronavirus-covid-19/news/news/2020/3/who-announces-covid-19-outbreak-a-pandemic (Accessed on 24 November 2020).

World Health Organisation (WHO). 2020b. *SAVE LIVES: Clean Your Hands*. Available from: https://www.who.int/infection-prevention/campaigns/clean-hands/en/ (Accessed on 24 November 2020)

Principles of wound care

Aby Mitchell

The maintenance of skin integrity and the retention of its protective barrier are major components of basic nursing care. Wound management is predominately a nurse-led discipline yet despite the emergence of new technologies and research into the field of acute and hard-to-heal wounds (McCluskey and McCarthy 2012; Guest et al. 2015), wound care continues to be described as a high-cost and unreliable healthcare activity. Inappropriate or lack of treatment and confusion regarding the role of nurses in wound care lead to delayed healing, infection, preventable pain and a reduced quality of life (O'Brien et al. 2011; Guest et al. 2015). It is suggested that in the UK, approximately 2.2 million wounds were managed by the NHS in 2012/2013 (Guest et al. 2015). The total cost of managing these wounds is estimated at £5.3 billion inclusive of associated comorbidities. About 66% of the annual cost is estimated to be incurred in the community with the remainder in secondary care. This cost will potentially increase over the next 20 years due to an ageing UK population.

The nurse's role in wound care encompasses the initial holistic assessment of the wound and the individual. The nurse needs to develop the ability to make the correct clinical and cost-effective decisions about treatment based on evidence-based practice, while regularly evaluating and monitoring the progress of the wound. This chapter aims to assist you to develop knowledge and understanding of the breadth of issues involved with wound healing physiology and to apply this understanding to your practice.

Wound management is a vast topic with an ever-expanding and developing knowledge base, to which whole books and journals are dedicated. Therefore, although this chapter provides a foundation, further reading is necessary, and you need to continually update your knowledge base. The Cochrane Library and the National Institute for Health and Clinical Excellence (NICE) – discussed in Chapter 1 – are good sources. When in the practice setting, there are specialist nurses (e.g. tissue viability, vascular and dermatology nurses) and other members of the multidisciplinary team (MDT) (e.g. podiatrists) who will be valuable resources for your learning.

This chapter includes the following topics:

- The phases of wound healing
- Classification of wounds and wound closure
- Factors affecting wound healing
- Wound assessment
- Wound management.

DOI: 10.4324/9781003020660-13

Although you can study this chapter at any stage of your learning, you will find it most relevant to work through the sections when based in a setting where you have people with different wounds. This chapter will enable you to link wound care to platforms 1–4 of the NMC (2018a, 2018b) proficiencies for both nurses and nursing associates. There is no substitute for looking at real wounds and applying theory to practice. Chapter 12 is essential prior reading, when managing wounds, an understanding of how microorganisms are transmitted, and adherence to standard precautions and aseptic techniques, is paramount.

Box 13.1 Recommended biology reading

The following questions will help you to focus on the biology underpinning this chapter's skills. Use your recommended textbook to find answers to the following:

- What characteristics must skin possess?
- What are the major layers of the skin?
- Which layer is avascular?
- What are the major functions of the skin? What role does skin play in homeostasis?
- How does the skin protect itself against damage and infection?
- What factors can lead to a breakdown in skin integrity? What would the consequences be?
- What is the goal of wound healing? What factors influence the degree of scarring?
- How does age alter the skin's characteristics? Consider the skin at birth, adolescence, young adulthood and old age.
- How does the appearance of skin change, during illness, injury or stress?
- What factors are necessary to maintain normal healthy skin?

PRACTICE SCENARIOS

The following practice scenarios illustrate different situations where wound care is required and are referred to throughout this chapter.

Adult

Mrs Warner is 78 years old and has a history of **type 2 diabetes**, which is managed with oral hypoglycaemic medication. Since her husband died 2 years ago, she has lived alone with her two cats and has been treated for depression. After falling in her kitchen, she was unable to get off the floor and was found by a neighbour some hours later. After assessment in the emergency department, she was diagnosed with a stable fracture of her pelvis. She was also found to have an ulcer (open sore) on one of her toes, which had an offensive discharge. Her blood glucose was high. She was transferred to a ward for rehabilitation and pain management. A few days later, a large area of black necrotic (dead) tissue developed on her sacrum, and discoloured areas on both her elbows. These wounds appeared to have been caused by the period of prolonged pressure on the kitchen floor. Mrs Warner is keen to get home as soon as possible as she is worried about her cats. She normally smokes 10 cigarettes a day and is overweight. Her diet is high in fat and carbohydrates, and she rarely eats fruit or vegetables.

Learning disability

Susan is 32 years old and has a moderate learning disability. She lives in a small group home and was recently in hospital having her acutely inflamed appendix removed. She has been discharged home and has a small abdominal wound, which seems to be healing well. However, Susan is concerned about the wound and is worried about getting it wet when she showers and drying and dressing afterward in case she harms the wound. She is due to have her sutures removed by the practice nurse. The community nurse for learning disability is visiting regularly to give some support in this situation. Susan's keyworker is her **health facilitator**.

Mental health

Colin is 28 years old and is being treated as an inpatient in the acute mental health unit, after deterioration in his mental health, which has affected his self-care ability. He has a diagnosis of substance abuse and schizophrenia, which is currently being treated with **clozapine**. Colin requires careful blood monitoring, as clozapine can affect white blood cell levels. While on the unit, he complained of pain in his left upper buttock. A large, hot, swollen area was found, which was diagnosed as being an **abscess**. Colin says that he has had several of these swollen areas before. Incision and drainage took place in theatre, and he has now returned to the unit, with a pack in situ in the wound. Antibiotics have been prescribed.

THE PHASES OF WOUND HEALING

A wound can be defined as a disruption of normal anatomical structure and function that results from pathological processes beginning internally or externally to the involved organ (Lazarus et al. 1994).

This definition still remains relevant in 2020 and continues to be used in the literature.

Wound closure occurs in one of three ways (Wounds UK 2020a)

- Primary intention: the healing of wounds with minimal tissue loss.
- Secondary intention: the healing of wounds occurs when the sides of the wound are not opposed, healing occurs from the bottom up.
- Tertiary intention: the healing of wounds that is a combination of healing by primary and secondary intention.

Box 13.2 Learning outcomes

By the end of this section, you will be able to:

1. distinguish the phases of healing and recognise tissue appearance at each stage;
2. appreciate that healing does not in reality occur in a simple linear manner.

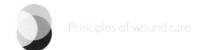

Learning outcome 1: distinguish the phases of healing and recognise tissue appearance at each stage

Wound healing is usually described in four distinct phases, but these descriptive models refer to the healing of acute wounds. Hard-to-heal wounds do not follow the normal sequence of events, so delays to the healing process are experienced. You may find different terminology being used to describe the phases. This chapter uses the approach that there are four interdependent phases during the wound healing process.

Haemostasis

Haemostasis is the process that causes bleeding to stop. Following initial wounding, blood loss is controlled by a complex series of events. Platelets become sticky and adhere to the wall of the blood vessel and each other forming a platelet thrombus. This acts as a temporary plug reducing blood flow out of the wound. The platelets also release serotonin and other chemical mediators, which results in vasoconstriction for a short period to create a haemostatic plug (Peate and Stephens 2019). In addition to minimising injury, this process initiates the inflammatory response.

The inflammatory phase

Inflammation is an innate response to tissue damage (Peate and Stephens 2019). Once haemostasis has been achieved, the blood vessels dilate to allow essential cells into the wound bed. The release of growth factors attract the migration of neutrophils, monocytes and macrophages to the wound bed, this process initiates the inflammatory phase. The primary function of these cells is to attract phagocytes to the inflamed area to kill bacteria and remove debris from dead and dying cells within the tissue spaces (Mitchell 2020). This process is known as phagocytosis. Increased blood flow, increases capillary hydrostatic pressure. The five cardinal signs of inflammation are heat, redness, pain, swelling and loss of function. The effectiveness of normal blood osmotic pressure increases capillary permeability, which leads to protein-rich fluid leaking onto interstitial tissue spaces (Mitchell 2020). As the fluid moves out of the capillaries, the viscosity of the blood increases, which slows down the flow. As a result, red blood cells clump together forcing white cells to move towards the endothelium of the vessels and causes swelling and pain. There is an increased demand for nutrients and oxygen in the damaged area increasing the person's metabolic rate which raises core temperature

The proliferative phase

The proliferation stage overlaps the inflammation stage as it starts to end. The focus of this stage is to rebuild tissue through three separate processes:

- **Granulation** leads to the formation of new blood vessels (angiogenesis), which deliver oxygen and nutrients to the healing tissues. Fibroblasts and endothelial cells are the primary cells in this phase. Fibroblasts from the surrounding tissue become activated by growth factors released in the inflammatory phase, enabling them to replicate and produce a collagen-rich matrix that builds elasticity and strength into the wound (Mitchell 2020). Granulation tissue is characterised by a reddish velvety carpet in the base of the wound. Unhealthy granulation tissue may be dark in colour and bleed easily, indicating possible infection and poor vascular supply to the tissue (Peate and Stephens 2019).

- **Contraction** is the approximation of the wound edges believed to be caused by the 'push' and 'pull' effect of the myofibroblasts.
- **Epithelialisation** resurfaces the wound by regeneration of epithelial cells.

The maturation phase

The maturation phase involves remodelling the tissue to form a scar. This phase can take a year or more as cellular activity reduces and the number of blood vessels in the wound decreases (Mitchell 2020).

Box 13.3 Activity: requirements for each stage of the healing process

ACTIVITY

Prepare notes on the phases of healing, which are outlined briefly above, from your recommended biology textbook. Focus your reading on the requirements for each phase of the healing process.

Your reading should have helped you to understand that the wound healing process is a complex interplay of events leading to complete healing.

Box 13.4 Activity: observation of phases of healing

ACTIVITY

Aim to observe an uncomplicated surgical wound, or a minor traumatic wound – this wound could even be a laceration on your own skin. Compare the appearance of the wound to the described criteria for different phases of healing. Discuss with a practitioner which phase of healing is predominant at present.

At different phases of wound healing, the tissue has a different appearance.

- When observed in the *inflammatory phase*, the wound appears swollen and red, and the surrounding tissue feels warm and can be painful. Recognising these signs (which occur due to local vasodilation) can be difficult at first. In the inflammatory phase, the wound is usually kept covered to prevent contamination.
- In the *proliferative phase*, signs of wound contraction commence. The appearance of tiny red buds is the first sign of primitive blood vessels emerging, acting as a transport system for nutrients, oxygen, cells and growth factors essential for connective tissue development (Peate and Stephens 2019). This friable tissue, which fills the deficit at the wound bed, is also referred to as granulation tissue. New epithelial cells divide and, migrate from wound edges and any remaining islands of epidermal cells that may encompass sebaceous glands and hair follicles.

- A wound in the *maturation phase* may remain in this phase for up to 2 years. It will appear smaller, and may be white and hard (scar tissue) and fixed to surrounding tissue, or similar in appearance to surrounding tissue, indicating a healed mature wound. The maximum tensile strength after injury is about two-thirds of its original strength (Peate and Stephens 2019).

- Colour of tissue on the wound is used to distinguish between viable and non-viable tissue. The presence of devitalised or non-viable tissue is a contributing factor to delayed wound healing (adapted from Atkin et al. 2019) (see Table 13.1, wound bed colour and tissue type).

ACTIVITY

Box 13.5 Activity: suture removal

Consider how the community nurse for learning disabilities might reduce Susan's anxiety about her wound and prepare her for suture removal.

The community nurse will need to have assessed Susan's cognitive and physical ability to care for her wound and would then be able to help Susan to understand the wound's healing and the care it requires.

The community nurse will work alongside Susan supporting her understanding. This support could be through advice to other professionals on the best method of communication, such as use of pictures or specific phrases. Susan may need reasonable adjustments to be able to have informed involvement in her care, such as: additional visits from the learning disability nurse to explain how the wound is healing and how to see if there is a problem; additional time from other professionals when meeting with Susan, to ensure she understands what they are doing; and support for Susan's carers so they can assist Susan if she needs support.

The nurse can use effective communication skills to ascertain Susan's understanding of the healing process, and her anxieties about this process. Perhaps using photos and pictures to support her understanding. The nurse could encourage Susan to look at the wound and point out the signs of healing, explaining about the sutures being removed when the wound is healed. Consent and informed choice is an important consideration when considering Susan's treatment plan. We cannot assume Susan lacks understanding to consent to procedures unless a mental capacity assessment is completed. It is expected that all reasonable actions have been taken to enable Susan to have an understanding of her condition and the treatment options.

Table 13.1: Wound bed colour and tissue type

Necrotic wound (black tissue)	Sloughy wound (yellow tissue)	Granulating wound (red tissue)	Epithelialising wound (pink tissue)	Infected wound (Green tissue)
Dead tissue – no healing has begun (Figure 13.1)	Made up of dead cells and occurs at the end of the inflammatory phase (Figure 13.2)	Occurs in the proliferation phase and leads to the formation of new blood vessels (Figure 13.3)	Occurs in the proliferation phase and resurfaces the wound (Figure 13.4)	Impedes wound healing and keeps the wound in the inflammatory phase

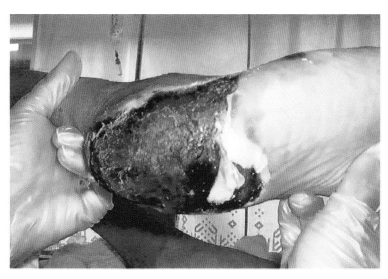

Figure 13.1: A diabetic ulcer that developed on this person's heel due to a combination of poor circulation and unrelieved pressure. The tissue bed is covered in hard black necrotic tissue. The wound will not heal until the devitalised tissue has been removed. Unfortunately, this ulcer could eventually lead to amputation of the individual's lower leg and foot.

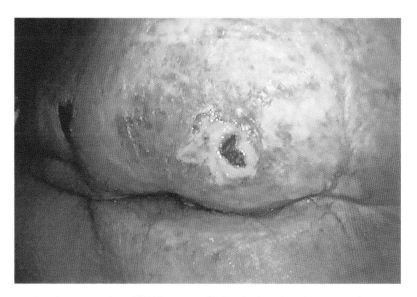

Figure 13.2: A pressure ulcer (EPUAP category 3) that developed on the sacrum of a person with multiple sclerosis. The wound bed is covered with yellow slough, except for a central necrotic area. Slough is soft necrotic tissue containing dead phagocytes, and the wound will not heal until this devitalised tissue is removed. Surrounding this ulcer are other areas of pressure damage, evidenced by discolouration (European Pressure Ulcer Advisory Panel (EPUAP) category 1) and superficial ulceration (EPUAP category 2).

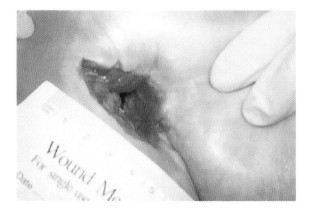

Figure 13.3: A pressure ulcer, which extends down to bone (EPUAP category 4), that developed on the sacrum of a person with a spinal injury. The ulcer was covered with 60% slough before debridement by maggots. The wound is now almost filled with red granulation tissue. This photo also shows how a ruler placed by the side of a wound before the photo can provide a more accurate record of its dimensions.

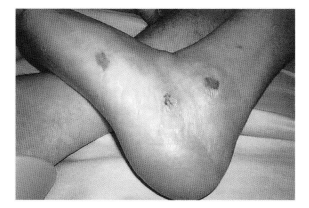

Figure 13.4: Pressure ulcers (EPUAP category 2) on the side of the foot/ankle of a person who has multiple sclerosis. They are now almost healed, with wound beds showing mainly pink epithelialising tissue.

Once Susan understands how the wound is healing, the nurse can then explain how to manage showering and give her practical advice about drying herself without rubbing the wound itself and about wearing clothing that will not rub the wound. The nurse must similarly ensure that Susan's carers understand these issues, so they can reinforce the information and be consistent in their reassurance and explanation.

The nurse can prepare Susan for her suture removal and will be able to ensure that the practice nurse removing Susan's sutures knows how Susan communicates and how she has been prepared. If there is anyone who has a healed surgical wound, perhaps Susan could, with the person's permission, talk to them. Actually, seeing a healed wound might help to allay her anxiety, if this is possible to arrange.

All the above-mentioned aspects should be incorporated in Susan's **Health Action Plan**.

Learning outcome 2: appreciate that healing does not in reality occur in a simple linear manner

Owing to several factors, wound healing is not always a straightforward process. A review of wounds caused by trauma, pressure or ulceration illustrates these issues. These wounds are considered in further detail in the 'Classification of wounds and their management' section.

Box 13.6 Activity: wound caused by trauma

If possible, select a person in your care with a wound caused by trauma, pressure or ulceration, in discussion with your practice mentor. Try to find out about the history of the wound and its healing process to date. Compare your investigations with the discussion below.

Trauma

Traumatic wounds are caused by a sudden or unplanned external insult and vary greatly in nature. Although minor wounds may heal in a straightforward manner, others involve extensive skin loss and contamination, which can affect the healing process and may require surgical intervention.

Pressure ulcers

Impaired circulation, shear or friction to the skin for even short periods is problematic in susceptible individuals, such as people who are frail, older or malnourished – consult Chapter 11 for a full discussion of pressure ulcers. Mrs Warner, as an older person, who also has diabetes, and had a period of immobility on a hard surface (the kitchen floor), is obviously a high-risk individual. The discoloured areas on Mrs Warner's elbows could potentially be a deep tissue injury and develop into necrotic ulcers similar to her sacral pressure ulcer.

Leg and foot ulceration

There are many causes of leg and foot ulceration, each having different distinguishing features, underlying pathology and treatment, but the majority are associated with circulatory problems. For example,

- *diffusion* – problems arise when the distance between the capillary and tissue cells is increased (e.g. by oedema);
- *perfusion* – occurs when there is arterial or venous insufficiency.

Currently, the national guidelines for leg ulcer care are produced by The National Institute for Health and Care Excellence (NICE) (NICE 2020a) and Wounds UK (2016, 2019). Treatment and management of leg ulcers has recently changed with the introduction of the CQUIN (2020) and Lower Limb Assessment Essential Criteria (2020–2021) (Wounds UK 2020b).

A leg ulcer is defined as a break in the skin below the knee, which has not healed within 2 weeks (NICE 2020a). It is estimated there are at least 730,000 individuals with leg ulcers in the UK, equating to 1.5% of the adult population (Guest et al. 2015). A venous leg ulcer occurs in the presence of venous disease and is the most common type of leg ulcer (NICE 2020a). Venous leg ulcers typically occur in the gaiter area of the leg (from the ankle to mid-calf). The estimated prevalence of venous leg ulcers in the UK is between 0.1% and 0.3%, and this increases with age with a 12-month recurrence rate of between 26% and 69% (NICE 2020a).

It is estimated that 70–90% of ulcers are venous in origin and 25% are arterial (Peate and Stephens 2019), but the ulcer can be of mixed aetiology too. Useful overviews of lower leg ulceration can be found in wound care at a glance – Peate and Stephens (2019). There are also many articles devoted entirely to leg ulcers and their management. See Figure 13.5.

Pressure ulcers (PUs) are caused by tissue damage when the blood supply to an area of skin is impaired because of significant pressure; they are often preventable (NICE 2014). The total cost of pressure ulcer treatment in the UK is estimated to be £1.4 million every day (NHS 2019).

In 2013, over 3.2 million adults were diagnosed with diabetes, with prevalence rates of 6% and 7% in England and Wales (NICE 2019c). It is estimated that 169,000 people have diabetic foot ulcers, which equates to 5% of adult diabetic individuals having a foot ulcer (Guest et al. 2015). These are complex wounds and cause unacceptably high levels of morbidity and mortality (Bilous and Donnelly 2010). The mean cost of a diabetic wound over 12 months is estimated at £7800 (Guest et al. 2018).

Figure 13.1 shows how severe these ulcers can potentially be. Diabetes care in the NHS costs approximately £10 billion (diabetes.org.uk 2014). Common problems include infection, osteomyelitis, neuropathy, peripheral arterial disease, Charcot arthropathy and amputation (NICE 2019a). Education and empowerment are

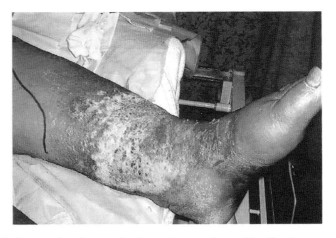

Figure 13.5: A venous leg ulcer that has been a long-standing problem for the person concerned. There are large areas of yellow slough and areas of red granulation tissue covering the wound. The lower foot looks oedematous, and there is hard scaly skin (hyperkeratosis) present. The surrounding skin also looks red, suggesting cellulitis.

essential to ensure that foot ulceration is reduced in people with a high-risk; this approach is being supported by the development of multidisciplinary care pathways within NHS acute care (NICE 2019c). However, Mrs Warner's depression could affect her ability to carry out this aspect of self-care.

You should now be aware that some wounds progress in a complicated manner owing to underlying health problems. These complex wounds often necessitate an MDT approach in diagnosis and management, with investigations performed to ensure accurate identification of the problem.

A scar is the end result of healing, but the formation of a mature scar can be a slow process. A scar is the product of many cells. However, specialist myofibroblast cells have a key role in healing, by shrinking the wound by contraction. Note that 75% of normal wound healing is by contraction, which results in a smaller, less visible scar. A scar initially consists of raised vascularised tissue – hence the red colour. Gradually, the redness disappears as the number of blood vessels reduces, and the colour changes to white. As noted, the new tissue will not be as strong as previously and may predispose an individual such as Mrs Warner to increased risk of pressure ulcer damage.

Some individuals have problems with hypertrophic scars and keloids. Although hypertrophic scars regress, keloid scars do not. Management of both of these problems requires a specialist and MDT, for both the physical and the psychological problems that may accompany them.

Hypertrophic scar

A raised, healed red scar that is uncomfortable and tight. This is caused by an increased deposition of collagen within the area of the original wound (Berman et al. 2017).

Keloid

A firm mass of scar caused by excessive collagen deposition, but it extends outside the wound boundaries (Rabey et al. 2017).

Summary

- Wound healing is a complex process involving phases of healing through which the wound must pass to heal adequately.
- The process is theoretically sequential, but in reality, parts of different phases occur concurrently.
- The end result is a scar of uncertain appearance and weakened structure in comparison with surrounding undamaged tissue.

CLASSIFICATION OF WOUNDS AND WOUND CLOSURE

Wounds are often divided into **acute** and **chronic**. Acute wounds result from surgery or trauma and usually heal relatively quickly with minimal need for external interventions, and proceed through an orderly and reparative process, if no complications occur (Lazarus et al. 1994). Chronic wounds, now referred to as 'hard-to-heal' wounds, are wounds that fail to proceed through an orderly, timely reparative process. These wounds do not follow a normal sequence of events and consequently, delays in the healing process are experienced (Mitchell 2020). Burns, due to the area of tissue damage, often behave more like hard-to-heal wounds. Such wounds include leg ulcers, PUs, diabetic foot ulcers, malignant wounds and any non-healing acute wound. They are usually caused by underlying health problems, including age, heart disease, diabetes mellitus, peripheral arterial disease and neuropathy (Escandon et al. 2011; Siddiqui and Bernstein 2010) and also social and psychological problems. Haemostasis may be absent from the process, and the individual's ability to heal is often impaired, with the inflammatory response being continually stimulated by the underlying disease process, resulting in a prolonged and excessive inflammatory phase of wound healing (Peate and Stephens 2019).

Learning to classify wounds will enable you to appreciate issues affecting their management, thus planning more effective care. There are a variety of ways of classifying wounds; this chapter uses a simple classification based on the cause.

Box 13.7 Learning outcomes

By the end of this section, you will be able to:

1 distinguish between acute and hard to heal;
2 discuss the principles of wound closure for different types of acute and hard-to-heal wounds.

Learning outcome 1: distinguish between acute and hard to heal.

Box 13.8 Activity: classification of wounds

ACTIVITY

Table 13.2 shows a classification of wounds, and Box 13.10 shows a classification of surgical wounds. Working from these tables, how would you classify the wounds of Mrs Warner, Susan and Colin?

Table 13.2: Wound classification

Classification	Types of wound	Causes and features
Acute	Penetrating wounds	Causative objects include missiles (e.g. bullets, explosion debris) or hand-held objects (e.g. knives, billiard cues)
		High infection risk.
Acute	Lacerations	Healing affected by the cause (whether it is a clean wound or is contaminated by dirt/debris), age of the wound and the individual. Wounds involving the eyes and joints are priorities.
Acute	Abrasions	Caused by the body being dragged against an abrasive surface, removing surface epithelium. Can be very painful and sensitive as nerve endings are exposed. If not meticulously cleaned, 'tattooing' results from dirt trapped in the dermis and epidermis, which is almost impossible to remove (Evans and Jones 1996).
Acute	Bites	Common cause of wounds; most are caused by dogs, but human bites are also common. High infection risk owing to the large number of microorganisms found in mouths.
Acute	Surgical	As these wounds are planned, risks (e.g. of infection) can be reduced to a minimum. Infection rates vary according to the type of surgery (see Box 13.10).

(Continued)

Table 13.2: **(Continued)**

Classification	Types of wound	Causes and features
Acute	Burns	Can be thermal (caused by flame, hot fluid or radiation), chemical (acid or alkali) or electrical. Can damage the epidermis only (superficial), the epidermis and the dermis (partial thickness) or extend into deeper tissue (full thickness). The extent of the burn is very important to assess, as fluid resuscitation may be needed.
Hard to heal	Venous leg ulcers	Caused by damage to the venous system in the leg, especially the valves, causing pooling and distending of vessels; by-products of this process cause tissue damage and ulcer formation.
		Risk factors include varicose veins and rheumatoid arthritis.
		Ulcers are usually shallow and situated in the gaiter area, with irregular edges.
		Pain may be severe, dull or aching.
Hard to heal	Arterial leg ulcers	Occur when impaired blood supply due to various causes leads to areas of tissue damage, as the blood vessel supplying the area becomes occluded. Ischaemic pain occurs and the ulcers tend to be small and deep with well-defined borders, situated at distal body locations (e.g. toes).
Hard to heal	Diabetic neuropathic or neuroischaemic foot ulcers	Chronic hyperglycaemia causes impairment of the nerve supply to the foot and lower limb; the resulting loss of sensation can lead to pressure damage, repeated trauma and/or penetration by foreign bodies. These ulcers are neuropathic in origin.
		In neuroischaemic ulcers, the combination of neuropathy and arterial disease produces a very complex wound with a poor prognosis.
Hard to heal	Pressure ulcers	Prolonged pressure on the skin produces obstruction of small vessels, resulting in damage of tissue, and sometimes deeper tissues, owing to lack of blood supply. Shearing and friction also contribute to their development.
Hard to heal	Infection-induced	Opportunistic organisms gain access through the skin via a small wound, and produce an ulcer.
		Tropical ulcers are one of the most common forms.
Hard to heal	Ulcers caused by cancer	Referred to as fungating wounds, these can complicate cancers in various areas of the body.
		They present as a rapidly growing fungus or with a cauliflower-like appearance, which may ulcerate.

You should have identified that Mrs Warner's sacral wound is a pressure ulcer and her toe wound is probably a hard-to-heal diabetic foot ulcer. Susan and Colin both have acute surgical wounds. However, although Susan's is a clean-contaminated wound, Colin's is a dirty wound as it is leaking seropurulent exudate (see Table 13.3). Figure 13.6 shows the wound of a man who had a hip replacement 10 days previously and has now had his skin closures removed. This wound would be categorised as a clean surgical wound. Now, try using the table to classify wounds of individuals in the practice setting, in the following activity.

Wounds are not always easy to categorise. All surgical wounds are at risk of complications such as dehiscence, haematoma, poor or abnormal scar formation, incisional hernia and surgical site infection (SSI) (Wounds UK 2020). These wounds

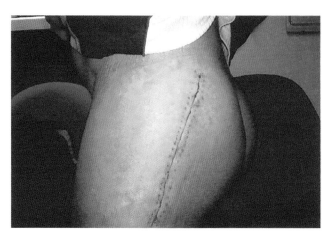

Figure 13.6: The hip wound of a man who had a total hip replacement.

Box 13.9 Activity: cross category wounds

ACTIVITY

With reference to Tables 13.2 and 13.10, explore the nature and cause of wounds within your practice setting. Do all the wounds clearly fit into a category type? Are there any wounds that started as acute, and have ended up as hard to heal? If so, why?

---

can start as acute but quickly become hard to heal. The underlying reasons are not always clearly understood but often relate to the person's physical health. Surgical wounds can be divided into four different classifications that determine the post-operative risk of SSI (see Box 13.10).

Box 13.10 Surgical wound classifications (NICE 2019a)

Clean: an incision in which no inflammation is encountered in a surgical procedure, without a break in sterile technique, and during which the respiratory, alimentary or genitourinary tracts are not entered (e.g. wound heals by primary closure).

Clean-contaminated: an incision through which the respiratory, alimentary, or genitourinary tract is entered under controlled conditions but with no contamination encountered (e.g. a surgical wound at risk of infection due to location).

Contaminated: an incision undertaken during an operation in which there is a major break in sterile technique or gross spillage from the gastrointestinal tract, or an incision in which acute, non-purulent inflammation is encountered (e.g. elective colorectal surgery). Open traumatic wounds that are more than 12–24 h old also fall into this category.

(Continued)

Box 13.10 (Continued)

Dirty or infected: an incision undertaken during an operation in which the viscera are perforated or when acute inflammation with pus is encountered (e.g. emergency surgery for faecal peritonitis), and for traumatic wounds if treatment is delayed, there is faecal contamination, or devitalised tissue is present (e.g. PUs, burns, faecal peritonitis).

Figure 13.7 shows an abdominal wound, 5 days after surgery. The distal part has broken down due to infection and the clips have had to be removed early.

A SSI is defined as a post-surgical infection that can affect either the incision or deep tissue at the operation site. There are three types: superficial incisional, deep/open incisional and organ space incisional (Wounds UK 2020a).

- Superficial incisional infection involves skin and subcutaneous tissue within 30 days of a procedure or up to 1 year for people receiving an implant.
- Deep/open incisional infection involves muscle and facial layers within 30–90 days of procedure.
- Organ/space incisional infection involves any part of the anatomy that is opened or manipulated during the surgical procedure within 30–90 days of the procedure (Wounds UK 2020a).

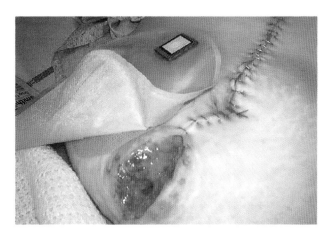

Figure 13.7: The abdominal wound of a woman who has had an abdominoperineal resection, with colostomy formation, for ulcerative colitis. The colostomy has been sited very close to the wound. The photo was taken on the fifth post-operative day. The wound had started to ooze a seropurulent exudate from the distal part of the wound, and had dehisced. The clips from this area have been removed. Towards the top of the wound and the central area, there is slight inflammation. In the dehisced area, small patches of red granulating tissue can be seen, but other areas look unhealthy. There is a dark centre to this area, which was found to be a sinus.

The following should not be considered to be related to SSI:

- Inflammation in response to surgery (early post-operative period)
- Erythema (discoloration associated with the individual's healing process)
- Mechanical (clean) dehiscence
- Stitch abscess.

(Wounds UK 2020a)

Table 13.3 Signs and symptoms of superficial, deep/open and organ/space incisional infection

	Pain/fever	Visible evidence of infection at site			Infection type	Pathologies
Superficial incisional infection	Increased pain, tenderness at the surgical site	Swelling and induration at site	Heat and redness at site	Purulent (discharge containing pus) drainage	Superficial wound abscess *(characterised by* **cellulitis** *limited to wound and adjacent soft tissue)*	
Deep/open incisional infection	Increased pain at site, wound dehiscence and unexpected **post-operative fever**	Spreading induration and swelling	Erythema and heat at site	Purulent discharge from incision	Deep wound **abscess** *(characterised by separations of the edges of incision exposing deeper tissues)* **or fasciitis**	Pathological blood test findings (elevated C-reactive protein, white blood counts, erythrocyte, sedimentation rates, pro-calcitonin)
Organ/ space incisional infection	**Post-operative fever**		Evidence of infection involving the organ or body space **seen on examination during surgery**	Purulent drainage from a drain through the skin into the organ or body space	Organ or body space abscess	Positive result of blood cultures, deep tissue biopsies, surgical sampling or pathological blood test findings (as in deep SSI)

Adapted from Wounds UK (2020a).

Risk factors associated with SSI include:

* Obesity
* Diabetes mellitus
* Current or recent smoking
* Emergency surgery
* Age > 65 years
* Extended duration of surgery
* Inadequate surgical closure
* Peri-operative hypothermia
* Surgery type (e.g. colorectal surgery).

Learning to identify surgical site infections and causative factors will help with preemptive measures, treatment and management.

Learning outcome 2: discuss the principles of wound closure for different types of acute and hard-to-heal wounds

Wounds may be closed through:

* primary closure;
* early (delayed primary) closure, that is, 4–6 days (performed before there is visible granulation tissue);
* late (secondary) closure, that is, 10–14 days;

- grafting using skin or artificial skin products;
- no closure (leaving the wound to heal by granulation).

Figure 13.6 shows a good example of a surgical wound that has healed by primary intention. Although the wound in Figure 13.7 was planned to heal by primary intention, the lower part may have to heal by secondary intention unless the wound is reclosed after the infection has cleared. **T**ertiary intention consists of wound closure via surgical reconstruction techniques.

ACTIVITY

Box 13.11 Activity: how wounds are closed

Try to find out how and when wounds are closed by observing in practice and asking practitioners. Consider

- a surgical wound (such as Susan's abdominal wound);
- a traumatic wound;
- a hard-to-heal wound (such as Mrs Warner's pressure ulcer).

Also, find out how long closure materials (clips, staples or sutures), if present, are left in the wound before removal. Does the site of the wound have any effect on this?

Surgical wounds

Clean or clean-contaminated wounds are managed by primary closure, using sutures, staples or clips, at the end of surgery. The aim is to protect the wound from the bacteria circulating in a hospital environment (Chapter 12 has more information on preventing infection) and promote the best cosmetic result. Thus, Susan's wound will have been managed by primary closure at the end of her operation, as were the wounds shown in Figures 13.6 and 13.7.

With contaminated or dirty surgical wounds, delayed primary closure may be preferable. In some cases, the wound may be left open, to heal by secondary intention. A dirty, infected wound, such as Colin's, will be left open to enable continuing drainage; closing the wound would allow buildup of exudate and a further abscess. When the infection is cleared, this wound may be reclosed by tertiary intention.

Traumatic wounds

Management of traumatic wounds depends on the degree of contamination (taking into account where and how the wound occurred); the extent of skin damage/skin loss; the site of the wound; and how long ago the injury occurred. A clean incisional wound, with little tissue damage, that occurred less than 6 hours previously (caused by a knife, for example) can be irrigated, debrided and managed by primary closure. However, if the injury is more than 6 hours old, or is heavily contaminated, for example, by soil, then primary closure should be delayed.

Bites should usually be left to heal by secondary intention or tertiary intention. These wounds are heavily contaminated owing to the type of bacteria and toxins present; exceptions are made where cosmetic effects are paramount, or restoring function takes priority.

Incised wounds and lacerations can be closed with tapes, sutures or tissue adhesive, the choice depending on factors such as size, depth and site. Tissue adhesive could be suitable for a small scalp wound, due to decreased procedure time and less pain, but should not be used for lacerations of the nostril, mouth or eye, where suturing is preferable to ensure accuracy of alignment.

If a person with a traumatic wound has delayed seeking attention, then prolonged bacterial invasion will have occurred. Usually, the wound will be cleansed with the aim of free drainage and/or detection of infection, followed by delayed primary closure by suturing at 4–6 days. Secondary closure should be used when a wound is heavily contaminated; although this leaves a broader scar than after primary (early or delayed) closure, it is still cosmetically preferable to that achieved through the healing of an open granulating wound.

Hard-to-heal wounds

Hard-to-heal wounds are usually healed by secondary intention. Granulation tissue fills the defect, and new epidermis covers the surface. This process is slow and time-consuming and provides poor protection against risks such as repeated pressure and infection. It can, nevertheless, provide a successful outcome. Mrs Warner's pressure ulcer will need to heal by secondary intention. When surgical excision of necrotic tissue is performed, as might occur with a pressure ulcer, the aim is also for healing to occur by secondary intention. Attempts to directly close large defects by bringing the edges of the wound together have often been unsuccessful, since the tension on the suture line pulls the wound apart. An alternative is to use surgical techniques such as skin grafting and skin flaps, examples of tertiary intention.

When to remove skin closures

The decision on when to remove skin closures depends on various factors;

* Site can affect healing rate. The face heals fast – sutures are often removed in 5 days. The feet heal more slowly, so sutures may be left in situ for 7–10 days.
* Factors such as ageing and diabetes can affect the rate of healing (see the 'Factors affecting wound healing' section).

People being discharged from hospital with skin closures in situ must be informed of exactly when and where the skin closures will be removed. Susan's sutures would probably be ready for removal at 7 days, and she can attend her local health centre for their removal by the practice nurse. Sometimes, it is necessary to arrange for the district nurse to visit a person's home for skin closure removal, for example, if it is difficult for the person to leave the house due to poor general condition or lack of mobility.

Summary

● Acute wounds usually heal uneventfully and quickly, but they can, in certain situations, be hard to heal.
● Hard-to-heal wounds frequently fail to heal in a timely and orderly manner.
● Different types of wounds are managed in different ways. In general, clean surgical wounds heal by primary direct closure, contaminated traumatic wounds heal by delayed primary closure and hard-to-heal wounds heal by secondary or tertiary intention.

FACTORS AFFECTING WOUND HEALING

There are a wide range of biological, psychological and sociological factors that influence wound healing. It is important to holistically identify factors that may affect wound healing for individuals when carrying out wound assessment (Peate and Stephens 2019). A multidisciplinary approach may be needed to address some of these factors. Individuals with acute wounds that are healing by primary intention usually require less input, but each individual should be assessed.

Box 13.12 Learning outcomes

On completion of this section, you will be able to:

1 explore the range of factors that can affect wound healing;
2 examine how a multidisciplinary approach can address factors affecting wound healing.

Learning outcome 1: explore the range of factors that can affect wound healing

Table 13.4 identifies general factors that can delay wound healing. When assessing a person with a wound, consider these questions:

* What underlying factors are interfering with wound healing?
* Does the person have an underlying condition that is delaying wound healing?
* Does the wound require debridement?
* Is the wound infected?
* What needs to be changed to move the wound healing process forward?

The following exercise is based on this framework.

Box 13.13 Activity: problematic wounds

With the guidance of your practice mentor, identify a person who (like Mrs Warner) has a problematic wound. Carry out the activity below.

- Look at their assessment documentation. Identify any factors that could influence wound healing (Table 13.4 will give you clues). Remember to consider the person as a whole, as well as their wound.
- Then ask yourself, can these factors be altered/changed? What action could help?

Table 13.4 includes factors that might have been identified for Mrs Warner. Compare the list you prepared for the person with this. You may well have identified a much wider range of issues, depending on the individual (also see Hess 2011; Mitchell 2020; Vowden 2011).

Table 13.4: Intrinsic and extrinsic factors for delayed wound healing

Intrinsic	Extrinsic
Oxygenation – oxygen is essential for cell metabolism and energy production. Hypoxic wounds are at increased risk of infection, reduced angiogenesis (the development of new blood vessels), reduced epithelialisation, fibroblast (connective tissue cell) proliferation, collagen synthesis and wound contraction	Age – cell regeneration slows down, skin elasticity is lost and collagen is reduced. *This is a factor that may influence Mrs Warner's wound healing*
Infection – infected wounds become 'stuck' in the inflammatory phase. The pathogenic microbes compete for nutrients and other resources. *This is a factor that may influence Mrs Warner's wound healing.*	Gender – oestrogen helps regulate a variety of genes associated with regeneration.
Venous insufficiency – increased venous pressure leads to a chronic inflammatory response over time. This can cause a breakdown of the tissue resulting in venous leg ulcers.	Poor dressing technique and wound management.
Comorbidities: Diabetes Chronic venous insufficiency Peripheral arterial disease Immune deficiency disorders Organ failure Are known to delay the healing process. In diabetes, narrowed blood vessels lead to decreased blood flow and oxygen to a wound. Elevated blood sugars decrease red blood cells, which carry nutrients to the tissue and lowers the efficacy of white blood cells (neutrophils and monocytes) to fight infection. *This is a factor that may influence Mrs Warner's wound healing.*	Lifestyle factors – alcoholism and smoking – smoking causes vasoconstriction that leads to hypoxia. Neutrophil and monocyte (cells that help prevent infection) activity are reduced and fibroblast proliferation and migration is reduced. Collagen is reduced in smokers, which means less tensile wound strength. Smoking impairs the cardiovascular system, delaying healing. It leads to inhibition of epithelialisation and a reduction in wound contraction. *This is a factor that may influence Mrs Warner's wound healing.* Alcoholism – diminishes host resistance making the body more at risk of infection.
Peripheral arterial disease – decreased blood flow to the lower extremities and wound. Reducing the amount of oxygen and nutrients to the wound bed. Figure 13.8 shows how a lack of blood supply affects skin and deeper tissues.	
Temperature – the cooler the wound, the longer it will take to heal. Higher temperatures promote vascular and arterial dilation.	Nutrition – is required to provide adequate support fort the increased energy demands of the healing process. The body requires 30–35 Kcal to heal a wound daily and 40 Kcal if the person is underweight. For adequate requirements for wound healing, see Table 13.6. *This is a factor that may influence Mrs Warner's wound healing.*

(Continued)

Table 13.4: **(Continued)**

Intrinsic	Extrinsic
Necrotic tissue or foreign bodies both prolong the inflammatory phase and increase infection risk. *This is a factor that may influence Mrs Warner's wound healing.*	Obesity – reduces the availability of oxygen to the wound. Skin folds can harbour bacteria and can cause damage to the skin by friction and pressure.
Dehydration – fluid is required for oxygen profusion, hydration of the wound bed, transportation of nutrients, as a solvent for minerals, vitamins, glucose and amnio acids and transport waste away from cells.	Pain – ineffective wound pain management can delay wound healing and contribute to lack of compliance.
Oedema – affects the permeability of vascular membranes. Also, fluid can leak into the surrounding skin.	Psychological factors – stress delays wound healing but altering the multiple physiological pathways required in the repair processes. Stress stimulates the hypothalamic-pituitary-adrenal (HPA) axis to produce stress hormones (cortisol and catecholamines), which activate a fight or flight response and prolong inflammation. Depression can affect the ability to self-care and manage long-term conditions. *This is a factor that may influence Mrs Warner's wound healing.*
	Steroids – the anti-inflammatory response of steroids reduces the inflammatory response, and affects the function of the macrophages, thus slowing healing.

Adapted from Mitchell (2020).

Colin has a long-standing mental health problem, and the discomfort associated with his wound may be a further source of stress. Susan, too, has been through a stressful experience. Now that she is back in her own environment with familiar staff members, it will be important to be supportive and reassuring. Thus, nurses should aim to relieve their stress and anxieties and help them to relax (see Chapter 2).

Exudate can be a major factor that influences wound healing. Where a moist wound bed is essential to wound healing too much exudate can lead to protein deficiency; moisture is associated with skin damage of the peri-wound (Mitchell and Hill 2020) and can negatively affect the person's quality of life (Wounds UK 2013). Table 13.5 shows the different types of wound exudate and the significance. Understanding exudate is an important factor in managing hard-to-heal wounds.

Chapter 5 highlights the need for an increased nutritional intake for wound healing. However, many people with hard-to-heal wounds, such as PUs, have poor nutritional intake and risk factors for malnutrition (Mitchell, 2018). Every person with a wound should be assessed nutritionally. Table 13.6 outlines the key nutrients required for wound healing and their role in the process.

Table 13.5: Descriptions of exudate and its significance

Type	Consistency	Colour	Significance
Serous	Thin, watery	Clear, straw-coloured	Often considered normal but increased volume may indicate infection (e.g. *Staphylococcus aureus*). May also be due to fluid from urinary or lymphatic fistula
Fibrinous	Thin, watery	Cloudy	May indicate the presence of fibrin strands, which would indicate a response to inflammation
Serosanguineous	Thin, slightly thicker than water	Clear, pink	Presence of red blood cells indicates capillary damage (e.g., after surgery or a traumatic dressing removal)
Sanguineous	Thin, watery	Reddish	Low protein content due to venous or congestive cardiac disease, malnutrition – or enteric or urinary fistula
Purulent	Viscous, sticky	Opaque, milky, yellow or brown, sometimes green	White blood cells, bacteria, slough or from enteric or urinary fistula. Bacterial infection (e.g. *Pseudomonas aeruginosa*)
Haemopurulent	Viscous	Reddish, milky	Established infection. May contain neutrophils, dying bacteria, inflammatory cells, blood leakage due to dermal capillaries, some bacteria
Haemorrhagic	Viscous	Dark red	Capillaries break down easily and bleed due to infection or trauma

Mitchell, A. 2020. Assessment of Wounds in Adults. *British Journal of Nursing*, Vol. 29, Number 20 Tissue Viability Supplement.

WUWHS (2007); Wounds UK (2013); Mitchell (2020).

Table 13.6: Nutrients required for wound healing and their function

Nutrient	Function	Dietary sources
Fat	Energy source; involves in formation of inflammatory mediators and clotting components; fat-soluble vitamins are essential for the building of new cell membranes in wound repair.	Butter, margarine, other spreading fats, oils, cream, full fat milk, cheese
Carbohydrate	Energy source for increased cellular activity during wound healing; in the absence of sufficient dietary or stored energy, the body utilises protein as an energy source.	Complex: bread, pasta, rice, noodles, scones, pancakes, potatoes. Simple: jam, sugar, biscuits, honey
Protein	Essential for building the new wound bed (collagen formation). Lack of protein decreases the synthesis of collagen and the production of fibroblasts.	Meat, eggs, cheese, milk, yogurt, fish, poultry, pulses, nuts
Vitamin A	Enhances the immune response; antioxidant; promotes collagen synthesis and epithelialisation.	Butter, margarine, other spreading fats, oils, milk, cheese, carrots, red peppers, tomatoes, eggs
Vitamin B complex	Assists formation of collagen mesh which supports new blood vessels as they move into granulating tissue.	Whole grains, breakfast cereals, milk and milk products, meat, fish liver

(Continued)

Table 13.6: **(Continued)**

Nutrient	Function	Dietary sources
Vitamin C	Assists formation of collagen mesh and angiogenesis; enhances iron absorption, promotes immune function.	Oranges, grapefruit, fruit juice, green vegetables, potatoes, strawberries
Vitamin E	With vitamin C, attacks damaging oxygen free radicals that are present in infected wounds and during the inflammatory phase of wound healing.	Vegetable oil, egg yolk, nuts, seeds
Vitamin K	Blood clotting.	Liver, green vegetables
Minerals: selenium, copper, manganese, zinc, iron	Fibroblast proliferation; collagen synthesis; improved oxygen delivery to tissue.	Selenium: Brazil nuts, meat, vegetables, fish, cereals Copper: meat, vegetables, cereals, tea, coffee. Manganese: tea, widely distributed in various foods Zinc: meat, milk, potatoes, bread Iron: red meat, liver, fortified breakfast cereals, eggs, pulses, green vegetables, sardines

Source: Adapted from Johnston, E. 2007. The role of nutrition in tissue viability. Wound Essentials 2: 10–21 and Wild et al. 2010, Basics in nutrition and wound healing.

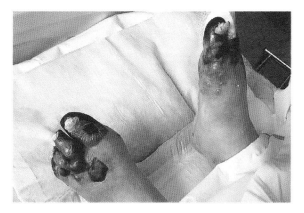

Figure 13.8: This person, whose feet are shown here, had a history of heart surgery and heart failure and lack of circulation to her feet. Over 2 weeks, she developed black necrotic toes, and the condition spread to the distal area of her feet owing to the lack of arterial circulation.

Learning outcome 2: examine how a multidisciplinary approach can address factors affecting wound healing

Addressing factors affecting healing requires MDT working, including relatives and the client, whose involvement is essential in the process of wound healing.

Box 13.14 Activity: members of MDT involved in wound healing.

ACTIVITY

Look back at Table 13.4 and list members of the MDT who might be involved in addressing the factors affecting Mrs Warner's wound healing. Make a note of what their specific roles might be.

Mrs Warner, who has hard-to-heal wounds, would require considerable multidisciplinary teamwork to address the factors affecting her wound healing. For example, you may have thought of some of the following; specialist nurse such as infection control nurse, Occupational Therapist, Social Worker, Dietician, Doctor and Podiatrist. If psychological adjustment relating to a wound is problematic, a psychologist's input is sometimes necessary. Voluntary organisations can also help to support individuals – Diabetes UK in Mrs Warner's case.

Summary

- A range of factors can interfere with the healing process of a wound. These factors relate to the individual's general health status, the condition of the wound and the care being received.
- Nurses should identify factors affecting wound healing in individuals and plan strategies to address them where possible, involving the MDT appropriately.

WOUND ASSESSMENT

When assessing a wound, you must consider the whole person, so factors that could influence healing such as their psychological and nutritional status, pain and medication must be addressed wherever possible (Mitchell 2020). This section prepares you to assess the wound itself, based on your knowledge of the phases of wound healing, the ability to classify wounds and an awareness of wider issues that affect wound healing. All these aspects underpin the assessment process. Useful articles relating to wound assessment include Ousey and Cook (2012) and Mitchell (2020).

Box 13.15 Learning outcomes

By the end of this *section, you will be able to:*

1 discuss the features of a wound assessment and how wound assessment tools/charts can be used;
2 record key information in a useful format that can be used to plan appropriate interventions.

Learning outcome 1: discuss the features of a wound assessment and how wound assessment tools/charts can be used

Wound assessment tools provide information on the wound. For example, the *Pressure Ulcer Classification Guide* produced by EPUAP is used to classify the degree of damage of PUs (see Box 13.16). Charts may include a diagram of the body for marking the location of the wound(s). The red–yellow–black (RYB) system (Gray et al. 2004) is based on assessing the condition of the tissue within the wound bed and has been incorporated in the wound assessment tool included in this chapter. Evaluating tissue type by a single variable such as colour has been described as subjective and limiting, but it can be used as a basis for selecting a dressing. If you look at Figures 13.1 through 13.5, you can see how the colours in the RYB system could be applied to these wounds (e.g. Figure 13.1: black).

Box 13.16 Pressure ulcer classification

- *Category 1.* Intact skin with non-blanching erythema of a localised area usually over a bony prominence. Discolouration of the skin, warmth, oedema, hardness or pain may also be present. Darkly pigmented skin may not have visible blanching.
- *Category 2.* Partial thickness loss of dermis presenting as a shallow open ulcer with a red pink wound bed, without slough. May also present as an intact or open/ruptured serum-filled or serosanguinous-filled blister.
- *Category 3.* Full thickness tissue loss. Subcutaneous fat may be visible but bone, tendon or muscle are *not* exposed. Some slough may be present. *May* include undermining and tunnelling.
- *Category 4.* Full thickness tissue loss with exposed bone, tendon or muscle. Slough or eschar may be present. Often include undermining and tunnelling.

Additional categories for the United States

Unstageable/unclassified: full thickness skin or tissue loss – depth unknown

Full thickness tissue loss in which actual depth of the ulcer is completely obscured by slough (yellow, tan, grey, green or brown) and/or eschar (tan, brown or black) in the wound bed.

Suspected deep tissue injury – depth unknown

Purple or maroon localised area of discoloured intact skin or blood-filled blister due to damage of underlying soft tissue from pressure and/or shear.

Source: European Pressure Ulcer Advisory Panel and National Pressure Ulcer Advisory Panel (EPUAP and NPUAP). 2009. *Treatment of Pressure Ulcers: Quick Reference Guide.* Washington, DC: NPUAP.

Other features that may be included in a wound assessment chart are listed below, in relation to Mrs Warner's sacral pressure ulcer. Note that she would require a chart for each of her wounds as each must be assessed separately.

- *Wound site.* A body map can be used to indicate wound site as well as writing 'sacrum' at the top of the chart.
- *Wound category.* Wound category relates to the wound classification discussed earlier. Mrs Warner's sacral wound will be recorded as a pressure ulcer and then graded using the EPUAP pressure ulcer classification system (Box 13.16 and Table 13.2).
- *Medication.* Mrs Warner could be taking medication that will affect wound healing.

Wound assessment

Holistic wound assessment is key to management and treatment of hard-to-heal wounds; however, there appear to be inconsistencies in wound care practice across the UK (Guest et al. 2015). The importance of wound assessment and the recognition of improving standards has been recognised by NHS England through the Implementation of a CQUIN indicator (Wounds UK 2018). Coleman et al. (2017) suggest a generic wound care assessment that considers general health information, wound baseline information, e.g. number of wounds and location, wound assessment parameters, e.g. size, tissue type and wound symptoms, e.g. pain, exudate and specialist referral required. The following assessment has been completed for Mrs Warner.

- Risk factors. Mrs Warner is a type 2 diabetic who smokes and suffers from depression.
- *Allergies.* Mrs Warner could have a known allergy to a dressing product, which should be noted.
- *Type/colour of tissue.* The type and colour of the tissue within the wound bed will assist in determining the treatment required to progress the wound. Black necrotic tissue (Mrs Warner's sacral pressure ulcer and Figure 13.1) and yellow sloughy tissue are considered to be non-viable tissue that require debridement. Red tissue is associated with a healthy granulating, well vascularised wound, with pink tissue indicating re-epithelialisation (Mitchell 2020; Ousey and Cook 2012). Bright red granulation tissue, which is friable and exuberant and associated with new areas of slough, increased exudate and malodour, could be signs of infection in a chronic wound (Mitchell 2020). The RYB system has been incorporated into the tool to assist in identifying the type of tissue within the wound bed.
- Black: necrotic tissue
- Yellow: sloughy tissue
- Red: granulating tissue
- Pink: epithelialisation
- Green: infected tissue.

The wound base may have several different types of tissue present. For example, Figure 13.5 shows a wound base that has both sloughy (yellow) areas and granulation tissue (red). Nurses assessing this wound would need to estimate the percentage of the wound bed covered with slough (yellow), and the percentage covered with granulation tissue (red) and record this on the chart. For Mrs Warner, the recording will be 100% necrotic (black), but in due course, as the wound progresses, there will be sloughy (yellow) areas, and then it is hoped some granulation tissue (red), and then areas that are epithelialising (pink).

- *Photograph.* Increasingly photos are used in wound assessment, but consent from the individual must be obtained in line with local policies (Ousey and Cook 2012). Often, a ruler is placed by the side of the wound when taking the photograph, showing the wound's size as well as its appearance (see Figure 13.3). Clearly, the sacral area would be a sensitive area to photograph and the reasons for doing so need careful explanation. However, the photos can be shown to Mrs Warner to help her to appreciate the nature of the wound, and how its healing is progressing.

- *Measurement.* The size is recorded in centimetres as width by length. Sometimes, a tracing is made, which creates a record of shape as well as size and this can be attached to the assessment tool.
- *Depth.* Depth is difficult to measure, but a wound probe or sterile wound swab can be used and then measured against a ruler. The depth of the wound can also be assessed through the identification of exposed structures such as tendon or bone (Mitchell 2020).
- *Pain.* Assessment of pain, using a number intensity scale where 1 is no pain and 10 is the worst pain imaginable, needs to occur before removing the dressing to establish whether Mrs Warner requires any analgesics and whether the current pain management strategy is effective. If the pain occurs only during dressing removal, a different product may be required. If the pain has increased and is associated with other signs and symptoms such as malodour, inflammation, increased exudate and delayed wound healing, a wound infection may be present (Mitchell 2020; Ousey and Cook 2012).
- *Infection.* The presence of infection can delay wound healing. In an acute wound, infection may be indicated by the presence of erythema (redness), swelling, localised heat and pain, purulent discharge and pyrexia (Ousey and Cook 2012). The identification of infection in hard-to-heal wounds is more challenging and frequently is associated with a general deterioration in the wound or the wound healing becoming stagnant. See Swanson, Grothier, and Schultz's (2015) document on wound infections.
- *Malodour.* A slight odour can occur due to wound occlusion and is associated with some types of dressing. However, an offensive odour is often a sign of infection. Necrotic wounds (Mrs Warner's sacral pressure ulcer) and fungating wounds are often malodorous. Assessing odour can help to identify infection, as one of a range of criteria, but also helps with dressing choice as some dressings are deodorising.
- *Swab taken.* Wound swabs taken should be recorded, but they have limitations. Chapter 12 discusses how and when to take wound swabs. The nurses must remember to check the results and discuss with the medical staff whether it is appropriate to treat the wound with antibiotics or with an antibacterial dressing containing substances such as iodine, silver or honey.
- *Exudate.* Exudate is fluid arising from the wound owing to increased permeability of capillaries. Exudate should be assessed for colour, consistency, odour and quantity (Wounds UK 2013). Estimating the amount of exudate (high, medium or low) is not easy, but a change in the volume or nature of the exudate could indicate an increasing bacterial load (Wounds UK 2013). The presence and extent of exudate will influence your dressing choice.
- *Colour of exudate.* The colour of the exudate will also indicate if infection is present in the wound (see the exudate descriptions in Table 13.5).

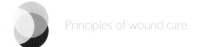

- *Condition of surrounding skin.* Condition of surrounding skin is important in considering the type of dressing to be used. For example, if the skin is moist/macerated, a more absorbent dressing to the wound bed may be needed. Also consider applying a barrier film such as Cavilon No-Sting Barrier Film beneath the dressing. If erythema (redness) or eczema is present, this could indicate an allergic reaction or that the dressing is being removed too frequently, causing trauma. Cellulitis or spreading erythema needs to be reported if it is a new feature as it indicates infection is present and systemic antibiotics are needed.

- *Wound edges.* In large and/or deep wounds, the edge of the wound may be undermined, whereby it is possible to reach underneath the edges of the wound. As the wound progresses to the proliferative phase, a shallow white/pink almost transparent border appears. This new epidermal tissue is fragile and easily removed. Edges that are rolled in can delay healing time. In hard to heal wounds, the edges can have a punched-out appearance, and small satellite wounds can be present. Wound edges that are hard and fibrous indicate a hard to heal wound.

Assessing a wound might also include any of the following considerations:

- *Is the wound open or closed?* How is the wound healing? Primary, secondary or tertiary intention? Susan's wound is healing by primary intention, but Mrs Warner's sacral wound is healing by secondary intention.

- *Extent of tissue involvement.* Does the wound involve epidermis, dermis, fat, fascia, muscle and/or bone?

- *Presence of foreign bodies.* Foreign bodies delay the healing process. Foreign bodies such as dirt or grit can also increase infection risk and lead to permanent marking.

- *Presence of a fistula or a sinus.* A fistula is an abnormal connection between two spaces such as skin surface and bowel. A sinus is a tract that ends in a blind cavity, and a sinus is frequently found in a deep pressure ulcer. A sinus should ideally heal from its base; if it heals first at the surface, fluid will accumulate within, promoting an abscess, which will subsequently break through to the surface. In Figure 13.7, the darkened central area of the dehisced part of the wound was found to be a sinus.

- *Wound drain and drain site.* Wound drains are inserted into some surgical wounds to promote the removal of fluid that would otherwise accumulate and form a potential growing medium for infection, or interfere with healing.

All wounds require a full holistic wound assessment and documentation in the person's notes. This would be appropriate and have been adequate for Susan's surgical

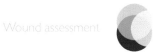

wound when she was in hospital, and for the wound shown in Figure 13.6, which is a straightforward clean surgical wound that healed without complication. The use of a wound assessment tool/chart requires the practitioner to document additional details, for example, if the wound is not healing as expected, possibly reverting to a previous stage, wounds with problems, or where required as a legal record, for example, after an assault or suspected neglect/abuse. For the assessment of the person's wound in Figure 13.7, it should be documented that the wound is complicated by infection causing dehiscence. Mrs Warner's pressure ulcer and ulcerated toe (which could, as a diabetic ulcer, deteriorate) are both hard-to-heal and problematic wounds, which should be documented.

Leg ulcer assessment

All individuals presenting with a leg ulcer should be screened for arterial disease by Doppler ultrasound measurement of ankle brachial pressure index (ABPI) by competent staff alongside a thorough clinical investigation within 2 weeks (Wounds UK 2016). Often a specific leg ulcer assessment chart is used to record this assessment, which includes documenting assessment of factors affecting wound healing (e.g. smoking, nutritional status). The ABPI is calculated by dividing the brachial systolic blood pressure by the ankle systolic blood pressure. A normal ABPI reading is about 1 and if the reading is 0.8 or above (up to 1.3), compression therapy can usually be applied following a full holistic lower limb assessment (Wound UK 2019; Mitchell and Elbourne 2019). Compression therapy aims to provide graduated compression, with the highest pressure at the ankle and the lowest at the knee, thus returning blood from the lower limb and preventing pooling in distended lower leg veins. An arterial ulcer is caused by an inadequate arterial blood supply to the area, and a person suspected of having an arterial ulcer may require vascular surgery.

Note: Accurate assessment is essential. Applying compression to a limb with an arterial ulcer could potentially lead to loss of the limb affected.

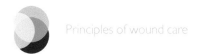

Learning outcome 2: record key information in a useful format that can be used to plan appropriate interventions

Box 13.18 Activity: evaluation of documentation

Review the documentation you completed using the wound assessment tool/ chart earlier, and consider this question: Is it specific and comprehensive enough to help you to plan the wound's management, and to promote continuity of care?

- The tools used are generally very wound-specific. They have to be simple to use, yet all-encompassing, but not so inclusive as to waste valuable time and deter use.
- These are legal documents. Have you accurately described the wound environment? Have you avoided the use of colloquialisms, such as 'wound bed appears fine' or 'copious amounts of exudate': what does 'fine' mean? How much is copious? Ensure that you use descriptive language that can be interpreted by anyone, not just yourself. This helps to promote continuity of care.
- A photograph of the wound provides a more objective record of the wound's status, alleviating potential variation in the use of descriptive terms and their interpretation.
- Has your assessment identified any problems with the current approach to wound management? For example, is the dressing allowing the wound to dry out, or the surrounding skin to become moisture damaged? Was the dressing painful to remove?

Box 13.19 Pregnancy and birth practice points: wound infection risk and recognition

There is a significantly increased risk of postpartum septicaemia, wounds can be abdominal or perineal and sepsis is still an important cause of maternal mortality. In the UK, there is an 8% risk of infection following lower segment caesarean section (LSCS), and antibiotic prophylaxis during the operation should be offered routinely (NICE 2019b). Usual practice is that prophylactic antibiotics are given when there is a complex perineal tear or at caesarean section. Prophylaxis reduces endometritis by 66–75% and also reduces rate of wound infection (Smaill and Gyte 2010). Remember that in addition to observing the wound assessing vaginal loss (colour, smell and amount) may be an important indicator that there is an infection. Often midwives will have a lower threshold of referral to specialists such as tissue viability as complex wound management is not part of usual care.

Women in the postnatal period should test for a full set of physiological vital signs if they have any symptoms or signs of ill health. These should be recorded and assessed against a Maternity Early Obstetric Warning System (MEOWS) chart.

Also read:

NICE. 2021. Caesarean Birth NICE guideline 192. Available from: www.nice.org.uk/guidance/ng192

MBRACCE. 2020. Saving Lives, Improving Mothers' Care. Available from: https://www.npeu.ox.ac.uk/assets/downloads/mbrrace-uk/reports/maternal-report-2020/MBRRACE-UK_Maternal_Report_Dec_2020_v10_ONLINE_VERSION_1404.pdf

Royal College of Obstetricians and Gynaecologists. 2015. The Management of Third- and Fourth Degree Perineal Tears. Available from: www.rcog.org.uk/en/guidelines-research-services/guidelines/gtg29/

Summary

- Wound assessment requires a holistic approach involving assessment of the whole person and the wound together.
- Wound assessment charts assist a systematic process and clear documentation of the wound's progress.
- Documentation important, for management as well as litigation reasons.
- Accuracy in recording assessment is an important skill to develop and does much to promote continuity of care, as well as a firm basis for planning interventions.

WOUND MANAGEMENT

You have already considered factors affecting wound healing and have identified that wound management must focus on both the wound and the person as a whole. It is important to be aware of the psychosocial effects of wounds so that you can be supportive; this is relevant to both acute and hard-to-heal wounds. The effects on body image of a wound can result in a range of psychological reactions, including a grief response, anxiety and depression (International Consensus 2012). The skin is 'a major factor in a person's body image', with denial, anxiety, pain, immobility and altered body image experienced by people with hard-to-heal wounds. Being aware of this can help health professionals to be understanding, and effective assessment can promote appropriate interventions, referrals and information provision (International Consensus 2012).

In this section, you focus on care of the wound itself, using a concept called wound-bed preparation (WBP). The focus of WBP denotes the importance of removing non-viable tissue (necrosis and slough) through cleansing/debridement, moisture balance, control of oedema and decreased bacterial burden (Ousey and Cook 2012) to promote healing.

Box 13.20 Learning outcome

By the end of this section you will be able to:

1. discuss how wound dressings are performed;
2. explain methods of debridement and cleansing;
3. identify a range of wound dressings and explain how a dressing is selected for an individual;
4. discuss ways of reducing pain and discomfort associated with wounds.

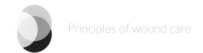

Learning outcome 1: discuss how wound dressings are performed

For information on aseptic technique, applied to wound dressings, see Chapter 12. A sterile technique has traditionally been used for wound care, but it may hold no advantage over a clean technique in hard-to-heal wounds. In essence, when using sterile technique, equipment, fluids and dressings are sterile, whereas with a clean technique, clean but non-sterile single-use gloves can be used, with tap water (that is safe enough to drink) used for cleansing (Fernandez et al. 2010).

Box 13.21 Activity: sterile technique

ACTIVITY

How do you think you might identify when a sterile technique would be essential and when a clean technique might be sufficient?

A sterile technique must be used if the person is immunocompromised or has undergone surgery, which carries a high infection risk. However, hard-to-heal wounds are likely to be colonised with bacteria, so a clean rather than sterile procedure may be sufficient.

Effective handwashing and gloving techniques are essential, whether a sterile or clean technique is used for wound care, and aprons should be worn too (see Chapter 12).

Learning outcome 2: explain methods of debridement and cleansing

Debridement

Debridement is the removal of non-viable tissue from the wound bed to promote wound healing (Vowden 2011). Hard to heal wounds can often contain sloughy or necrotic tissue, which acts as a barrier to wound healing and can harbour bacteria increasing the risk of malodour and infection. There are a range of debridement techniques used in the UK, which are discussed in Box 13.22:

- Autolytic
- Biological
- Enzymatic
- Surgical
- Sharp
- Mechanical
- Hydrosurgery.

Box 13.22 Methods of debridement

Autolytic debridement

- Autolytic debridement is the most conservative type of debridement. It is a natural process in which the body's own enzymes break down necrotic tissue. Moisture is created to rehydrate, soften and liquefy hard eschar and slough (Manna et al. 2020).

(Continued)

Box 13.22 (Continued)

- Indicated for non-infected wounds and enhanced by moist environment. This can be created, using dressings such as hydrogels, hydrocolloids and hydrofibre.
- *Hydrogels* – designed to donate fluid to the wound bed through their high water content, which rehydrate the eschar and slough, promoting autolysis (Cowan 2012).
- *Hydrocolloids* – contain gel-forming agents combined with elastomers and an adhesive matrix, which in the presence of exudate forms a moist gel (Cowan 2012).
- *Hydrofibre* – highly absorbent non-woven sheets or ribbon composed entirely of hydrocolloid fibre, which in the presence of exudate, converts to a soft moist gel (Cowan 2012).

Larval therapy

Larvae act by moving over the surface of a wound bed and secreting powerful enzymes that break down dead tissue into a liquefied solution, which they can then digest together with bacteria present in the wound (Manna et al. 2020). Larval therapy is quicker than autolytic debridement and is most effective where the devitalised tissue is not dry; frequently autolytic treatment is required initially to soften and liquefy the devitalised tissue before application (Gray et al. 2011). Larval therapy has also been demonstrated to reduce the bacterial burden of the wound bed and facilitate healing (Gray et al. 2011).

Sharp debridement

The removal of dead or foreign material just above the level of viable tissue using sharp instruments such as a scalpel, performed without anaesthetic by a doctor or an experienced nurse (Manna et al. 2020). It requires skill and knowledge of the anatomical structures and should be governed under strict local guidelines.

Surgical debridement

The excision or wide resection of necrotic tissue, often extending into the viable or healthy tissue. It is performed in the operating theatre by a surgeon (Manna et al. 2020). It is most suitable for large areas or in wounds that contain contaminated tissue or sepsis where rapid removal is required (Gray et al. 2011). This method of debridement can be costly, and risk of anaesthesia has to be considered (Gray et al. 2011).

Hydrosurgery

Hydrosurgery system is a safe, effective system that combines lavage with sharp debridement. This type of debridement has shown to be effective in removing damaged and necrotic tissues (Vowden 2011).

Wound debridement can lead to improved healing rates, reduced risk of infection and improved quality of life (Gray et al. 2011). It was identified earlier that Mrs Warner's sacral wound requires debriding of its necrotic tissue. Debridement can be carried out in several ways (Box 13.22). The choice of debriding agent should be according to the individual, wound and practitioner competence.

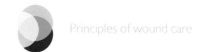

Dressings promoting autolysis and biosurgical methods (sterile maggots) may be more acceptable to individuals and less painful. Gray et al. (2011) provide an overview of the use and effectiveness of larval therapy. Figure 13.3 shows a deep sacral pressure ulcer the day after maggots had been removed after 3 days in situ. The ulcer, which was 60% covered with slough, is now about 85% granulation tissue. Vacuum-assisted closure uses negative pressure to remove slough and loosen necrotic tissue from the wound bed (Henderson et al. 2012). The use of honey in wound care has been well published. It has been found to have a debriding action as well as many other beneficial effects, for example, antibacterial activity (Grothier and Cooper 2011; Mitchell 2018).

> ### Box 13.23 Activity: wound cleansing
>
> You have probably seen wound cleansing carried out in practice. Think about the following: Why are wounds cleansed? How are wounds cleansed? What are wounds cleansed with? Compare your thoughts with the points below.

Purpose of wound irrigation

Wound irrigation is not always necessary and has sometimes been carried out ritualistically without sound rationale for practice (Peate and Stephens 2019). The aim of wound irrigation is to remove contaminated/foreign material from the wound bed, that is, slough, necrotic tissue, exudate and dressing debris. Nurses must decide whether this can be achieved by cleansing or debridement, as discussed earlier, is needed. In most cases simple tap water irrigation will remove the wound of contaminants and bacteria. In more complex wounds, such as new surgical wounds, if there is an underlying fracture or if the person's health is compromised, sterile saline is advisable (Peate and Stephens 2019).

Wound exudate is produced as a normal part of the healing process to prevent the wound bed from drying out, while facilitating the migration of cells and providing essential nutrients and growth factors. Inappropriate management of exudate can lead to skin damage and prolong wound healing (Wounds UK 2013). Enzymes in chronic wound exudate may cause skin stripping (excoriation) and requires wound cleansing to protect the peri wound (Wounds UK 2013). Further reasons for wound cleansing are so that the wound can be assessed and to maintain hygiene and enhance well-being, particularly when there is excessive exudate and malodour.

Cleansing methods

There are many different options for wound cleansing and the criteria for choosing should include the following:

* Acute or hard to heal wound
* Current infection, risk of infection or recurring infection

- Clinical efficacy
- Availability and cost effectiveness.

(Weir and Swanson 2019)

- **Irrigation.** Irrigation of wounds is often considered preferable to swabbing and maybe essential to rid the wound of contaminants. In most cases, simple tap water irrigation is sufficient, in cases where there is an underlying fracture, or if the person's general health is compromised, sterile saline is advised (Peate and Stephens 2019). Frequency of irrigation should depend on the clinical presentation of the wound. Unnecessary irrigation can delay wound healing by damaging new granulation and epithelial cells. Avoid using gauze swabs for irrigation as these cause trauma and pain in wound contact and spread the bacteria around the wound without removal. Irrigating fluid should simply be poured over the wound (Peate and Stephens 2019).
- **Bathing.** Individuals with leg ulcers find it can be comforting, and psychologically enhancing, to bathe their legs in a lined bucket, which can then be disposed of afterwards. The same principle can be used for a sacral pressure ulcer. In addition, to the therapeutic and hydrating effect of soaking legs in buckets, wound cleansing softens any residual exudate and reduces infection. It is important not to use any traditional soaps that tend to be alkaline. These are detrimental to the skin barrier function and damage corneocytes (found in the stratum corneum), increasing dryness and creating friction (Mitchell and Liumigusin 2020). A skin cleanser with a pH range similar to normal skin is preferable. Avoid aggressive cleansing as this can increase frictional forces and abrade skin (Mitchell 2020). If there is no wound infection present, cleaning of the bath with normal detergent is adequate but if the wound is infected, the bath should be cleaned with hypochlorite solution. This would be necessary, therefore, if Colin has a bath, which could well be a soothing method of wound cleansing for him.

Wound cleansing solutions

Although a wide selection of solutions have been used to cleanse wounds, normal saline is often considered the solution of choice, as it is isotonic and non-toxic to healing tissue (Gouvela and Miguens 2007). Several studies have shown the effectiveness of tap water, distilled water, boiled water and antibacterial solutions in lowering bacterial counts and reducing infection. The consensus on which cleaning agent is most effective remains debatable and requires further investigation (Probst 2020). Solutions used for cleansing/irrigating should be used at body temperature if possible, thus reducing the cooling of the wound bed, which adversely affects healing. The use of antiseptic cleansing agents is rarely indicated for routine wound cleansing.

Wounds UK (2020a) has published a Best Practice Statement reviewing the use of antiseptics and antimicrobials in wound healing. The main use of these products should be to treat wound infection, and their use should be avoided if no infection is

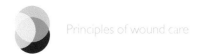

present. Traumatic wounds are likely to be contaminated with bacteria, and it would be appropriate to use antiseptics/antimicrobials in these wounds.

Learning outcome 3: identify a range of wound dressings and explain how a dressing is selected for an individual

Before considering which dressing to apply, have a look at some dressings in your clinical area. What are the attributes of these dressings and can these be influenced by the nature and condition of the wound (wound related) – for example, increased exudate.

Box 13.24 Activity: selecting dressings

ACTIVITY

Go back to the wound you assessed earlier. How might you select a dressing? Discuss with a practitioner how a specific dressing is chosen for an individual. There may be local clinical guidelines and, if so, try to locate them.

There are many dressings available in the UK, which can be categorised as in Table 13.7. Things to consider when deciding upon a dressing include the following:

- Does the wound require a dressing at all?
- What is the purpose of the dressing?
- Promotion of autolytic debridement or granulation formation?
- Absorption or rehydration?
- Reducing the bacterial burden?
- Controlling moisture levels?
- Appropriate size of dressing
- Availability
- Ease of application and removal
- Comfort
- Frequency of dressing changes
- Dressing efficacy
- Cost

Your choice of dressing should be informed by your wound assessment, taking into account the safety and efficacy of the wound care product. Consider the stage of wound healing, type and colour of tissue, site of wound, pain relief and amount of exudate.

Gray et al. (2009) have further developed the concepts of WBP into Applied Wound Management (AWM) to provide a systematic and practical approach to wound management, assisting with establishing the immediate treatment goals. The concept utilises three different continuums each relating to a wound parameter, namely, viability of the tissue, presence of infection and levels of exudate. Focusing on these areas will help you to determine whether the dressing has the required properties to debride or promote healing, whether infection needs to be targeted and the level of absorbency that needs to be controlled. Always consult the manufacturer's instructions when applying dressings.

Table 13.7: Wound dressings

Dressing type	Examples	Uses	Contraindications	Cautions
Simple absorbent dressings (island dressings)	Cosmopor E Mepore Opsite Plus	Wounds healing by primary intention (e.g. straightforward surgical wound).	None	Gentle removal for friable skin
Superabsorbent dressings	Cutisorb Ultra Eclypse Sorbion sachet S Zetuvit	Venous leg ulcers, PUs, diabetic foot ulcers, abdominal wounds. Any highly exuding wounds.	None	Review regularly to avoid MASD
Hydrocolloids	Granuflex Comfeel Duoderm Hydrocoll Tegaderm hydrocolloid	Suitable for clean, granulating wounds or sloughy/necrotic wounds. They are principally indicated for low to moderately exuding wounds. For example, PUs, leg ulcers, surgical wounds, dehisced wounds, traumatic wounds, ruptured blisters.	Heavy exuding wounds Infected wounds Risk of gas gangrene	Diabetic foot ulcers
Alginates	ActivHeal alginate Kaltostat Sorbsan	Moderately to heavily exudating wounds, including infected, sloughy, and granulating and epithelialising wounds. Can be used to loosely pack puncture and cavity wounds. Not suitable if the wound is completely dried out.	None	Senstivities Must be covered with an insulating dressing
Antimicrobials	Bactigras (Chlorhexidine) Acticoat, Aquacel Ag and Allevyn Ag adhesive (silver) Inadine, Iodosorb and Iodoflex (iodine) Coviden Kendall AMD Suprasorb X+PHMB (PHMB) Medihoney	All hard to heal and acute wounds that are critically colonised or infected.		Should be reviewed every 2 weeks
Film dressings	Bioclusive Hydrofilm Opsite Tegaderm	Primary wound closure (e.g. straightforward surgical wound). To protect skin susceptible to damage from shearing; superficial abrasions.	None	Superficial wounds of all types and on vulnerable skin or scar tissue
Foams	Allevyn Biatain Tielle Mepilex Border (soft silicone)	Suitable for wounds with low to moderate exudate levels. They can be applied under compression therapy, although this is likely to adversely affect the absorbent capacity.	None	Sensitivities Avoid direct application to dry wounds

(Continued)

Table 13.7: **(Continued)**

Dressing type	Examples	Uses	Contraindications	Cautions
Hydrogels	Intrasite Conformable (impregnated dressing) ActivHeal Hydrogel (gel) Hydrosorb (hydrogel sheet)	Hydrogels are suited to the management of dry or low exuding wounds. Will usually require a secondary dressing.	Heavily exuding wounds Infected wounds Risk of gas gangrene	Diabetic foot ulcers
Negative pressure wound therapy (NPWT)	KCI Vacuum-Assisted Closure (VAC) Smith & Nephew Renasys Go	NPWT is suitable for acute, hard to heal and traumatic wounds, as an adjunct to surgery, and for salvage procedures such as wound dehiscence.	Malignancy of the wound Untreated osteomyelitis Nonenteric or unexplored fistulas Placement of NPWT on exposed blood vessels, organs or nerves.	People on anticoagulants or platelet aggregation inhibitors People with inadequate tissue coverage over vascular structures Exposed bone or tendon
Non- adherent	Mepitel Urgotulle	Non-adherent dressings are suitable to prevent dressings adhering to the wound bed.	None	May not achieve the aim of a moist wound healing environment
Odour control	Carboflex Clinisorb	Malodorous wounds, including fungating tumours.		

Source: Adapted from Peate and Stephens (2019) Wound care at a glance.

NICE (2020c) reviewed the evidence for post-operative dressings in preventing SSI, concluding that it is generally accepted good clinical practice to cover the wound with an appropriate interactive dressing (a semipermeable film membrane with or without an absorbent island) for a period of 48 h, unless there is excess wound leakage or haemorrhage. Susan's wound dressing could, therefore, have been removed after 48 h and the wound left open, but it is important to understand how Susan feels and to determine whether she would feel more comfortable and less worried with a film dressing left in place. Orthopaedic surgery, such as hip and knee replacements, tends to be complicated by inflammation, fluid collection and blister formation. The increased incidence of wound blistering in individuals with orthopaedic needs may be caused by dressings applied over a joint for a long time causing friction.

Dressings for diabetic foot ulcers must be chosen with particular care as excess moisture and occlusive environments can cause bacteria to multiply quickly, and spread infection. People with diabetes do not display the classic signs of infection, and their circulation can be affected by peripheral arterial disease. Historically, hydrocolloid dressings have been avoided in people with diabetes, favouring antimicrobial products such as iodine and honey. Dumville et al. (2017) has reviewed their use and suggest that the use of an antimicrobial dressing instead of a non-antimicrobial dressing may increase the number of diabetic foot ulcers healed and there is probably little difference between the risk of adverse events between systemic antibiotic and antimicrobial treatments for diabetic foot ulcers.

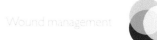

There are constantly new products being developed. This chapter has incorporated available systematic reviews, clinical guidelines and Best Practice Statements, but there are many more in progress; check the Cochrane Library, NICE, Wounds International and Wounds UK for their latest publications.

All individuals need education about their wound care and dressings. Such education has already been discussed a little in relation to Susan and her wound.

Box 13.25 Activity: preparation for discharge home

If you were being discharged home with a dressing in situ, or had had a dressing applied by the community nurse, what sort of things would you want to know?

You would probably want to know some of the following:

- Can I get the dressing wet? If not, how can I manage activities such as washing?
- When should the dressing be redone, and by whom?
- What should I do if the dressing becomes loose, uncomfortable, too tight, falls off or soaks through?
- What should I expect of the wound? For example, when will it heal?
- Will the wound be painful? If so, how can I deal with this?
- How will I know if the wound is becoming infected?
- Are there any special instructions I should follow?

Education should involve relatives and carers as applicable. For Susan, her carers should have educated before her discharge, and explanations given to Susan using appropriate communication methods. This information is also important to people receiving inpatient care to allay anxiety, build confidence and promote self-care. Written information can back up verbal instructions; it is difficult for people to retain a lot of new information, particularly when under stress. Written individual information should be readable, understandable and culturally relevant to be effective in promoting self-care and relieving anxiety (International Consensus 2012).

Leg ulcer bandaging

Compression bandaging should be first-line treatment to optimise treatment for people with venous leg ulcers, chronic venous insufficiency and oedema (Wounds UK 2016). Treatment of venous disease is aimed at correcting, as far as possible, incompetent values. Compression therapy supports the veins and valves to push the venous blood up the leg towards the heart, reducing congestion in the capillaries and veins. At the same time, the extra fluid from the tissue is squeezed back into the veins, reducing oedema. The increased blood velocity ensures that more nutrients reach the tissues to improve the skin condition, reduce dryness and restore elasticity. The compression is applied so that the pressure at the ankle is higher than the pressure at the knee, that is, graduated according to Laplace's law. There are many different types of compression therapy (see Table 13.8).

There are various different treatment options suitable for individuals depending on the clinical scenario, for example, exudate levels, distorted limbs. Table 13.9 is a guide to the different compression options.

The required amount of pressure applied to the limb to achieve therapeutic levels is determined by the person's underlying pathologies and their ability to tolerate the compression as it can be extremely painful (Wounds UK 2016). Before selecting a compression bandage, each person should be individually assessed and their lifestyle considered. Table 13.10 considers compression options based on clinical scenario.

Table 13.8: Types of compression therapy

Compression system	Advantages	Disadvantages
Compression hosiery kits (use first-line if possible)	Does not require training/high level of skill to apply Delivers constant compression levels Encourages self-care Cost-effective Delivers compression to the foot Allows people to wear preferred clothes and footwear	Unsuitable for unusual limbs Not suitable for rapid decreasing limb sizes Does not contain exudate and will require an additional dressing
Compression wraps	Allows for easy adjustment if limb size changes Facilitates self-care Delivers compression to the foot	Application technique can reduce level of compression applied Not practical for highly exuding wounds
Compression bandages	Adaptable to fit unusual-shaped wounds. Suitable for most limb sizes can facilitate most volume reduction and reshaping	Level of compression applied dependent on technique Some bandage systems do not involve compression from the foot upwards. This can lead to pooling oedema in the foot, reduced mobility and delayed wound healing around the malleolus These bandage systems can be bulky, which may limit footwear and clothing

Adapted from Wounds UK (2016) Best Practice Statement Holistic management of Venous Leg Ulceration.a

Table 13.9: Compression options

Elastic bandages	Properties	Inelastic bandages	Properties
Long stretch	Contain elastomeric fibres that are able to stretch over 100% of original strength Generally applied at 50% stretch Low static stiffness index therefore exert a more constant pressure	Short stretch	Contain few of no elastic fibres Commonly applied at 100% stretch Higher static stiffness index generating higher working pressures on movement and lower resting pressures
Multilayer	Function in a similar way to inelastic systems due to the number of layers		

Adapted from Wounds UK (2016) Best Practice Statement Holistic management of Venous Leg Ulceration.

Table 13.10: Compression options depending on clinical scenario

Clinical presentation	Hosiery	Wraps	Bandages
Normal leg shape	√	√	√
Low to moderate exudate	√	√	√
Individual able to self-care	√	√	X
Person has additional support, i.e. relative/carer	√	√	X
Presence of oedema	X	√	√
High levels of exudate	X	X	√
Deep skin folds	X	X	√

Adapted from Wounds UK (2016) Best Practice Statement Holistic management of Venous Leg Ulceration.

There is strong evidence to support the use of hosiery kits as the first compression option except in people who do not meet the criteria. Healing rates for hosiery kits are comparable to compression, can be applied by individuals, relatives and carers and provide a more cost-effective option (Wounds UK 2016).

Compression bandaging should only be applied by a trained practitioner who is deemed competent with the appropriate skill level. The recommended standards are mild (<20 mmHg), moderate (≥20–40 mmHg), strong (≥40–60 mmHg) and very strong (>60 mmHg). The standard for venous leg ulcers is ≥40 mmHg. However, compression should be used only in the absence of significant arterial disease, so as discussed earlier in this chapter, arterial blood supply must first be assessed.

In addition to the previously mentioned guidelines, the most useful documentations on compression are Wounds UK (2016) Holistic Management of Venous Leg Ulceration Treatment and Wounds UK (2019), addressing complexities in the management of venous leg ulcers. Compression therapy needs to be continued after healing, to manage venous insufficiency, without compression, the underlying problem – venous hypertension – will return, and a leg ulcer will form once more (Wounds UK 2016). Therefore, education and involvement are essential.

You should get the opportunity to observe leg ulcer bandaging in practice, possibly at a clinic, or with the district nurse. Try to find out about a local leg ulcer clinic, and arrange a visit.

Learning outcome 4: discuss ways of reducing pain and discomfort associated with wounds

Unfortunately, individuals often associate their wounds with pain; this pain can be based on physical or psychological reasons. Pain in wounds is defined as 'a noxious symptom or unpleasant experience directly related to an open skin ulcer' (World Union of Wound Healing Societies (WUWHS) 2004). Any care relating to wounds can cause fear and distress, whether it is the removal of a surgical drain, a dressing change or removal of skin-closing devices such as staples, clips or sutures. A person with a traumatic wound experienced pain when the injury occurred, so the thought of having a wound dressing could be distressing. Pain assessment and measurement are fundamental in trying to establish the cause of pain and how to manage it effectively. Table 13.11 provides a summary of factors contributing to pain associated with

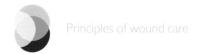

Table 13.11: Causes of wound pain and measures to minimise pain and trauma to the tissues and the surrounding skin

Cause of wound pain	Issues to consider and ways of minimising pain
Wound cleansing and debridement	Gentle irrigation of the wound with warm normal saline or tap water
	Restrict the use of antiseptics to contaminated traumatic wounds
	Plan and organise dressing changes to reduce prolonged exposure to air
	Avoid wiping gauze or cotton across the wound bed
Wound management products: areas to consider	Select the correct dressing for the conditions at the wound bed, related to tissue type and level of exudate present. Does the dressing need to absorb exudate or donate fluid?
	Hydrogels and hydrocolloids will cause maceration to the periwound area if used on heavily exudating wounds, extending tissue damage and increasing pain levels
	Alginates and hydrofibre will adhere to wounds with low exudate, causing pain and trauma upon removal
	Avoid adhesive dressings on people with very fragile skin, an excoriated periwound area or those on long-term steroid treatment
	Some dressings such as honey products can create an osmotic pull on the wound bed, which some people find extremely painful
	Antibacterial dressings containing iodine and silver can cause increased pain
	Refrain from changing the dressing too frequently if not indicated
	Always remove dressings as per the manufacturer's instructions
Treatments	Compression therapy can be extremely painful
	Negative pressure wound therapy (NPWT) can increase pain and can cause tissue trauma upon removal
	Larval therapy can increase pain
Emotional and social aspects	Increased pain may be related to how the person perceives their wound and the effect it has upon their lives, so nurses should empathise and help alleviate their anxieties
	Malodour may contribute to these negative feelings
Disease processes	Identify and treat clinical wound infection as this may cause pain at the wound bed
	Associated diseases may contribute to pain, such as peripheral vascular disease, ischaemia, rheumatoid arthritis, osteoarthritis, diabetic neuropathy, phantom limb pain, oedema, cellulitis, cancer, eczema

Source: Adapted from Hollinworth, H. 2005. The management of patients' pain in wound care. Nursing Standard 20(7): 65–70.

wounds, and possible solutions. Jenkins (2020) examines the principles of wound pain assessment, and Chapter 9 considers assessment and management of pain in detail.

Analgesia before dressing changes may be required. Opiates are necessary if the pain is severe; otherwise, non-steroidal anti-inflammatory drugs or simple analgesics are suitable. Sufficient time should be allowed for them to take effect before removing the dressing and commencing any treatments. Nitrous oxide (Entonox) also can help some people. Other pain reduction strategies include use of relaxation and distraction.

ACTIVITY

Box 13.26 Activity: strategies for wound care

Drawing on the material in this section, identify possible strategies for wound care for Mrs Warner, Colin and Susan. Remember to consider debridement, cleansing, wound dressing choice and pain management.

Table 13.12 presents points that you might have identified.

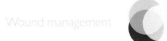

Table 13.12: A possible wound management strategy for Colin, Mrs Warner and Susan

	Colin	Mrs Warner	Susan
Wound type	Dirty surgical wound on buttock	1. Necrotic sacral pressure ulcer 2. Infected diabetic neuropathic ulcer on toe	Clean-contaminated surgical wound on abdomen
Debridement needed?	Surgical debridement performed	1. Yes, identify an appropriate option for this individual (see Box 13.22)	Not required
Cleansing?	Yes, bathing, showering or irrigation with warm saline	1. Could bath or shower, or the wounds could be irrigated with warm saline when the dressings are renewed 2. Consider use of antiseptic for infected toe ulcer (Wounds UK 2011)	Not required Can bath or shower as she wishes
Which dressing?	Pack wound with alginate or hydrofibre and cover with a foam dressing	1. Sacrum: Dress with a hydrogel covered with a hydrocolloid to initiate autolytic debridement. Once the tissue has liquefied, apply larval therapy. 2. Toe: Dress with an antimicrobial dressing with foam as a secondary dressing	Not necessary after first 48 h, but Susan may find it more comfortable or acceptable if her wound is covered with a film dressing until her sutures are removed
Pain management	Assess pain Information giving and explanations Regular analgesics (e.g. non-steroidal anti-inflammatory drugs) The alginate or hydrofibre dressing should be comfortable to wear and painless to remove	Assess pain Information giving and explanations Hydrogel, hydrocolloid and foam dressings are all comfortable to wear and should be painless to remove if the manufacturers' recommendations are followed; regular analgesics if needed (neuropathic ulcers are usually painless)	Assess pain information giving and explanations Regular analgesics may be needed Remove film dressing with care, following manufacturers' recommendations; removal of skin closures will need careful preparation, reassurance and support

 Box 13.27 Children and young people: practice points – wound dressing application

Children can find the process of a wound dressing distressing; fear and pain are potential problems. Hospital play specialists have knowledge and skills to support children during such clinical procedures.

The type of dressing used should be carefully chosen, to minimise pain on removal; dressings with silicone adhesive facilitate a non-traumatic removal. Probst (2020) provides detailed chapters on wound care in babies, young children, teenagers and young adults. For further information and guidance, see:

Probst, S. 2020. *Wound Care Management. A Person-centered Approach*, 3rd edn. London: Elsevier, Section 2, Chapters 4–6, pp. 61–104.

Summary

● Wound assessment must precede effective wound management, which requires the application of suitable cleansing methods, the most appropriate dressing to cover the wound and pain-relieving strategies.

● Application of these skills in the care of each individual is the product of knowledge and experience.

CHAPTER SUMMARY

This chapter has aimed to introduce an understanding of how wounds heal, with an emphasis on the systemic nature of wound healing, and the range of factors that may impair wound healing. An awareness of how wounds can be assessed and managed, taking into account their underlying causes, has also been promoted. The chapter emphasised an individualistic and holistic approach to wound care and discussed different options available for managing wounds.

You have been encouraged to take the opportunity to apply knowledge to practice and to start to gain experience in observing wounds and identifying their stage of healing. Involving the person and their families, working with the MDT, accessing expert knowledge and being aware of the need to continually update have all been addressed. This chapter did not attempt to include specialist knowledge – further in-depth reading in relation to individual topics such as leg ulcers, PUs and burns should be undertaken where applicable.

To conclude, an understanding of wound care is important for all nurses and nursing associates. This chapter has introduced key principles to act as a foundation for future learning.

REFERENCES

Atkin, L., Bucko. Z., Conde Montero, E. et al. 2019 Implementing TIMERS: The Race against Hard-to- heal Wounds. *Journal of Wound Care* 28(suppl 3a): 1–49.

Berman, B., Maderal, A. and Rapheal, B. 2017. Keloids and hypertrophic scars: Pathophysiology, classification, and treatment. *Dermatologic Surgery* 43(suppl 1): 3–18.

Bilous, R. and Donnelly, R. 2010. *Handbook of Diabetes.* Oxford: Wiley-Blackwell.

Coleman, S., Nelson, A., Vowden, P. et al. 2017. Development of a generic wound care assessment minimum data set. *Journal of Tissue Viability* 26(4): 226–40.

Cowan, T., ed. 2012. *Wound Care Handbook 2012–2013*, 5th edn. London: Mark Allen Healthcare.

Dumville, J., Lipsky, B., Hoey, C. et al. (2017) Topical antimicrobial agents for treating foot ulcers in people with diabetes. *Cochrane Systematic Review.* Available from: https://doi.org/10.1002/14651858.CD011038.pub2 (Accessed on 5 May 2021).

Escandon, J., Vivas, A.C., Tang, J. et al. 2011. High mortality with patients with chronic wounds. *Wound Repair and Regeneration* 19(4): 526–8.

European Pressure Ulcer Advisory Panel and National Pressure Ulcer Advisory Panel (EPUAP and NPUAP). 2009. *Treatment of Pressure Ulcers: Quick Reference Guide.* Washington, DC: NPUAP.

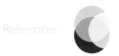

Evans, R.C. and Jones, N.L. 1996. The management of abrasions and bruises. *Journal of Wound Care* 5: 465–8.

Fernandez, R., Griffiths, R. and Ussia, C. 2010. Water for wound cleansing. *Cochrane Database of Systematic Reviews* 2. Art. No.: CD003861. doi: 10.1002/14651858.CD003861. pub3

Gouvela, J.C. and Miguens, C. 2007. Is it safe to use saline solution to clean wounds. *EWMA Journal* 7(2): 7–12.

Gray, D., Acton, C., Chadwick, P. et al. 2011. Consensus guidance for the use of debridement techniques in the UK. *Wounds UK* 7(1): 77–84.

Gray, D., White, R., Cooper, P. et al. 2004. The wound healing continuum, an aid to clinical decision making and clinical audit. *Applied Wound Management Supplement. Wounds UK* 1(1): 9–12.

Gray, D., White, R., Cooper, P. et al. 2009. An introduction to applied wound management and its use in the assessment of wounds. *Wounds UK* 5(4): 4–9.

Grothier, L. and Cooper, R. 2011. Medihoney dressings made easy – products for practice. Wounds *UK* 6(2). Available from: http://www.wounds-uk.com (Accessed on 19 January 2013).

Guest, J., Ayoub, N., McIlwraith. T. et al. 2015. The health economic burden that wounds impose on the National Health Service in the UK. *British Medical Journal Open* 5(12). Available from: https://bmjopen.bmj.com/content/5/12/e009283 (Accessed on 19 May 2021)

Guest, J.F., Fuller, G.W. and Vowden, P. 2018. Diabetic foot ulcer management in clinical practice in the UK: Costs and outcomes. *International Wound Journal* 15(1): 43–52.

Henderson, V., Timmons, J., Hurd, T. et al. 2012. NWPT in everyday practice made easy. *Wounds International* 1(5). Available from: http://www.woundsinternational.com (Accessed on 19 May 2021).

Hess, C.T. 2011. Checklist for factors affecting wound healing. *Advances in Skin and Wound Care* 24(4): 192.

Hollinworth, H. 2005. The management of patients' pain in wound care. *Nursing Standard* 20(7): 670.

International Consensus. 2012. Optimising wellbeing in people living with a wound. *Wounds International.* Available from: http://www.woundsinternational.com (Accessed on 19 May 2021).

Jenkins, S. 2020. The Assessment of Pain in Acute Wounds (Part 1). *Wounds UK* 16(1): 26–33.

Johnston, E. 2007. The Role of Nutrition in Tissue Viability. *Wound Essentials* 2: 10–21.

Lazarus, G.S., Cooper, D.M., Knighton, D.R. et al. 1994. Definitions and guidelines for assessment of wounds and evaluation of healing. *Archives of Dermatology* 130: 489–93.

Manna, B., Nahirniak, P., and Morrison, C. 2020. *Wound Debridement.* Ncbi.nlm.nih.gov. Available from: https://www.ncbi.nlm.nih.gov/books/NBK507882/ (Accessed on 13 November 2020).

McCluskey, P. and McCarthy, G. 2012. Nurses' knowledge and competence in wound management. *Wounds UK* 8(2): 37–47.

Mitchell, A. 2018. Adult pressure area care: Preventing pressure ulcers. *British Journal of Nursing* 27(18).

Mitchell, A. 2020. Wound assessment: Acute and chronic wounds. To be published December 2020.

Mitchell, A. and Elbourne, S. 2019. Lower limb assessment. *British Journal of Nursing* 29(1): 18–21.

Mitchell, A. and Hill, B. 2020. Moisture- associated skin damage: An overview of its diagnosis and treatment. *British Journal of Community Nursing* 25(3): 12–18.

Mitchell, A. and Liumigusin, D. 2020. Assessment and Management of Hypergranulation Accepted for publication BJN.

Mitchell, T. 2018. Use of Manuka honey for autolytic debridement in necrotic and sloughy wounds. *Journal of Community Nursing* 32(4): 1–5.

National Health Service. 2019. *The Atlas of Shared Learning: React to Red; Reducing Pressure Ulcers in Care Home Settings.* Available from: https://www.england.nhs.uk/atlas_case_study/react-to-red-reducing-pressure-ulcers-in-care-home-settings/ (Accessed 3 November 2021).

National Institute for Health and Clinical Excellence (NICE). 2014. *Pressure Ulcers: Prevention and Management, Clinical Guideline [CG179].* London: NICE.

National Institute for Health and Clinical Excellence (NICE). 2019a. *Surgical Site Infection: Prevention and Treatment of Surgical Site Infection.* Clinical Guidelines 74. London: NICE.

National Institute for Health and Clinical Excellence (NICE). 2019b. *Caesarian Section Guidelines.* London: NICE.

National Institute for Health and Clinical Excellence (NICE). 2019c. *Type II Diabetes in Adult Management.* London: NICE.

National Institute for Health and Clinical Excellence (NICE). 2020a. *Leg Ulcer – Venous.* London: NICE.

National Institute for Health and Clinical Excellence (NICE). 2020b. *Pressure Ulcers: Prevention and Management.* London: NICE

National Institute for Health and Clinical Excellence (NICE). 2020c. *Preventing and Treating Surgical Site Infections.* London: NICE.

Nursing and Midwifery Council. 2018a. Standards of proficiency for registered nurses. Available from: https://www.nmc.org.uk/standards/standards-for-nurses/standards-of-proficiency-for registered-nurses/ (Accessed on 13 November 2020).

Nursing and Midwifery Council. 2018b. Standards of proficiency for nursing associates. Available from: https://www.nmc.org.uk/standards/standards-for-nursing-associates/standards-of-proficiency-for-nursing-associates/ (Accessed on 13 November 2020).

O'Brien, M., Lawton, J.F., Conn, C.R. et al. 2011. Best practice wound care. *International Wound Journal* 8(2): 145–54.

Ousey, K. and Cook, L. 2012. Wound assessment: Made easy. *Wounds UK* 8 (2). ISSN 1746-6814: 1:4.

Peate, I. and Stephens, M. 2019. *Wound Care At A Glance.* 2nd ed. Wiley-Blackwell. Chichester.

Probst, S. 2020. *Wound Care Nursing E-Book: A Person-Centered Approach*, 3rd edn. Online: Elsevier.

Rabey, N., Goldie, S. and Price, R. 2017. 5-Fluorouracil for keloid scars. *Cochrane Database of Systematic Reviews.*

Siddiqui, A.R. and Bernstein, J.M. 2010. Chronic wound infection: Facts and controversies. *Clinics in Dermatology* 28: 519–26.

Smaill, F.M. and Gyte, G.M.L. 2010. Antibiotic prophylaxis versus no prophylaxis for preventing infection after cesarean section. *Cochrane Database Systematic Reviews* 1. Art. No: CD007482. doi:10.1002/14651858.CD007482.pub2.

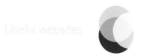

Swanson, T., Grothier, L. and Schultz, G. 2015. Chair International Wound Infection Institute, Nurse Practitioner Wound Management, South West Healthcare, Warrnambool, Australia; 2. Consultant Nurse Tissue Viability/Service Manager, Tissue Viability Centre, Provide CIC, St Peter's Hospital, Maldon, UK 3. Professor, Department of Obstetrics and Gynecology, Institute for Wound Research, University of Florida, Gainesville, USA Wound infection made easy.

Vowden, P. 2011. Hard-to-heal wounds made easy. *Wounds International* 2(4). Available from: http://www.woundsinternational.com

Weir, D. and Swanson, T. (2019) Ten top tips for wound cleansing. *Wounds International* 10(4): 8–11.

Wild, T., Rahbarnia, A., Kellner, M., Sobotka, L. and Eberlein, T. 2010. Basics in nutrition and wound healing. *Nutrition* 26(9): 862–6.

World Union of Wound Healing Societies (WUWHS). 2007. *Wound Exudate and the Role of Dressings. A Consensus Document.* London: MEP. Available from: http://www.woundsinternational.com (Accessed on 13 November 2020).

World Union of Wound Healing Societies. 2004. Principles of Best Practice: Minimising Pain at Wound Dressing-Related Procedures. A Consensus Document. Available from: https://www.woundsinternational.com/resources/details/minimising-pain-wound-dressing-related-procedures-wuwhs-consensus-document (accessed on 15 October 2020).

Wounds UK. 2013. Best Practice Statement. Effective exudate management. Available from: www.wounds-uk.com (Accessed on 13 November 2020).

Wounds UK. 2016. Best Practice Statement: Holistic management of venous leg ulceration. Available from: www.wounds-uk.com (Accessed 13 November 2020).

Wounds UK. 2018 Best Practice Statement: Improving holistic assessment of chronic wounds. Available from: www.wounds-uk.com (Accessed on 13 November 2020).

Wounds UK. 2019. Best Practice Statement: Ankle brachial pressure index (ABPI) in practice. Available from: www.wounds-uk.com (Accessed 13 November 2020).

Wounds UK. 2020a. Best practice statement: Post-operative wound care – reducing the risk of surgical site infection. Available from: www.wounds-uk.com (Accessed on 13 November 2020).

Wounds UK. 2020b. Update CQUIN 2020–2021. Available from: https://www.wounds-uk.com/news/details/update-cquin-202021-news (Accessed on 13 November 2020).

USEFUL WEBSITES

European Pressure Ulcer Advisory Panel: www.epuap.org
European Wound Management Association: www.ewma.org
World Wide Wounds: www.worldwidewounds.com
Wounds International: www.woundsinternational.com
Wounds Research: www.woundsresearch.com
Wounds UK: www.wounds-uk.com

Assessing and responding to sudden deterioration in the adult

Sue Maddex

The ability to recognise, monitor, interpret and respond to changes in a person's health status are core nursing skills. The Nursing and Midwifery Council Future Nurse Standards of Proficiency for Registered Nurses (2018a) and Standards of Proficiency for Nursing Associates (2018b) highlight many clinical skills that are required of the practitioner in this instance. These skills are addressed in this chapter.

Historically, several publications of National Institute for Health and Care Excellence (NICE 2007), the National Patient Safety Agency (NPSA 2011) and the National Confidential Enquiry into Patient Outcome and Death (NCEPOD 2012) highlight that practitioners require training, education and direction while acquiring these assessment skills. Practitioners need to be able to review and address care deficits and improve the care of people who are deteriorating to ensure that the best outcome for the individual is achieved. In 2007, NICE developed a guideline recommending that healthcare professionals should monitor individuals to identify those whose health may deteriorate suddenly. NICE's (2007) aim was to assist practitioners in recognising how to respond to the risk factors seen in people when they are deteriorating. These risk factors include changes in vital signs, individual assessment and escalation procedures. The NPSA (2011) identified that some improvements had been developed in recognising and responding to a person who was deteriorating but acknowledged that many challenges remained. NCEPOD (2012) provided a detailed review of the situation, finding a succession of system and performance failures that compromised individual safety and well-being throughout the care pathway. The report revealed that systems sometimes leave junior staff to assess and that early warning systems sometimes failed to track the deterioration of vital signs effectively and trigger an emergency response. Clearly, some improvements have been made to assist practitioners in their assessment and management of a person who is deteriorating. Many trusts have embarked on developing training for their staff to develop their skills and have linked with higher educational institutes who have further developed education courses in critical care and deterioration care management. Together they continue to strive to achieve programmes of study that are robust and address the deficits of managing a person whose condition is

DOI: 10.4324/9781003020660-14

deteriorating. Nationally, the development of the National Early Warning Scores (NEWS1) by the Royal College of Physicians (RCP 2012) aimed to promote a tool that could be used to assess a person's vital signs parameters and escalate individuals who were deteriorating. Latterly, the NEWS2 was further developed by the Royal College of Physicians in 2017 and 2020. The scoring tool incorporates the use of physiological and neurological parameters that are used to score a person's health or deterioration (see Chapter 4 for more details of using this scoring system tool). The development of this national tool has been a major step forward in enabling practitioners to use a common language and scoring system when communicating their concerns about potential deterioration. Previously, tools were developed locally and not necessarily transferrable between wards and departments. Some further issues existed with the community setting not using escalation tools that were congruent with hospital settings and vice versa. The NEWS2 tool is now incorporated in many electronic online systems both in the community and hospital setting. This tool can be used to track deterioration and encourage the healthcare practitioner to report observed changes and is a trigger system for escalation. In the recent COVID-19 pandemic, the NEWS2 scoring system has enabled practitioners to recognise and respond to individuals at risk of deterioration and ensure a timely response was initiated (RCP 2020). NICE (2020a) suggests improvements are still on going from their original review in 2007 (CG 50). They support the use of NEWS2 in addressing, recognising and responding to a person who is deteriorating. Other recommendations include increasing the level of monitoring of individuals regarding their vital signs review and the recording and interpretation of data obtained by these systems. Consideration should also be given to reviewing the use of paper charts versus electronic systems incorporating NEWS2 scoring to evaluate which system provides a satisfactory clinical response for the person. The use of pre-hospital NEWS2 scoring systems and strategies for their escalation and use are also areas that are currently under review. Once a NEWS2 score has been obtained, the importance of the response time to an individual who is unwell and deteriorating is still a matter of concern. The need for a graded response to deterioration was addressed by the Royal College of Physicians (2017) who, adding to their original work of NEWS scoring added an escalation tool. They also offered further guidance on communication and escalation processes recommending that escalation tools were incorporated in vital signs monitoring and are used for the subsequent handover of the individual. This has added structure to escalating the deterioration of an individual to relevant parties. Subsequently, the use of NEWS2 and escalation tools has assisted in ensuring the timely transfer of an individual to the appropriate care facility. NICE, Medtech Innovation Briefing 205 (Available from: https://www.nice.org.uk/advice/mib205/chapter/The-technology), regarding NEWS2 systems, details current systems that are used and brings together current thinking about NEWS2 and electronic systems used for escalation. It highlights how technology can assist in vital signs reporting and how physiological parameter measurements have the potential to be recorded more frequently and reviewed more often using such systems. The use of NEWS2 scoring and its associated technological devices is an ever-changing area of practice. Training, education and research continue in these areas to develop more strategies to care for the individual who is deteriorating. Hence, the importance of this chapter's topic to explore these issues and continue the conversation.

This chapter addresses the immediate recognition, response and care of an adult person when their condition is deteriorating. The chapter explores skills relevant to managing airway obstruction, breathlessness, circulatory problems and disability assessment and unconsciousness. Some relevant skills are discussed in the other chapters of this book, so you can refer to them as appropriate. Chapter 4 includes monitoring vital signs (temperature, pulse, respiration, oxygen saturation and blood pressure) and neurological assessment including ACVPU and the GCS.

This chapter includes the following topics:

- Recognising and responding to people who are deteriorating: an overview
- Airway management problems and related skills
- Breathing problems and related skills
- Circulatory problems and related skills
- Disability and unconsciousness and related skills
- Exposure and review of the person.

Box 14.1 Principles of biology

At the beginning of Chapter 4, there were questions related to biology underpinning the measurement of vital signs. Check those again to ensure that you understand the principles. The following questions will help you to focus on the biology underpinning this chapter's skills. Use your recommended textbook to find out:

- What is homeostasis?
- Why is glucose important to the body?
- What is the role of insulin in the body?

Airways and breathing

- What are the structures of airways?
- How is oxygen transported in the body?
- What role do cilia play?
- How does the respiratory system respond to respiratory tract infection?
- What other situations could cause respiratory distress or dysfunction?
- Where is bronchial smooth muscle located?
- What is the consequence of bronchoconstriction?
- Where are the pleural membranes? What functions do they have?
- What is surfactant? How does it prevent lung collapse?
- How can lung function be assessed? What factors could affect lung function?
- What do you understand by the term acid–base balance?

(Continued)

Box 14.1 (Continued)

Circulation

- How is blood pressure controlled within the body, and how might this be affected if a person is in shock?
- What are baroreceptors and where are they found in the body?
- What is the basic structure of the heart? Name its layers.
- What is the electroconduction system of the heart?
- What is the function of the sino-atrial node?

Nervous system

- What is the role of the medulla oblongata in the body?
- Describe the structure of the brain.

PRACTICE SCENARIOS

The following scenarios illustrate situations where sudden deterioration in a person's condition might occur in different settings. These scenarios will be referred back to throughout the chapter.

Adult community setting: airway obstruction

Mrs Mary Wyatt, aged 89 years, is resident in a care home. She has a history of Parkinson's disease and sometimes has difficulty eating. Today, during lunch, she started to choke on a piece of meat. Staff initially encouraged her to cough but Mary was becoming tired and her colour was deteriorating. The staff attempted first aid which included back blows in an attempt to clear her airway obstruction, which was not successful, and they called an emergency ambulance. The ambulance crew have used suction and administered oxygen therapy. Mary has now arrived in the emergency department, where a team of staff are awaiting.

Mental health setting: breathing problem

Tina Lunn is 58 years old and has a long history of mental illness. She has been admitted to an acute mental health unit owing to her deteriorating mental state. She is known to have asthma, has becotide (a corticosteroid) and salbutamol (a bronchodilator) inhalers and takes oral prednisolone (also a corticosteroid). The staff are encouraging her to manage her asthma, to monitor her peak flow and take her inhalers as prescribed. However, one morning after a restless night, her respiration is so laboured that she has difficulty completing sentences and she is very distressed and wheezy. Her peak flow is about half her normal measurement. A salbutamol nebuliser (prescribed on an as-required basis) is administered via oxygen with some effect. The doctor diagnoses a chest infection and asks for a sputum specimen to be collected.

Adult hospital setting: circulatory problem

Sira Patel, a 67-year-old woman, has just returned from the operating theatre after undergoing a left total hip replacement. She is known to have atrial fibrillation, which is managed with 62.5 micrograms of digoxin daily. The anaesthetist has requested that she has cardiac monitoring for the first 24 h postoperatively and will have a 12-lead electrocardiogram (ECG) performed the following morning. She has PCA in progress, and oxygen is being delivered at 5 l/min via a face mask. She also has an intravenous infusion in progress. While conducting her postoperative observations, you find that her blood pressure has decreased, her heart rate is increasing and is irregular and her respiratory rate is also rising. Furthermore, she has excessive drainage from her wound.

Learning disability setting: impaired conscious level

Enid Campbell is a 52-year-old woman with a severe learning disability and very limited verbal communication. She lives in a group home. She is overweight and was diagnosed with type 2 diabetes 6 years ago. It was initially treated with oral hypoglycaemic agents; however, owing to her blood glucose level being persistently high, she was started on insulin injections, which are administered by her carer. This morning the community nurse for learning disability is visiting to advise on her hydration and nutrition. When the nurse arrived, Enid's carers reported that a short while ago, Enid slumped forward in her wheelchair and seemed unable to hold herself up. Some twitching of her right arm and leg was noticed. Enid has no history of epilepsy. When a staff member spoke to her, she was initially unable to respond but is now responsive though 'not her usual self'. The carer checked her blood glucose and it was within Enid's usual range. Her general practitioner (GP) has been contacted and is on her way to Enid's home.

EQUIPMENT REQUIRED FOR THIS CHAPTER

Find out what equipment is available within your skills laboratory or your practice area for monitoring acutely ill individuals. In particular, look for:

* Resuscitation Council (UK 2021a, 2021b) guidelines (available on www.resus.org.uk or via app on a smartphone/tablet application);
* Cardiac monitoring equipment three-lead or five-lead;
* Twelve-lead ECG machine;
* National Early Warning Score (NEWS2) chart or electronic device able to record and escalate vital signs;
* Peak flow meter;
* Blood glucose monitoring equipment.

RECOGNISING AND RESPONDING TO PEOPLE WHO ARE DETERIORATING: AN OVERVIEW

The NCEPOD's (2012) *Time to intervene* report found that survival to discharge after in-hospital cardiac arrest was 14.6%. In addition, hospital cardiac arrest is common, and sadly, it is associated with a high mortality rate (Andersen et al. 2019). Respiratory or cardiac arrest is often proceeded by a period of slow physical and progressive physiological derangement that may be poorly recognised and treated (Resuscitation Council 2021b). This deterioration is usually preceded by changes in the physiological parameters that represent failing respiratory, cardiovascular and neurological systems, for example, increased respiratory rate, increased heart rate and evidence of new confusion or reduced levels of consciousness. Recognition of these changes and early intervention in dealing with these changes appropriately can help prevent further decline or even death. Traditionally, the identification of critically ill and deteriorating individuals relied on clinical intuition (Benner 2001; Melin-Johansson et al. 2017). Although a controversial subject area, nurses value their intuition in a variety of clinical settings and report it is more than simply a gut feeling (Melin-Johansson et al. 2017). However, articulating what nurses see in their everyday practices and validating intuitive grasps can often be challenging. The introduction of physiological 'track-and-trigger' systems such as the NEWS2 has enabled staff to identify those at risk and assist in the early detection of critical illness to support practitioners in making decisions regarding the person's care. The total reliance upon NEWS scoring alone should be avoided and in the decision-making process, it should be used alongside other clinical indicators such as appearance of the individual, co-existing medical conditions, altered physiology and previous medical history. Familiarity with these assessment skills will enable you to develop confidence in your decision-making strategies. As healthcare practitioners, you will be responsible for caring for people who become acutely ill, so learning about the use of track-and-trigger assessment NEWS2 tools is essential.

Note: The assessment and management of individuals who are critically ill have been constantly under review so you must keep abreast of new documents and guidelines that may influence your practice.

Decisions about resuscitation

The cessation of breathing and heartbeat in a person is a natural process of dying (Resuscitation Council 2021b). For a person who experiences sudden cardiac or respiratory arrest, cardiopulmonary resuscitation (CPR) can be effective in improving the chances of recovery for the person who is deteriorating. In some situations, however, due to gradual deterioration, CPR cannot be effective and may be detrimental to the individual's wishes or failing health condition. People who, due to their condition, will not benefit from resuscitation attempts may have a 'Do not attempt resuscitation' (DNAR) request signed. The British Medical Association, Resuscitation Council and Royal College of Nursing offer practitioner guidelines relating to how these decisions are made and by whom. Decision frameworks and consideration of healthcare team views should be used to assist in planning the best outcome. These decisions, however, are complex and require a great deal of knowledge and skills to ensure the optimum outcome for the person is achieved. Senior clinicians should be involved in these processes and assist and guide junior healthcare practitioners to develop their own decision-making skills. The individual's best interests should be paramount in any decision-making process regarding CPR and DNAR.

Recommended Summary Plan for Emergency Care and Treatment (ReSPECT) pathway

To assist individuals and healthcare professionals to have difficult conversations regarding cessation of treatment and end-of-life care, a ReSPECT pathway (2020) has been developed and amended recently. This pathway enables individual wishes and preferences to be documented. It supports practitioners to explore and review the desired care and treatment for a person. Where no explicit decision has been made in advance, there should be an initial presumption in favour of resuscitation; see: https://www.resus.org.uk/respect for further guidance. Please also review your local trust/clinical area protocol for current recommendations for performing CPR and ReSPECT pathway advice (2020). All care establishments that face decisions about attempting CPR should have a policy about CPR decisions (Resuscitation Council 2021b). It is important to familiarise yourself with these procedures and seek senior advice regarding deployment of such pathways.

Soft signs of individual deterioration in the decision-making process

Recognising that a person does not appear to be their normal self is something that is a key skill of many healthcare professionals. Carers are in a unique position to be close to a person both physically and psychologically at often difficult times for a person. Staff caring for an individual over a period of time often see or feel that something is not quite right but find it difficult to articulate their feelings of 'all is not well.' Intuition is said to play a part in any health care professional's role and can provide important information in the detection of deterioration of the individual's health (Romero-Brufau et al. 2019). It is often reported by staff to explain a reason for a telephone call or an escalation of concern and documented in the person's notes prior to their physical deterioration. This is referred to as intuition. Benner et al.'s (2009) model of skills acquisition purports that intuition is a way of knowing and that nurses develop these skills as they progress from novices to become expert practitioners. Douw et al. (2015) explain how a practitioner's intuition develops over a period of time within their role. In essence, less experienced practitioners may not see the same deterioration signs as those that experienced practitioners begin to see. Indications of worry or concerns by significant others and carers plays an important part in recognising deterioration of an individual. An ability to see what is happening and responding to these signs is crucial to ensure an individual is cared for rapidly and effectively. While physiological parameters of NEWS2 changes can be charted and responded to, early deterioration signs should also be noted and charted in similar ways. The soft signs of deterioration are often missed until extensive physiological changes are seen and should be escalated in the same way as physiological parameters. You need to ensure that you report these feelings and findings to seniors so that a review of your suspicions can occur and never be afraid to say you feel something is not quite right with someone in your care. It is important also to acknowledge that paid and unpaid carers may also feel intuitively that something may be of concern and these need to be listened to.

Douw et al. (2015) in their systematic review identify 170 signs and symptoms of deterioration, which include some soft signs of deterioration. They categorise these into 10 general indicators. These are:

1. Changes in respiration – with an inability to speak, the presence of noisy breathing or altered respiratory noises.
2. Changes in circulation – impaired peripheral perfusion, cold extremities, tachycardia, pale and clammy features.
3. Temperature changes – evidence of rigors, hypo or hyperthermia.
4. Unexpected trajectory – not progressing as care staff feel they should i.e. expected recovery time from events does not follow normal pattern of events.
5. Individuals themselves indicating they feel unwell or not quite right.
6. Subjective nurse observation and nurses who remain convinced that something is wrong without a rationale.
7. Nurses feeling something is wrong without a rationale – intuitive grasp that all is not well as seen by the nurse.
8. Changes in mental state – new confusion outside of those of dementia, verbal impairment, vague, slow speech and reactions.
9. Agitation – reduced mobility, restlessness, reluctance to get out of bed.
10. Pain – new and increasing pain in the absence of new injury and trauma.

Being able to recognise and respond to these soft signs of deterioration can significantly reduce hospital admissions for many. Consideration of these soft signs of deterioration along with vital signs monitoring using NEWS2 can significantly improve the outcome or enable appropriate end-of-life care provision.

Box 14.2 Learning outcomes

By the end of this section, you will be able to:

1. explain the components of a NEWS chart or e-observation system, understand how scores are calculated and decide the action to be taken
2. discuss how to use a communication tool in the acute/emergency setting
3. appreciate the key aspects of an ABCDE approach for assessing and managing an acutely unwell person
4. locate and recognise emergency equipment.

Learning outcome 1: explain the components of a NEWS2 chart or e-observation system, understand how scores are calculated and decide the action to be taken

While this is addressed in detail in Chapter 4, a quick overview is offered here. NEWS2 is an evaluation tool based on six physiological parameters: respiratory rate, SpO_2, pulse rate, blood pressure, temperature and ACVPU score (RCP 2017). The NEWS2 allocates points to measurements outside the 'normal' parameters, alerting staff to the individual's deteriorating condition. These tools are used in primary care, for ambulance service assessments and in hospital (RCP 2017). They can be used for anywhere there are concerns about their health, such as post operatively, following severe trauma or if there is a serious acute medical condition.

The use of physiological track-and-trigger systems is effective in reducing mortality and morbidity of those who are acutely ill as well as preventing admissions to the intensive therapy unit (ITU). The National Institute for Health and Clinical Excellence (NICE 2007, 2011, 2016a; NHS Choices 2015) recommends their use to monitor all adults in acute hospital settings and if detected early enough, simple interventions such as fluid or oxygen administration can help prevent further deterioration. Knowing when to intervene is, however, a skill that requires practice to anticipate and judge what is required and when. Developing this kind of skilled know-how and intuitive grasp of a situation can be imperative to improve outcomes. Benner (2001), Odell et al. (2009) and Turan et al. (2019) highlighted how intuition is used in becoming a competent practitioner. Clinical decision-making is part of this process in which intuition contributes and adds to the depth of nurses' ability to detect deterioration in an individual. Healthcare professionals having an idea that something is wrong or about to happen and a feeling that guides an individual to make choices about their actions can assist decision-making processes. Pretz and Folse (2011) explain how intuition can be part of this process. The NEWS2 score is sometimes used to validate this intuition by confirming that all vital signs parameters are not within normal limits. The use of the NEWS2 can help early detection and management, but this is a tool to assist decision-making by the senior care team. As with any tool in clinical practice, the value and constraints of the NEWS2 should be appraised.

NOTE when using NEWS2 with individuals who are diagnosed with COVID-19, any increase in oxygen requirements should trigger an escalation even if there is no significant increase in the NEWS2 score (RCP 2020).

Box 14.3 Activity: NEWS2 (National Early Warning Score)

Within your clinical area, find out what NEWS2 chart/electronic device is used and identify what protocol should be followed to ensure that the appropriate staff are called to assist. Try calculating the NEWS2 for individuals who are not acutely unwell and observe the differences that the scores reveal.

Use this link to find the NEWS2 chart for reference: https://www.rcplondon.ac.uk/projects/outputs/national-early-warning-score-news-2

Although the level of response is dependent on the facilities available, the RCP (2017) outlines the following actions when using the NEWS2:

- A **low score** (score of 1–4) should prompt assessment by a competent registered nurse who should decide whether to change the frequency of clinical monitoring or initiate an escalation of clinical care.
- A **medium score** (score of 5–6) should prompt an urgent review by a clinician competent in the assessment of acute illness – usually a ward-based doctor or acute team nurse, who should consider whether escalation of care to a team with critical care skills is required (i.e., critical care outreach team).
- A **high score** (score of 7 or more) should prompt emergency assessment by a clinical team/critical care outreach team with critical care competencies and usually transfer of the individual to a higher dependency care area.

The RCP (2017) advises that the NEWS2 tool should NOT be used in children under the age of 16, or women who are pregnant, because the physiological response to acute illness can be modified in children and by pregnancy. However, modified tools may be used; see 'Practice points' boxes at the end of this section.

Using technology to assist you with assessment

Increasingly, healthcare practitioners can use technology to assist them in assessing acutely ill or individuals who may be deteriorating. Smartphone applications, web devices and handheld bedside computers, and for example, e-observations, are available to assist in recording and analysing data from observations. Ensure that you discuss these applications and devices within the clinical area and use only accredited and trusted sources for these purposes. Many systems that are designed specifically for practice areas work well with trust protocols to enable informed decisions to be made about individual care. These also incorporate NEWS2 systems to prompt all healthcare professionals involved in care to respond appropriately in a timely manner. There can however be no replacement for observing and assessing individuals visually yourself and learning key skills that alert you to signs of a person's deterioration. You will use and develop these skills further throughout your career.

Box 14.4 Activity: identifying electronic devices used to record data

In your practice area, identify which electronic devices are used to record an individual's data and ensure that you receive adequate training to use them.

ACTIVITY

Learning outcome 2: discuss how to use a communication tool in the acute/emergency setting

Gaining assistance early is essential to help manage a clinical emergency. Effective communication is the cornerstone of good healthcare but is difficult to master (Pritchard 2010).

Ineffective or poor communication can hinder the escalation process resulting in an untimely response to a person who is deteriorating. The Royal College of Nursing (RCN 2019) and NHS Improvements (2020) recommend the use of communication tools, for example, SBARD. These tools aim to help improve communication amongst health care professionals and ultimately improve outcomes. They facilitate handovers and escalation when referring the person on to other members of the healthcare team.

Box 14.5 Activity: communication tools available

When you are next in clinical practice, find out what communication tools are being used as there are a variety of tools available.

ACTIVITY

An example of a communication tool is SBARD (Situation–Background–Assessment–Recommendation, Decision). A communication tool helps practitioners escalate concerns, focus on conversations in often difficult circumstances and convey a message to summon help quickly. Box 14.7 displays the SBARD tool with examples of information for each component. National Health Service Trusts have developed their own versions of the tool, but the principles of using this communication tool remain.

Box 14.6 Activity: Mrs Patel's scenario

Reread Mrs Patel's scenario, presented at the start of this chapter, and identify the vital signs you will assess to complete her NEWS2. Then consider how a healthcare worker might use SBARD (Box 14.7) when contacting the doctor to seek help with Mrs Patel.

ACTIVITY

The **situation** you would want to report would be Mrs Patel's NEWS2 score with any potential areas of concerns. For example, a respiratory rate of 30. You would also note her excessive wound drainage. In explaining the **background**, you would include her recent surgery and current treatment (e.g. oxygen, PCA, cardiac monitoring), her history of atrial fibrillation and its treatment. Your **assessment** might include your concern that she is developing shock due to excessive bleeding. Your **recommendation** is likely to be that you request an immediate visit.

Decision, in this section would consist of you documenting any conversations that have taken place regarding Mrs Patel's care and amending her care plan accordingly.

Ensure that you understand these tools so that you can use them to assist you in everyday situations when asking for help. Using them regularly in everyday situations can assist in refining these key skills. This will help if you need to use them effectively in an emergency situation.

Box 14.7 The SBAR (D) communication tool

Situation – explain the reason for calling: your location, the reason you are calling about and their diagnosis, the issue of concern, for example, NEWS2, pain, wound drainage, urine output.

Background – supporting background information – further information: reason for admission and treatment, mental status, skin (e.g. pale, clammy), oxygen therapy.

Assessment – state what your assessment is, for example, 'I think the problem is …' or state that you do not know what the problem is but the person is deteriorating.

Recommendation – state your recommendation for intervention, treatment, for example, 'I would like you to see her now'. Clarify whether any further tests should be carried out or treatment changed.

Decision – what decision has been agreed? Note any conversations that have taken place and document in the care plan. Available from: https://www.england. nhs.uk/wp-content/uploads/2021/03/qsir-sbar-communication-tool.pdf.

Learning outcome 3: appreciate the key aspects of an ABCDE approach to assessing and managing an acutely unwell person

When a person is acutely ill or at risk of deterioration, it is vitally important that they have an initial assessment and are frequently reassessed to evaluate interventions used and to ensure there is no further deterioration. Immediate assessment involves the ABCDE approach:

Catastrophic haemorrhage

Catastrophic haemorrhage is characterised by major bleeding involving limbs or pulsatile arterial bleeding. It is seen as a leading cause of morbidity and mortality in trauma cases in both military and civilian settings (Winstanley et al. 2019). When caring for a person who has deteriorated, the initial assessment should include a review of any evidence of catastrophic bleeding. Initial assessment should be conducted to ascertain the extent of injury and/or insult to body, leading to haemorrhage. Recognising and responding to sudden deterioration in an individual due to haemorrhage is key to increasing their chances of survival. Many lessons have been learned from conflicts of war and civil unrest regarding the use of limb tourniquets and haemostatic agents to improve survival chances in cases of severe blood loss. NHS England (2020) produced guidance regarding major incidents and mass casualty events in light of recent events that have required intervention by healthcare practitioners. Nickson (2019) highlights the goals of management in a situation where there is catastrophic haemorrhage are to find the source of bleeding and STOP the bleeding. Once bleeding is stemmed, transferring the person to the right location for the treatment of catastrophic haemorrhage is key to increasing their chances of survival. Many pre-hospital settings and clinical areas have a major haemorrhage protocol that is activated in such cases, which enables healthcare practitioners to follow a decision-making tree to ensure the person receives optimal care at this stage.

Review the following list now to help you with learning and recognising how to approach an assessment of a person who is deteriorating.

- Catastrophic haemorrhage control
- Airway (consider cervical spine protection)
- Breathing
- Circulation
- Disability (involves assessment of neurological status)
- Exposure (enables a full examination to be undertaken).

Cervical spine protection

In the event of suspected trauma, the cervical spine should be immobilised as per national and local trust trauma guidelines. This is achieved usually through the use of a rigid cervical collar with head restraint.

This order of assessment and interventions is used because airway obstructions kill faster than disordered breathing, which in turn kills faster than haemorrhage or cardiac dysfunction. Resuscitation Council (2021b) advocates the use of ABCDE approaches in any clinical emergency for immediate assessment and treatment. They add that high-quality ABCDE skills amongst all team members can save valuable time and improve team performance, which should in turn influence outcomes for the individual. Remember that you can use the ABCDE system in any location: on the street, in a person's home or within the hospital situation.

NICE (2016a) advocates this systematic approach and states that it can also be used for initial assessment and management of major trauma. The Resuscitation Council (2021b) offers guidance regarding the ABCDE approach outlining underlying principles for all deteriorating and critically ill individuals.

Extensive bleeding in trauma can cause rapid deterioration and much has been learned from military combat where personnel have often experienced life-threatening and life-changing injuries. Catastrophic haemorrhage is one of the most common and potentially preventable causes of traumatic death. Winstanley et al. (2019) explain how it is the leading cause of morbidity and mortality in trauma. They explore the use of haemostatic dressings to arrest bleeding. Levy et al. (2021) identify how direct pressure, wound packing and limb tourniquets can be used in haemorrhage situations to improve individual outcomes. These tourniquets should be used with caution and practitioners should have adequate education to apply and remove these devices.

Airway: does the person have a patent airway? (with cervical spine protection)

A patent airway is essential to ensure that there is adequate oxygen circulating in the body. The aim of this assessment is to obtain and maintain a clear and patent airway, using airway adjuncts to sustain this if necessary. If the airway is compromised – or a potential for compromise – is present, you must protect and maintain it, otherwise hypoxic brain damage will occur. When a person becomes unconscious, there is a reduction in their muscle tone, so the tongue can fall back and occlude the airway. Blood, secretions and vomit may also be present. There are various airway adjuncts available, which are discussed later. If someone needs help to maintain a patent airway, they must be constantly observed to ensure the airway does not become occluded. It is imperative to ensure the safety of all practitioners during airway management techniques. Aerosol-generated procedures should be carried out with the correct level of personal protection equipment (PPE). The World Health Organization (2020) offers guidance in view of recent pandemic experiences of COVID-19. They highlight that staff should be adequately protected, using the appropriate level of PPE if necessary. Staff should be limited to who is present during airway management techniques, including intubation. Chun Hei Cheung et al. (2020) recommended that airway devices should be chosen for their purpose required and equipment should be risk assessed and the procedure should be as risk averse as possible. Merelman and Levitan (2020) discuss the management of a high-risk airway. They highlight how airway management is a cause of anxiety in emergency situations and how competent airway management is based upon training, practice and dedication to excellence. Skilled practitioners with appropriate skills should be used to ensure that the person's airway is obtained, supported and maintained.

Breathing: is the individual breathing? If so, is it sufficient?

Once the airway is established and secured, an evaluation of the person's breathing is necessary. At this stage, it is important to try to identify hypoxia and rectify this. Hypoxia that is undetected and untreated can lead to further rapid deterioration in their condition. To establish oxygenation of the body, a review of the person's oxygen saturation via a SpO_2 probe can be conducted. A rapid assessment of respiratory rate and rhythm, any presence of hypoventilation or hyperventilation can assist in identifying any deterioration of the person's breathing. These findings should be recorded on the NEWS2 system. If breathing is compromised, then supplementary oxygen by nasal cannulae, non-rebreather oxygen mask, bag-valve-mask (BVM) ventilation or mechanical ventilation should be applied if current protocol recommends this use. Oxygen administration is considered later in this chapter. Risks of oxygen devices should be considered. Bosson (2020) explains that BVM ventilation is an essential part of airway management allowing oxygenation and ventilation until a definitive airway can be established. However, aerosol particles can pose a risk to the healthcare professional during such procedures and appropriate

Bag-valve–mask (BVM)

A handheld device used to provide ventilation to a person who is not breathing or breathing inadequately.

PPE should be used during these processes. Establishing and maintaining an adequate airway is essential as failure to do so can lead to organ failure and cardiac arrest and is a major contributing factor to home and hospital deaths (Brady and Burns 2019). Learning these skills and practising these to maintain competency is essential.

There are many airway manoeuvres that can assist in airway management. Basic airway maintenance techniques include considering position of the tongue and soft tissue obstruction of the hypopharynx in an unconscious person. This can be corrected by chin lift, jaw thrust (Resuscitation Council 2021a). Definitive airways, for example, intubation and supraglottal devices should be used for an apnoeic individual who have the inability to maintain their own airway or when basic airway adjuncts fail.

In some people who present with head injury, for example, suspected base of skull fracture, basic airway adjuncts are ill advised. Fabich et al. (2020), in their case report, highlight that an emergency airway plan is crucial to survival and that successful airway management requires planned team actions. They explore how even in traumatic military situations where facial gunshot wounds were seen, planning is key to increase survival chances.

Circulation: what do you note about the individual's circulation? Is it sufficient?

When airway and breathing are established and maintained, assessment of the circulation is key. The assessment of circulation allows the practitioner to review capillary refill time (CRT), heart rate, blood pressure, ECG and urine output, which are then charted on the NEWS2 score system. Circulatory assessment must be performed systematically and rapidly in someone who is acutely ill. If perfusion is compromised, then hypoxia and tissue damage occur quickly. Restoring adequate circulating blood volume is essential if oxygen deficit and inadequate tissue perfusion are present. Three of the most common indicators of inadequate circulatory function are hypotension (low blood pressure), tachycardia (increased heart rate) and oliguria (decreasing urinary output). The pulse rate may rise for various reasons and is not necessarily specific to hypovolaemia (low blood volume). Various pre-existing medical conditions or medications may cause tachycardia, for example, Mrs Patel who has a cardiac conduction disturbance.

Note: A person with a high spinal cord injury may have bradycardia, not tachycardia. A simple assessment of circulation can be obtained from CRT (see later in the chapter).

Blood pressure data can be misleading or unreliable. However, typical compensatory mechanisms used to maintain perfusion to the heart and brain may produce a normal systolic pressure. Loss of up to 15% of the circulating volume (700–750 mL for a 70 kg individual) may produce few obvious symptoms, while loss of up to 30% of the circulating volume (1.5 L) may result in mild tachycardia, tachypnoea and anxiety (Bonanno 2012). Hypotension, marked tachycardia (pulse rate 110–120 bpm) and confusion may not be evident until more than 30% of the blood volume has been lost, while loss of 40% of circulating volume (2 L) is immediately life-threatening

(Bonanno 2012). If hypotension is present, it requires immediate attention and treatment. Systolic blood pressure measurement and analysis is now advocated in the NEWS2 scale (RCP 2017) to indicate altered pathophysiology.

Disability: is the person conscious? Assess the level of consciousness

A rapid neurological evaluation is conducted once the airway is secured, breathing is adequate and circulatory issues have been dealt with. To do this, the individual's level of consciousness can be assessed using a rapid assessment ACVPU tool within an initial assessment. This scale enables the practitioner to gain a quick assessment of their neurological status as opposed to the GCS, which offers a more in-depth assessment but takes longer to conduct.

> **ACVPU tool**
>
> A = Alert
> C = new confusion
> V = (responds to) Voice
> P = (responds to) Pain
> U = Unresponsive

Once conducted, the assessment results are added to the NEWS2 score. The GCS, as described in Chapter 4, is used once the initial assessment is conducted if a neurological deficit is suspected or diagnosed. You should also check the pupil's reaction to light (see Chapter 4). Pupillary responses can give important information about the causes of neurological problems. If the pupils are both dilated, it can denote stress or fear, and can also indicate that sympathetic stimulants have been taken (e.g. tricyclic antidepressants, adrenaline). If the pupils are both constricted, it can indicate that opiates have been taken (e.g. morphine) or that the brain stem has been affected (https://www.glasgowcomascale.org/). However, a dilated pupil on one side can indicate a unilateral space-occupying lesion such as a haematoma, tumour or abscess, which is a medical emergency.

A decreased level of consciousness may indicate cerebral injury. Factors such as hypoxaemia, hypovolaemia, alcohol and/or drugs may also alter the level of consciousness. Generally, if the GCS is less than 8, the level of consciousness is severely compromised, and they will require help to maintain their airway. It is also important to undertake a blood glucose recording (discussed later in this chapter).

Exposure: look for other information that will assist you in finding the cause of deterioration

During this stage of the assessment, the aim is to review the individual for any signs of further injury or identify any drains or dressings or wounds that may be causing deterioration. For example, wounds that look infected may be a source of sepsis. Dressings that are oozing and have lots of blood loss can be an indication of hypovolaemia. At this stage in the assessment, the individual should be completely undressed to be thoroughly examined. In acute deterioration or traumatic injury, it may be necessary to cut off the clothes. Consent to this should be obtained where possible and the dignity of the person must be protected, and they should not be exposed unnecessarily but covered as soon as the assessment of this section is completed. During this stage, the temperature is recorded and charted on the NEWS2 system. Indications of hypothermia and pyrexia would require further investigation and treatment. The individual could be warmed with blankets or other warming devices to prevent the rapid onset or continued state of hypothermia.

Initial treatments using blankets should however always be done with caution as it is important that a person is warmed up gradually to prevent further insult on the body systems. When combined with rapid infusions of cold fluids or blood products and exposure, hypothermia can have potentially fatal results, if left untreated. Hypothermia can be classified as mild (32–35°C), moderate (28–32°C) and severe (less than 28°C) (Nickson 2019). It can be associated with impaired thermogenesis and decreased levels of consciousness due to hypoxia. Cardiac arrhythmias may be seen as the heart is fragile due to the lack of circulating blood leading to potential coagulopathies and higher mortality (Zafren and Crawford Mechem 2020). The individual who is cold can be very sensitive to movement as all organs suffer a degree of blood reduction and movement can dislodge clots thus causing further deterioration. Careful handling of the individual is required and change in position restricted until an initial assessment is carried out. Generally, people with hypothermia should be constantly assessed and a process of active warming (a process that transfers heat to the individual) should be commenced (NICE 2016a). The warming process will take some time and can take the form of a resuscitative process, passive warming or consist of peripheral active warming depending on the person's condition. Gradual warming should be carried out, thus minimising the risks to vital organs. Sudden warming of an individual is to be avoided (Li 2019; NICE 2016b; Nickson 2019). Monitoring of skin and core temperature is recommended to avoid this occurring.

During this section of the assessment, the capillary blood glucose is assessed (described later in this chapter) to ascertain signs of further deterioration and potential causes of ill health. This is noted by the practitioner and handed over to a senior clinician or dealt with immediately at the bedside if it falls below normal limits or is raised above the known highest parameter.

Remember: Always reassess ABCDE regularly and do not progress from one stage to another until you have dealt with the first.

Learning outcome 4: locate and recognise emergency equipment

In any new clinical area where you are working, always familiarise yourself with emergency equipment and its location. Emergency equipment must be checked regularly to ensure it remains in working order, and it should be rechecked after each usage. The necessary equipment might be on a resuscitation (cardiac arrest) trolley, or the items – including oxygen, suction and defibrillator (see Box 14.9) may be available in separate locations. The Resuscitation Council (UK) (2021b) advises on appropriate equipment for pre-hospital situations, cardiac arrest trolleys and clinical areas.

Box 14.8 Activity: emergency equipment

ACTIVITY

Locate the emergency equipment and ask a member of the team to check the equipment with you. This will assist in you becoming familiar with this equipment.

Box 14.9 The automatic external defibrillator or defibrillator

Locate the AED in your clinical area and become familiar with its operation. A defibrillator is a device that delivers electrical current across the myocardium. It is used when the heart is suffering from disorganised electrical activity (e.g. ventricular fibrillation). By passing electricity through the heart in a controlled dose, the heart can be stopped briefly with the intention of restoring organised spontaneous electrical activity (see www.resus.org.uk).

The shock is administered by charging up the defibrillator to the appropriate dosage, placing the paddles or attaching pads on the person's chest and pressing the discharge button. People using defibrillators require specialist training as it is a complex and potentially dangerous skill. There are AEDs available that can automatically recognise rhythms and give instructions for defibrillation. These are becoming increasingly available both inside and outside the hospital setting.

Box 14.10 Children and young people: practice points – assessment in emergencies

If faced with a sick child, remember to use an ABCDE approach and act upon your findings until skilled help arrives. If you are required to care for children, you must become familiar with the PEWS chart in use and seek advice from your practice healthcare professional to develop confidence in assessing children using an ABCDE approach. In practice areas that care for children, there will be a separate paediatric resuscitation trolley.

Useful resources

The Department of Health's website (www.spottingthesickchild.com) aims to support healthcare professionals in the assessment of acutely ill children.

For resuscitation advice visit: www.resus.org.uk

See also:

Glasper, A., Coad, J. and Richardson J. 2015. (eds.) Paediatric early warning scores. In: *Children and Young People's Nursing at a Glance*. Chichester Wiley: Blackwell, 24–25.

Box 14.11 Pregnancy and birth: practice points assessment in emergencies

Pregnancy and birth for the majority of women is a normal, physiological process. However, some women may develop unexpected complications and specialist care is required. Severely ill pregnant mothers may be cared for in a variety of non-midwifery settings; theatre; theatre recovery; general high-dependency unit (HDU); and intensive care unit (ITU). Care must be managed safely by the multidisciplinary team, including specialist medical staff, anaesthetists, obstetricians and midwives. Detecting signs of deterioration in the physical health of pregnant mothers can be difficult due to an altered physiology, and it is important to identify warning signs of impending collapse (see Chapter 4 on measuring and monitoring vital signs).

In an emergency, the mother and unborn child must receive appropriate, timely and specialised care immediately. Remember to stay calm and try to identify and treat the underlying cause; the initial assessment and management priorities for caring for a deteriorating pregnant mother and her resuscitation follow an ABCDE approach, with some adaptations and additional skills needed. An unconscious woman if over 20 weeks gestation should be positioned in the left lateral position or the uterus should be gently displaced manually to the left to relieve aortocaval compression.

For further information on special circumstances, guidance available from: https://www.resus.org.uk/library/2021-resuscitation-guidelines/special-circumstances-guidelines (Accessed on 22 May 2021).

AIRWAY MANAGEMENT PROBLEMS AND RELATED SKILLS

There are many reasons why a person's airway becomes compromised, including infection, smoke inhalation, allergic reaction, foreign body obstruction or trauma. Foreign bodies may cause either a mild or a severe airway obstruction and are usually inhaled bits of food such as meat, boiled sweets and fruit, or vomit or blood. Acute allergic reactions (e.g. a bee sting, peanuts, penicillin) can cause the trachea or throat to swell until it is closed.

Box 14.12 Learning outcomes

By the end of this section, you will be able to:

1 recognise the signs of an obstructed airway and take appropriate action;
2 identify and discuss the different types of airway adjuncts available;
3 explain reasons for oxygen administration and discuss how it can be delivered safely through different delivery devices;
4 discuss how suction equipment is used in practice.

Learning outcome 1: recognise the signs of an obstructed airway and take appropriate action

An airway can obstruct very suddenly, so it is important to be able to recognise the signs and act on them. Your mandatory basic life-support training will address this topic. Visit www.resus.org.uk for up-to-date guidelines on airway management.

Box 14.13 Activity: Mary Wyatt's scenario

ACTIVITY

Looking at Mary Wyatt's scenario, how do you think care home staff knew she had an obstructed airway? What first aid should the staff have attempted?

Resuscitation Council (UK)

The Resuscitation Council's evidence-based guidelines are reviewed approximately every 5 years. Current guidance available from: Resuscitation Council (UK) 2021b. *Resuscitation Guidelines.* http://www.resus.org.uk/pages/guide.htm.

Mary was eating at the time and she may have clutched her neck. The Resuscitation Council (UK) (www.resus.org) suggests that in mild airway obstruction, the person is able to speak, breathe and cough, and can verbally respond to the question: 'Are you choking'? However, with a severe obstruction (as in Mary's case), she would not have been able to speak but might have nodded and her attempts at coughing would have been silent.

- To recognise an airway obstruction, the recommended method is 'look, listen and feel' (www.resus.org.uk)
- **Look to see whether there are any chest and abdominal movements**. In normal respiration, the chest and abdomen move outwards during inspiration and inwards during expiration, but with respiratory compromise, there is a seesaw pattern of movements. Other signs include using accessory muscles: neck and shoulders and a pulling in of the trachea.
- **Look at the person's colour**. As hypoxia develops, the peripheries gain a grey/blue tinge (cyanosis). Peripheral cyanosis is seen in areas like hands and toes. Central cyanosis (blueness in the tongue and lips) is a late sign of airway obstruction. However, in people with darker skin, cyanosis may look grey or whitish, while the areas around the eyes can appear grey or bluish.
- **Listen for sound of breathing**. Normal breathing should be quiet – noise indicates a partially obstructed airway. Respiratory sounds can indicate the position of the obstruction:
  - *Stridor*, a high-pitched sound usually heard during inspiration, is due to partial blockage of the trachea, larynx or pharynx.
  - *Gurgling* can indicate fluids such as blood or vomit in the upper airways.
  - *Snoring* indicates partial blockage of the pharynx usually by the tongue or soft palate.
  - *Expiratory wheeze* can be heard when the airways collapse during expiration (e.g. asthma).
- However, a silent chest is a bad sign too as it indicates a totally occluded airway.
- **Feel**. Feel for breath by placing your cheek or your hand close to the person's mouth. You should be able to feel the air movement at the mouth. Resuscitation Council (2021a) explains how during the COVID-19 pandemic, the look, listen and feel approach has been conducted at a 2-m distance if level 3 PPE is not worn.
- COVID ALERT. When dealing with a person who has or is suspected of having COVID-19, any aerosol-generating procedures (AGP) are a potential risk so staff should wear appropriate personal protective equipment level 3. This includes gloves, full-face visors and fluid repellent gowns. The person's face should be covered with a mask or cloth in a community setting or first aid situation. This is done to protect the rescuer from aerosol-generated situations. Airway adjunct

insertion, suctioning and airway manoeuvres should be carried out by practitioners who are wearing L3 PPE. For current guidance, please see: Statement on COVID-19 in relation to CPR and resuscitation. Available from: https://www.resus.org.uk/covid-19-resources/covid-19-resources-general-public/resuscitation-council-uk-statement-covid-19 (Accessed on 9 June 2021).

Airway opening

You will learn airway opening in your mandatory basic life-support sessions and review these in your clinical areas. In recent events of the COVID-19 pandemic, all aerosol-generated procedures should be carried out wearing appropriate PPE. The steps to follow are discussed below to offer an overview of the procedure. Please ensure that you review national guidelines and local clinical protocols prior to attempting any of these procedures and seek guidance from appropriate senior practitioners:

- If it is possible, turn the individual onto their back.
- To perform a **head tilt and chin lift**, rest one hand on the person's forehead and place the fingertips of your other hand on to the chin, taking care not to press on the soft tissue under the chin, which can obstruct the airway. Gently push down on the forehead and lift up the chin to open the airway.
- A **jaw thrust** may be used if there is suspected neck injury. This is a procedure that will be performed by experienced trained practitioners. An overview is given here, so that you understand the process. To perform this manoeuvre, the practitioner will kneel (or stand if the individual is on a bed) near the top of their head. They will grasp the angles of the lower jaw on both sides with their fingers and lift. This displaces the mandible (jawbone) forward while tilting the head backward.

Dealing with someone who has an airway obstruction can be alarming. If the person is showing signs of a mild airway obstruction, they should be encouraged to cough to help clear their airway. You should observe them closely in case they deteriorate and require intervention.

If (as in Mary Wyatt's case) the airway obstruction is severe or their cough becomes ineffective, you should help them to clear the airway. It is important to remain calm, talk to the person and explain what you are doing, as struggling to breathe can be a very frightening experience. The Resuscitation Council (UK) explains the steps to take.

- Give up to *five* sharp blows between the shoulder blades using the heel of your hand. Stand behind the person and lean them forward, so when the object is dislodged, it will come out of the mouth and not back down the airway.
- If these back blows are unsuccessful, give up to *five* abdominal thrusts. Stand behind the person and put both arms around their upper abdomen. Make a fist with one hand and place it in between the navel and the bottom end of the sternum. Clasp the other hand around it and pull sharply inwards and upwards. Ensure that you do not have your face directly behind their head as the movement can cause their

head to move upwards, causing you an injury. If the person is seated or small you, may need to kneel behind them.

- If after five abdominal thrusts the object has still not been expelled, then give further back blows and abdominal thrusts until the object is expelled.
- If the person loses consciousness, support them to the floor and begin basic life support (see the guidelines at www.resus.org.uk).

What you are attempting to do is to increase the intrathoracic pressure, thus forcing the object out – similar to the effect of coughing. As there is risk of internal damage, the person should always be medically assessed following abdominal thrusts.

Box 14.14 Activity: different types of airway adjuncts

Try to look at different types of airway adjuncts. Which ones have you seen in practice? How do you think they would be used?

Learning outcome 2: identify and discuss the different types of airway adjuncts available

You may have identified any of the airway adjuncts summarised in Table 14.1. The paramedics attending Mary Wyatt may have inserted one of these. You might have seen these devices used in emergency situations or in the operating theatre. There are other methods to help secure an airway, including endotracheal tubes and tracheostomies. All airway adjuncts must be inserted by trained professionals who will have learned how to select the correct size for each individual and how to insert them safely. In a situation where a person's airway is compromised, it is imperative that their airway is cleared as rapidly as possible and that their oxygen levels are monitored and maintained.

Box 14.15 Activity: airway adjuncts available and their location

When next in your clinical area, find out what airway adjuncts are available and their location. Ensure that you can recognise these pieces of equipment. Ask a member of the team for guidance, if necessary.

Ensure you follow current national guidance and work within local trust protocols to keep safe and to minimise the risk to self and to other people.

Learning outcome 3: explain reasons for oxygen administration and discuss how it can be delivered safely through different delivery devices

Breathing normally involves a process of inspiration and expiration. This is achieved by expansion of the thoracic cavity and air being forced down into the lungs. The oxygen we need is gained from the atmospheric air around us. Oxygen constitutes approximately 21% of air at sea level. Oxygen therapy is the administration of extra

Table 14.1: Airway adjuncts

Basic oropharyngeal airway

A rigid curved plastic tube used for unconscious people

The mouth is checked to ensure that nothing could be pushed back during insertion

Inserted upside down until it has passed the teeth to prevent the tongue being pushed back, then rotated into the correct position

If any signs of gagging or straining occur, it must be removed immediately

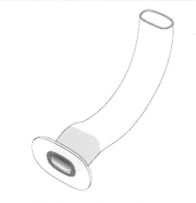

Figure 14.1: Basic oropharangeal airway.

Nasopharyngeal airway (NPA)

Can be used when an oropharyngeal airway cannot be tolerated, or inserted (e.g. when there are facial injuries or clenched jaws)

Should not be used if there is a suspected basal skull fracture, owing to risk of penetrating the brain tissue.

The NPA, once in place, can be used for suctioning

However, the vagus nerve can be stimulated, producing bradycardia – in which case, suctioning should stop and senior staff should be alerted

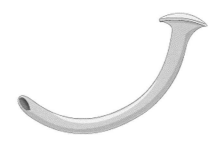

Figure 14.2: Nasopharangeal airway.

Laryngeal mask airway (LMA)

Has an inflatable cuff that is inserted into the pharynx

When the tube is inserted, the cuff is inflated, creating an airtight seal

Bag-valve apparatus and oxygen can be attached to ventilate the person, which has been shown to reduce risk of gastric regurgitation (Resuscitation Council (UK))

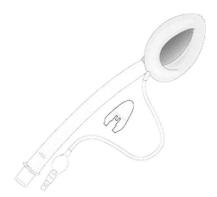

Figure 14.3: Laryngeal mask airway.

Supraglottic device

This is a soft gel, non-inflatable airway device. It is a colour-coded device that allows sealing of the pharyngeal, laryngeal and peri-laryngeal structures.

Further guidance regarding establishing and maintaining an airway can be found on www.resus.org.uk. These skills range from simple BLS techniques to advanced skills and will be dependent upon your role as to whether you are expected to perform these skills; therefore, it is important to check with your local clinical setting.

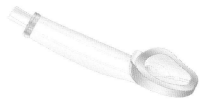

Figure 14.4: Supraglottal device.

NB: Please review current guidance from COVID guidance before attempting any airway procedures in your clinical area. Available from: https://www.resus.org.uk/about-us/news-and-events/resuscitation-council-uk-position-covid-19-guidance-september-2020 (Accessed on 9 June 2021).

oxygen to enable a higher inspiration of oxygen than that achieved during normal breathing. Oxygen delivery equipment is essential in emergency situations and is available in all acute settings and many community care environments too. Oxygen delivery relies on a patent airway.

Oxygen therapy may be a short-term measure in acute illness or long-term therapy for chronic respiratory disease. For all individuals, other than in an emergency situation, oxygen concentration is prescribed (see www.bnf.org) to achieve specified target oxygen saturation measurements, British Thoracic Society (BTS; 2017).

Hypercapnic respiratory failure

Hypercapnic respiratory failure

Involves inadequate gas exchange by the respiratory system where there is a build-up of carbon dioxide.

For most acutely ill adults, the target oxygen saturation is 94–98%, but it is 88–92% for people at risk of hypercapnic respiratory failure (O'Driscoll et al. 2017). Correct procedures and local guidelines must be followed for oxygen delivery. Refer to BTS guidelines (2017) for use of oxygen therapy.

Box 14.16 Activity: the benefits of oxygen therapy

ACTIVITY

Reflect upon a situation when you have seen oxygen therapy being used within the hospital or community. When might people benefit from oxygen therapy?

Hypoxaemia

Low O_2 tension or partial pressure of O_2 (PaO_2) in the blood.

BTS guidelines (2017) advise that oxygen is a treatment for hypoxaemia, not breathlessness, so oxygen saturation measurements should guide whether oxygen is administered. You may have thought of the following situations where hypoxaemia might occur:

- After a general anaesthetic;
- In emergency situations such as cardiac or respiratory arrest, shock and airway obstruction (as with Mary Wyatt);
- In chest injuries following trauma;
- In acute respiratory disease (e.g. asthma, as with Tina);
- In chronic respiratory conditions such as COPD and cystic fibrosis where long-term oxygen therapy may be needed, usually for a minimum of 15 h per day;
- In heart disease where cardiac output is reduced (e.g. myocardial infarction).

Myocardial infarction

A myocardial infarction (MI) occurs when there is interrupted blood supply to the myocardium, causing death of tissue and usually resulting in severe chest pain which may radiate to the arms, jaw and/or neck, often accompanied by sweating. 'Heart attack' is the lay term for this condition.

Oxygen supplies

In hospital, oxygen is obtained either from a wall-mounted piped oxygen supply or on rare occasions a cylinder (black with white shoulders). If cylinders are used, the dial showing the remaining oxygen must be inspected regularly as they can run out quite quickly. It is also imperative that equipment is checked to ensure good working order.

Delivery devices

Different concentrations of oxygen are administered according to clinical need, which affects oxygen administration devices used. For example, for someone like Tina, who is very breathless and mouth breathing, a mask must be used. Nurses must record details of oxygen concentration, delivery device and commencement and termination of therapy, and sign for oxygen administration on the drug chart at each drug round (BTS guidelines 2017).

ACTIVITY

Box 14.17 Activity: oxygen delivery devices

Either in your clinical setting or in the skills laboratory, look at oxygen delivery devices. How do you think different concentrations are achieved?

Choice of oxygen delivery system

Oxygen therapy can be delivered at varying concentrations, often measured in percentages (e.g. 24%, 28%, 35% and 40%); please refer to BTS (2017) for further information. The oxygen flow is measured in litres per minute using a flow meter. Devices include simple oxygen masks, Venturi masks, nasal cannulae, high flow nasal cannula and non-rebreathing masks (Figure 14.5). These devices are disposable and packaged separately and each individual has their own equipment. Masks should be cleaned regularly, especially if the person has a productive cough (please refer to manufacturer's guidelines for cleaning instructions and recommended length of use). If a mask or nasal cannulae is worn for an extended period, there is a risk of pressure ulcer development, particularly on the bridge of the nose or behind the ears. Therefore, masks and cannulae must be correctly applied, a good fit, and replaced regularly.

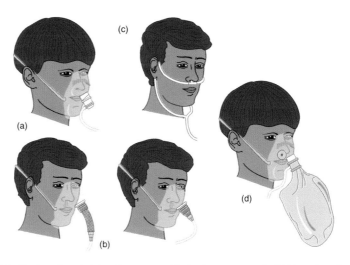

Figure 14.5: Devices for administering oxygen: (a) simple oxygen mask, (b) Venturi masks, (c) nasal cannulae and (d) non-rebreathing mask.

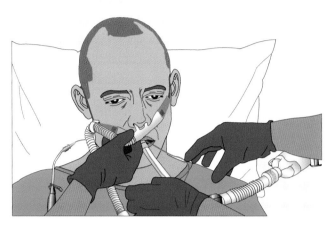

Figure 14.6: High flow nasal cannula diagram (HFNC).

O'Driscoll et al. (2017) suggest the following options for stepping up or down oxygen doses:

- Venturi 24% mask at 2–4 L/min or nasal cannulae at 1 L/min
- Venturi 28% mask at 4–6 L/min or nasal cannulae at 2 L/min
- Venturi 35% mask at 8–10 L/min or nasal cannulae at 4–6 L/min
- Venturi 40% at 10–12 L/min or simple face mask at 5–6 L/min
- Venturi 60% at 12–15 L/min or simple face mask at 7–10 L/min
- Non-rebreather mask at 15 L/min.

Nasal cannula that deliver high flow oxygen are now increasingly used and can be an effective treatment when weaning people off high levels of oxygen.

Each device will now be considered in more detail.

Nasal cannulae

These may be used for people with acute or chronic respiratory disease where low levels of oxygen are required. They are well tolerated and administer oxygen directly into the nostrils. Oxygen flow is adjusted using the oxygen flow meter. Estimated oxygen concentration in the range of 25–40% can be obtained using a flow rate of 2–6 L per minute. However, flow rates of more than 4 L per minute are not recommended due to the drying effect on the nasal mucosa (BTS 2017). Administration may not be very accurate, as oxygen intake can vary. Sharma et al. (2020) explain how traditional nasal cannula can be useful to deliver 4–6 L of oxygen. To make the nasal cannulae fit closely, move the ends of the tubes through the horizontal piece of tubing across the nose and also the adaptor on the tubing below the chin. With nasal cannulae, people can eat, drink and talk more easily than with masks and procedures such as mouth care can be carried out without disrupting oxygen administration and can be more comfortable if oxygen is delivered on a long-term basis. Some individuals find an oxygen mask claustrophobic. Materials like Softech® make the cannulae easy to tolerate and comfortable to wear (see www.teleflex.com).

High flow nasal cannula

Where low flow nasal cannula devices are not successful or poorly tolerated due to an individual's worsening condition, high flow oxygen nasal cannula are available, for example, optiflow. These are non-invasive devices that warm and humidify HFNC air/oxygen blends. HFNC is used to treat hypoxia where poor success has been seen using low flow oxygen nasal cannula and can deliver up to 100% humidified and heated oxygen at a rate of 60 L/min. HFNC can be used in acute hypoxemic respiratory failure, some people with COPD, sleep apnoea, acute heart failure, respiratory failure following surgery and individuals who cannot be intubated (Sharma et al. 2020). High flow nasal cannula can offer humidification and warming of inspired air, which is extremely important to improve comfort and compliance of use for an individual (Koczulla et al. 2018). These devices have been useful in the COVID-19 pandemic where people have required long-term oxygen therapy. The lasting effects of contracting COVID-19 are yet to be examined in the literature.

Simple face mask

Sira Patel is currently receiving oxygen via a simple face mask. These are referred to as Hudson, medium concentration (MC) or semi-rigid. To make the mask fit comfortably, the strap should be adjusted to fit behind the ears. The oxygen amount delivered is adjusted by using the flow meter and the exact amount delivered depends on the rate and depth of breathing. If an individual is breathing rapidly, large amounts of room air are drawn into the mask. This mixes with the oxygen therefore diluting the concentration (Olive 2016). Oxygen can be delivered at 4–15 L/min, achieving concentrations of 35–70% (see manufacturer's guidelines for the mask you are using). Rates of below 4 L/min should not be used as, with a low flow rate, rebreathing of carbon dioxide may occur due to exhaled carbon dioxide accumulating within the mask (O'Driscoll et al. 2017).

Venturi mask system

In the Venturi system, the oxygen concentration is not significantly affected by the rate and depth of breathing and a set concentration can thus be achieved (Pennisi et al. 2019). The mask is supplied with different coloured fittings, each clearly marked with an oxygen percentage and the required flow rate. The device ensures that oxygen flow is accurately diluted with entrained air. You can thus administer the exact percentage prescribed by fitting the correct device and setting the correct flow rate.

Non-rebreathing masks

These have a large reservoir for oxygen with valves to allow the individual to inhale only oxygen and prevent it from mixing with expired gases. Oxygen concentration is determined by the flow meter. They can provide up to 85% oxygen (Gwinnutt 2016), particularly for short periods of time, for example, postoperatively or in an emergency such as Mary's. The valve on the mask must be pressed to enable the chamber to fill with oxygen prior to applying the mask to the person's face.

Other oxygen delivery devices

Some people need additional technology to deliver oxygen to them and assist their breathing; Box 14.19 summarises the use of these devices.

Hazards of oxygen therapy

Box 14.18 Activity: hazards arising from oxygen therapy

Can you think of any hazards that might arise from oxygen therapy?

The two main hazards are fire and the delivery of oxygen to people with chronic pulmonary disease who retain carbon dioxide.

Fire hazard

You have probably attended fire lectures or completed an e-learning activity where the fire triangle was outlined. Can you remember the three factors necessary for fire? Oxygen, fuel and heat are needed; if one of these is missing, the fire cannot start or will quickly go out. Oxygen supports combustion and thus enhances the inflammable properties of other materials such as cigarettes, grease and oil (Roots 2016). Administration of oxygen could therefore be a fire hazard.

Box 14.19 Other devices to deliver oxygen: CPAP, NIPPV, and ventilation

Continuous positive airway pressure (CPAP)

This breathing support system is a machine that delivers positive airway pressure through a mask and tubing. The mask is tight fitting, is not easily tolerated and compliance to the treatment can be difficult to achieve. It is primarily used in cases of obstructive sleep apnoea, pneumonia and correcting hypoxia in type 1 respiratory failure. It works by splinting the airway open.

Non-invasive positive-pressure ventilation (NIPPV) or Bilevel Positive Airway Pressure (BiPAP trademark)

This process involves positive-pressure ventilation, and it offers the person a support to their breathing. Its aim is to deliver air with added oxygen through a tight-fitting mask or similar device. It is usually used in type 2 respiratory failure where hypercapnia is seen and is useful in the treatment of COPD with respiratory acidosis. It is valuable in weaning individuals off tracheal intubation ventilation as a support to breathing until they are able to function without support.

Ventilation

A mechanical ventilator machine can support or replace a person's breathing when they are experiencing extreme respiratory dysfunction or is unable to breathe due to injury or disease. The individual is intubated via the nose or mouth and attached to the ventilator machine. Mechanical ventilation is used

(Continued)

Box 14.19 (Continued)

after a full respiratory assessment indicates no other alternatives to assist breathing. People receiving this type of treatment may be cared for in a high-dependency acute area or ICU or in theatre.

The use of ventilator support has had unprecedented use during the COVID-19 pandemic with many people requiring airway support.

Box 14.20 Activity: precautions to reduce the risk of fire during oxygen therapy

ACTIVITY

What precautions will be needed to reduce the risk of fire during oxygen therapy?

You may have thought of:

- Displaying No Smoking signs.
- Removing devices that can spark.
- Educating individuals and relatives about the risk of smoking during oxygen administration and alcohol-based sprays (e.g. in perfume).
- Knowledge of fire procedure and equipment.
- Oxygen cylinders in the home should be kept away from gas fires, naked flames and hot radiators (NHS 2020).

People who retain carbon dioxide

Normally, rising levels of CO_2 stimulate respiration. However, some people with chronic respiratory disease may continuously have a high level of CO_2 in their blood and therefore their chemoreceptors are no longer stimulated by this. For these individuals, who retain CO_2, the less important hypoxic drive predominates, which means that breathing is only stimulated by lack of oxygen and they are referred to as being **hypercapnic**. However, oxygen therapy can improve the individual's outcomes. O'Driscoll et al. (2017) reported improved survival rates in people with COPD who have long-term oxygen therapy. People with chronic respiratory disease are, therefore, normally prescribed less than 28% oxygen (via a Venturi mask) or 2 L/min (via nasal cannulae) initially and would only be prescribed a higher amount if indicated by arterial blood gas analysis or pulse oximetry (O'Driscoll et al. 2017). They should carry an oxygen alert card to inform health care professionals of their oxygen requirements (O'Driscoll et al. 2017, NHS 2020).

Box 14.21 Activity: adult with hypoxia and confusion who is not tolerating oxygen therapy

ACTIVITY

If an adult with hypoxia and confusion is not tolerating oxygen therapy, what could you do?

People who understand how and why they need oxygen are more likely to tolerate it so clear explanations are necessary. An adult who is confused due to hypoxia may resist oxygen therapy, and careful management of these people is required to prevent sudden deterioration. Repositioning can improve breathing and ventilation, for example, sitting upright in a chair or in bed, will be helpful. Nasal cannulae rather than a mask may be better tolerated. Support and explanations from a familiar relative or significant other may help. If a person with learning disabilities needs oxygen therapy, you must consider their level of understanding and learning ability. Demonstration of the mask/cannulae in position on a carer or nurse, and an explanation of the associated sensations and sounds, may be reassuring. People who experience claustrophobia also require support to be able to accept the close-fitting oxygen mask. Many people who are short of breath feel afraid and anxious, so a relaxed approach, distraction techniques and an ability to communicate calmly are essential to support them effectively.

Humidification of oxygen devices

The use of oxygen can have a drying effect on the upper airway. The National Heart, Lung and Blood Institute (2020) reports that oxygen therapy can cause dryness, bloody nose, skin irritation and mucus dryness. Dryness of nostrils and mouth can be prevented through good oral hygiene, application of aqueous cream and adequate fluid intake. However, the use of petroleum jelly should be avoided because of its potentially flammable nature (NHS 2020). Oxygen administered for more than a short period of time can be humidified, particularly if the concentration administered is high, for example, over 35%, or at a rate of 4 L per minute or above (O'Driscoll et al. 2017).

ACTIVITY

> ### Box 14.22 Activity: humidification equipment
>
> Locate humidification equipment either in the skills laboratory or in the clinical setting. What sort of water is to be used and why? What hazards might be associated with humidification equipment?

Humidification provides a moist environment and so may encourage bacterial growth. Sterile water should be used to minimise bacterial contamination. Humidifiers should be used according to the manufacturer's instructions.

Learning outcome 4: discuss how suction equipment is used in practice

If the airways become obstructed by secretions, blood or vomit, a suction device should be used. However, suctioning is a traumatic procedure and can have some limitations such as producing hypoxia and bradycardia. Sinha and Fitzgerald (2020) highlight that the risk and benefits should be calculated for the individual. It is important to assess the person during and after the suctioning and ensure that any oxygen device is repositioned immediately. Suctioning should only be done if clinically indicated.

Suctioning devices can be wall mounted or portable and have a negative-pressure regulator so that the degree of suction can be altered accordingly. The amount of suction required depends on the viscosity of the secretions but the recommended amount is between 100 and 150 mmHg (Main and Denehy 2016).

ACTIVITY

Box 14.23 Activity: locating a suction device

While in the clinical setting, locate a suction device. With a member of the team, check whether it is working efficiently. What attachments are there, and which might you use for Mary?

To collect the debris, it will also have a reservoir, which must be kept clean and clear. A correct sized tubing should be connected, with enough length to reach and a suitable suction tip selected. This can be a wide bore rigid tip, for example, a Yankauer sucker, which can be used to clear vomit or secretions from the mouth, or a soft flexible catheter that can be used in conjunction with an airway adjunct. In Mary's case, a Yankauer sucker could have been used in an attempt to remove the piece of meat initially. When she had an airway inserted, *it would then* be possible to insert a flexible suction catheter down the airway as well as use the Yankauer sucker to clear her mouth. Box 14.24 outlines the procedure for suctioning the mouth.

Box 14.24 Procedure for suctioning the mouth – this procedure carries a high risk from aerosol-based transmission

- Aerosol-generating events such as this procedure should be done following trust clinical guidelines. Appropriate PPE equipment must be worn by the healthcare professional. Procedure should only be conducted when deemed safe and necessary.
- Check whether the suctioning equipment is functioning correctly and collect other equipment.
- Maintain standard infection control precautions throughout; wear PPE.
- Explain the procedure and gain consent if able to do so. Consider implied consent in those who are unresponsive, sedated or unconscious.
- Connect one end of the suction connecting tubing to the machine's suction post and the other end to a clean catheter or Yankauer sucker.
- Set the suction machine pressure at the recommended amount.
- Prepare the person for the procedure and if possible, ask them to open their mouth, so that you are able to see where the secretions are.
- Insert the catheter or sucker into the mouth but do not apply suction.
- Gently withdraw the catheter while applying suction.
- Clean the catheter by sucking through some clear water.
- Repeat the procedure, if necessary.
- Dispose of the used equipment appropriately.
- Make sure the person is comfortable after suctioning.
- Assess the individual to ensure that they have suffered no adverse effects from the suctioning.

All suctioning equipment should be checked daily along with emergency equipment, before and after use to ensure its proper working. A suction device should only be used by staff who have had appropriate training.

Box 14.25 Children and young people: practice points – airway management

Choking is common in small children and often characterised by respiratory distress associated with coughing, gagging and/or stridor. Choking in children mainly occurs during feeding or playing. For guidance on choking management, see: www.resus.org.uk

In areas where children are cared for, there will be airway adjuncts, oxygen and suction equipment in smaller sizes to cover all ages.

Further reading

Glasper, A., Coad, J, and Richardson J. (eds.). 2015. Infant Resuscitation and Young Person Resuscitation. In: *Children and Young People's Nursing at a Glance*. Chichester: Wiley Blackwell, 44–7.

Macqueen, S., Bruce, E.A. and Gibson, F. 2012. Resuscitation practices. In: *The Great Ormond Street Hospital Manual of Children's Nursing Practices*. Chichester: Wiley-Blackwell, 681–4.

Box 14.26 Pregnancy and birth: practice points – airway management and choking

Managing the pregnant mother's airway requires unique consideration and skill due to the anatomical and physiological changes in pregnancy.

For further reading see: OAA DAS Obstetric Airway Guidelines. Available from: https://www.oaa-anaes.ac.uk/OAA_DAS_Obstetric_Airway_Guidelines (Accessed on 9 June 2021).

For women in the third trimester who are choking, if back blows are unsuccessful, **do not** use abdominal thrusts but alternate backslaps with chest thrusts: see NHS What should I do if someone is choking. Available from: https://www.nhs.uk/common-health-questions/accidents-first-aid-and-treatments/what-should-i-do-if-someone-is-choking/ (Accessed on 9 June 2021).

Summary

- When dealing with a person who is deteriorating, it is vital to seek help immediately.
- Recognising an airway obstruction and dealing with it quickly and effectively can prevent further deterioration.
- Oxygen therapy is given to treat hypoxaemia and must be given in accordance with recommended guidelines using an appropriate delivery device.
- Suction should be used to clear secretions from the airway but should only be performed by an appropriately trained person.

BREATHING PROBLEMS AND RELATED SKILLS

Breathing problems resulting in tachypnoea (rapid breathing) and dyspnoea (difficulty in breathing) can indicate significant disease. Wheatley (2018) notes how the person's respiratory rate is the first parameter to rise when they are deteriorating. The Royal College of Nursing (RCN 2017) identified that people with learning disabilities have increased health needs compared with the wider population. People with learning disabilities are at risk of respiratory tract infections caused by aspiration or reflux if they have swallowing difficulties. There are many causes of breathing problems; some originate from the respiratory system (e.g. asthma, COPD), but other causes are due to problems with other body systems, for example, heart or renal failure.

All people who experience acute breathing problems should be evaluated by a healthcare professional immediately. There are a range of skills needed to assess and care for people with breathing problems. Many are included elsewhere in this book and in other sections of this chapter; you will be referred to these during this section.

> **Box 14.27 Learning outcomes**
>
> By the end of this section, you will be able to:
>
> 1 discuss the signs and symptoms of a person who is having difficulty breathing;
> 2 outline assessment skills, investigations and interventions for a person with an acute breathing problem;
> 3 measure and record a person's peak expiratory flow rate;
> 4 describe how sputum expectoration can be encouraged and sputum specimens collected.

Learning outcome 1: discuss the signs and symptoms of a person who is having difficulty breathing

> **Box 14.28 Activity: symptoms of a person having difficulty breathing**
>
> What are the signs and symptoms of a person who is having difficulty breathing? Consider a person, like Tina, who is acutely breathless – her scenario will give some clues.

ACTIVITY

You may have considered the following:

- Tachypnoea (rapid breathing)
- Tachycardia (rapid pulse)
- Noisy breathing, for example, wheezing
- Cyanosis
- Delayed CRT (see explanation later in this chapter)
- Inability to speak in full sentences
- Use of accessory muscles for breathing
- Coughing
- Pursed lips

- Flared nostrils
- The person may lean forward and hold their chest
- Confusion or disorientation if hypoxic.

In extreme situations, people who have breathing difficulties will continue to deteriorate despite healthcare interventions. Their respiratory muscles become fatigued as they fail to sustain respiratory function. Oxygen therapy or mechanical support (artificial ventilation) may not maintain adequate gaseous exchange. Healthcare professionals should explain the seriousness of the situation to the individual, family and significant others, giving time, support and understanding to make decisions about their own or their family member's care. People in this situation may deteriorate very quickly. If the respiratory system suddenly ceases, then apnoea occurs, and respiratory arrest follows. Resuscitation Council (UK) (2021b) guidelines should then be followed. Immediate causes of respiratory failure will be considered and treated accordingly.

Learning outcome 2: outline assessment skills, investigations and interventions for a person with an acute breathing problem

Individuals with acute breathing difficulties (like Tina Lunn) can use up considerable energy in trying to breathe and are often extremely anxious and frightened. Prompt and careful assessment and management of their breathlessness must occur. You should adopt a calm and confident approach to help alleviate their fears. Chapter 2 addresses communication in detail.

Box 14.29 Activity: assessment skills for an individual with an acute breathing problem

ACTIVITY

What assessment skills, investigations and interventions will be carried out to assess and care for an individual with an acute breathing problem? Tina Lunn's scenario will give some clues.

As discussed earlier, using an ABCDE framework will promote a systematic approach. You might have included the following.

Assessment

- airway patency (see earlier section);
- observation of effort, depth, rhythm and sound of breathing (see Chapter 4);
- pulse oximetry for measuring oxygen saturation (see Chapter 4);
- blood pressure and pulse measurement (see Chapter 4);
- capillary refill assessment (discussed later in this chapter);
- peak flow measurement (discussed later in this section);
- observation of sputum and sputum specimen collection (discussed later in this section);

- cardiac monitoring and electrocardiogram recording (discussed later in this chapter);
- temperature measurement (see Chapter 4) – as infection may be an underlying cause.

Investigations
- chest X-ray;
- blood tests – specifically venous blood gas or arterial blood gas analysis (see Box 14.30).

Interventions
- oxygen therapy (see the previous section);
- administration of inhalers and nebulisers (see Chapter 10);
- positioning in an upright position to aid lung expansion.

Observation of respiration and other vital signs are relevant to all the individuals in this chapter's scenarios. Mrs Patel may have a chest X-ray performed if there is concern about her developing a chest infection or heart failure. If Tina's condition does not improve with the nebulisers and oxygen prescribed, she might need to have a chest X-ray, which could require her being transferred to the emergency department at a different hospital. Mrs Patel, Mary and Tina may have blood gas analyses performed and all will require oxygen therapy. Tina will have her peak flow rate recorded, and a sputum specimen needs to be collected.

Learning outcome 3: measure and record a person's peak expiratory flow rate

Peak expiratory flow rate (PEFR) is a simple test of lung function. The peak flow meter measures an individual's ability to exhale. PEFR is recorded in litres per minute and is the maximum flow rate achieved on forced expiration, when starting at full inspiration. As previously identified, Tina is an asthmatic, so the measurement of her PEFR is particularly helpful. Asthma leads to a reduction of lung volume and variable obstruction of the airways. Asthma UK (a charity that supports people with asthma – see www.asthma.org.uk) recommends that people with asthma monitor their PEFR regularly. It is particularly useful for people who have difficulty recognising that their asthma control is worsening. See Asthma UK: manage your symptoms. Available from: https://www.asthma.org.uk/advice/manage-your-asthma/ (Accessed on 9 June 2021).

Venous blood gas analysis (VBG)

Venous blood gas analysis can be used in an emergency situation. They offer initial indications to healthcare practitioners about the respiratory and metabolic status of the individual. VBG reviews carbon dioxide and pH levels and is obtained from a sample taken via venepuncture. The blood test is analysed for acid–base balance. It is important to ascertain your local policy regarding your role and collections of this sample. Venous blood is obtained using venepuncture techniques and the sample is analysed to review treatment and management of acid–base balance in the body.

Capnography

This handheld device or monitor wave offers a non-invasive way to assist in the interpretation of the person's gaseous exchange. The capnography device fits to an intubation tube to give these results. Capnography offers the practitioner immediate results at the bedside until further analysis is available. The device is used in an emergency resuscitation situation and during anaesthesia and sedation events. It can advise practitioners regarding the individual's breath to breath carbon dioxide levels, the level of exhaled breath and their respiratory rate. The normal level ranges from 35 to 45 mm Hg. Arterial blood gases (ABGs) and VBGs sampling in an emergency situation can take time to obtain a specimen and analysis, so this device can assist in early recognition of gaseous exchange issues.

Box 14.30 Arterial blood gas analysis

- Arterial blood gas (ABG) is a blood test performed on arterial blood.
- Its purpose is to measure oxygen, carbon dioxide, bicarbonate levels and hydrogen concentration (pH) levels in the blood, thus providing an overview of the person's gaseous exchange, respiratory status and acid–base balance.
- The body's ability to regulate acid–base balance is crucial for survival; enzymes essential for biochemical reactions in cells function best within certain ranges of pH. Thus, impairment of body functions results from abnormal acid–base balance.
- The results of blood gas analysis affect treatment such as administration of medicines to adjust acidosis and oxygen therapy.

Procedure

- Taking an arterial sample of blood is an advanced skill that is carried out by a healthcare professional who has received appropriate training – doctors or registered nurses with additional education.
- Radial and femoral arteries are commonly used.
- The test can be painful and individuals undergoing the test need support.
- Local anaesthesia should be used, except in emergencies or if the person is unconscious or anaesthetised (O'Driscoll et al. 2017).
- After the needle has been withdrawn, pressure needs to be applied for about 5 min to prevent bleeding.
- The sample is analysed, and its components can offer vital evidence of
- well-being.
- People requiring regular blood gas analysis (e.g. those who are being mechanically ventilated) will have an arterial line setup, from which blood can be extracted when necessary.

See Kaufman, D. 2020 for more information Interpretation of ABGs. Available from: https://www.thoracic.org/professionals/clinical-resources/critical-care/clinical-education/abgs.php (Accessed on 9 June 2021).

Understanding peak expiratory flow rate measurement

Peak flow measurements are essential to know how well a person is able to blow air out of their lungs. Peak flow meters can be used by people with asthma to monitor and manage their condition and are often available on prescription. The readings are usually noted by the person and a diary kept of their readings. In an emergency situation when an individual experiences an asthma attack, it is important to know if they are responding to treatment such as nebulisers. So, a peak flow reading before and after a drug dose via nebuliser can assist in seeing improvement.

There are several types of peak flow meters available; the same peak flow meter should be used for a particular individual to ensure consistency. Figure 14.7 shows a peak flow meter that adheres to EU standard EN 13826 (see www.peakflow.com for details). Electronic peak flow meters are now available, and many people have their own devices. The standard meter measures up to 1000 L/min but low reading or paediatric meters are also available. These should be used for children and adults with widespread airways disease.

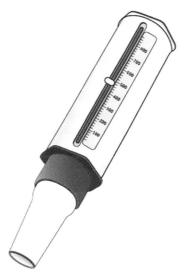

Figure 14.7: A peak flow meter that adheres to EU standard EN 13826.

Box 14.31 Activity: peak flow meter and mouthpiece

Access a peak flow meter and mouthpiece. Using the instructions and diagrams in Box 14.32, measure your PEFR, noting the measurements. Now work through the instructions/questions below:

1 Try measuring your PEFR while in a semi-upright position. How does it compare with your original reading? What does that tell you about positioning of s prior to PEFR measurements?
2 What would you do if a measurement seemed low?
3 How could PEFR measurements be recorded?
4 How often might PEFR be measured?

ACTIVITY

Points that you may have considered:

1. PEFR measurements can be misleading if the person is not positioned upright and does not use the correct technique.

2. If a low reading is obtained, you should confirm that the person's position and technique are correct. Then, as with any other observation, you would report the abnormal measurement to a senior clinician. Little can usually be deduced from a single PEFR measurement as a series is required to produce a comprehensive picture. However, a single low reading may need a quick response. Obviously, the person's general condition and other observations will be considered too.

3. In hospital, PEFR is often recorded simply as a figure at the bottom of the observation chart. There are special charts available, particularly for ongoing monitoring; these are often used for home PEFR monitoring.

4. Generally, twice-daily (morning and early evening) measurements are sufficient, except during acute episodes. PEFR measurements are often necessary to monitor medication effects, for example, inhaled bronchodilators. The PEFR is then measured before and 30 min after medication (when the medication is having the maximum effect).

Box 14.32 Measuring peak expiratory flow rate

- With the mouthpiece attached, hold the peak flow meter with the scale uppermost and the pointer at zero.
- Stand upright. Take a deep breath, close your lips around the peak flow meter and blow as hard as possible as if blowing birthday candles out.
- Take note of the reading and return the pointer to zero.
- Repeat the test twice more, taking note of each reading. Record the highest result.

What are normal PEFRs?

People are normally advised about their baseline PEFR, according to age, height and gender. European standards, EN 13826, for measuring PEFR (see www.peakflow.com), offer a chart for average PEFR readings. Generally, an adult should achieve 400–600 L/min, but males achieve a higher figure than females, and greater height increases the measurement. Even in individuals without asthma, there are variations in the measurement, with the morning figure being lower, and the highest being achieved in early evening. This tendency is likely to be exaggerated in people with asthma such as Tina. NICE (2020b) recommends that everyone who has asthma should be aware of their own personal PEFR values and judge their deterioration or improvement on their own values rather than relying on predicted values. It also recommends these values should form part of the person's asthma action plan, which is the personal plan for managing asthma, developed with the healthcare team. Tina may have her own asthma action plan and her PEFR should be compared with her 'normal' value and her immediate care should be based upon this plan.

Box 14.33 Activity: PEFR measurement

Why might teaching people who have asthma to measure their PEFR be useful in managing their condition?

You may have considered:

- To find out how well their asthma is controlled.
- Regular measurements may reveal a gradual (and possibly asymptomatic) deterioration, which requires action (e.g. change of medication) to prevent an acute episode. If the reading falls below 80% of an individual's best level, then preventive medicine (usually an inhaled steroid) should be increased (see www.asthma.org.uk).
- Without PEFR monitoring, people can be unaware of worsening symptoms; the measurement may fall by up to 50% before symptoms are noticed.
- Circumstances affecting measurements may be identified (e.g. contact with a cat), thus enabling asthma triggers to be recognised.
- The measurement may indicate the severity of the asthma at that particular time. The lower the measurement, the narrower the airways. A measurement of below 50% of the baseline requires immediate medical attention.
- To monitor how any change in medication is affecting respiratory status.

British Thoracic Society/Scottish Intercollegiate Guidelines Network (BTS/SIGN 2019) emphasises that teaching people to use inhalers and volumatic spacer devices and monitoring their PEFR should be only part of a comprehensive asthma management programme. This should also include instruction about avoiding asthma triggers, correct use of medication, identification of warning signs of worsening asthma and what action to take. Ongoing education and monitoring can be achieved through attending asthma clinics where the correct technique in PEFR measurement can be checked. Manual dexterity and coordination for using peak flow meters needs to be assessed. Asthma UK recommends that individuals keep a peak flow diary to identify significant issues or readings. The diary also offers the person and the healthcare team an overview of what is happening in their lungs, how effective medications are in treating breathlessness and average PEFR readings over a given period of time.

Spirometry

It is a test that can help diagnose lung function and identify how respiratory disease affects the lungs that uses a spirometer, a device consisting of a mouthpiece attached to a machine that measures the amount of air exhaled.

Despite the potential benefits of PEFR monitoring, long-term levels of use can be low, even in motivated people who have taken part in an educational programme. However, the introduction of electronic devices coupled with asthma health educational sessions at asthma clinics are just some of the steps that have been taken to improve this situation. Haynes (2018) identifies that in primary care settings, spirometry is used for the diagnosis and management of asthma and COPD. This assessment can take place in the community setting to ensure that individuals are fully aware of their diagnosis and can monitor the effects of their treatment and spirometry offers further objective feedback.

Learning outcome 4: describe how sputum expectoration can be encouraged and sputum specimens collected

The production of mucus by the respiratory tract acts as a moisturiser and helps protect the vital organs from drying out. Adults normally produce about 1–1.5 L per day of mucus in the respiratory tract, but it goes unnoticed as it is usually swallowed (Fahy and Dickey 2010). Mucus can trap particles of dust, allergens and smoke to further protect the body from harm. In those with cystic fibrosis, excess mucus is seen in the airways and a respiratory infection will exacerbate mucous production. The mucus clogs the airway and makes breathing out problematic for the person (see What Is Cystic Fibrosis. Available from: https://www.cff.org/What-is-CF/About-Cystic-Fibrosis/, Accessed on 9 June 2021). Smoking can also stimulate excessive mucus production. The mucus expectorated from the lungs is termed 'sputum'. Sputum consists of lower respiratory tract secretions, nasopharyngeal and oropharyngeal material (including saliva), microorganisms and cells (Rubin 2009). Clearance of secretions is very important to maintain a clear airway and reduce the risk of infection (Rubin 2009). However, individuals may deny the existence of sputum due to social stigma or lack of awareness, for example, in cases such as cystic fibrosis or those who smoke excessively. Some, particularly women, feel embarrassed to expectorate, and they are more likely to swallow their sputum.

ACTIVITY

Box 14.34 Encouraging expectoration of sputum

How can you encourage Tina to expectorate her sputum?

First, Tina needs to understand why it is important to clear her secretions. She will be able to cough more easily if in a well-supported, upright position, and a sputum pot and tissues should be provided. If she is well hydrated, her sputum will be less thick and therefore easier to cough up. A dry mouth makes expectoration difficult, and infected sputum can taste unpleasant. Therefore, you should provide mouth care or assist Tina to go the bathroom. Privacy should be given if there is embarrassment, and nurses should ensure that they do not show distaste even though they may feel it.

ACTIVITY

Box 14.35 Activity: normal vs abnormal sputum

How would you describe normal sputum? What do you think might cause sputum to look abnormal?

Sputum (or mucus) is odourless, clear and thin, but people who have respiratory disease may expectorate sputum, which is altered in colour and consistency. When assessing, it is important to identify what the individual's sputum is like normally. Signs of respiratory infection are sputum, which is green, yellow or rust in colour, and it may be odorous. Purulent green sputum in people with an acute exacerbation of their COPD is highly associated with infection (www.blf.org.uk). A *pseudomonas* infection produces thick green sputum with a characteristic odour.

A stringy mucoid specimen often occurs with bronchial asthma (www.asthma.org). If blood is present, the sputum will be rust or red in colour and is termed haemoptysis. It may be a sign of infection but can also occur in cancer, heart failure and pulmonary embolus. Haemoptysis can be distressing and it is important to check whether it has actually come from the lungs and has not been vomited (haematemesis) or come from the nose (epistaxis). Haemoptysis is worsened by vigorous coughing, chest trauma, chest physiotherapy, anticoagulant therapy and activity. When assessing the amount being produced, it is best to ask in terms of teaspoons, tablespoons or cups. Individuals may comment on the sputum's taste, which may be unpleasant if infected or salty with cystic fibrosis.

When sputum is being produced, especially in suspected respiratory disease, a specimen is often required for laboratory examination. You will remember that Tina has been asked to produce a sputum specimen as she may have a chest infection. The goal of sputum collection is to gain a fresh, uncontaminated specimen of secretions from the tracheobronchial tree (Warrell et al. 2012). The lower respiratory tract can be colonised by many different bacteria; collection of a sputum specimen can help identify which bacteria are causing an infection.

Box 14.36 Activity: sputum specimen

Why might a sputum specimen need to be sent to the laboratory?

A sputum specimen may be sent for microbiological examination if infection, including tuberculosis (TB), is suspected. It may also be sent for cytology – examination for abnormal (e.g. cancerous) cells. Box 14.37 outlines the equipment needed, and the procedure and additional points are discussed below.

Box 14.37 Key points in collecting a sputum specimen

Equipment needed

- A sterile specimen container with a leak-proof lid or cap, and tissues.

Key points

- An early-morning specimen is best, as bacteria counts are probably highest then.
- Careful explanation is needed.
- The mouth should be rinsed with water and teeth brushed to prevent contamination with oral microbes.
- The sputum should be expectorated directly into the labelled container and the lid reapplied immediately.

When a sputum specimen is collected, it must come from the lower airways rather than being cleared from the throat or saliva. This needs to be explained carefully to the person, taking into account level of understanding. You can explain that the specimen must come from the 'windpipe'. Sputum is usually more viscous and purulent than saliva; if the specimen appears to be saliva, it should be discarded. A physiotherapist can assist people who have difficulty expectorating.

When sputum is being sent for testing for TB, the specimen should be at least 10 ml. Three early-morning specimens taken on different days are required as *Mycobacterium tuberculosis*, which causes TB, may only be present in small numbers, particularly in the disease's early stages (Shepherd 2017). As *Mycobacterium tuberculosis* has very resistant cell walls, it is stained using a special dye that cannot be removed by acid or alcohol. This method is termed the 'acid-fast bacilli' or AFB test (Shepherd 2017). Most bacteria grow within 24–48 h, but the *Mycobacterium tuberculosis* can take up to 6 weeks to grow (Wilkins et al. 2010). Nevertheless, microscopic examination of the sputum can lead to an initial tentative diagnosis.

Box 14.38 Children and young people: practice points – breathing problems

Assessment and management of airway and breathing in infants and children is significantly different in comparison with adults due to the anatomical and physical features. Children are more likely to suffer a respiratory arrest, whereas adults are more likely to suffer a cardiac arrest.

For respiratory assessment see:

Veal, Z., McAlinden, O. and Crawford, D. 2018. Care of children and young people with respiratory problems In: Price J. and McAlinden O. (eds.) *Essentials of Nursing Children and Young People*. London: Sage, 270–84.

Royal College of Nursing (RCN). 2017. Standards for assessing, measuring and monitoring vital signs in infants, children and young people. Available from: https://www.rcn.org.uk/professional-development/publications/pub-005942 (Accessed on 9 May 2021).

Resuscitation Council (UK): Paediatric Life Support. Available from: https://www.resus.org.uk/training-courses/paediatric-life-support (Accessed on 9 June 2021).

For PEFR measurements in children see:

Gormley-Fleming, E. and Martin, D. (eds.). 2018. Peak expiratory flow. In: *Children and Young People's Nursing Skills at a glance*. Chichester: Wiley, 56–57.

A free to use online learning resource called Spotting the Sick Child is recommended for professionals.

See here: https://spottingthesickchild.com/

Summary

- There are many reasons for acute breathing problems. These situations can be frightening and so a calm, confident approach is necessary.
- You need to understand the assessment skills, investigations and interventions that may be needed and develop your skills to assist people with acute breathing problems.

- Peak flow measurements are important indicators of respiratory function, particularly in people who have asthma. They must be recorded accurately and consistently, as they may influence treatment.
- Nursing measures can encourage expectoration of sputum, which can then be observed for colour, consistency, amount and odour.
- Careful explanations can help ensure that an uncontaminated sputum specimen is obtained.

CIRCULATORY PROBLEMS AND RELATED SKILLS

An effective circulation requires a functioning cardiovascular system and adequate blood volume. A range of symptoms result when abnormalities occur, so effective assessment skills and interventions are needed to support individuals with circulatory problems.

Box 14.39 Learning outcomes

By the end of this section, you will be able to:

1 identify common causes of acute circulatory problems and key aspects of assessment;
2 describe the term 'capillary refill time' and be able to perform the skill;
3 attach an individual to a cardiac monitor and recognise sinus rhythm;
4 outline how a 12-lead electrocardiograph is recorded.

Learning outcome 1: identify common causes of acute circulatory problems and key aspects of assessment

There are many causes of circulatory problems.

Box 14.40 Activity: Mrs Patel's circulatory problem

ACTIVITY

With regard to reading Mrs Patel's scenario. Can you identify possible causes of a circulatory problem?

You read that Mrs Patel has an abnormality in her heart's conduction system (atrial fibrillation), which will affect her circulation. You also know that she would have lost blood from her circulation during surgery and is continuing to do so. A reduction in blood volume (due to fluid loss or haemorrhage) can lead to hypovolaemia and then shock. Shock is a complex condition leading to a cascade of physiological reactions in the body. It is caused by an underlying medical condition or trauma; if left unmanaged, it can be life-threatening. Your biology book will give a detailed explanation – see Box 14.41 for a few key points.

In shock, there is a reduction in the person's cardiac output and significant changes occur in their vital signs. It is important to find the cause of shock and treat it quickly. Mrs Patel has a lot of drainage from her wound and changes in her vital signs. Thus, her rate of intravenous fluid administration may be increased to boost the circulating fluid volume, or a blood transfusion may be commenced (see Chapter 10).

Anaphylactic shock is caused by an allergic reaction, when a person is exposed to and reacts to a trigger that causes airway compromise, breathing difficulties and circulatory compromise. This is often associated with urticaria (raised itchy rash). The incidence of allergic reaction within the United Kingdom (UK) is increasing and related fatalities have been reported. The Resuscitation Council (UK) (see www.resus.org.uk) produces guidelines to help practitioners recognise and respond to allergic reactions immediately. Please refer to these guidelines for up-to-date information on actions and drugs of choice in dealing with this emergency situation.

Box 14.41 Shock: key points

- Shock is a potentially recoverable but significant reduction in circulating blood volume that leads to inadequate tissue perfusion.
- The inability to deliver oxygen and nutrients to body tissues leads to metabolic and functional impairment and hypoxia.

Types of shock

- Hypovolaemia – low blood volume.
- Cardiogenic shock – due to the heart's inability to pump blood around the body efficiently (e.g. following MI).
- Anaphylactic shock – a severe allergic reaction (see 'Preventing and managing anaphylaxis' in Chapter 10).
- Septic shock – occurs in severe infection. The systemic inflammatory response causes vasodilatation of peripheral blood vessels, increased capillary permeability and thus extravascular fluid loss.
- Neurogenic shock – rapid loss of vasomotor tone leads to vasodilation and a severe decrease in blood pressure.
- Emotional shock – emotion triggers or past events can stimulate the parasympathetic nervous system leading to vasovagal syncope (unconsciousness). Spontaneous recovery usually occurs within a few minutes.

How will you know a person is in shock?

There are four stages of shock: initial, compensatory, progressive and refractory (Summers 2020) (Garretson and Malberti 2007).

- *Initial* – the body shows signs of reduced cardiac output.
- *Compensatory* – the body attempts to restore homeostasis and improve tissue perfusion.
- *Progressive* – the body loses its ability to compensate, bringing about acidosis and electrolyte imbalance.
- *Refractory* – irreversible cell damage occurs and the body's organs are affected.

As the person's condition deteriorates, their vital signs may change. You may notice changes in the persons NEWS2 scoring. This will include potential changes in the persons ACVPU scale, changes in respiratory heart rate and blood pressure. These changes are due to physiological changes in the body that result in physical changes in the person's body. The body first tries to compensate by moving fluids around from within the cells to the circulation, attempting to maintain blood pressure in a normal range. However, there may be a slight rise in the heart rate. As the body loses the ability to compensate, respiratory rate rises as the body tries to apply as much oxygen as possible on to the remaining red blood cells and deliver them to the cells. As this body mechanism fails, the body becomes overwhelmed. Acidosis and electrolyte imbalance follow, with the individual becoming cold, clammy, less responsive and confused. Eventually, the body becomes overwhelmed and death will occur if these signs of deterioration are not seen and treated appropriately.

ACTIVITY

Box 14.42 Development of shock
Look back at Mrs Patel's scenario. Are there any indications that she is developing shock?

In the scenario, Mrs Patel has lost a lot of blood, so she will start to show signs of shock at an early stage. Her heart and respiratory rates are rising and her blood pressure is falling. There may also be evidence of Mrs Patel becoming confused or less responsive. However, Mrs Patel's body has an ability to compensate for a short time during shock responses, and each person responds to shock differently.

Assessment and management of an individual who is in shock should follow a systematic ABCDE approach, as discussed earlier in this chapter. Measuring vital signs and calculating a NEWS2 score – including CRT, conscious level (ACVPU), heart rate, blood pressure and urine output – are all important for people in shock. When the body is under threat and fluids are lost, the renal system attempts to rectify this by diminishing the amount of fluid the body loses or excretes. Thus, the individual in shock may have a urinary catheter inserted, with hourly urine measurements being recorded (see Chapter 6 for urinary catheterisation procedure). To further assist with monitoring, those who are critically ill might have a central venous pressure line inserted and/or an arterial line.

Central venous pressure line (CVP)

A central venous catheter might be inserted when a person is showing signs of deterioration. This is to facilitate central venous pressure (CVP) monitoring. Typically, a CVP line is inserted into the jugular, subclavian or brachial veins; the catheter tip will lie in the superior vena cava. CVP monitoring assists in assessment of circulating blood volume and identification of circulatory failure. CVP measurements must be interpreted in conjunction with other vital signs and NEWS scoring, with the trends of all observations and findings assessed rather than a single measurement being acted upon. If Mrs Patel continued to deteriorate, CVP monitoring might be commenced as it would help to carefully manage fluid replacement while preventing overloading her – a particular danger with her cardiac condition. CVP monitoring is an advanced skill: https://www.oxfordmedicaleducation.com/clinical-skills/procedures/central-line/ explains this procedure in detail central line (central venous catheter) insertion.

The use of a CVP line and its measurement in guiding fluid management is debated by De Backer and Vincent (2018). While they acknowledge this procedure is a frequently used variable to guide fluid management, they highlight how many have challenged its use. However, De Backer and Vincent (2018) recognise the value of such a reading to assist in fluid replacement therapy of a person who is critically ill. Complications from the insertion of a CVP line include infection, embolus or haemorrhage, so it is imperative that this line is handled carefully and its use is monitored throughout.

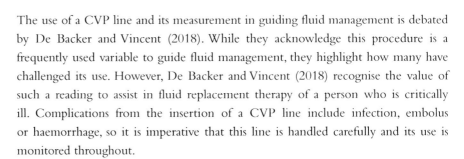

Box 14.43 CVP measurements and their indications

When in the practice setting, identify whether anyone is having their CVP measured. Ask a healthcare professional to explain why they are having CVP monitoring and how this procedure is carried out. Discuss what the CVP measurements indicate about their condition.

Arterial line

An arterial line is inserted into an artery. As with central lines, this is an invasive procedure with potential complications, many of which are similar to those associated with central lines. The main reason for inserting an arterial line is to allow continuous arterial blood pressure monitoring and arterial blood sampling. Arterial BP recordings have greater accuracy than the non-invasive methods for BP recording (Pierre and Keenaghan 2020). This is due to arterial lines allowing direct measurement via the cannula placed in the artery. A variety of arterial sites may be used to achieve this recording (e.g. radial, brachial and femoral). This is an advanced skill carried out by qualified practitioners; however, you may be required to assist with this procedure.

Box 14.44 Activity: arterial line management

In your practice area, identify if anyone who has arterial lines in situ. Ask a healthcare professional to explain how these lines are managed according to trust policy.

Learning outcome 2: describe the term 'capillary refill time' and be able to perform the skill

To assess CRT, cutaneous pressure is exerted on the person's fingertip for 5 s and released. The finger should be held at heart level or just above and the pressure should be enough to cause blanching (Resuscitation Council 2021a). The test indicates capillary perfusion. Normally, CRT is less than 2 s. Situations where CRT is increased include shock, dehydration, aortic aneurysm, aortic occlusion, cardiac tamponade, hypothermia and Raynaud's syndrome.

Raynaud's syndrome

A condition causing constriction of small blood vessels, usually in the hands and feet.

Box 14.45 Activity: capillary refill

ACTIVITY

Depress the tip of your finger for 5 s, then release the pressure and watch the blood return to your capillaries. Now, repeat the test and time the return of the blood to your finger. This should be less than 2 s, usually the time it takes you to say 'capillary refill'.

Learning outcome 3: attach an individual to a cardiac monitor and recognise sinus rhythm

You read that Mrs Patel had a cardiac monitor attached postoperatively. The paramedics would have attached cardiac monitoring to Mary, which will be continued on her arrival at the hospital. Cardiac monitoring is carried out for many acutely ill individuals and where heart rhythm is, or may become, abnormal (e.g. cardiac conditions, electrolyte imbalance, poisoning, hypothermia). You may have seen this equipment on placement or in the skills laboratory.

Box 14.46 Activity: cardiac monitoring equipment

ACTIVITY

When you are next in your practice area, see what types of cardiac monitoring equipment are available. How many leads are attached to the person and where?

You may have observed three or five leads being attached for monitoring. With three-lead monitoring, there are three standard bipolar leads, I, II and III: red, yellow and green (or black) (see Figure 14.8). With five-lead monitoring, lead colours can vary so check the equipment coding and seek guidance as required. The monitor leads are connected

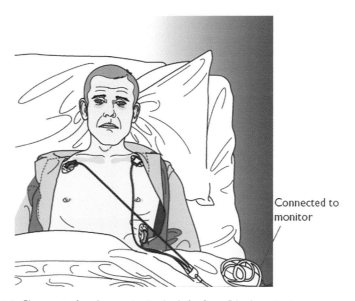

Connected to monitor

Figure 14.8: Placement of cardiac monitoring leads for 3- or 5-lead monitoring.

to adhesive electrode pads placed on the individual's chest. The cardiac monitor detects voltage differences within the body surface and amplifies and displays these as a signal (Hampton and Hampton 2019). The device can offer useful information to healthcare professionals, such as indicating myocardial ischaemia and cardiac arrhythmias.

Box 14.47 outlines key points for cardiac monitoring. The ECG produces a graphic recording of the heart's electrical impulses producing a PQRST complex (Hampton and Hampton 2019). Figure 14.9 shows the PQRST complex and briefly identifies what each part of the complex denotes (see Hampton and Hampton 2019 for more detail).

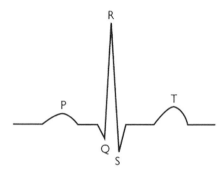

P wave: represents atrial depolarisation prior to atrial contraction.
QRS: represents depolarisation of the ventricles prior to ventricular contraction:
– **Q:** the first downward deflection
– **R:** the first upward deflection
– **S:** the first downward deflection following the R wave
T wave: the next positive wave which shows ventricular repolarisation.

Figure 14.9: The PQRST complex.

Box 14.47 Cardiac monitoring: key points

- First establish the individual's identity and rationale for cardiac monitoring.
- Inform the person about the procedure and gain their cooperation and verbal consent.
- Check that the person does not have a cardiac pacemaker in situ. If they do, seek advice before connecting any monitoring equipment, as some devices can interfere with cardiac pacemakers.
- Assemble all equipment: cardiac monitor and ECG leads, skin-pad electrodes, alcohol wipe and razor.
- Ensure that the skin is clean and free from grease as the electrodes will not adhere to the chest fully otherwise. With consent, shave or trim any chest hair to ensure that the electrodes will stick.
- Place electrodes on the chest (see Figure 14.8).
- Turn on the monitor and adjust the setting to lead I, II or III as directed. Lead II is usually chosen as it shows a positive R wave and a clear P wave.
- Check whether the person is comfortable and that the cardiac monitor is recording. Take note of the rate and rhythm of the heart and report if there is an abnormality. If unsure, ask a senior colleague to review with you.
- Record that you have commenced cardiac monitoring in the relevant notes.

Once connected to a monitor, you may observe that the individual has a 'normal' heart rhythm (sinus rhythm), portraying that electrical impulses are travelling from the SA node to the atrioventricular node, down the septum of the heart, into the Bundle of His and then the left and right bundle branches and the Purkinje fibres. If you need to remind yourself about this physiology, read about the heart's conduction system in your biology book. However, Mrs Patel's heart rhythm is known to be atrial fibrillation.

ACTIVITY

Box 14.48 Activity: Mrs Patel's pulse

Look at the two rhythm strips in Figure 14.10 that show sinus rhythm and atrial fibrillation. What differences can you see? Look at the following for each strip:

- the rate – frequency of the complex;
- the regularity of each complex occurring;
- whether P waves are present and precede each QRS.

Now, think about what you would feel if taking Mrs Patel's pulse. How might it differ from the pulse of a person with sinus rhythm?

You will have noticed that, unlike in sinus rhythm, in atrial fibrillation, 'P' waves cannot be identified. This is because the atria are 'fibrillating' rather than contracting, and the impulses are conducted through the atrioventricular node irregularly, so the QRS complexes appear irregularly. You will see that the QRS complexes occur more frequently as often uncontrolled atrial fibrillation leads to a more rapid heart rate. If you were feeling Mrs Patel's pulse, it would feel irregularly irregular. This observation is an important indicator of atrial fibrillation and it should be reported. In this section, you have learned how to attach a cardiac monitor, how to observe a rhythm strip and how to recognise one common arrhythmia, atrial fibrillation.

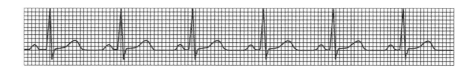

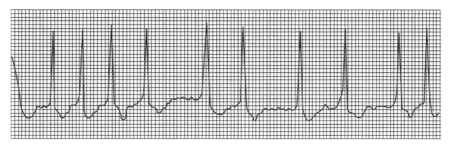

Figure 14.10: Comparison of sinus rhythm and atrial fibrillation.

Box 14.49 Activity: attaching a cardiac monitor to a colleague

ACTIVITY

You may be able to practise attaching a cardiac monitor to a colleague in the skills laboratory. If so, ask them to move around and then to simulate cleaning teeth. Note how this muscle movement affects the cardiac monitor's rhythm display.

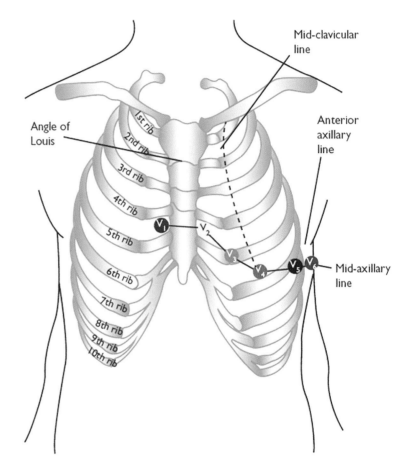

Figure 14.11: Placement of chest leads for 12-lead ECG.

There are many textbooks, websites and applications that look in detail at interpreting arrhythmias, so access them for further reading about arrhythmias.

Remember: Observing a cardiac monitor is no substitute for observing the person. The observations previously discussed – vital signs and capillary refill – must also be carried out during your assessment.

Learning outcome 4: outline how a 12-lead electrocardiograph is recorded

The 12-lead ECG is a useful diagnostic tool and can comprehensively illustrate the individual's heart rhythm and rate.

ACTIVITY

> ### Box 14.50 Activity: ECG recording
>
> Mrs Patel is to have an ECG recorded as she is known to have atrial fibrillation. In what other situations might an ECG be recorded? Think back to when you have seen an ECG recorded in practice.

ECGs are often recorded as a routine investigation before anaesthesia, particularly in older people, to identify myocardial ischaemia, in people with electrolyte imbalances and when the heart may be affected by drugs. The ECG is also recorded in emergency situations, for example, individuals who have collapsed, and people with a history of a fall. Therefore, Enid might have an ECG recorded, either in the community, when her GP visits, at the health centre by the practice nurse or if she is referred to a hospital.

Electrical impulses precede cardiac muscle (myocardium) contraction, so this electrical impulse is captured and recorded in an ECG. Waveforms vary in different leads placed on the person's body, and the ECG records the conduction of electrical impulses through the heart from different points. Think of taking a picture with a camera and obtaining a 360° view of the person's heart from various positions around their bed. For more detail about the physiology underpinning ECGs and their interpretation, refer to your physiology textbook and specialist cardiology books (e.g. Iaizzo 2015). This section focuses on the practice of recording an ECG; Box 14.51 provides key practice points for recording ECGs.

Placement of the 4 ECG leads on the limbs

The 12-lead ECG uses 10 electrodes (sometimes referred to as 'leads') to obtain the reading: 6 are placed on the person's chest and 1 on each of the 4 limbs. All ECG machines use the same principle of recording electrical impulses from the heart but more wireless machines are now available. The placement of these electrodes offers 12 views of electrical activity in different areas of the heart – hence, the name 12-lead ECG.

The four limb leads (which are labelled) are placed as follows:

- RA on right arm;
- LA on left arm;
- LL on left leg;
- RL on right leg – this plays no part in the actual reading other than providing an earth.

> ### Box 14.51 Recording ECGs: key points
>
> - Assemble the equipment: ECG machine, alcohol wipes, tissues, razor (to trim chest hair, if necessary), disposable pre-gelled electrodes.
> - Identify the individual, explain the procedure and gain their verbal consent.
> - Ensure the person's privacy and dignity is maintained during the procedure.
> - Position the individual in a semi-recumbent position if their clinical condition allows; otherwise, record the ECG in the position they are comfortable in.
>
> *(Continued)*

Box 14.51 (Continued)

- Plug in the ECG machine to the DC power supply or ensure that the machine's battery is fully charged.
- Perform hand hygiene.
- Clean the person's skin, where the electrodes are to be applied, with an alcohol wipe and remove excess chest hair if the electrodes will not adhere to the skin.
- Apply the electrodes to the limbs and chest: for chest lead positions, see Figure 14.11.
- Connect the ECG leads to these electrodes, placing the lead box on the abdomen.
- Switch on the ECG machine, check calibration of the machine and ECG size.
- Set the paper speed at 25 mm/s unless otherwise instructed.
- Enter the person's name, date of birth, date and time of procedure if the ECG machine has these facilities.
- Inform them you are going to now record the ECG and advise them not to move, speak or cough but to breathe normally. Print the ECG. Remember that movement will affect the reading and be seen as an artefact on the ECG, and then the test will have to be repeated.
- Advise the individual that you have completed the test. Attempt to reassure them as this may be an anxious time.
- Advise that the ECG will now be reviewed by a nurse or doctor trained in this procedure. Do not make any attempt to offer a diagnosis at this stage and avoid suggesting the test was 'all right' as they may misinterpret this as an indication that their ECG shows no signs of disease or problem.
- Labelling – If this has not been entered before the procedure, note the person's details now on the ECG printout. Do not allow anyone to remove the ECG from the machine before you label it. Record if they have chest pain or not at this stage. If this is a serial ECG, also write the number on it. If it was a 15-lead ECG, note this too.
- Disconnect the ECG leads from the individual, make them comfortable and assist them to redress, if necessary.
- Document that you have recorded an ECG.
- Clean the ECG machine before returning it to its storage place and reconnecting it to the DC power supply.
- Show the ECG to a competent practitioner and assist in any treatment that is now required.

If the individual is an amputee, place the electrode on the stump.

The placement of these leads forms six standard leads: three bipolar leads (I, II, III) and three augmented vector leads (aVR, aVL, aVF). These limb leads record electrical activity in the following areas:

- I, II and aVL – the lateral aspect of the heart;
- III and aVF – the inferior aspect of the heart;
- aVR – the right atrium.

Placement of the four limb leads on the torso

In some clinical situations, the limb leads may be placed on the torso when the limbs cannot be used. There will be a difference in the depth and height of the waves recorded if leads are placed on the torso rather than the limbs that will affect the reading of the ECG. Ask a member of the team to show you the differences in what you see. You may have observed a shift in the cardiac axis to the right, a smaller R wave in lead 1 and smaller Q waves in the inferior leads.

Placement of the six chest leads

The six chest leads provide the other six views and are colour-coded and labelled: red (V1), yellow (V2), green (V3), brown (V4), black (V5) and purple (V6). These leads are placed on the torso (see Figure 14.11):

- V1 – at the fourth intercostal space, approximately 1–2 cm right of the sternum;
- V2 – at the fourth intercostal space, approximately 1–2 cm left of the sternum;
- V4 – at the left side of the chest at the fifth intercostal space on the mid-clavicular line;
- V3 – midway between V2 and V4;
- V5 – at the fifth intercostal space at level of V4 (anterior axilla, halfway between V4 and V6);
- V6 – at the same level as V4 and V5, at the mid-axilla line.

These chest leads record electrical activity in the following areas (see Hampton 2008):

- V1 and V2 – right ventricle;
- V3 and V4 – septum and anterior wall of the left ventricle;
- V5 and V6 – anterior and lateral walls of left ventricle.

Box 14.52 Activity: intercostal spaces on the chest

ACTIVITY

Look at Figure 14.11 and try feeling for the fourth and fifth intercostal spaces on your own chest in front of the mirror.

Using additional electrodes for the 15 lead ECG recording

The ECG lead placement can be extended to improve the views of the heart. In some instances, in practice, you may see 15-lead ECGs being recorded using extra lead placements. These additional leads sometimes used in ECG recordings are:

- Posterior leads: V7, V8, V9: these are positioned in order following V6, along the 5th intercostal space.
- Right-sided leads: Leads can be placed on the right side of the chest to enable better views of the right ventricle. These are placed in a 'mirror image' of the left chest leads and will be labelled accordingly: V2R, V3R, V4R, V5R and V6R. Not all of these will necessarily be used – V4R is most often used in practice.

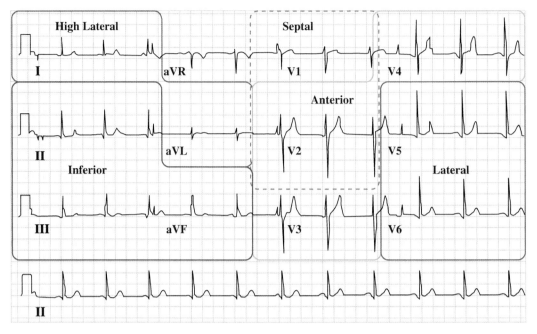

Figure 14.12: The 12-lead ECG and what it can show.

You must ensure that the ECG is labelled to indicate the additional leads used. Where additional leads are placed may vary so follow local policy and guidance.

Now review the ECG above and see if you can identify where the leads are situated on the individual and what areas of the heart they review.

What the ECG shows you

The ECG looks at the heart regions through a variety of leads.

- I and AVL – high lateral
- II and III and aVF – inferior
- V2, V3 and V4 anterior
- V1 and V2 septal
- V5 and V 6 lateral
- Leads I, II and III can tell you about cardiac axis.

How to read an ECG in a systematic way

Try to adopt a systematic approach as you review the ECG. It is significant to note here that if the individual is symptomatic at any stage of your review, this should be acted upon immediately and the appropriate care given, e.g. basic life support, analgesia or senior review. Otherwise, continue as follows.

Firstly establish the person's name, date of birth and identification/hospital number to ensure this ECG refers to the correct individual.

Now looking at the ECG, you will see a series of large and small squares. Think of this as a graph that plots the heart's electric conduction system and captures a moment in time, to tell us what the heart is doing in 1 min. This graph has X and Y axes.

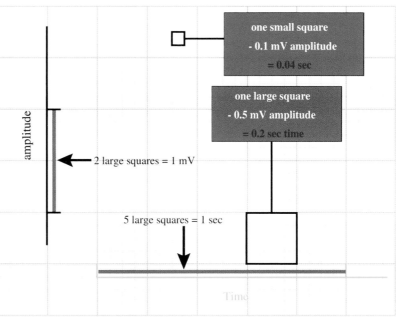

Figure 14.13: Time and voltage.

ECG Complex
Showing Time and Voltage Scales

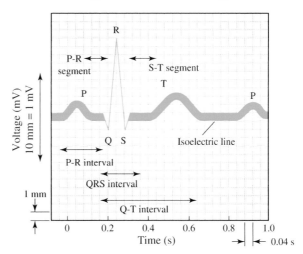

Figure 14.14: ECG complex time and voltage.

The vertical (*X* axis) shows amplitude/voltage, while the horizontal (*Y* axis) shows time.(see Figures 14.13 and 14.14)

The graph and the squares

Each square represents time.

One small square = 0.04 second

5 small squares (1 large square) = 0.2 second

5 large squares = 1 second

30 large squares = 6 seconds

300 large squares = 60 seconds

The paper speed of an ECG runs at 25mm/s.

Now look at the rhythm strip on the ECG

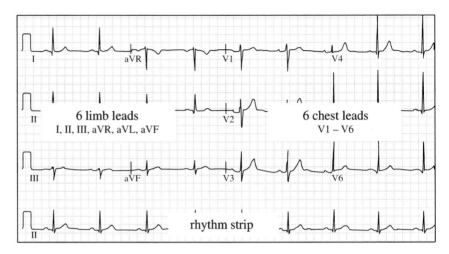

Figure 14.15: The 12-lead ECG (1).

Next look at the rhythm strip

Ask yourself does this look like a regular rhythm? (as shown above)

OR does it look irregular? (as shown below (see Figure 14.16))

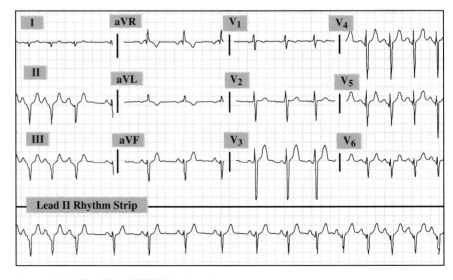

Figure 14.16: The 12-lead ECG(2) rhythm strip.

Remember that the squares/blocks indicate time along the Y axis.

Now look at the overall picture on the graph

(see Figures 14.17 and 14.18)

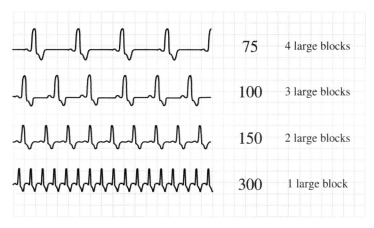

Figure 14.17: Calculating the heart rate.

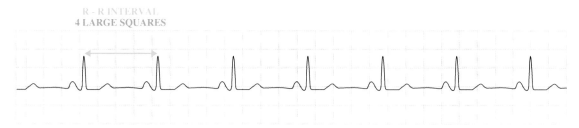

Heart Rate = 300 ÷ (number of large squares in one R - R interval)

$$300 \div 4 = 75 \text{ BPM}$$

Heart Rate = 75 BPM

Figure 14.18: Heart rate is 75.

Step 1 Interpreting regular or irregular rhythm

Regular rhythm

Look at the heart rate, e.g. 75.

Measure heart rate by counting number of large squares between successive QRS complexes and divide by 300, e.g. 300 divided by 4 = 75.

Irregular rhythm

Measure heart rate by counting the number of QRS complexes in a 6-s interval and multiply by 10.

10 QRS = 6 s (30 large squares)

100 QRS complexes 60 s (300 large squares)

Step 2 Calculating rate

Rate – is it normal, fast or slow. Use a normal sinus rhythm ECG to get started here and see the difference in a slow or fast rhythm.

Regular or irregular rhythm.

P waves – are they present?

Do they appear before an QRS complex?

QRS is the complex narrow (normal) or broad (prolonged).

Step 3 cardiac axis

Cardiac axis offers us an overall direction of electrical activity on the heart.

Normal, leftward, rightward or indeterminate. Normal axis of the heart is from −30 to +90 degrees.

Start by looking at Leads I and II. Ask yourself do they travel in the same direction? That is, are they both positive above the isoelectric line?

Lead I up, lead II up = normal

Or do they have lead I up, lead II down? = left axis deviation

Lead I down, lead II up? = right axis deviation

Step 4 P waves

The P wave is indicative of atrial activity. It shows us depolarisation of the left and right atria. It is concerned with atrial contraction. If a P wave is present, it indicates atrial activity. If no P waves are present, this would indicate a more serious situation of a broad, prolonged complex.

Step 5 P–R interval

The P wave should ideally be followed by a QRS complex, as that of our normal sinus rhythm ECG. The P–R interval is a timed event and is normally between 0.12 and 0.20 seconds. This represents the time interval from atrial activity to the start of ventricular activity. If this section of the ECG is affected, it can indicate heart block. These heart blocks range from first degree, second degree, type I and type 2 and third degree or complete.

Step 6 QRS complex

In a healthy heart, the electrical impulses spread over the ventricles and ventricular depolarisation occurs. This is seen as a QRS complex. This should be reviewed for its width, height and shape. Width is narrow or broad, height is small or tall, morphology is about the individual complex. If this wave pattern becomes wide, it can be an indication that a problem is occurring with depolarisation. Issues with muscle activity can be an indication of electrolyte imbalance, toxicity and poisoning.

Q waves can be seen in isolation and can be normal. However, a full lead of Q waves on an ECG is a cause for concern indicating that a previous MI or acute cardiac event has occurred. This related to previous medical history, can assist the practitioner in answering any concerns about the ECG findings.

Step 7 ST segment

In a normal ECG, it is along the isoelectric line. The ST segment is referred to as being normal, elevated or depressed. It is where ventricular depolarisation and repolarisation occur. This segment of the ECG indicates acute MI, left or right bundle branch issues or pericarditis. This ST elevation can be seen in various leads and can give the healthcare practitioner an indication that the heart is affected in specific areas. For example, V1 and V2 relate to the septum and indicate septal changes. V3 and V4 relate to the anterior area of the heart and indicate anterior changes. Leads I, aVL, V5 and V6 relate to the lateral area of the heart and indicate lateral changes and Leads II, III and aVF relate to the inferior area of the heart and indicate inferior changes. These changes in an ECG will also be accompanied with symptoms of chest pain, nausea, and in certain situations, may be a precursor to acute coronary syndrome or eventual death. It is imperative that the individual's symptoms are immediately reviewed and that local protocols are followed, so that immediate intervention can occur thus improving outcome and survival.

Step 8 T waves

The T wave represents ventricular repolarisation. It is normally a gradual upstroke and a rapid downstroke. The T can however be affected in some individuals, for example, those who have ischaemia of the myocardium or coronary heart disease. Changes in this wave require further investigation and treatment.

Learning to approach ECGs in a systematic way will assist in your knowledge and skills of interpretation. Look at as many ECGs as you can in a clinical area and look at the individual to see what signs and symptoms they display in comparison with their ECG.

Monitoring devices used after initial ECG recording – telemetry

Once an ECG has been performed, it may be necessary to observe and monitor vital signs including their heart rhythm on a continuous basis. The development of telemetry devices has enabled individuals to be continually monitored while remaining mobile. Telemetry devices are small wifi/bluetooth devices that monitor ECG and also record respiratory rate, SpO_2. These devices can be used in the hospital setting or in the community. They enable the individual to be mobile and active while being monitored thus relieving them from bedside monitoring devices. The results can be fed back to a central device that is monitored by clinicians.

ACTIVITY

Box 14.53 Activity: ECG recording

If possible, while in your healthcare setting, observe an ECG being recorded and then record one under supervision. An ECG technician, or clinician, might be able to assist you with this activity. Look at the ECG recorded and observe the differences in how the PQRST complex appears in the 12 different views. In some practice areas, you may see a 15-lead ECG being recorded.

Use the step method to begin to identify the areas shown on the ECG and consider as many normal sinus rhythm ECGs as you can then move on to reviewing more complex ECGs.

Always continue to observe and assess at regular intervals, while people are in your care. ECGs are a tool for assessment and should not be viewed in isolation from vital signs and other individual observations.

Box 14.54 Children and young people: practice points – circulatory problems

For management of circulatory problems in children, see the following sources:

Glasper, A., Coad, J. and Richardson, J. (eds.). 2015. *Infant resuscitation and Young Person Resuscitation in Children and Young People's Nursing at a Glance.* Chichester: Wiley-Blackwell 44–47.

Royal College of Nursing (RCN). 2017. Standards for assessing, measuring and monitoring vital signs in infants, children and young people. Available from: https://www.rcn.org.uk/professional-development/publications/pub-005942 (Accessed on 9June 2021).

Resuscitation Council (UK): Paediatric Basic Life Support. Available from: https://www.resus.org.uk/library/2021-resuscitation-guidelines/paediatric-basic-life-support-guidelines (Accessed on 9 June 2021).

For ECGs in children, see:

Gormley-Fleming, E. 2010. Assessment and vital signs: A comprehensive review. In: Glasper, A. Aylott, M. and Battrick, C. (eds.) *Developing Practical Skills for Nursing Children and Young People.* London: Hodder Arnold, 109–148.

Summary

- Assessment of an individual's physiological parameters of pulse and blood pressure are important aspects of the ABCDE assessment.
- Recognising and responding to signs of shock in individuals is essential in nursing practice.
- Clinical skills such as measuring capillary refill are simple to learn and greatly assist in your assessment. Practice these skills and take time in refining them.
- Cardiac monitoring and the recording of a 12-/15-lead ECG are more complex skills that will require direct supervision at first, and then as you gain

knowledge and experience in a variety of settings, you will become competent in these skills and understand their significance.

UNCONSCIOUSNESS AND RELATED SKILLS

Our awake state is known as consciousness, while unconsciousness is defined as when an individual's awareness no longer exists. Normal reflexes protecting conscious individuals are lost and so healthcare professionals must maintain their safety and provide all care needed. For initial assessment of an unconscious person, look back to Chapter 4 for an overview of how to carry out a neurological assessment – ACVPU and the GCS – and ensure that you can conduct these assessments before continuing with this section as they are necessary for anyone with altered conscious level. There are many causes of unconsciousness including abnormal temperature, oxygen or blood glucose levels, infection (e.g. encephalitis, meningitis), drug intoxication, seizures, focal head injury (trauma), hypoxia, hypercarbia (high levels of carbon dioxide in the circulating blood) or vascular events (shock, stroke). Investigations will be conducted to determine the underlying cause. In this section, general care of an unconscious person is considered, followed by a review of blood glucose monitoring, which will be carried out for a person with altered consciousness and also management of seizures.

Box 14.55 Learning outcomes

By the end of this section, you will be able to:

1 appreciate the general care required for people who are unconscious;
2 discuss the principles of blood glucose monitoring;
3 explain how to deal with seizures.

Learning outcome 1: appreciate the general care required for people who are unconscious

Box 14.56 Activity: ability to self-care

Reflect on how unconsciousness will affect a person's ability to self-care. What general care might an unconscious person require?

You should have identified that an unconscious person's airway must be maintained, and oxygen and suction could be necessary (see earlier sections). The person will also need care to prevent complications of immobility (Chapter 11), personal hygiene care, including mouth and eye care (Chapter 7), care of their elimination (Chapter 6) and maintenance of their fluid and nutrition (Chapter 5). It is also important to consider whether they are experiencing pain and ensure their comfort (see Chapter 8 and 9 for more information).

Communication is vital when dealing with unconscious individuals. When people lose consciousness, they may still be aware of their surroundings and sensitive to touch and speech. Thus, Enid's carer should have talked to her calmly while she appeared unresponsive. It is very important to talk to individuals who are unconscious and to explain what you are going to do. Social conversation is also helpful so that the person is aware of your presence. Family members and significant others should be encouraged to talk to the unconscious person. They might need your help and support in doing this initially. Also having a role in the situation can calm the carer allowing health professionals to continue with important aspects of care. Having someone there who knows the person is valuable, however not if they are distracting from the care being given.

Learning outcome 2: discuss the principles of blood glucose monitoring

Hypoglycaemia or **hyperglycaemia** can cause unconsciousness. Glucose is generated in the body from the foods we eat and is circulated in the blood. Insulin is necessary to enable glucose to enter the cells to provide energy for cellular metabolism. Check your biology textbook or the Internet for a detailed explanation about this process. If glucose levels rise or fall outside the normal range (4–7 mmol/L; 3.6–5.8 mmol/L fasting), then the person's conscious level will be affected and they can become extremely unwell. Blood glucose monitoring is therefore often carried out by or for people known to have diabetes. However, other underlying medical conditions and traumatic incidents can affect a person's blood glucose levels without them having diabetes. So, most unconscious or medically unwell people will have their blood glucose levels assessed to identify if these are within the normal range. This test is referred to as a capillary blood glucose test (CBG).

Organisations have varying policies about who can carry out blood glucose monitoring, so you must go by local policy as to whether you can carry it out in practice. You must be trained how to use your organisation's particular blood glucose monitoring equipment.

ACTIVITY

Box 14.57 Activity: blood glucose monitoring

Find out about blood glucose monitoring in your own practice setting.
Investigate:

* what equipment is used;
* what training is given to use this equipment;
* whether there are training updates;
* who can carry out blood glucose monitoring.

The Diabetes UK website (www.diabetes.org.uk) is regularly updated and very informative about managing diabetes; ensure that you review this regularly as management interventions change rapidly. In particular, do look up recognition and management of hypoglycaemia on this website. Also, there are NICE guidelines about managing diabetes and more information is available via www diabetes.org.uk.

Blood glucose monitoring is part of the daily routine of many people with diabetes, who know their normal blood glucose levels and are aware of how to control their blood glucose. In Enid's instance, her carers know her usual blood glucose level and will be monitoring this, highlighting any abnormality to the health professionals. When a person becomes unwell due to infection, disease, trauma or a mental health problem, they may be unable to control their diabetes. Blood glucose levels are measured by carrying out a finger prick and gaining a blood sample, which is then analysed using a glucose meter. There are different types of glucose meters available. Alternatively, a blood sample can be taken to the biochemistry laboratory for analysing glucose levels. This test usually takes a little time to perform and is therefore not useful in an emergency situation. Treatment will need to be administered according to the blood glucose level. Box 14.59 lists key points in blood glucose measurement.

Box 14.58 Activity: reasons for blood glucose tests being inaccurate

Read Box 14.59 carefully and identify possible reasons for blood glucose tests being inaccurate. Now categorise these causes under the following headings: 'Problems with technique' and 'Problems with equipment'. What could be the consequences of obtaining an inaccurate blood glucose result – either too high or too low?

Box 14.59 Blood glucose monitoring: key points

Equipment

- Finger-pricking device, gauze/cotton wool for cleaning finger with water and drying, glucose meter, reagent strips

Technique

- Remember infection control: perform hand hygiene before the procedure and apply non-sterile gloves.
- The glucometer must be maintained and checked as per manufacturer's instructions and the strips should be correctly stored (airtight container) and in date. The user must be trained to use the specific meter and strips.
- Fingers used should be third, fourth or fifth on either side of the end of the finger – but not the top, as this is more painful. This gives 12 possible sites and the site should be rotated to avoid causing neurological damage over time with repeated finger pricks. The thumb and second finger are not used as these are most important for touch.
- If the hand is very cold, ensure that the individual is warm first.
- The finger site must be washed and dried with water as contamination by food, etc., can affect the accuracy of the test.
- The finger should not be squeezed/milked from the base.
- After the finger has been pricked, apply blood to the reagent strip and then insert the strip into the meter for reading, as per the manufacturer's instructions.
- Ensure safe sharps disposal, dispose of gloves and perform hand hygiene.
- Record the result in the person's notes.
- Show the results to a competent practitioner and assist in any treatments that are necessary.

You must pay attention to both technique and the equipment used to gain accurate results. Test strips and monitoring equipment must be in date and regularly maintained. Examples of technique error include failing to wash the finger (consider how the result might be affected if the person has just been eating grapes or chocolate), squeezing the finger leading to interstitial blood entering the blood sample and insufficient blood being obtained. Equipment problems can include reagent strips that have been exposed to air or are out of date, and a machine that has not been quality-checked as per manufacturer's instructions.

Gaining inaccurate results of any test is potentially very dangerous. Blood glucose monitoring directly affects treatment. For example, a sliding-scale insulin pump is adjusted according to the blood glucose result. If the result obtained was higher than it really is, the person might be administered more insulin than they really need, with the risk of developing hypoglycaemia. If the result is lower than it really is, the person might not be administered enough insulin and could become increasingly hyperglycaemic. Recording and reporting results from the test is important because, like other information obtained in assessment, it directly impacts on care. If a blood glucose result was very high or very low, immediate action might be necessary.

Box 14.60 Activity: blood glucose measurement within your organisation

ACTIVITY

Arrange to observe blood glucose being measured and, if allowed within your organisation's policy, and if you have been trained on the meter used, carry out blood glucose monitoring under supervision. Ensure that you document the result and discuss its implications with a member of the team.

Learning outcome 3: explain how to deal with seizures

A seizure is caused by a sudden burst of excess electrical activity in the brain, causing a temporary disruption in the normal message passing between brain cells, resulting in the brain's messages becoming halted or mixed up (see www.epilepsy.org.uk for more information). Some people experience a seizure on a one-off basis, where no diagnosis is given, and seizures can be caused by medical conditions in some instances. However, some people experience seizures on a regular basis and are then said to have epilepsy. People should be referred to as having epilepsy rather than being 'an epileptic', which is a label (www.epilepsysociety.org.uk). They may wear jewellery, alerting that they have epilepsy or carry a card indicating the medication they are prescribed.

All healthcare practitioners should be able to recognise and respond appropriately to a person experiencing a seizure. There are thought to be around 60 different types of seizures that vary in severity. Epilepsy has been estimated to affect 600,000 people in England. While epilepsy affects about 1% of the population, a third of people with learning disabilities have epilepsy; nearly half the people with severe learning disabilities have epilepsy. (www.epilepsy.org.uk).

NICE (2020c) addressed the importance of healthcare practitioners remaining up to date in the management of epilepsy. The updated guideline specifies the different drug options that doctor and nurse prescribers should prescribe, both according to type of seizure (i.e. when a diagnosis has not yet been confirmed) and according to the epilepsy syndrome.

Recognising the different types of seizures can help the person experiencing the symptoms gain the correct help and medications to stabilise their condition. Epilepsy types include focal onset or auras, generalised onset, combined generalised and focal onset and unknown onset (Scheffer et al. 2017). The basic seizure classification is related to:

- Where the seizure begins in the brain (onset)
- Level of awareness during seizure
- Other features of seizure, e.g. movement.

Seizures are usually classified by signs and symptoms that the person displays during this time.

Focal seizures start in and affect one part of brain but sometimes two (bilateral) tonic – clonic.

Warming sensations or aura can sometimes accompany this.

Focal aware seizures (FAS)

The person is aware and alert and aware something has happened to them afterwards.

Focal impaired awareness seizures (FIAS) affect one large part of the brain, and as conscious level is affected, the person may appear confused.

Focal to bilateral tonic–clonic seizure

The person is unconscious and will convulse and shake (tonic–clonic) seizure.

Generalised onset

This affects both sides of the brain, the person appears unconscious and will not remember what has happened to them.

Clonic seizures – characterised by repeated jerky movements that are seen on one side or part of the body or both sides depending on where the seizure starts in the body.

Myoclonic seizures – muscle jerking is seen here with uncontrollable movements.

Absence seizures – seen in children more than adults, characterised by frequent absent or vague periods in the child's activities.

Unknown onset – unclassified if a clinician has not got enough detail regarding the seizure.

For further information, please visit International League against Epilepsy (www. ilae.org) and Epilepsy Foundation (www.epilepsy.com).

Status epilepticus

A single seizure that lasts 30 min or longer; or a series of seizures without consciousness being regained in between (see http://www.epilepsy.org.uk/info/treatment/status-epilepticus).

When a person with epilepsy has a seizure, it should always be treated as an emergency situation and prompt action should be taken in a systematic manner. Some people who experience epileptic seizures have prolonged episodes; these are known as status epilepticus.

Convulsive stages and interventions

Immediate care

A person should be assessed using an ABCDE approach (see the earlier section) and interventions as per Resuscitation Council (UK) guidelines should be followed as required. Drug therapy may be needed; for example, buccal diazepam may be given or midazolam may be administered rectally by an appropriately trained person (see Chapter 10).

During the seizure, **do**:

* protect the person from further harm and provide privacy;
* maintain their airway (see earlier section);
* stay with the person and reassure them by speaking calmly.

During the seizure, **do not**:

* restrain the person in any way;
* put any object in the person's mouth;
* attempt to rouse the person.

Subsequent care

Monitoring using the ABCDE approach must continue, with recording of vital signs and consideration of possible causes of the seizure. After convulsions have ceased, move the individual into the recovery position to protect their airway (see www.resus.org.uk for further details of this position). Sometimes, incontinence occurs during a seizure, so be sensitive and promote dignity.

Hospitalisation usually follows if the person does not recover spontaneously. At this stage, maintenance of vital signs (as discussed in Chapter 4) should continue. Assessment of ABGs, monitoring of blood glucose levels, cardiac monitoring and recording of a 12-lead ECG, as discussed earlier in this chapter, will be carried out as indicated. Prolonged seizures may require medical review and alteration of medications may occur.

See NICE (2020c) Clinical Guideline 137 for full details about the management of people with epilepsy.

Wearable or bed seizure detection devices

Devices worn by a person on the wrist, like a watch or placed on a person's mattress can detect seizure activity and record this activity via an app alerting carers or clinicians to a person who is having a seizure. The data collected from these devices can inform healthcare professionals about the future care required for a person who experiences epilepsy.

Box 14.61 Children and young people: practice points – neurological problems

The NICE (2020c) guideline 137 covers epilepsy in children as well as adults.

Febrile seizures may occur in children aged from 6 months to 6 years, with one-third of children who experience them going on to have subsequent seizures (NICE 2018).

NICE. 2018. Clinical Knowledge Summary: Febrile seizure available from: https://cks.nice.org.uk/topics/febrile-seizure/

For blood glucose monitoring in children, see

Gormley-Fleming, E. 2010. Assessment and vital signs: A comprehensive overview. In: Glasper, A., Aylott, M. and Battrick, C. (eds.) *Developing Practical Skills for Nursing Children and Young People.* London: Hodder Arnold, 109–47.

For neurological care in children, see

Allen, K. J. 2012. Neurological care. In: Macqueen, S. Bruce, E.A. and Gibson, F. (eds.) *The Great Ormond Street Hospital Manual of Children's Nursing Practices.* Chichester: Wiley-Blackwell, 436–71.

Box 14.62 Pregnancy and birth: practice points – neurological problems

- An unconscious woman in her third trimester of pregnancy should be positioned on her left side to reduce aortocaval compression The Royal College of Obstetricians and Gynaecologists update (2021) Epilepsy in Pregnancy Guideline No. 68 137 covers in detail joint working and the care of women with epilepsy pre-conceptually, during pregnancy and in the postnatal period.
- Tools such as ROSIER (Recognition Of Stroke In the Emergency Room) and FAST (Face, Arms, Speech Test) are suitable for pregnant mothers.
- Rarely, pre-eclampsia in pregnancy can lead to eclampsia, which is a type of seizure that is life-threatening to the mother and baby.

For further information:

- Special Circumstances Guidelines: https://www.resus.org.uk/library/2021-resuscitation-guidelines/special-circumstances-guidelines#specific-health-conditions
- Pre-eclampsia: https://www.rcog.org.uk/en/patients/patient-leaflets/pre-eclampsia/
- Royal College of Obstetricians and Gynaecologists: Epilepsy in Pregnancy (2016) Available from: https://www.rcog.org.uk/en/guidelines-research-services/guidelines/gtg68 (Accessed 9 June 2021).

Summary

- People who are unconscious need support and monitoring of their airway, breathing and circulation as well as pressure area care, support for hygiene, elimination and nutrition, and comfort and communication.
- Blood glucose monitoring can assist in identifying the cause for a person's deterioration. This skill should be observed in your practice setting, and appropriate training on using specific equipment should be obtained before practising this skill. Local policies must be adhered to.
- Dealing with seizures and recognising the stages of convulsion and responding appropriately are important skills for all nurses.

CHAPTER SUMMARY

In this chapter, we have reviewed how to recognise, respond to, and manage the person who is deteriorating. Recognition of a person's deterioration has been addressed by reviewing how the NEWS2 score can be used as a tool to indicate how a person requires further intervention and care. The systematic ABCDE assessment approach was discussed and aspects of this assessment strategy have been discussed. Appropriate emergency skills and care interventions have been highlighted and further reading opportunities suggested to ensure you are conversant with the potential causes of individual deterioration. The ABCDE tool can be used for assessments that are required to be performed rapidly in pre-hospital and hospital settings. Due to the emergency situation, it may not be possible to discuss with your colleagues what is happening in the clinical area. Try to find an opportunity to review emergency assessments with your colleagues after the event when you will be able to learn more about the situation and the person's assessment and management. Attend debriefing events or staff teaching sessions if possible, to reflect in and on your actions in these events. The ABCDE assessment forms part of many escalation systems. Try to familiarise yourself with your local organisation's electronic devices and methods of record-keeping and protocols. It can take considerable time to become confident in these assessment skills. The recognition, assessment and management of the person who is deteriorating remains a challenge for all healthcare practitioners. Practise your skills of assessment regularly, learn how to observe for signs of deterioration. These include both soft signs and physiological signs. Measure vital signs accurately and communicate your findings immediately using a communication tool to escalate your concerns. Recognising, responding and managing a person who is deteriorating can be a challenge for many healthcare providers. Recent pandemics have taught us much about caring for a person who is deteriorating and hopefully provided new information to improve individual care in this field. This field of healthcare is an ever-changing situation where new challenges and technology can be used to improve future person-centred care and outcomes.

I acknowledge the contribution of Tracey Valler-Jones to previous editions of this chapter regarding care of the person whose condition is deteriorating.

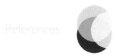

I dedicate this chapter to all the individuals, families and significant others who have experienced first-hand the devastating effects of deterioration during the COVID-19 pandemic and to the practitioners who have worked tirelessly to provide care and whose knowledge and skills have been tested each day.

REFERENCES

Andersen, L. Holmberg, M. Berg, K. et al. 2019. In Hospital cardiac arrest: A review. *JAMA* 321: 1200–10.

Benner, P. 2001. From Novice to Expert Excellence and power in *Clinical Nursing Practice Commemorative Edition*. USA: Pearson Education.

Benner, P. Tanner, C. and Chesla, C. 2009. *Expertise in Nursing Practice: Caring, Clinical Judgement and Ethics*. New York: Springer.

Bonanno, F.G. 2012. Shock-A reappraisal: The holistic approach. *Journal of Emergencies, Trauma and Shock* 5 (20): 167–77.

Bosson, N. 2020. Bag valve mask ventilation techniques. Available from: https://emedicine. medscape.com/article/80184-technique (Accessed on 21 April 2020).

Brady, M. and Burns, B. 2019. Airway Obstruction. Available from: https://www.stat-pearls.com/articlelibrary/viewarticle/17310/ (Accessed on 28 April 2020).

British Thoracic Society. 2017. BTS guidelines for oxygen use in healthcare and emergency settings Available from www.brit-thoracic.org.uk (Accessed on 21 April 2020).

British Thoracic Society/Scottish Intercollegiate Guidelines Network (BTS/SIGN). 2019. *Guidelines on the Management of Asthma*. Available from: www.brit-thoracic.org.uk (Accessed on 21 April 2020).

BTS/SIGN. 2019. Asthma guideline quick reference guide. Available from: www.brit-thoracic.org.uk (Accessed on 21 April 2020).

Chun-Hei Cheung, J., Tin Ho, L., Cheng, J., Cham, E. and Lam, K. 2020. Staff safety during emergency airway management for COVID 19 in Hong Kong. *The Lancet*. https://doi.org.10.1016/S2213–2600 (2)300084-9.

De Backer, D. and Vincent, J. L. 2018. Should we measure the central venous pressure to guide fluid management? Ten answers to 10 questions *Critical Care* 22(1): 43.

Douw, G. Holwerda Schoonhoven, L. 2015. Nurses worry or concern and early recognition of deteriorating patients on general wards in acute care hospitals: A systematic review *Critical Care* (London England) 19(1): 230.

Fabich, R., Franklin, B. and Langan, N. 2020. Definitive management of a traumatic airway: Case report. *Military Medicine* 185(1–2): e312–316. https://doi.org/10.1093/milmed/usz167

Fahy, J. and Dickey, B. 2010. Air mucus function and dysfunction. *New England Journal* 363(23): 2233–47.

Garretson, S. and Malberti, S. 2007. Understanding hypovolaemic, cardiogenic and septic shock. *Nursing Standard* 50(21): 46–55.

Gwinnutt, C. 2016. *Clinical Anaesthesia*. Oxford: Blackwell Publishing.

Hampton, J. 2008. *ECG Made Easy*, 7th edn. London: Churchill Livingstone

Hampton, J. and Hampton, J. 2019. *ECG Made Easy*, 9th edn. London: Churchill Livingstone.

Haynes, J. 2018. Basic spirometry testing and interpretation for the primary care provider *Canadian Journal of Respiration Therapy* 54(4). doi: 10.29390/cjrt-2018-017.

Iaizzo, P. 2015. *Handbook of Cardiac Anatomy and Physiology and Devices*, 3rd edn. London: Springer.

Koczulla, A., Scheenberger, T. and Gloeckl, R. 2018. Long term oxygen therapy. *Dtsch Arztebl Int.* 115(51–52): 871–877. doi: 10.3238/arztebl.2018.0871 (Accessed on 21 April 2020).

Levy, J.M., Pasley, J., Remick, K.N., Eastman, L., Margolis, A.M., Tang, N. and Goolsby, C.A. 2021. Removal of the prehospital tourniquet in the Emergency Department. *Journal of Emergency Medicine* 60 (1): 98–102.

Li, J. 2019. Hypothermia treatment and management. Available from: https://emedicine. medscape.com/article/770542-overview (Accessed on 28 April 2020).

Main, E. and Denehy, L. 2016 *Physiotherapy for Respiratory and Cardiac Problems in Adults and Paediatrics*, 5th edn. Edinburgh: Churchill Livingstone.

Melin-Johansson, C. Palmqvist, R. Ronnberg, L. 2017 Clinical intuition in the nursing process and decision making _A mixed studies review. *Journal of Clinical Nursing* 26(23–24): 3936–49.

Merelman, A. and Levitan, R. 2020. A modern approach to basic airway management. *Journal of Emergency Medical Services* 4(43). Available from: https://www.emsairway. com/2018/11/14/a-modern-approach-to-basic-airway-management/ (Accessed on 30 April 2021).

National Confidential Enquiry into Patient Outcome and Death (NCPEOD). 2012. Time to intervene. Available from: https://www.ncepod.org.uk/2012cap.html (Accessed on 5 February 2021).

National Health Service Improvements. 2020. SBAR communication tool – Situation, background, assessment, recommendation. Available from: http://www.improvement. nhs.uk (Accessed on 4 February 2020).

National Heart, Lung and Blood Institute. 2020. Explore oxygen administration. Available from: http://www.nhlbi.nih.gov/ (Accessed on 30 April 2020).

National Institute for Health and Clinical Excellence (NICE). 2007. *Acutely Ill Patients in Hospital: Quick Reference Guide*. Clinical Guideline 50. London: NICE.

National Institute for Health and Care Excellence (NICE). 2016a. Major trauma: Assessment and initial management NICE guideline [NICE guidelineG39]. Available from: https://www.nice.org.uk/guidance/ng39 (Accessed 5 February 2021).

National Institute for Health and Care Excellence (NICE). 2016b. Hypothermia: Prevention and management in adults having surgery. Clinical guideline CG65) Available from: https://www.nice.org.uk/guidance/cg65 (Accessed January 2021).

National Institute for Health and Care Excellence (NICE). 2020a. *Surveillance of Acutely Ill Adults in Hospital: Recognizing and Responding to Deterioration* (Clinical guideline CG50). London: NICE.

National Institute for Health and Clinical Excellence (NICE). 2020b. Asthma: Diagnosis and monitoring and chronic asthma management (NICE guideline 80). (Accessed on 5 February 2021).

National Institute for Health and Care Excellence (NICE). (2020c) Epilepsies: The Diagnosis and Management. Clinical Guidelines 137. Available from: https://www.nice.org. uk/guidance/cg137 (Accessed 8 February 2021)

National Patient Safety Agency (NPSA). 2011. *Safer Care for the Acutely Ill Patient: Learning from Serious Incidents*, 5th report. London: NPSA.

Nickson, C. 2019. Hypothermia Life in the fast lane. Available from: https://litfl.com/ hypothermia/ (Accessed on 28 April 2020).

Nickson, C. 2019. Major Haemorrhage in Trauma. Available from: www.litfl.com (Accessed on 27 December).

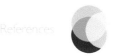
Nursing and Midwifery Council (NMC). 2018a. Standards of proficiency for registered nurses. Available from: www.nmc.org.uk (Accessed on 24 April 2020).

Nursing and Midwifery Council (NMC). 2018b. Standards of proficiency for nursing associates 10 October Available from: www.nmc.org.uk(Accessed on 24 April 2020).

O'Driscoll, B.R. Howard, L.S. and Davison, A.G. 2017. BTS guideline for emergency oxygen use in adult patients. *Thorax* 72(Suppl) il–i89 May.

Odell, M. Victor, C. and Oliver, D. 2009. Nurses' role in detecting deterioration in ward patients: Systematic literature review. *Journal of Advanced Nursing* 65(10): 1992–2006.

Olive, S. 2016. Practical procedures: Oxygen therapy. *Nursing Times* 112(1–2): 12–14.

Pennisi, M. Congedo M. Bello, G. et al. 2019. Early nasal high flow versus venturi mask oxygen therapy after lung resection: A randomized trial. *Critical Care* 23(68). https://doi.org/10.1186/s13054-019-2361-5.

Pierre, L. and Keenaghan, M. 2020. Arterial lines. Available from: www.ncbi.nlm.nih.gov (Accessed on 30 April 2020).

Pretz, J. Folse, V. N. 2011. Nursing experiences and preference for intuition in decision making. *Journal of Clinical Nursing* 20: 2878–2889.

Pritchard, M.J. 2010. How effective communication skills can reduce anxiety in elective surgical patients. *Nursing Times* 107(3): 22–3.

Recommended Summary Plan for Emergency Care and Treatment ReSPECT. 2020. *Decisions Relating to Cardiopulmonary Resuscitation Guidance*, 3rd edn. Available from: https://www.resus.org.uk/sites/default/files/2020-06/ReSPECT-Patient-Guide.pdf (Accessed on 9 June 2021).

Resuscitation Council (UK). 2021b Resuscitation guidelines. Available from: https://www.resus.org.uk/library/2021-resuscitation-guidelines (Accessed on 9 June 2021).

Resuscitation Council. 2021a. Cardiopulmonary resuscitation: Standards for clinical practice and training. Available from: http://www.resus.org.uk/pages/standard.pdf (Accessed on 5 May 2021).

Romero-Brufau, S., Gaines, K., Nicolas, C.T. et al. 2019. 'The fifth vital sign? Nurse worry predicts inpatient deterioration within 24 hours', *JAMIA Open* 2(4): 465–70. doi: 10.1093/jamiaopen/ooz033.

Roots, D. 2016. The London Approach to reducing home oxygen related harm: Shared responsible oxygen prescribing and risk assessment. Available from: https://www.networks.nhs.uk/nhs-networks/london-lungs/network-events/OxygenRiskAssessmentandResponsiblePrescribing.Nov2016.pdf (Accessed on 4 June 2020).

Royal College of Nursing (RCN). 2019. Communication-tools and interventions. Available from: www.rcn.org.uk (Accessed on 28 April 2020).

Royal College of Physicians (RCP). 2012. *National Early Warning Scores: Standardising the Assessment of Acute Illness Sensitivity in the NHS*. Available from: http://www.rcplondon.ac.uk (Accessed on 2 February 2013).

Royal College of Physicians (RCP). 2017. National early warning scores 2(NEWS2). Available from: https://www.rcplondon.ac.uk/projects/outputs/national-early-warning-score-news-2 (Accessed on 2 November 2021).

Royal College of Physicians. 2020. *NEWS2 and Deterioration in COVID-19*. Available from: http://www.rcplondon.ac.uk/news/news2-and-deterioration-covid-19 (Accessed on 5 February 2021).

Rubin, B.K. 2009. Physiology of airway mucus clearance. *Respiratory Care* 47: 761–8.

Scheffer, I. Berkovic, S. Capovilla, G. et al. 2017. ILAE classification of the epilepsies: position paper of the ILAE commission for classification and terminology. *Epilepsia* 58(4): 512–21.

Sharma, S., Danckers, M., Sanghavi, D. and Charkraborty, R. 2020. High flow nasal cannula. Available from: www. ncbi.nlm.nigh.gov (Accessed on July 2020).

Shepherd, E. 2017. Specimen collection 4: Procedure for obtaining a sputum specimen. *Nursing Times* 113(10): 49–51.

Sinha, V. and Fitzgerald, B. 2020. Surgical airway suctioning. Available from: www.ncbi.nlm.nih.gov (Accessed on 15 July 2020).

Summers, R. 2020. Pathophysiology and treatment of hypovolaemia and hypovolaemic shock. *Nursing Standard* 35(3): 77–82. doi: 10.7748/ns.2020.e10675

Turan, N., Ozdemir Aydin, G., Ozsaban, A., Kaya, H., Aksel, G., Yilmaz, A., Hasmaen, E. and Akkus, Y. 2019 Intuition and emotional intelligence: A study in nursing students. *Cognet Psychology* 6: 1633077. www.doi.org/10.1080/23311908.2019.1633077

Warrell, D., Cox, T. and Firth, J. 2012. *Oxford Textbook of Medicine*, 5th edn. Oxford: Oxford University Press.

Wheatley, I. 2018 Respiratory rate 5: Using this vital sign to detect deterioration. *Nursing Times* (online) 114(10): 45–46.

Wilkins, R.L., Dexter, J.R. and Heuer, A.J. 2010. *Clinical Assessment in Respiratory Care*, 6th edn. St. Louis: Elsevier Mosby.

Winstanley, M., Smith, J. and Wright, C. 2019. Catastrophic haemorrhage in military trauma patients: A retrospective database analysis of haemostatic agents used on the battlefield. *BMJ Military Health* 165(6). http://dx.doi.org/10.1136/jramc-2018-001031.

World Health Organisation. 2020. Technical specifications of personal protective equipment for COVID-19. Available from: https://www.who.int/teams/health-product-policy-and-standards/assistive-and-medical-technology/medical-devices/ppe/ppe-covid (Accessed 2 November 2021).

Zafren, K. and Crawford Mechem, C. 2020. Accidental hypothermia in adults. Available from: https://www.uptodate.com/contents/accidental-hypothermia-in-adults#! (Accessed on 1 November 2021).

USEFUL WEBSITES

- Asthma UK: www.asthma.org.uk
- British Lung Foundation: www.blf.org.uk
- British National Formulary: www.bnf.org/bnf
- British Thoracic Society: www.brit-thoracic.org.uk
- Diabetes UK: www.diabetes.org.uk
- Epilepsy Action: www.epilepsy.org.uk
- Resuscitation Council (UK): www.resus.org.uk
- Peak flow information: www.peakflow.com

Managing care at the end of life

Scott Elbourne and Gavin Walker

Palliative and end-of-life care (EoLC) is an important aspect of nursing. Around 500,000 people die in England every year, excluding the Covid-19 pandemic, and it is expected that, by 2040, this will rise to 590,000 (Dying Matters 2020). The main aetiology of death is stroke and heart failure; however, one in four people in the UK will die of cancer (Office for National Statistics [ONS], 2020). It should also be appraised that due to an increasing and ageing population, a significant proportion of older adults will be living with comorbidity and therefore an increase in deaths due to comorbidity and frailty will likely pertain as a leading cause of mortality in the coming years (National Institute for Health and Care Excellence [NICE], 2016). In response to this, nurses need to be managing and delivering services that can identify and care for people who require palliative care and are likely to be approaching the end of their lives (Mitchell and Elbourne 2020; NICE 2019). This chapter will explore the principles and practice of palliative care and EoLC. Biopsychosocial aspects of death, dying and bereavement will be explored alongside the communication skills that enable comprehensive holistic assessment, advance care planning (ACP) and comfort care.

The chapter includes the following topics:

End-of-life care:

- The differences between palliative care and EoLC
- Assessment skills
- Communication skills – difficult conversations
- Advance care planning
- Symptom control
- Ethical principles for EoLC
- Last offices
- Grief and bereavement.

DOI: 10.4324/9781003020660-15

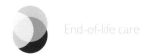

PRACTICE SCENARIOS

The following scenarios illustrate the palliative and EoLC needs of two individuals. These two scenarios have been chosen to reflect the differing palliative care and EoLC needs of a person with malignant disease (cancer) and non-malignant disease (Alzheimer's). They will be referred to throughout this chapter.

Adult

William Newton, who likes to be called 'Bill', is a retired accountant aged 73. He is terminally ill with a history of oesophageal cancer and metastases in his lungs. He is cared for by his wife at home with the support of community nurses and the Macmillan nurse. He is taking regular oral morphine for pain control. He has a very low haemoglobin (Hb) and has been admitted for a blood transfusion. He is weak, breathless and his general condition is poor. He has a **body mass index (BMI)** of 16. He can swallow only very small amounts of liquidised food and drink. He has some of his own teeth but also a partial denture, which he likes to wear, although it is now ill-fitting. His tongue appears coated, and his mouth is dry.

Mental health

Alzheimer's disease

Alzheimer's disease is the most common cause of dementia, affecting around 496,000 people in the UK. The term 'dementia' describes a set of symptoms, which can include loss of memory, mood changes and problems with communication and reasoning.

Osteoarthritis

A joint disease caused by cartilage loss in a joint. Pain and stiffness are symptoms.

Violet Davies, aged 76 years, has moderate Alzheimer's disease. She has been admitted to a care home for respite as her husband is physically and emotionally exhausted and needs a break. He has refused help in the past as he has been determined to look after his wife, but he has now agreed to take a holiday visiting friends. Violet is physically well, but she is also known to have osteoarthritis in her right hip and knee. She looks permanently worried and is agitated; she keeps repeating the same phrase over and over. Mr Davies looks shaky and tearful at the thought of leaving his wife for a week.

PRINCIPLES OF END-OF-LIFE CARE

Box 15.2 Learning outcomes

By the end of this section, you will be able to:

1. Discuss the differences/similarities between palliative care and EoLC.
2. Explore the different approaches to palliative care and EoLC.
3. Communicating with people who are receiving unwelcome news and strategies for having difficult conversations with individuals, families and carers.
4. Explore the benefits of ACP to enable people to plan their future care to meet their individual needs, wishes and preferences.

Learning outcome 1: discuss the differences/similarities between palliative care and end-of-life care

To ensure we are giving high quality care, we need to undertake a thorough assessment of the person's needs. The needs of people who are palliative or end of life can be similar; however, there are some differences. To understand these needs, we first need to appraise if the person has palliative care or EoLC needs.

Palliative and end-of-life care

The term 'palliative care' is sometimes referred to as EoLC; however, there are subtle differences between the two, which can lead to confusion. The term 'palliative care' is derived from the Latin word *palliare* meaning 'to cloak'. This notion could be perceived as protecting or shielding the individual. However, the term 'palliative' in medicine, also refers to the need to identify and manage the underlying symptoms of a life-limiting disease, rather than the disease itself, referring to the uncurable nature of the disease. It should not be assumed that a person is imminently dying when they are diagnosed with a life-limiting disease. People can live many years with incurable illnesses, particularly with today's advancements in treatments that can stem the rate of progression in some diseases. Furthermore, palliative care should focus on a person's quality of life, rather than quantity, and should attempt to address their holistic needs, such as psychological, social and spiritual, and not exclusively on their physical symptoms (Mitchell and Elbourne 2020). The World Health Organization (2020) provides what is often referred to as the definitive explanation of the meaning of palliative care:

Palliative care is an approach that improves the quality of life of patients and their families who are facing the problems associated with life-threatening illness. It prevents and relieves suffering through the early identification, correct assessment and treatment of pain and other problems whether physical,

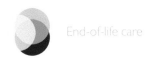

psychosocial or spiritual. Available from: https://www.who.int/news-room/fact-sheets/detail/palliative-care (Accessed on 24 June 2021)

The term 'end of life' is often referred to by health professionals as the terminal stage of a person's illness, whereby the person would be considered to be actively dying or in the last months, weeks, days and hours of their lives. The General Medical Council (2010) defines EoLC as 'the care that is required during the last 6–12 months of life, regardless of the individual's diagnosis'. The terms 'palliative' and 'end of life' may be even more unclear for individuals and families, and it could be argued that such discussion about definitions for them are meaningless and what is important is access to the right support, at the right time according to their needs.

Marie Curie (2018) gives us an idea of the types of individual support required for those whose needs are palliative or are at the end of their lives. You will notice that the emphasis in their definition is supporting quality of life and recognising that the transition between palliative and end of life is identifying who might be in the last year of their lives and therefore ensuring that their care needs are met (Mitchell and Elbourne 2020).

Palliative care is treatment, care and support for people with a life-limiting illness. The aim of palliative care is to support the person to have a good quality of life, which includes being as well and active as possible for the time the person has left. This can involve:

- planning for future care with a detailed advance care plan that expresses the person's individual needs and wishes
- controlling physical symptoms such as pain
- emotional, spiritual and psychological support needs
- social care needs including assistance with washing, dressing or eating
- support for the person's carers, family and friends.

Similarly, EoLC also focuses on treatment, care and support, but it is for people who are thought to be in the last year of their life. This includes people with:

- advanced, progressive, incurable conditions
- frailty and comorbidity that place them at increased risk of dying within the next 12 months
- existing conditions whereby they are at risk of dying suddenly from acute crisis (NICE, 2019)
- life-threatening acute conditions caused by sudden catastrophic events (General Medical Council UK 2010, p 8).

ACTIVITY

Box 15.3 Palliative care or end-of-life care needs?

Review the scenarios at the start of this chapter. What are the key differences between Violet's and Bill's care needs and how might these differences help to identify if a person has palliative care or EoLC needs?

- Violet has **Alzheimer's disease**, which is a progressive and life-limiting illness. Violet is physically well at present; however, it is not uncommon for people with non-malignant diseases, such as Alzheimer's, to have 'peaks and troughs' in their health status due to unpredictable episodes of acute illness, e.g. urine and chest infections. Individuals with Alzheimer's often have unpredictable disease trajectories, meaning it is not always easy to identify when their disease is progressing from having palliative care needs, to requiring EoLC. Signs and symptoms of such a decline in disease trajectory can include further deterioration in mental health, less physical activity and not wanting to eat or drink. However, for Violet, a change in mental and physical health, e.g. agitation, less physical activity, and poor appetite, could be related to pain from her arthritis, which she may not be able to communicate to her husband and carers. It is important not to make assumptions about the reasons underlying a change in Violet's behaviour. We know that Violet is currently physically well; however, her husband is physically and emotionally exhausted and is now struggling to care for her needs at home. On understanding this, we should anticipate that Violet's Alzheimer' disease might be progressing and that she may need a significant increase in her care needs following a comprehensive holistic assessment. It is also important to look for signs and symptoms of other disease processes, e.g. cancer and infection, which could be masked by the Alzheimer's disease, which could also explain a sudden deterioration in health.

- Bill has terminal cancer; he may have lived for many years with this life-limiting disease. However, Bill is now showing typical signs and symptoms of disease progression, e.g. increased pain, weight loss, exhaustion and reduced swallow reflex. People with cancer, who have been diagnosed as palliative, often follow predictable disease trajectory when compared with a non-malignant disease, such as Alzheimer's. Healthcare workers will often look for indicators such as increasing pain, weight loss, reduced physical activity and reduced appetite to anticipate the increasing needs of someone who is declining and in need of symptom control. Bill has been admitted into hospital for symptom control of his shortness of breath and physical weakness, secondary to his low Hb. Whilst Bill is in hospital, it would be important to carry out a holistic assessment. Areas of concern outlined in Bill's scenario such as his pain, loose dentures, sore mouth, weight loss and poor swallow reflex would be identified, and possible interventions could be discussed with Bill to help improve his quality of life. Bill would be considered palliative; however, his decline could be indicating a transition towards end of life.

We can see that both Violet and Bill have differing needs at present even though they could be both considered palliative. This highlights the importance of holistic assessment in understanding the individual's needs to ensure they are cared for appropriately.

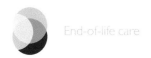
Summary
- The terms 'palliative' and 'end of life' could be viewed as care approaches that focus on improving quality of life and planning for a peaceful dignified death – both terms are mutually inclusive and share the same ethos and principles.

Learning outcome 2: explore the different approaches to the delivery of palliative and end-of-life care

Person-Centred Care – Holistic assessment

Holistic assessment is the core element to a clear and robust plan of care that when disseminated across health and social care services can support and facilitate robust communication between professionals to enable the co-ordination and delivery of care that is focused on person, carer and family (Garbutt 2018). The key components of providing the right care at the right time for people at the end of life is early identification of their needs and effective communication between all involved (Mitchell and Elbourne 2020). To this end, many organisations have systems that allow providers and commissioners of care to identify individuals who are palliative and might be entering into the last 6–12 months of life to ensure their needs are met throughout their care journey (Garbutt 2018). To enable the identification of care needs, it is vital to undertake a holistic assessment. For people who have learning disabilities, it would be good practice to involve the learning disability nursing team, either through the learning disability liaison nurse in a hospital or directly with the team, depending on your local service provision. They will support you communicating with the person and their family and carers (NHS 2017a). See also: www.bild.org.uk/wp-content/uploads/2020/01/Improving-End-of-Life-Care-for-LD-Jan-2019-FINAL-1.pdf.

There is an abundance of health and social care guidelines, policy and law related to care provision for those who require palliative care or EoLC, but before we review this, it is vital to appraise and understand the needs of the person through a detailed holistic assessment. Person-centred care is a vital component of good palliative care. It promotes the importance of viewing each individual holistically and acknowledges the biopsychosocial impact of a person's illness on their psychological, emotional, social and spiritual well-being. Effective biopsychosocial care is dependent on an approach to assessment that identifies these issues and acknowledges them equally alongside the medical, symptom and treatment-related aspects of care (Engel 1977). According to the National End of Life Care Programme (2010), holistic assessment is vital to identify where a person's needs are currently not being addressed and indicates where other health and social care professionals could be involved to address this. Individual preferences and wishes can also be highlighted, enabling the person to be more in control of what is happening and therefore promoting dignity and choice (National Palliative and End of Life Care Partnership 2015). The Holistic Common Assessment tool (see Table 15.1) provides guidance for holistic assessment of the supportive and palliative care needs of adults. All people who have been recognised to be approaching the end of their life should be offered this type of biopsychosocial assessment (National End of Life Care Programme 2010).

As previously mentioned above, there are milestones on an individual's disease trajectory within a person's EoLC journey that may indicate when an assessment is appropriate. A structured approach to holistic assessment is valuable at key points in a person's care pathway:

1. at diagnosis of a life-limiting illness,
2. when a person shows signs of health deterioration,
3. when the person is identified as approaching the end of life or
4. when the individual is thought to be entering into the dying phase (actively dying).

As you can see, there are multiple opportunities to undertake holistic care assessments, it could be that an assessment is undertaken at each of these stages or preferably, continuously throughout the individual's journey. However, it can be difficult or potentially harmful initiating these conversations, and it is important to recognise the right time for the individual to have these conversations as this can be just as important as having the conversation itself – see Chapter 2 Communication: a person-centred approach.

The following holistic assessment can be carried out by any professional who knows the person, their condition and its management and has the appropriate skills to ensure each person is seen as an individual (End of Life Care Strategy 2008; National End of Life Care Programme 2010; National Palliative and End of Life Care Partnership, 2015). The below is an outline of the topics covered in the assessment, many service providers will use a paper or electronic format to undertake the assessment that will cover each domain with questions to guide and support health professionals through the assessment with individuals, carers and families.

Psychosocial assessment at the end of life, points to remember:

- **Consent is necessary to the assessment process** – We must ask for consent to undertake any assessment or treatment plan (Consent and **best interests** are discussed later in this chapter).
- **Assessment should be led by individual concerns** – What needs does the person have, not what we think they need, although it is ok to make suggestions.
- **It should be carried out *with* the person and families not *on* them** – they should be at the centre of the discussion – active listening skills are key (see Chapter 2, Communication: a person-centred approach).
- **It should be done in a conversational style rather than viewed as a series of boxes that must be ticked** – it can be helpful to take notes rather than trying to complete the assessment tool at the time which can be completed in full after the assessment. Be sure to inform them that you will be taking notes, but this will not distract them from the conversation.
- **Helping individuals to assess their own needs should be central to the process** – everyone has different needs, we must be careful not to impose what we think they need, although suggestions can be made.

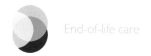

Table 15.1: The common holistic tool

Domain 1: Background information and assessment preferences	**Demographic** and contact details, history of illness, treatment plan, professional involved, next of kin.
	Consent to assessment, previous assessments undertaken, preferences for setting of assessment and family involvement.
Domain 2: Physical well-being	Impact of illness on physical well-being, symptoms such as pain, nausea and breathlessness, effect on sleep, energy levels, nutrition, weight loss.
Domain 3: Social and occupational well-being	Type of accommodation, who they live with, level of dependency and sources of help with shopping, meal preparation, etc.
	Work and financial issues, family and close relationships, needs related to children (talking to them about death).
Domain 4: Psychological well-being	Mood, anxiety, adjustment to worsening illness or treatment, knowledge/understanding of disease/ treatment, sources of emotional support, unresolved concerns, coping strategies and strengths, perception of the future.
Domain 5: Spiritual well-being and life goals	Identification of views on faith or belief, impact of illness on faith/belief, practical support or other needs related to religion or spiritual matters (contact with faith leader, opportunity/space to pray).
	Discussion of important life goals or exploring what endows life with meaning and purpose.

National End of Life Care Programme (2010).

- **Professionals undertaking assessment should have reached an agreed level of competency in key aspects of assessment** – It is important to be competent and confident in undertaking holistic assessments. However, be assured that it takes time and experience to feel comfortable having discussions regarding palliative care and EoLC needs.
- **Individual preference for communicating with professionals, their family and friends should be considered** – As previously mentioned, recognising the right time to initiate EoLC discussions can be difficult – be guided by the verbal and non-verbal cues. Some people will want to have these discussions at the point of diagnosis, others may initiate these discussions when their health deteriorates, and others may not want to have these discussions at all or would prefer these discussions to be held on their behalf with a carer/family member.

(National End of Life Care Programme 2010)

A comprehensive holistic assessment affords health and social care professionals the opportunity to understand the needs of the person and their families/carers. In doing so, we can support the notion of providing EoLC that promotes a 'good death'.

The End-of-Life Care Strategy

In 2008, the *End-of-Life Care Strategy* (Department of Health 2008) undertook a systematic review of how people died in the United Kingdom and provided a quality framework to evidence how they and their families should be cared for. The strategy is subject to annual reviews of progress against its stated aims to improve EoLC provisions. The strategy identified a dearth of public discussion around death, highlighting that even clinicians had difficulties in initiating end-of-life discussions and identifying people advancing toward the end-of-life. There was a significant absence of individual and carer satisfaction in the quality of EoLC, with 54% of complaints in acute hospitals related to care of the dying/bereavement support (Healthcare Commission, 2007). The strategy placed an emphasis on improving education and training around EoLC for all practitioners to achieve the aim of allowing more people to die in the place of their choice. Research highlighted by Dying Matters showed disparity between where people would wish to die and their preferred place of care, and actual place of death (Shucksmith et al, 2013). This research found that around 70% of people would choose to die at home; however, 50% of people were dying in hospital.

However, there appears to be a downward trend in people dying in hospital. According to Public Health England (2018), in 2004, 57.9% died in hospital, whereas in 2016, this number had fallen to 46.9% with more people dying at home (23.5%) or in their preferred place of care, i.e. a nursing home (21.8%) or hospice (5.7%). However, there was significant variation across the country by district and local authority, with the proportions of deaths in hospital ranging from 34.2% to 63.1% (Office of National Statistics, 2020).

Box 15.4 Activity: providing end-of-life care in hospital and community settings

- Why do you think more people are dying in their preferred place of care?
- What are the challenges of providing EoLC in the hospital and community settings?

We can examine the answers to the above activity by exploring government policy and national guidelines that have helped to shape palliative care standards in the United Kingdom:

Ambitions for palliative and end-of-life care: 2015–2020

In 2015, the Ambitions for EoLC were introduced, not to replace the EoLC strategy and the improvements that followed, but to build upon its commitment to improving EoLC through national partnership. The National Palliative End-of-Life Care Network (2015) proposes six ambitions for improving palliative and EoLC as a framework for local implementation, whereby individuals and organisations can lay these foundations on their own or collectively:

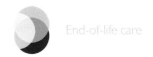

1. each person is seen as an individual
2. each person gets fair access to care
3. maximising comfort and well-being
4. care is coordinated
5. all staff are prepared to care
6. each community is prepared to help.

Each of the six ambitions is accompanied with a statement to give focus to the ambition in practice from the viewpoint of the person nearing the end of life. The attention is on the experience of the dying person; however, each of the ambitions should also be viewed as an ambition for carers, families and, where appropriate, for people who have been bereaved. The impetus is for open and honest conversation and the importance of integrated care delivered by compassionate, caring and competent health and care staff (The National Palliative End-of-Life Care Network, 2015). These ambitions support the continued implementation of the Gold Standards Framework (GSF) and ACP, which will now be explored.

The Gold Standards Framework

The EoLC strategy states that all organisations commissioning EoLC provisions are required to utilise a systematic approach to care through the implementation and use of evidence-based, quality-assured tools to promote effective EoLC. The GSF (2006) is a good example of such a tool. The GSF aims to improve palliative care and EoLC provided by health and social care professionals in the community by actively identifying or 'caseload finding' individuals who might be nearing the end of life. Once an individual is identified, the health and social care team can undertake a holistic assessment to support a plan of care.

The GSF focuses on enabling continuity of care, teamwork, advanced planning, symptom control and person-centred support, which is inclusive of carers and family. The GSF guides health professionals with prompts and tools to help them identify when someone may be entering the end-of-life phase of their illness, i.e. the last 6–12 months of their lives.

Prognostic Indicator Guidance

There are several indicators that suggest someone may be entering the last 6–12 months of life. These range from quite general indicators to much more specific ones relating to specific conditions and the physical changes that occur as it progresses.

The **surprise question**: would you be surprised if this person were to die in the next 6–12 months?

This is a question based on professional intuition and encourages the practitioner to think about how an individual is coping day to day with an advancing disease. By looking at the context of:

- Individual choice: someone with advanced disease makes a choice for comfort care only
- Individual need: they are in special need of supportive or palliative care

- Clinical indicators: general predicators of end-stage illness and cancer-specific indicators (any person whose cancer is metastatic or inoperable) (Gold Standards Framework Prognostic Indicator Guidance 2006; Garbutt 2018).

General predictors of end-stage illness

- **Multiple co-morbidities** – several disease processes, can be both chronic and acute.
- **Weight loss: greater than 10% weight loss over 6 months** – fat loss and muscle wasting (cachexia) become apparent. It can be subtle at first, for example, you may notice that clothes are not fitting, but later weight loss can be visually obvious and upsetting to the person and their family.
- **General physical decline** – mobility problems are often pronounced, and there will be a higher risk of falls. General lethargy/weakness leads to the person becoming chair/bed bound.
- **Dependence in most activities of daily living (ADLs)** – e.g. washing and dressing, managing medications, self-feeding, getting to the bathroom.
- **Repeated unplanned/crisis admissions** – a clear plan of care and understanding of the person's wishes and preferences can prevent admissions; nevertheless, they are a good indication that their illness is either uncontrolled or advancing. Some people are admitted for symptom control, e.g. pain management or reversible conditions secondary to the main illness, e.g. hypercalcaemia (high calcium levels) due to bone cancer or in Bills Scenario, his low Hb.

Box 15.5 Activity: assessing the predictors in Bill and Violet's scenarios

ACTIVITY

Think back to Bill's scenario, how many of the above general predictors does he have?

Would you be surprised if Bill were to die within the next 12 months?

Does Violet have any of the above predictors? Could Violet's current condition be easily confused with someone who is showing signs of end-stage illness?

If we were to undertake a holistic assessment with Bill, we would find, as already mentioned in the scenario, that Bill has increasing pain, loose dentures due to weight loss, sore mouth and poor swallow reflex. We may find that Bill is struggling with ADLs and has become more bed/chairbound over the past few weeks. Although Bill's health may have deteriorated due to the low Hb, we should consider that the above symptoms are good prognostic indictors for end-stage illness and an EoLC plan, if not already in place, should be discussed with Bill, his family and communicated to all health and social professionals caring for Bill. It is likely that Bill would die within the next 12 months and that this was probably identified by his GP, district nurse or palliative care nurse before his admission for the blood transfusion.

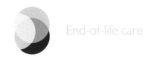

In Violet's scenario, we know that she is currently well. Her arthritis often exacerbates causing pain and discomfort, which may affect her cognitive status, nutrition and mobility. As previously mentioned, people with Alzheimer's often have unpredictable disease trajectories, meaning it is not always easy to identify when their disease is progressing from having palliative care needs, to requiring EoLC. It is not uncommon for those with dementia to have many of the above prognostic indicators that can make it difficult to comprehend if a person is approaching end of life. The importance here is to monitor Violet's health closely, preferably by a team of professionals who know her well. Relatives can often notice small changes in their loved one's health, and their opinions should always be heard. It is difficult to say if Violet would likely die in the next 12 months; it is possible that health professionals may consider the surprise question and may refer to the GP for Violet to be placed on the Gold Standards Framework Register. This ensures that Violet's needs are monitored closely with a plan of care that can be revised in line with her physical and mental health at the time of ongoing assessment.

Box 15.6 Activity: resources for end-of-life care for people with dementia

Access the following sites and look at the resources available for EoLC for people with dementia:

https://www.alzheimers.org.uk/get-support/help-dementia-care/end-life-care

My future wishes ACP for people with dementia in all care settings (NHS England 2018) https://www.england.nhs.uk/publication/my-future-wishes-advance-care-planning-acp-for-people-with-dementia-in-all-care-settings

---

Disease trajectories

Different diseases progress at different rates and have periods of stability punctuated by exacerbations where the person's condition will deteriorate.

Malignant diseases such as cancer often follow a predictable trajectory of deterioration, which therefore makes care planning easier to anticipate. However, some illnesses can be problematic in predicting time frames of mortality, particularly if the person has non-malignant life-limiting illnesses. For example, chronic obstructive pulmonary disease, where it can be challenging to appraise if the person is having an acute exacerbation or if they are at the end of life (Cohen-Mansfield et al. 2018). Similarly, a person with dementia may have a longer, slower and unpredictable trajectory, with often unnoticeable changes that over time means that they will become weaker, more dependent and more prone to opportunistic infections or other problems such as difficulty swallowing, poor nutritional intake and mobility problems (Garbutt 2018). Therefore, it is important to understand that some people might only receive EoLC in their last weeks, days or hours and as such, every effort should be made to ensure that wishes and preferences, such as the person's preferred place of care or advance decisions to refuse treatment, are sensitively discussed and documented in advance care plans as early as possible with the individual and their family members (Macmillan Cancer Support 2019; Mitchell and Elbourne 2020; National Palliative and End of Life Care Partnership, 2015).

Disease trajectories and prognostic indicators are useful adjuncts to anticipating the needs of the person; however, everyone with life-limiting illnesses will at some point experience a deterioration in their condition that will require EoLC. The onus is on health professionals to identify the triggers, such as recurrent exacerbations, repeated hospitalisations, deterioration in general condition, weight loss, increasing lethargy and dependence. In doing so, health professionals will employ an attitude of anticipation that informs proactive planning, rather than reactive care, which often has poorer outcomes. ACP can facilitate open discussions and proactive care planning of future needs, wishes and preferences of the person (Macmillan Cancer Support 2017; Thomas et al. 2016).

Learning outcome 3: communicating with people who are receiving unwelcome news and strategies for having difficult conversations with individuals, families and carers

Breaking unwelcome or bad news is often medical staff's role, but increasingly specialist nurses and other healthcare professionals are involved. Nurses should understand how to facilitate the situation to minimise distress for the person and their relatives. It is often at times of intimate contact (e.g. bed-bathing) that searching questions are asked. Bad news can be defined as any news that adversely and seriously affects how an individual views their future (RCN 2015).

Giving bad news is often cited as the most difficult part of the healthcare professional's role and can engender feelings of guilt, distress and fear for one's own mortality. Healthcare staff may sometimes avoid telling the whole truth either because they fear the person's reactions, or those of their relatives, or they fear acknowledging their own feelings. Although it can be distressing to receive bad news, it is rarely acceptable to withhold the truth from them. Society holds the belief that truth is a fundamental and valued principle and is essential for establishing effective relationships. Furthermore, people need correct information for making informed choices in decision-making (NHS England 2017b). Current government strategy has recognised the importance of people participating in decisions about their care and treatment, and the phrase 'no decision about me without me' sums up this person-centred approach (NHS England, 2017b, 2019; DH 2012).

People generally want to be told the truth, and the Code (NMC 2018) states that nurses and nursing associates must be open and honest. Arguments relating to deception in healthcare stress the importance of respecting the person's autonomy. This respect involves acknowledging aspects such as individual preference and establishing an environment of trust that enables the individual to feel accepted, respected and involved in their care (Birkhäuer et al. 2017).

Glaser and Strauss (1968 cited in Andrews and Nathaniel 2015) describe four different aspects related to awareness in the context of dying:

- Closed awareness: the person is not aware of their impending death.
- Suspicion awareness: the person is not sure they are dying but suspect that staff believe they are.

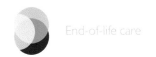

- Mutual pretence: everyone knows the person is dying but pretend otherwise.
- Open awareness: the person and staff acknowledge that the person is near to the end of life.

It is challenging to have clear decisions in EoLC and nursing staff have a role to play in contributing to these decisions. Awareness context can help to guide discussions and to focus care for the individual (Andrews and Nathaniel 2015). Sometimes staff are faced with family asking that the person is not told of their diagnosis or that they are terminally ill (or the person may not want family to be told). This may be out of a sincere wish to save the person distress. Twycross and Wilcock (2016) outline the importance of open dialogue and that sharing of truth does not mean there is no hope. It is the individual not the family who make decisions in relation to sharing information and ethical considerations of confidentiality are clear that relatives can only be given information with the permission of the person being cared for. Generally, if these situations are handled sensitively and with compassion, effective relationships can be developed and maintained.

Sivell et al. (2015) emphasises the importance of conducting discussions and interviews in a sensitive and structured way to elicit information about the person's beliefs, attitudes and values. A supportive environment helps the person to disclose their concerns, enabling nurses to adapt information according to individual emotional needs.

Buckman's (2005) Setting, Perception, Invitation, Knowledge, Empathy, Strategy and Summary (SPIKES) strategy centres on addressing and recognising the emotional aspects of the person's experience.

Setting – ensuring privacy, adequate time, set up of room, removing the chance of interruptions, listening mode.

Perception – how the person views the seriousness of their situation and the language and vocabulary they use to describe it.

Invitation – finding out how much the person would like to know about their situation.

Knowledge – giving a warning that you are going to give bad news, using similar language and avoiding technical jargon.

Empathy – listening for and identifying emotions and their source and acknowledging these emotions and sources.

Strategy and summary – checking understanding, summarising and allowing time for questions and clarification.

Although SPIKES is directed primarily towards medical staff, it provides valuable insight for nurses dealing with individuals at this sensitive time.

ACTIVITY

Box 15.7 Activity: breaking bad news

Think of a situation when someone has been given bad news. Write down some of the factors you would need to have considered had you been the one breaking the bad news.

You may have considered the following:

Setting – Where would you give the bad news? Was there somewhere private?

Perception – How serious did you think the person thought their condition was?

Invitation – Were they asked about what they wanted to know? How would you do this?

Knowledge – Did you think about the words and language you might use and how you might ascertain their current understanding?

Empathy – What emotions might you expect and how do you think you would respond?

Strategy and summary – How did you check understanding and did you consider making arrangements for future meetings?

Buckman (2005) suggests that if breaking bad news is perceived to have been handled insensitively, it can have adverse long-term consequences for the person in adjusting to the illness, and for the family in their bereavement. Therefore, nurses have a role to play in ensuring that breaking difficult news is handled sensitively and that sufficient time is given to the process including any follow-up.

Learning outcome 4: Explore the benefits of ACP to enable people to plan their future care to meet their individual needs, wishes and preferences.

Advance care planning

ACP is a voluntary discussion about future care, wishes and preferences between an individual and their care providers. ACP identifies how an individual wishes to be cared for before they lose capacity to make decisions. Such decisions can include, but not limited to, where a person may wish to die, their views on treatments and interventions and who they may wish to make decisions on their behalf should they become incapacitated, with an emphasis on maintaining dignity. It is important to note that these conversations are not limited to health professionals and can be undertaken by any member of the multidisciplinary team who is competent to have these discussions with individuals (Garbutt 2018; Mitchell and Elbourne 2020).

It is important to acknowledge that not everyone will want to have these discussions; however, for some, it will be a crucial way of maintaining control and autonomy of their care options. We discussed earlier in this chapter the best time to undertake a holistic assessment with people who have been diagnosed with a life-limiting illness; the same principles apply to advance planning. A structured approach to ACP is valuable at key points in a person's care pathway, some people will want to discuss their wishes and preferences at the point of diagnosis of a life-limiting illness, others may wish to wait until such a time that their health deteriorates. Whilst sharing of their preferences as soon as possible should be encouraged, we must be careful not to push these discussions with people who are not ready, as this can be potentially harmful. It is important that health professionals have refined communication skills in recognising the right time to initiate these discussions. We should also remember that ACP discussions are an ongoing process throughout the person's journey towards

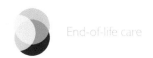

end of life and they may wish to revisit their wishes and preferences and should be facilitated to do so (Pfeifer and Head 2018).

An ACP can be documented in multiple forms – it could be a verbal discussion; it could be recorded using a video camera; some people will choose to write their own advance care plans that are witnessed by their family and a professional and it can also be documented in an individual's healthcare records by a member of the multidisciplinary team. However, it is important that all conversations are clearly and explicitly documented to ensure that all members of the multidisciplinary team are aware of the ACP to ensure that the individual's wishes are realised (Marie Curie 2020).

Some individuals will often ask for family and friends to be involved in their ACP, whilst this is encouraged, it can also be problematic, particularly, if the individual's wish for EoLC is dependent on their family and friends. A good example of this is when someone wishes to die at home; family and friends may be anxious about their abilities to cope with caring for them, particularly if they are unaware of health and social services that are available to support them. It is important to appraise and discuss with the person, family and friends any challenges they foresee with this and any practical solutions to support them. This might include formal carers, specialist palliative care nurses and district nurses who can provide excellent home care and can support the family and friends to fulfil the individual's wishes of dying at home. The value of an ACP is that it opens discussions between the person, their family and the professionals involved in their care. If preferences are unknown, families and professionals are left to try to guess what a person may have wanted (Garbutt 2018). Equally, some people may change their minds about a decision they have made, and this is often true when their illness progresses. Therefore, it is important to regularly review and document the ACP with them to ensure that their wishes and preferences coincide with what they are thinking and feeling at the time (Thomson et al. 2021).

ACP promotes the person-centred care approach and thus forms a significant part of the holistic care approach discussed earlier in this chapter. It can support the person to ask questions about their prognosis, how their health might change over the course of their illness and who will be there to support them and their family. ACP is invaluable to professionals who can anticipate future care needs therefore ensuring that the care they provide is proactive and not reactive. Understanding the wishes and preferences of the individual, and their family and carers ensures that the person stays in control even when they become too ill to tell us what they want, it also ensures that health professionals are aware of how to proceed if someone does have a crisis and therefore lessens the emotional burden on the family and friends who may be asked to make **best-interest** decisions at a time when they are trying to cope with the emotion of their loved one dying (Garbutt 2018).

For people living in social care accommodation, residential care or supported living, the support needs of the carers (paid or unpaid) also need to be considered. Carers may be involved in the person's care throughout but would not have had the education or training in regard to palliative care practices to understand the relationship between ACP, mental capacity, best-interest decision-making, advance decision to refuse treatment (ADRT) and lasting power of attorney (LPA).

Mental capacity

The Mental Capacity Act (MCA) was introduced in 2005 and came in full force in 2007. It aims to protect individuals who lack capacity to make decisions for themselves. The MCA safeguards the individual to ensure that the decision-making process remains focused on their best interests and that their wishes and preferences remain at the core of the decision-making process. The MCA empowers individuals to plan for the future in the event that they may lose capacity and makes clear who should be involved in decision-making and what the process should entail (Garbutt 2018).

The MCA 2005 is underpinned by five key principles:

1. A person must be assumed to have capacity unless it is established that he lacks capacity
2. A person is not to be treated as unable to make a decision unless all practicable steps to help him to do so have been taken without success
3. A person is not to be treated as unable to make a decision merely because he makes an unwise decision
4. An act done, or decision made, under this Act for or on behalf of a person who lacks capacity must be done, or made, in his best interests
5. Before the act is done, or the decision is made, regard must be had to whether the purpose for which it is needed can be as effectively achieved in a way that is less restrictive of the person's rights and freedom of action.

The application of the MCA to EoLC is imperative, as the progressive nature of life-limiting illnesses will undoubtedly lead to a person losing capacity to make decisions at some point in the future (Garbutt 2018).

Best-interest decision-making

If an individual is assessed as having lost capacity and their wishes and preferences are unknown, then there is an expectation that health professionals along with the views of the family will make a decision that this is in the **best interests**. The MCA 2005 says that any previously stated views and preferences must be considered when making such a decision. It could be that they have previously mentioned their views or preferences about their care, but perhaps they did not want to formally document this on an ACP or perhaps their health deteriorated sooner than anticipated. Should a decision need to be made in the **best interests** of the individual, there should be a discussion with all key people involved in their care, e.g. carers, relatives, friends or a person who has been given LPA (Garbutt 2018). Ultimately, the decision would be the responsibility of the person who understands the implications of various courses of action, ensuring that the decision that is made is not more burdensome to the person. An example of this could be admitting them into hospital for intravenous antibiotics for an infection when the outcome would probably be futile and the person might die in hospital, when they had mentioned that they would wish to die at home (Mitchell and Elbourne 2020). For more information on mental capacity

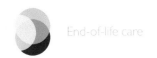

and best-interest decisions, see Chapter 3. Fundamentals of mental health assessment for non-mental health practitioners.

Lasting power of attorney

Individuals can choose to appoint another person as their LPA who can make decisions on their behalf when they are unable to do so (Marie Curie 2020). There are two areas in which a person can act as an LPA:

1. Care and Welfare
2. Finance and Property.

An LPA can act on the individuals' behalf for their care and welfare only at the point when the individual is unable to make decisions for themselves (incapacitated). An LPA for finance and property, once registered, can act at any time on behalf of the individual, if they have been given permission by the individual to do so. Identifying if an LPA has been appointed by an individual should be shared with all those responsible for the individual's care. Holistic assessment and ACP discussions are useful adjuncts to identifying an LPA (Garbutt 2018).

The preferred priorities for care

The preferred priorities for care document is a useful adjunct to documenting ACP discussions. The document supports holistic assessment, which is inclusive of socioeconomic circumstances and further ensures that the person has a format to detail their wishes and preferences. The document also details services that they are accessing or may need to access in the future, which includes an ongoing needs assessment to ensure care needs are reassessed as required. The document is used across the domiciliary setting including nursing homes and residential homes and has become more commonplace in acute hospitals (Garbutt 2018).

Advance decisions to refuse treatment

An ADRT replaces previously used terms such as 'living wills' and 'advance directives'. This document is a statement of wishes and preferences made to refuse certain treatments in a specific situation. The ADRT ensures that the person has communicated what treatments they would not want to receive at the point they are unable to speak for themselves, examples include:

- If your illness is incurable and all possible treatments have been explored, you would not want to be kept alive with artificial feeding or intravenous fluids.
- You are in the last few days of life and have an infection, you would not want to be given antibiotics, particularly if this means an admission into hospital.
- Do not attempt resuscitation (DNAR) (Resuscitation Council UK 2016).

The ADRT can only be used if the person has become incapacitated, until such a time consent applies for individuals to accept or refuse treatment. An ADRT is legally binding and forms an integral part of an ACP empowering individuals to document their wishes and preferences regarding treatment (Macmillan Cancer Support 2019).

Recommended summary plan for emergency care and treatment form

People can also complete a recommended summary plan for emergency care and treatment (ReSPECT) form with a clinician. These forms are not legally binding as ADRTs are; however, their aim is to develop a shared understanding about their condition between the healthcare professional and the individual, the outcomes they value and those that they fear and then how treatments and interventions, such as cardiopulmonary resuscitation (CPR) fit into this. It supports the important principle of personalised care and forms another integral part of ACP (Resuscitation Council UK 2019).

Box 15.8 Activity: advance care planning discussions

ACTIVITY

- How would you feel about having ACP discussions with someone you were caring for?
- When do you think would be the best time to have these discussions with individuals?

We can imagine a scenario related to Bill for example – when he was admitted into hospital, his wife informed the nursing team that he had an ADRT. He had been admitted a couple of times previously for pain control and his low Hb. Bill had deteriorated markedly since his last admission and was now too unwell to discuss his wishes and preferences, so the doctor discussed the ADRT with Bill's wife who was LPA and his daughter. The ADRT stated that Bill did not want to be resuscitated should he suffer a cardiac arrest, but he would have treatments if it would improve his quality of life. Bill's wife and daughter were informed that the blood transfusion had not had the desired effects in controlling his symptoms and that the palliative care team were managing his pain and breathlessness with good effect via a syringe driver. The medical team reviewed the ADRT and were happy to respect it. Bill was at the end of life and his family were asked about his preferred place of care. Bill's wife stated that he wanted to die at home and necessary arrangements were made to discharge Bill into the care of the GP and district nurse team. The advantages of these conversations having taken place ensures continued individualised care.

As healthcare professionals, we must be sure that what is written in an ADRT form meets the essential criteria to uphold its validity:

1. Has the person lost capacity?
   All attempts must be made to assess an individual's ability to make an informed decision but if capacity is in question, then discussion must take place with family and/or LPA.
2. Is the decision valid?
   Have they changed their mind or done or said anything that might be inconsistent with the ADRT?

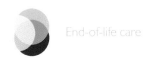

3. Is the advanced decision applicable?

Does the ADRT specify which treatment the person wishes to refuse and is the treatment in question specified in the ADRT?

4. Does the decision refer to life-sustaining treatment?

Does the ADRT clearly refer to a decision by the person to refuse life-sustaining treatment? Is it signed by the person and by a witness?

(Garbutt 2018; NHS England 2018)

Summary

- If breaking bad news is perceived to have been handled insensitively, it can have adverse long-term consequences for individuals and their family in adjusting to the illness.
- Nurses have a role to play in ensuring that breaking difficult news is handled sensitively and that sufficient time is given to the process including any follow-up.
- A comprehensive holistic assessment affords health and social care professionals the opportunity to understand the needs of the person and their families/carers. In doing so, we can support the notion of providing EoLC that promotes a 'good death'.
- Every effort should be made to ensure that wishes and preferences, such as the person's preferred place of care or advance decisions to refuse treatment, are sensitively discussed and documented in advance care plans as early as possible with the person and family members.
- The MCA safeguards the individual to ensure that the decision-making process remains focused on their best interests and that their wishes and preferences remain at the core of the decision-making process.

SKILLS FOR END-OF-LIFE CARE

Box 15.9 Learning outcomes

By the end of this section, you will be able to:

1. Identify and support the care needs of those in their last few days of life
2. Reflect on the process of "last offices": Care of the body after death
3. Describe the principles of loss, grief and bereavement.

Learning outcome 1: identify and support the care needs of those in their last few days of life

Care in the last few days of life
Diagnosing dying: signs and symptoms of approaching death

It is an important skill for nurses to be able to recognise when someone is approaching end of life or is actively dying. It is imperative that nurses are capable of identifying clinical indications of the dying process to support the person and family members effectively. Once we have identified that they are dying, we need to have honest and appropriate conversations with them or with family members, if they are acting on their behalf, to ensure we proceed with their wishes and preferences, e.g. where the person wishes to die (Kennedy et al. 2014).

Predicting when someone might die is difficult and is often poorly judged. Families will often ask health professionals to give them an indication of when their relative might die. It is important not to guess or to be persuaded into giving an answer that can be incorrect. Experienced health professionals who are competent in recognising signs and symptoms of active dying, might be able to give indications of hours, days or weeks (Mitchell and Elbourne, 2020). It would be appropriate to explain the unpredictability of the situation and support the family with focusing on the present and how they could assist in supporting the person's comfort and dignity (Garbutt 2018). The common signs and symptoms that signify when someone is actively dying include:

Signs and symptoms of approaching death:

* Tiredness and weakness
* Reduced interest in getting out of bed
* Needing assistance with all personal care
* Less interest in things happening around them
* Diminished intake of food and loss of ability to swallow
* Drowsy or reduced cognition
* May be disorientated in time or place
* Difficulty concentrating
* Colds hands and feet
* Bladder and bowel problems (retention of urine or constipation)
* Unable to cooperate and converse with family/carers
* Difficulty swallowing routine medicines
* Respiratory changes – breathlessness (dyspnoea).

(Marie Curie 2020; Mitchell and Elbourne 2020)

Common signs and symptoms in the last 48 hours of life – active dying

* Pain
* Restlessness/agitation
* Upper airway secretions
* Nausea and vomiting.

What do we mean by a good death?

Box 15.10 Activity: a good death

ACTIVITY

* What would be your idea of a good death?
* Have you witnessed a death where you felt the care was less than ideal?

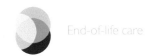

The concept of a 'good death' may seem incomprehensible to many, particularly, if they are in good health. However, how and where people wish to die is important to individuals, particularly when this subject is broached during EoLC discussions. In today's modern world, the notion of what represents a good death might vary according to culture, religion or non-religious views (O'Gorman 1998). The 'modern West' which comprises individualistic societies such as ours in the UK, will often agree a less than ideal death is often one without autonomy, for example, someone who has Alzheimer's disease, who is unable to communicate his or her own wishes (Garbutt 2018). Arguably, our society's concept of a 'good death' is characterised by choice and control, e.g. dying in one's own home with loved ones around for comfort, free of pain, agitation and fear, and possibly a death that was anticipated, allowing for time to prepare, but not one that came after a sustained period of suffering and loss of independence. The London End of Life Clinical Network (2015) promotes the following attributes required for any service providing EoLC to support the notion of a good death.

- Access to psychological and spiritual support
- Tailored symptom control, e.g. pain management
- Timely assessment and provision of services
- Care, which is competent, confident, compassionate and personalised
- Joined-up, coordinated services and pathways that are easy to access and navigate
- A supportive culture that fosters excellence, confidence, innovation and education in all staff.

We will now explore some of the above points in more detail through the appraisal of guidelines, policy and law that supports people, their families/carers and health professionals to provide care provisions that support a 'good death'.

Symptom control at end of life

Psychological and spiritual support

Psychological distress is an understandable and natural reaction to living with a life-limiting illness and nurses and nurse associates need to acquire skills that demonstrate a person-centred compassionate, listening approach. This is even more crucial in what may be the last few days of someone's life. Psychological support should encompass general emotional support as well as the recognition of when a person needs more specialised input from other professionals (Johnson et al. 2015). Recognition of anxiety and/or depression is important, and when delivering EoLC, there will often be sensitive conversations with individuals and those close to them. Being able to initiate, facilitate and respond in these sensitive situations is very important and relies on open and honest communication. Taking time to reassure and prepare relatives for what happens when their loved one is dying can reduce their fears and anxiety: the care of the family is central to good holistic care of the person (see also Chapter 2: Communication: a person-centred approach).

Some people may become withdrawn in the last few weeks of their life and whilst this may not be detrimental to them, if there is underlying psychological distress, this could have a negative effect on acceptance of treatment and on their families (Twycross and Wilcock 2016).

Another aspect of care that nurses and nurse associates need to be aware of is to address a person's spiritual needs and Quinn (2020) suggests that healthcare staff should understand and acknowledge spirituality, which includes 'spiritual joy' and 'spiritual pain'. Spirituality has been defined as a concept that '…encompasses the search for meaning, personal values and development, a sense of connection to something bigger than ourselves…' (Twycross and Wilcock 2016 p. 57).

For some, spirituality is linked to their religious beliefs; however, many people who have no religious affiliation still have spiritual needs and it is essential to explore whether or not faith and religion are important for the individual.

Spirituality, therefore, can include anything that brings meaning to someone's life and may be guided by their beliefs and values and links to their hopes, dreams, joys and sorrows (Quinn 2020). In a busy hospital environment, it may be difficult for people to discuss their fears and concerns, so it is important to try to provide quiet and private spaces. Quinn (2018) suggests that spiritual pain is often revealed through the kind of questions that are asked:

For example:

- Why has this happened to me?
- What has my life meant?
- How will I be remembered?
- What is the point of everything?
- I have regrets – can I put them right?

The person in spiritual pain may feel despair or a sense of hopelessness so exploring their feelings can lead to the provision of the appropriate support. Sometimes just being there and listening can be the most supportive way to offer compassionate individual care.

Tailored symptom control

Pain

It is important to ensure that symptoms of pain are anticipated and addressed proactively. It is important for staff caring for those at the end-of-life to have skills in recognising when an individual is in pain, particularly if they are unable to communicate their pain or discomfort. Signs of pain can include non-verbal signs such as grimacing and verbal signs such as groans or moans (Farrell and Paice 2019). Family and friends who know the person well are often able to tell when they are in pain, especially if they have been their main carer – it is important to listen to their concerns and if appropriate, administer analgesia (Marie Curie 2020). Sometimes relatives can confuse pain with agitation and vice versa, which may elicit similar symptoms as described above, this can also be challenging for health professionals to ascertain. A thorough assessment is needed to deduce if they have pain, are agitated, or both, to ensure correct management of these symptoms (Garbutt 2018). See Chapter 9 for more on assessing and managing pain.

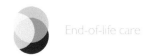
Restlessness/agitation

Restlessness and agitation are typical symptoms associated with someone who is actively dying. Signs can include restless legs, arms waving in the air, picking at the bed covers, moaning and facial expressions that convey discomfort (Mitchell and Elbourne 2020). Before the use of medication is considered to treat these symptoms, all reversible causes should be excluded or managed, examples of common reversible causes of agitation include:

- Pain
- Urinary retention
- Full rectum
- Nausea
- Cerebral irritation
- Anxiety and fear
- Side-effects of medication
- Poor positioning.

(Farrell and Paice 2019)

If the reversible cause cannot be found, then treatment for restlessness and agitation often requires the use of anxiolytic (anti-anxiety) and/or sedative medication.

Upper airway secretions

Upper airway secretions can accumulate when someone is too weak to expectorate. This is a common symptom at the end of life and is often referred to as the 'death rattle', owing to the moist, noisy breathing that can be heard. The sound of these secretions is distressing for family members who may be concerned that their loved one's airway is blocked and they cannot breathe. It is important to explain to the family that the person can still breathe and if they are unconscious, they may be unaware, which can give reassurance that they are not in discomfort. If possible, upper airway secretions should be anticipated, as once established, they are more difficult to remove than prevent (Garbutt 2018). Repositioning can help, but if treatment is required, antimuscarinic drugs such as hyoscine butylbromide or glycopyrronium can be given subcutaneously to prevent exacerbation of secretions (Mitchell and Elbourne 2020).

Nausea and vomiting

Nausea and vomiting are common symptoms in people who are at the end of life. The cause of nausea and vomiting can be challenging to identify; common causes include gastric stasis, bowel obstruction, medication and metabolic disorders such as hypercalcaemia and renal failure. However, when a person is actively dying, it may be difficult to investigate the cause or can be inappropriate to do so (Garbutt 2018). In these circumstances, broad-spectrum anti-emetics such as cyclizine and levomepromazine can be given via a subcutaneous injection and/or subcutaneously, via a syringe driver over 24 h to manage the symptoms (Mitchell and Elbourne 2020).

Other comfort measures

Symptom control is an important intervention to ensure that the person is kept as comfortable as possible in their last few weeks of life. However, we should not neglect other essential nursing skills such as personal care to promote their comfort and dignity. Comfort measures such as washing, mouth care and changing of incontinent pads can ensure a good level of hygiene (see Chapter 7: Meeting hygiene needs and Chapter 8: Promoting comfort and sleep). Pressure relieving mattresses can help to reduce the risk of pressure ulcers in people who are bed bound and can further support comfort (see Chapter 11: caring for people with impaired mobility for more on pressure area care). It is normal in the dying process for the swallow reflex to reduce that at this point, the person will not want fluids and/or food. At this stage, people rarely ask for fluids or food, but the family and carers may be concerned that their loved one is suffering (Garbutt 2018). It important to inform them that this is normal and is not causing discomfort to them and that if they were to be given fluids or food, this would probably cause more discomfort as the body would be unable to digest the contents. This could lead to nausea and vomiting as well as the risk of aspiration (Mitchell and Elbourne 2020).

Syringe drivers

A syringe driver is useful for symptom control when oral administration is not possible and repeated subcutaneous injections or administration of medication by other routes is inappropriate, ineffective or impractical. Although syringe drivers are primarily used in EoLC, they may also be appropriate for people who are not imminently dying. Consider using a syringe driver for the following:

- Persistent vomiting
- Reduced consciousness
- Dysphagia
- Weakness
- Bowel obstruction or malabsorption
- Significant tablet burden
- Unwilling to take tablets by mouth
- Unable to absorb oral medications
- Following head and neck lesions or surgery
- Death rattle when someone is unconscious
- Poor symptom control with oral drugs
- To improve comfort. (O'Brien 2012; NHS Scotland 2014; Stevens 2015)

The goals for administering medication using a syringe driver should be discussed and any concerns addressed. It is important to explain to the individual and their family members that although the syringe driver may allow symptoms associated with the dying process to be helped, it will not expedite the dying process. Individuals and family members should be assured that the decision to start a syringe driver is not irreversible and if symptoms improve, this may be stopped (Thomas and Barclay 2015). See Table 15.2 for advantages and disadvantages of using syringe drivers in EoLC.

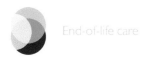

Table 15.2: Advantages and disadvantages of syringe drivers in EoLC

Advantages	Disadvantages
Repeated injections are not required	Staff training required
Symptom control with a combination of drugs	Possible inflammation and pain at infusion sites and increased risk of infection
24 h symptom control and comfort without peaks and troughs	Skin site availability may become a problem if the person is emaciated.
Only needs reloading once every 24 h	Requires daily visits from district nurses and other health professionals
The person can remain ambulant	
	Not all drugs can be administered via a syringe driver

The most common portable syringe driver nurses will encounter in use in the UK in homes and care settings requires refilling every 24 h and administers consistent therapeutic drug levels, set in millilitres (mL) per hour. Safety features include a mechanism to stop the infusion if the syringe is not properly and securely fitted, alarms that activate if the syringe is removed before the infusion is stopped, and an internal log to record pump activity.

Medications suitable for syringe drivers

An understanding of the drugs that can be used in syringe drivers and the therapeutic effects is an essential component of EoLC (Table 15.3). Nurses must always safeguard the interest of those in their care by only accepting responsibility for duties that they are competent and able to practise safely without supervision (Nursing and Midwifery Council 2018). It is suggested that theoretical knowledge alone is insufficient and nurses must be deemed competent through locally agreed competency frameworks that incorporate best practice and requirements for continuous training (O'Brien 2012). Many medications are mixed with water for injection (sterile water) or normal saline (NaCl 0.9%). Sterile water is compatible

Table 15.3: Common medicines used in syringe drivers and indications

Drug	Indications	Dose
Opioids for pain relief		
Diamorphine	Opioid-responsive pain, breathlessness	5–10 mg/24 h, if no opioid before
5 mg, 10 mg, 30 mg, 100 mg, 500 mg powder ampoules		Can be diluted in a small volume
		Preferred for high opioid doses
Morphine sulphate	Opioid-responsive pain, breathlessness	5–10 mg/24 h, if no opioid before
10 mg, 30 mg in 1 ml 60 mg in 2 ml		First-line opioid analgesic
Oxycodone	Opioid-responsive pain, breathlessness	2–5 mg/24 h, if no opioid before
		Second-line opioid analgesic if morphine/diamorphine not tolerated

(Continued)

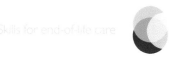
Table 15.3: (Continued)

Drug	Indications	Dose
Anti-emetics		
Cyclizine 50 mg in 1 ml	Nausea and vomiting due to mechanical bowel obstruction, raised intracranial pressure and motion sickness	50–150 mg/24 h Can cause redness, irritation at the site Incompatible with normal saline, always use water for injection
Haloperidol 5 mg in 1 ml 10 mg in 2 ml	Opioid for metabolic-induced nausea, delirium	2–10 mg/24 h
Levomepromazine 25 mg in 1 ml	Complex nausea, terminal delirium/agitation	5–25 mg/24 h as anti-emetic 100 mg/24 h as sedative Initially 12.5–50 mg/24 h, titrated according to response (doses above 25 mg should be given under specialist supervision) Second-line sedative if midazolam ineffective If purple or yellow discolouration discard – this can be caused by light exposure
Metoclopramide 10 mg in 2 ml	Nausea and vomiting (peristaltic failure, gastric stasis/outlet obstruction)	30–100 mg/24 h
Anticholinergics		
Glycopyrronium bromide 200 mcg in 1 ml 600 mcg in 3 ml	Chest secretions or colic	0.6–1.2 mg/24 h for bowel colic and excessive secretions Second-line; non-sedative Longer-duration action than hyoscine
Hyoscine butylbromide (Buscopan) 20 mg in 1 ml	Chest secretions, bowel obstruction (colic, vomiting)	60–300 mg/24 h for bowel colic 20–120 mg/24 h for excessive respiratory secretions First-line; non-sedative
Hyoscine hydrobromide 400 mcg in 1 ml 600 mcg in 1 ml	Chest secretions	1.2–2 mg/24 h for bowel colic and excessive secretions Third-line; sedative Can precipitate delirium
Sedatives		
Midazolam 10 mg in 2 ml	Myoclonus, seizures, terminal delirium/agitation	Initially 10–20 mg/24 h, adjusted according to response; usual dose 20–60 mg/24 h 20–40 mg/24 h for convulsions in palliative care
Steroids		
Dexamethasone 3.3 mg in 1 ml	Brain metastases, nausea and vomiting, anorexia, bowel obstructive symptoms, emergency management of suspected superior vena cava obstruction (SVCO) or malignant spinal cord compression (MSCC)	Dose depending on indication, ranges from 2 to 16 mg for emergency management of SVCO or MSCC. Contact specialist palliative care team for advice

Source: Joint Formulary Committee, 2020; NHS Scotland, 2020

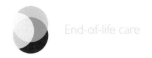

Table 15.4: Drug compatibility

Name of drug	Morphine sulphate	Diamorphine	Oxycodone
Cyclizine[a]	✓	✓	✓
Haloperidol	✓	✓	✓
Glycopyrronium	✓	✓	✓
Hyoscine butylbromide	✓	✓	✓
Hyoscine hydrobromide	✓	✓	✓
Levomepromazine	✓	✓	✓
Metoclopramide	✓	✓	✓
Midazolam	✓	✓	✓

[a] Use water for injection as diluent for cyclizine.

Source: Joint Formulary Committee (2020), NHS Scotland (2020)

with most medicines except levomepromazine, ondansetron, hyoscine butylbromide and octreotide, which should be diluted with normal saline. One of the advantages of syringe drivers is that two or more drugs (occasionally up to four) can be mixed together and infused. Knowledge of compatibility of drugs is essential (Table 15.4) and observation of physical compatibility such as precipitation, discolouration or cloudiness of the infusion mixture is important (Thomas and Barclay 2015). Always seek pharmacy advice for three or more drugs and follow local procedure guidelines.

Setting up a syringe driver

Equipment

- Syringe driver
- Luer lock syringes – manufacturers recommend the size of the syringe that should be used with their devices. Syringe drivers are calibrated in millilitres per hour. It is important to establish the final volume required in the syringe before choosing the size
- Drug label
- Butterfly needle or infusion set cannula
- Transparent surgical dressing
- Syringe driver case and battery
- Subcutaneous infusion set
- Water for injection or normal saline
- Medicines
- Sharp's box
- Prescription and monitoring chart
- Non-sterile gloves
- Skin cleansing agent.

Procedure

Explain the rationale for setting up the syringe driver and the procedure to the person and relatives

- Obtain consent
- Wash hands
- Check individual name and NHS number
- Ask the person if they have any known allergies
- Check the battery for the syringe driver. If the battery is below 40% at the start of the infusion, discard and use a new battery
- Set rate – this is the rate at which the syringe plunger will be moved forward by the motor in millilitres per hour (McKinley T34). Special attention should be paid to the rate if the machine has returned from servicing
- Test the start button – this must be tested before administering the infusion. Press the start/test button and hold it down. Releasing the button starts the syringe driver. If the alarm does not sound, the system is not safe to use (O'Brien 2012)
- Establish the final volume required in the syringe. It is considered good practice to make the solution as dilute as possible to reduce the likelihood of problems with drug compatibility and minimise site irritation. Check with compatibility tables and pharmacist if advice is needed (NHS Highland and NHS Greater Glasgow and Clyde 2007)
- Select syringe size. Make sure that the syringe is a good quality and Luer lock type (attached by twisting action) to avoid disconnection (O'Brien 2012). The dimensions of syringes will vary depending on the manufacturer
- Draw up the medication – make sure to check which diluent to use and drug compatibility
- Write the medication on the label along with date, time and signature of nurse
- Prime the line and extension set. This must be primed to the tip of the needle (O'Brien 2012). This needs to be done manually and prior to needle/cannula insertion. Measure the volume prior to priming to the set. This will ensure that correct concentration levels are administered as prescribed. If replenishing the driver, the infusion will finish early the following day. If the prescription is changed, the line needs to be re-primed (NHS Highland and NHS Greater Glasgow and Clyde 2007)
- Re-explain procedure and check that the person is in a comfortable position
- Wash hands and put on gloves
- Use skin cleansing agent to decontaminate the skin around insertion site using skin cleansing agent (Gabriel 2015) and allow 30 s to dry (see Box 15.11 for suitable and unsuitable infusion sites)
- Gently pull the protective sheath away from the stylet
- Keep the skin taut over the insertions site and insert at a 45-degree angle
- Insert the needle/cannula into subcutaneous fat to enhance absorption of medication
- Remove stylet and dispose of immediately in a sharp's container
- Connect primed infusion set and start infusion
- Cover cannula with a transparent surgical dressing
- Ensure that the device is not placed too far above the level of the infusion site. This will increase the risk of a bolus delivery (O'Brien, 2012)

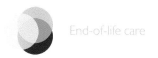

- Place the syringe driver into a locked box to avoid the pump being tampered with or damaged during infusion
- Dispose of equipment as per organisational policy
- Remove gloves and wash hands
- Ensure that the person is comfortable
- Check the last service date of the syringe driver. Record the serial number of the syringe driver, record the syringe make and size. Document the flow rate in millilitres per hour, battery percentage, diluent name and batch number. Record the drug name and batch number, total volume in the syringe (ml) of drugs and diluent. Document the site used and appearance, syringe and signature of persons preparing and checking the syringe driver (NHS Highland and NHS Greater Glasgow and Clyde, 2007)
- The pump should be checked at each visit in the community and primary care settings and every 4 h in hospital and hospice settings. Record the time and date of check
- Check the infusion site for: redness, swelling, discomfort/pain, leakage of fluid
- Record any findings. It may be necessary to re-site the cannula if the infusion site has been compromised.

Box 15.11 Suitable and unsuitable infusion sites

- Skin folds – the infusion site cannot be easily observed and the device cannot be safely secured. There is also a potential risk of impaired absorption
- Limb oedema/lymphoedema – this is an infection risk and can impair absorption
- Previously irradiated skin – impaired blood supply could reduce absorption, increased infection risk and damage to dry/delicate skin
- Bony prominences – reduced subcutaneous tissue, impaired absorption and device difficult to safely secure
- Near joints/areas of flexion – uncomfortable for the individual and a greater potential for the device to become dislodged
- Dry skin areas – increased potential for skin breakdown and risk of infection
- Infected/broken skin – increased risk of infection

Summary

- Palliative and EoLC are essential parts of nursing care. With more people choosing to die at home, it is important that nurses are competent in managing this process.
- End-of-life care should always be person-centred and include ACP when considering treatment.
- Syringe drivers are useful when the oral route of administration is not possible, or absorption of medication is not optimal. It is important that discussions about medication management occur throughout the dying process and are tailored to meet individual needs.

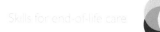

- Symptom control is an important intervention to ensure that the person is kept as comfortable as possible in their last few weeks of life. However, we should not neglect essential nursing skills such as personal care to promote their comfort and dignity.

Learning outcome 2: reflecting on the process of last offices: Care of the body after death

This section explains the care of the body after death. The term 'last offices' (thought to be derived from military/religious practices) does not encompass the multicultural society that we live in today and does not cover the differing nursing tasks involved; therefore, the term 'care of the body after death' is more appropriate (National End of Life Care Programme (NEoLCP), 2010). There are a variety of points to consider when assessing the extent of the care required. The practice of preparing the body of a person who has died for removal to the mortuary or undertaker is the last caring act that nurses can perform for them, and it may be regarded as an expression of holistic care and respect.

Reflect on the rationale for the care of the body after death

The care of the body after death is part of a long human tradition in the ritual of marking the transition between life and death (Anderson, 2017). For families, seeing their loved one looking clean and well cared for may help the grieving process. It is also important that the body does not pose a risk to staff who come into contact with it. After death has apparently occurred, it must be confirmed, usually by a doctor, or senior nurse, as locally agreed policy permits (NEoLCP/NNCG(PC) 2010). The family, if not present, must be informed as soon as possible. In cases where death is expected, families may be asked whether they wish to be informed immediately if the death occurs at night or would prefer to wait until morning.

Box 15.12 Activity: what happens to the body after death?

ACTIVITY

What difference might the care setting and the circumstances of a death make to what happens to the body after death?

If Bill dies in an acute care setting, care of the body after death will be carried out by nursing staff; his body will initially be moved to the hospital mortuary by porters and at a later stage collected by an undertaker. However, if he dies at home, care of his body after his death may be minimal before his body is removed by an undertaker. After death in a non-acute care setting, for example, a care home or hospice, local policies affect procedures, but again the body is likely to be removed by an undertaker. In some instances, legal constraints dictate what care may be given. For example, after an unexpected death or a death that takes place within 24 h of an operation, in England, the coroner's office must be informed and a post-mortem may be required (NEoLCP/NNCG(PC) 2011).

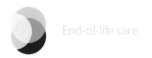

Box 15.13 Activity: hazards a body may present

What hazards may a body present to those who handle it after death?

There may be leakage of body fluids or a risk from sharp objects such as cannulae attached to the body (also see Chapter 12: Infection control and prevention). There will also be moving and handling issues. Therefore, staff caring for a body after death should take appropriate measures to prevent problems arising.

Religious and cultural factors affecting the performance of care of the body after death

Regardless of the deceased person's cultural and religious background, privacy and dignity must be maintained for them and their family. Drawing the curtains around the bed in an open ward is the least requirement. Where possible, the body may be moved to a side room for greater privacy, and to minimise distress to others.

The person's religious and cultural background must be considered at this point. Many of the world's major religions have specific rules and rituals concerned with death, for example, about who can touch the body. However, it is important not to assume that the person or their families will wish these rules to be followed to the letter (Anderson 2017; NEoLCP/NNCG(PC) 2011). As with all human activities, there are many shades of opinion and belief. Ascertaining these beliefs in advance, if possible, is part of sensitive, holistic care. The person was once alive and must be treated with dignity, and it is important that the environment, actions and behaviour of the staff convey respect (NEoLCP/NNCG(PC) 2011).

Box 15.14 Activity: differing needs of cultures and religions

Find out the differing needs of cultures and religions in relation to the care of the body after death.

You will find that there are particular practices associated with different religions and cultures. Nurses should familiarise themselves with these practices so that all interventions are spiritually and culturally acceptable and do not cause offence. It is important to find out what the person's preferences and wishes are before death, and these should always take priority (Anderson 2017). Many of the world's major religions have specific rules and rituals concerned with death, for example, about who can touch the body. However, it is important not to assume that the person or their families will wish these rules to be followed to the letter.

Some examples of different care needs after death include:

Islam: Family members will stay with the dying patient and perform last rites. The person's head should point towards Mecca. Ideally, the body should not be touched by non-Muslims after death, but if they must be touched, gloves should be worn.

Hinduism:

The family may wish to inform a Hindu priest. The body must not be touched by non-Hindu, hence gloves must be worn. Relatives of the same sex may wish to wash the body – preferably in water mixed with water from the River Ganges (some may prefer nurses to do this). Family may wish to stay during last offices. If possible, the eldest son should be present.

There are many different religions and whilst the healthcare professional cannot know details of all, it is important to find out as much as possible in relation to individuals in our care to meet their needs. For further information, see: http://www.ijern.com/journal/April-2014/05.pdf

Box 15.15 Activity: reflecting on experiences of care when someone has died in a clinical setting

Have you been present when someone in hospital, unit or a care home resident, has died? Did the other inpatients/residents show awareness of what had occurred? What comments did they make? How can you respond?

In most settings other than the person's own home, there will be other inpatients or residents around. At least some of them will be aware of the event and may ask, directly or indirectly, about the deceased person. It is important to answer questions sensitively and honestly, but without revealing confidential details.

Box 15.16 Activity: expectations of religious/cultural background

Regarding Bill, who can be expected to die fairly soon, what would you expect his religious/cultural background to be?

From his name, you might assume that he will have a Western/Christian background, but such assumptions can be dangerous; always ask and do not assume. Among Christian religions too, there are variations, with different religious practices around the time of death.

Box 15.17 Activity: contacting religious leaders for advice

Do you know how to contact the local chaplain, rabbi, imam or other religious leaders, so that you can gain advice about any special requirements at the time of death and when carrying out care of the body after death?

Nurses need to be aware of how to contact local religious leaders, as referring to, and liaising with them may be an important contribution to people's spiritual support. You may find there is a folder produced by the hospital chaplaincy with contact

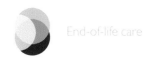

details and information regarding different religions. In many instances, if they follow a particular religion, individuals and their families will have their own contacts.

The procedure for care of the body after death, with attention to safety and dignity

Immediate care after death

In whatever setting, when a death takes place, there are a few actions that should be carried out very soon afterwards, within 2–4 h to preserve their appearance, condition and dignity (NEoLCP/NNCG(PC) 2010).

Close the eyes by gently applying pressure to the eyelids for about 30 s.

Lay the person down flat, leaving one pillow, and straighten the body and limbs into neutral positions as soon as possible.

Insert dentures, if usually worn (e.g. with Bill, we know he likes to wear his denture).

Close the mouth and support the jaw with a pillow, to ensure it remains closed.

The body starts to become rigid soon after death and all these actions become more difficult to perform later.

In a hospital setting, it is usual to leave the body for about an hour before full care after death is carried out. During this period, the family may visit and sit with the person, holding their hand if they wish. Therefore, immediately after death, the surrounding environment should be tidied up, equipment removed and the bed linen attended to so that the person looks peaceful and comfortable. Families need to be given time and support and will, before they leave, need written information about what to do next (e.g. when and how to collect property, register the death, arrange the funeral) (NEoLCP/NNCG(PC) 2011).

Care of the body after death procedure

Before commencing the procedure, you should gather the equipment required, including items for washing the person (see also Chapter 7: Meeting personal needs: hygiene).

Box 15.18 Activity: additional items required

ACTIVITY

What other items do you think might be needed in addition to those mentioned in Chapter 7 (Box 7.9).

If the person is not to wear their own nightclothes, a shroud (long white gown) might be required. Local hospital policies vary on this issue; however, sometimes, hospital nightclothes are used if a person's own are not available as some people consider shrouds, which were traditionally used, to be upsetting to families.

The person's property should be listed and packed ready for collection by the family, so the appropriate documentation (Property Book) will be needed. If the person has a wound, a waterproof dressing is required. If there are tubes to be left in, spigots will be needed to plug these. Additional name bands and identity labels may be necessary according to the setting and local policy. A disposable receiver may also be required.

The procedure described below includes usual practice, but must always be guided by local policy, people's individual circumstances and particular religious and cultural requirements. Sometimes, a family member of the deceased may wish to be involved, perhaps helping with washing or hair brushing. Ensure privacy as previously described. Two nurses are usually required for this procedure due to moving and handling needs but also for the emotional support.

Protect yourself against possible infection by using plastic apron and gloves (see Chapter 12 on preventing cross-infection). For people with communicable diseases, the existing infection control measures should continue.

Wash the person as described in 'Bathing a person in bed', as culturally appropriate.

Cover any wounds with waterproof dressings. Check local policy relating to removal of drains, tubes, cannulae or catheters. If a post-mortem is to take place, these materials should be left in unless advised otherwise but can be spigotted. If no post-mortem is going to be performed, these tubes can usually be removed, but always check if unsure.

If leakage from any orifice seems likely to continue, insert packing, according to local policy, or an incontinence pad can be applied.

Manually express the urinary bladder into a disposable receiver, if necessary and as per local policy.

Place a clean sheet under the person, using safe moving and handling techniques.

Remove and/or record the whereabouts of any jewellery, as previously discussed, with family (or the person). Recording should always be done in the presence of a witness. Jewellery left on the body should be secured with tape to prevent it being lost.

Dress the person in clean personal clothing or a shroud according to local policy and the family's wishes and brush the person's hair.

Shaving a deceased person whilst they are still warm can cause bruising and marking, which will show up days later. Usually, the funeral director will attend to shaving (NEoLCP/NNCG(PC) 2011).

Clean the mouth and replace any dentures.

If the family have not yet viewed the body, this could be an appropriate point for them to do so.

Attach identification labels to the person according to local policy.

Wrap the body in a clean sheet, securing it with tape but not too tight to prevent leaving marks.

A body bag may be necessary if there are infection control issues. Consult the local infection control policy or contact the infection control nurse for advice.

Dispose of the used equipment according to infection control principles and wash your hands.

Make a list of, and store, property and jewellery according to local policy, in the presence of a witness. When packing soiled clothing, ask sensitively if the family would like them included or disposed of safely.

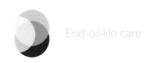

Arrange for the porters to collect the body, or the undertaker in a residential setting.

ACTIVITY

Box 15.19 Activity: comparing local policy on the care of the body after death

Find and compare the local policy on care of the body after death with what you have read above.

As with any other clinical practices, there will be a local policy, probably developed by a multidisciplinary group including the hospital chaplaincy, which takes the local situation into account.

 Box 15.20 Children and young people: practice points – EoLC

For all aspects of EoLC for children, including care after death:

See:

Clarke, S. 2013. Children and young people with life limiting conditions. In: Thurston C. (ed.) *Essential Nursing Care for Children and Young People. Theory, Policy and Practice.* Oxon: Routledge, 318–60.

Macqueen, S., Bruce, E.A. and Gibson, F. 2012. Palliative care. In: *The Great Ormond Street Hospital Manual of Children's Nursing Practices.* Chichester: Wiley-Blackwell, 577–96.

Also see: 'Together for short lives' Available from: http://www.togetherforshortlives.org.uk/ (Accessed on 22 May 2021).

 Box 15.21 Pregnancy and birth: practice points – pregnancy loss and stillbirth

Nursing staff may be directly involved with pregnant or recently delivered mothers in a variety of healthcare settings. In gynaecology or surgical wards, women may experience spontaneous abortion (miscarriage), termination of pregnancy (TOP) for fetal anomaly or evacuation of retained products of conception after delivery. Intensive care unit (ITU) staff may provide care for critically ill women after obstetric emergencies or severe illness/accident and on rare occasions, deal with a maternal death. Community nurses may work alongside practice nurses, performing blood tests or baby immunisations.

Whatever the context of care, the approach must be compassionate, considerate and respectful.

Read the following and consider how it makes you feel:

It should have been the happiest day
To remember all our life
But joy has turned to heartache
No breath, no beat, no life. (Anon)

For further suggested reading to support mothers and families through pregnancy loss or stillbirth, see:

Pregnancy Loss and the Death of a Baby: Guidelines for Professionals, available from the Child Bereavement Charity at www.childbereavement.org.uk/

Other useful websites:

www.winstonswish.org.uk (Winston's Wish-charity for bereaved children)

www.miscarriageassociation.org.uk (Miscarriage Association)

www.fsid.org.uk (Foundation for Sudden Infant Death)

www.uk-sands.org.uk (Support for bereaved parents)

Summary

- Meeting the hygiene needs of a person who has died in a safe and culturally sensitive way is an essential part of nursing care.
- The extent to which care of the body after death is carried out may vary according to the setting and will be influenced by local policy and the individual family.

Learning outcome 3: describe the principles of loss, grief and bereavement

When a person is dying, a profound series of emotions and reactions occur for the individual and all those involved in their care (Garbutt 2018). This section aims to describe the nature of these emotions and reactions with theoretical models and coping strategies for bereavement, loss and grief.

Definitions

- **Loss** is the feeling of anguish after the death of a loved one or something of value (Murray Parkes 2006a, 2006b).
- **Grief** is an intense psychological response of pain and sadness experienced after the loss of a loved one (Walter and McCoyd 2009).
- **Bereavement** is the process of mourning a lost relationship and is the period during which signs and symptoms of grief are made visible, e.g. depression (Buglass 2010).

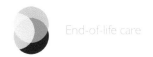

Models of bereavement, loss and grief

There are several theoretical models of loss and grief that have attempted to understand the complex nature of the emotions that we experience when we are bereaved. One such model was developed by Elizabeth Kubler-Ross in 1969 in her seminal work on the five stages of grief. Kubler-Ross worked with terminally ill people and noted that the medical profession was underprepared to care for them and their families who were experiencing grief. Kubler-Ross (1969) argues that individuals experience grief by going through five stages of emotion:

- Denial – 'this isn't happening to me' – Individuals may disagree with a diagnosis they have been given or family members may refuse to accept that their loved one has died.
- Anger – 'why has this happened to me' – once individuals have accepted that they cannot stay in denial, they often elicit anger towards the situation or at others close to them.
- Bargaining – people will often struggle to find meaning in the situation, they may reach out to others for understanding. Feelings of guilt often prevail here, and bereaved individuals might ask 'why them, and not me?'
- Depression – is often closely associated with grief; individuals may experience a number of overwhelming emotions such as sadness, emptiness, hostility, despair and hopelessness.
- Acceptance – this is where individuals enter a period of reality and understanding of the situation, whilst they may never accept their loved one has died; they learn to live with their loss and accept their new reality.

Other researchers have also contributed to the development of models to illustrate the grieving process, such as John Bowlby and his four stages of grief model (Bowlby 1961) and Colin Murray Parkes' phases of grief theory (Murray Parkes 1998). However, these models have faced criticism for their linear structure with others arguing that individuals might not have a smooth transition from one stage to the next; they might skip a stage or find that they have regressed back a few stages on their journey to acceptance. Some they may go through all these stages in a day and their experience may see-saw between these stages. There is also an argument that individuals may never accept the loss of a loved one but learn to live with this loss (Illich 1975; Parker 2007). Interestingly, Worden (1991) suggests that those who are bereaved need to work through a series of 'tasks' rather than stages to find acceptance, e.g. accept the reality of the loss, experience the pain of grief and adjust to an environment with the deceased missing. Completing these tasks highlights the importance of the bereaved undertaking an active process to reach a state of acceptance and that grief is central to the process.

Symptoms of bereavement, grief and loss

Bereavement, grief and loss can cause various symptoms that can affect individuals in different ways.

Common symptoms include:

- Shock, numbness, disbelief and confusion – these feelings can often be the initial reaction to loss. Some individuals describe a feel of 'being in a daze'
- Profound sadness, crying and depression
- Anxiety
- Feeling tried or exhausted
- Anger – sometimes towards the person who has died or the reason for your loss
- Guilt – individuals can often feel guilty about something they may have said or did not say to their loved one, or not being able to prevent their loved one from dying.

(NHS 2019a)

The above symptoms may not be present all the time and sometimes strong feelings may appear unexpectedly. Think back to the five stages of grief model (Kubler-Ross, 1969) and the series of 'tasks' model (Worden, 1991); it was proposed that individuals who are bereaved will often experience various stages/phases of grief that encompass many of the above symptoms and that to find acceptance, individuals will need to work through specific 'tasks' such as learning to adjust to a new environment without the presence of their loved one. There are self-help strategies and services that aim to support individuals in coping with grief, which will now be discussed.

Coping with bereavement

- Talking with family and friends can be a vital source of support during bereavement. It could be that they are also feeling grief and that you are having a shared experience, or they have experienced grief in the past and can support you.
- Talking with a health professional or bereavement counsellor who can provide you with a holistic care plan to support you through your bereavement.
- Referral for psychological therapy – Cognitive Behavioural Therapy (NHS 2019b).
- Accessing the six ways to feel happier – simple lifestyle changes to help you feel more in control and able to cope (NHS 2019c).
- Peer support sessions – where individuals use their own experience to support each other, which can be accessed on the Mind website (MIND 2021).
- Access mental well-being audio guides for low mood and depression, anxiety control training, sleep problems and unhelpful thinking (NHS 2021).
- Mindfulness training or meditation to help support you to live in the moment at your own thoughts and feelings, and to the world around you to improve your mental health and well-being (NHS 2018).

Summary

- It is important to not use too many coping strategies all at once. The key is to find which coping mechanism works for you, small targets that can be easily achieved often have better outcomes.
- It is important for individuals not to focus on situations they cannot change, but to invest their time and energy into improving their health and well-being.

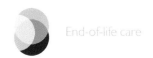

● Individuals can often feel very alone when coping with bereavement, but it is important that they are made aware that grief is a normal response after a loss and that support is available for them.

CHAPTER SUMMARY

Palliative care and EoLC are an essential part of nursing care and should always be person-centred and include ACP when considering treatment. Nurses have a role to play in ensuring that breaking difficult news is handled sensitively and that sufficient time is given to the process including any follow-up. A comprehensive holistic assessment affords healthcare and social care professionals the opportunity to understand the needs of the individual and their families/carers. In doing so, we can support the notion of providing EoLC that promotes a 'good death'. Every effort should be made to ensure that wishes and preferences, such as the person's preferred place of care or advance decisions to refuse treatment, are sensitively discussed and documented in advance care plans. The MCA safeguards the individual to ensure that the decision-making process remains focused on their best interests and that their wishes and preferences remain at the core of the decision-making process. Syringe drivers are useful when the oral route of administration is not possible, or absorption of medication is not optimal. It is important that discussions about medication management occur throughout the dying process and are tailored to meet individual needs. The extent to which care of the body after death is carried out may vary according to the setting and will be influenced by local policy and the individual family. Individuals can often feel very alone when coping with bereavement, but it is important that they are made aware that grief is a normal response after a loss and that support is available for them. Palliative and EoLC are synonymous and as such should be viewed as care approaches that focus on improving quality of life and planning for a peaceful dignified death – both terms are mutually inclusive and share the same ethos and principles.

REFERENCES

Alzheimer's Society. n.d. End of life care. Available from: https://www.alzheimers.org.uk/get-support/help-dementia-care/end-life-care (Accessed on 18 April 2021).

Anderson, B. 2017. Facilitating person-centred after-death care: Unearthing assumptions, tradition and values through practice development. *International Practice Development Journal* 7(1). https://doi.org/10.19043/ipdj.71.006

Andrews, T. and Nathaniel, A. 2015. Awareness of dying remains relevant after fifty years. *Grounded Theory Review* 14(2): 3–10.

Birkhäuer, J., Gaab, J., Kossowsky, J. et al. 2017. Trust in the health care professional and health outcome: A meta-analysis. *PloS One* 12(2). doi:10.1371/journal.pone.0170988

Bowlby, J. 1961. Processes of mourning. *International Journal of Psychoanalysis* 42: 317–339.

Buckman, R. 2005. Breaking bad news: The S-P-I-K-E-S strategy. *Community Oncology* 2. doi: 10.1016/S1548-5315(11)70867-1

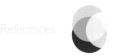

Buglass, E. 2010 Grief and bereavement theories. *Nursing Standard* 24(41): 44–47.

Cohen-Mansfield, J., Skornick-Bouchbinder, M. and Brill, S. 2018. Trajectories of end of life: A systematic review. *The Journals of Gerontology* 4(73): 564–72.

Department of Health. 2008. *End of Life Care Strategy: Promoting High Quality Care for Adults at the End of their Life*. London: Department of Health.

Department of Health. 2012. No decision about me without me. Available from: http://data.parliament.uk/DepositedPapers/Files/DEP2012-1873/LiberatingtheNHS-Nodecisionaboutmewithoutme.pdf (Accessed on18 April 2021).

Dying Matters. Frequently asked questions. 2020. Available from: https://www.dyingmatters.org/page/frequently-asked-questions (Accessed on 10 September 2020).

Engel, G. 1977. The need for a new medical model: a challenge for biomedical science. *Science* 196: 126–9.

Farrell, B. and Paice, J. 2019. *Oxford Textbook of Palliative Nursing*, 5th edn. Oxford: Oxford University Press.

Gabriel, J. 2015. Syringe drivers: Their key safety features. *International Journal of Palliative Nursing* 21(7): 328–330. https://doi.org/10.12968/ijpn.2015.21.7.328

Garbutt, D. 2018 End of life care. In: Peate, I. and Wild, K. (eds.) *Nursing Practice: Knowledge and Care*. Oxford: Wiley Blackwell, 404–427.

General Medical Council. 2010. Treatment and care towards the end of life: Decision making. Available at https://www.gmc-uk.org/ethical-guidance/ethical-guidance-for-doctors/treatment-and-care-towards-the-end-of-life (Accessed on 22 December 2020).

Gold Standards Framework. 2006. Prognostic Indicator Guidance to aid identification of adult patients with advanced disease in the last months/year of life, who are in need of supportive and palliative care. Version 2.25 Prognostic Indicator Paper. Available from: https://www.palliativecareggc.org.uk/wp-content/uploads/2015/12/gsf-prognostic-indicators.pdf (Accessed 13 May 2021).

Healthcare Commission. 2007. *Spotlight on Complaints. A Report on Second-stage Complaints about the NHS in England*. London: Healthcare Commission. Available from: https://delta.bipsolutions.com/docstore/pdf/15763.pdf (Accessed 10 September 2020).

Illich, I. 1975. The medicalization of life. *Journal of Medical Ethics* 1(2): 73–7.

Johnson, A., Rees, J., Delduca, C. and Criddle, R. 2015. Psychological support: Sharing good practice. Available from: https://www.macmillan.org.uk/documents/aboutus/health_professionals/macvoice/psychological-support-sharing-good-practice.pdf (Accessed on 24 June 2021).

Joint Formulary Committee. 2020. British National Formulary. Available from: https://bnf.nice.org.uk/guidance/prescribing-in-palliative-care.html (Accessed on 13 May 2020).

Kennedy, C., Brooks-Young, P., Brunton Grey, C. et al. 2014. Diagnosing dying: And integrative literature review. *British Medical Journal Supportive and Palliative Care* 4: 263–70.

Kubler-Ross, E. 1969. *On Death and Dying*. London: Tavistock.

London End of Life Clinical Network. 2015. What is a good death? Available from: http://www.londonscn.nhs.uk/publication/what-is-a-good-death (Accessed 22 December 2020).

Macmillan Cancer Support. 2017. No regrets. How talking more openly about death could help people die well. Available from: https://www.macmillan.org.uk/_images/no-regrets-talking-about-death-report_tcm9-311059.pdf (Accessed on 22 March 2020).

Macmillan Cancer Support. 2019. *Advanced Decision to Refuse Treatment*. Available from: https://www.macmillan.org.uk/cancer-information-and-support/treatment/if-you-

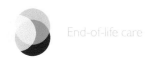

have-an-advanced-cancer/advance-care-planning/advance-decision-to-refuse-treatment (Accessed on 23 December 2020).

Marie Curie. 2018. What are palliative care and end of life care? Available from: https://www.mariecurie.org.uk/help/support/diagnosed/recent-diagnosis/palliative-care-end-of-life-care (Accessed on 13 May 2021).

Marie Curie. 2020. Planning your care in advance. Available from: https://www.mariecurie.org.uk/help/support/terminal-illness/planning-ahead/advance-care-planning (Accessed on 23 December 2020).

Marie Curie. 2020. Signs that your loved one might be dying. Available from: https://www.mariecurie.org.uk/help/support/being-there/end-of-life-preparation/signs-of-dying (Accessed on 23 December 2020).

Mental Capacity Act. 2005. *Code of Practice (2007)*. London: TSO.

MIND. 2021. Peer support. Available from: https://www.mind.org.uk/information-support/drugs-and-treatments/peer-support/finding-peer-support/ (Accessed on 10 February 2021).

Mitchell, A. and Elbourne, S. 2020. Advance care planning and syringe drivers. *British Journal of Nursing* 29(17): 1010–15.

Murray Parkes, C. 1998. *Coping with Loss*. Oxford: Wiley Blackwell.

Murray Parkes, C. 2006a. *Love and Loss. The Roots of Grief and Its Complications*. Hove: Routledge.

Murray-Parkes, C. 2006b. Symposium on complicated grief. *Journal of Death and Dying* 51(1): 1–7.

National End of Life Care Programme. 2010. *Holistic Common Assessment of Supportive and Palliative Care Needs for Adults Requiring End of Life Care*. Available from: https://www.bl.uk/collection-items/holistic-common-assessment-of-the-supportive-and-palliative-care-needs-of-adults-requiring-end-of-life-care#

National Health Service. 2018. Mindfulness. Available from: https://www.nhs.uk/mental-health/self-help/tips-and-support/mindfulness/ (Accessed 5 April 2021).

National Health Service. 2019a. Grief after bereavement or loss. Available from: https://www.nhs.uk/mental-health/feelings-symptoms-behaviours/feelings-and-symptoms/grief-bereavement-loss/ (Accessed 10 February 2021).

National Health Service. 2019b. How it works – cognitive behavioral therapy (CBT). Available from: https://www.nhs.uk/mental-health/talking-therapies-medicine-treatments/talking-therapies-and-counselling/cognitive-behavioural-therapy-cbt/how-it-works/ (Accessed on 10 February 2021).

National Health Service. 2019c. How to be happier. Available from: https://www.nhs.uk/mental-health/self-help/tips-and-support/how-to-be-happier/ (Accessed on 10 February 2021).

National Health Service. 2021. Mental wellbeing audio guides. Available from: https://www.nhs.uk/mental-health/self-help/guides-tools-and-activities/mental-wellbeing-audio-guides/ (Accessed 10 February 2021).

National Institute for Health and Care Excellence. 2016. Multimorbidity: Clinical assessment and management. NICE guideline NG56. Available from: https://www.nice.org.uk/guidance/ng56 (Accessed on 22 December 2020).

National Institute for Health and Care Excellence. 2019. End of life care for adults: service delivery. NICE guideline NG142. Available from: https://www.nice.org.uk/guidance/ng142/chapter/Recommendations (Accessed on 22 December 2020).

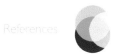

National Palliative and End of Life Care Partnership. 2015. Ambitions for palliative and end of life care: A national framework for local action 2015–2020. Available from: https://www.nationalvoices.org.uk/sites/default/files/public/publications/ambitions-for-palliative-and-end-of-life-care.pdf (Accessed on 12 June 2021).

NHS England. 2017a. Delivering high quality end of life care for people who have a learning disability. Available from: https://www.england.nhs.uk/publication/delivering-high-quality-end-of-life-care-for-people-who-have-a-learning-disability/ (Accessed on 18 April 2021).

NHS England. 2017b. Person-centred approaches: A core skills and education training framework. Available from: https://skillsforhealth.org.uk/wp-content/uploads/2021/01/Person-Centred-Approaches-Framework.pdf (Accessed on 18 April 2021).

NHS England. 2018. My future wishes: Advance care planning for people with dementia in all care settings. Available from: https://www.england.nhs.uk/publication/my-future-wishes-advance-care-planning-acp-for-people-with-dementia-in-all-care-settings/ (Accessed on 18 April 2021).

NHS England. 2019. NHS long-term plan. Available from: https://www.longtermplan.nhs.uk/ (Accessed on 18 April 2021).

NHS Highland, NHS Greater Glasgow and Clyde. 2007. Syringe pump guidelines CME McKinley T34 (ml/hour): For use within Argyll and Bute CHP and Clyde. Available from: https://www.palliativecareggc.org.uk/wp-content/uploads/2013/10/T34Guideline_Oct2016.pdf (Accessed on 13 May 2021).

NHS Scotland. 2014. End of life care: Scottish palliative care guidelines. Available from: https://www.palliativecareguidelines.scot.nhs.uk/guidelines/end-of-life-care.aspx (Accessed on 13 May 2021).

NHS Scotland. 2020. End of life care: syringe pumps. In: Scottish Palliative Care Guidelines. (updated version of guideline published 2014). Available from: https://tinyurl.com/y4w7u8rs (Accessed on 13 May 2021).

Nursing and Midwifery Council (NMC). 2018. *The Code: Professional Standards of Practice and Behaviour for Nurses, Midwives and Nursing Associates.* London: NMC. Available from: tinyurl.com/zy7syuo (Accessed 10 September 2020).

O'Gorman, S.M. 1998. Death and dying in contemporary society: An evaluation of current attitudes and the rituals associated with death and dying and their relevance to recent understandings of health and healing. *Journal of Advanced Nursing* 27: 1127–35.

Office for National Statistics (ONS). 2020. Leading causes of death, UK: 2001–2018. Registered leading causes of death by age, sex and country. Available at: https://tinyurl.com/yxc5unu4 (Accessed on 22 December 2020).

Parker, G. 2007. Is depression over-diagnosed? Yes. *British Medical Journal* 335(7615): 328–329.

Pfeifer, M. and Head, B.A., 2018. Which critical communication skills are essential for interdisciplinary end-of-life discussions? *AMA jJournal of eEthics.* 20(8): 724–731.

Public Health England. 2018. (National End of Life Care Intelligence Network). Statistical commentary: End of life care profiles, February 2018 update. Available from: https://tinyurl.com/y9hzbss4 (Accessed 10 September 2020).

Quinn, B. 2018. Making sense of pain and loss: searching for meaning while living with cancer. *Cancer Nursing Practice.* 17 (5) 29-36.

Quinn, B.G. 2020. Responding to people who are experiencing spiritual pain. *Nursing Standard.* doi:10.7748/ns.2020.e11523.

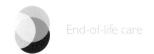

Resuscitation Council UK. 2016. Decisions relating to cardiopulmonary resuscitation. Available from: https://www.bma.org.uk/media/1816/bma-decisions-relating-to-cpr-2016.pdf (Accessed on 23 June 2021).

Resuscitation Council UK. 2019. Resuscitation Council UK introduces version 3 of ReSPECT form. Available at: https://www.resus.org.uk/about-us/news-and-events/resuscitation-council-uk-introduces-version-3-respect-form (Accessed on 23 December 2020).

Royal College of Nursing (RCN). 2015. Breaking bad news: Supporting parents when they are told of their child's diagnosis. Available from: http://londonneonatalnetwork.org.uk/wp-content/uploads/2015/09/RCNBreakingBadNewsSupportingParents.pdf (Accessed on 30 April 2021).

Shucksmith, J., Carlebach, S. and Whittaker V. 2013. Dying: Discussing and planning for end of life. *British Social Attitudes* 30. Available from: https://www.dyingmatters.org/sites/default/files/BSA30_Full_Report.pdf (Accessed on 10 September 2020).

Sivell, S., Prout, H., Hopewell-Kelly, N. et al. 2015. Considerations and recommendations for conducting qualitative research interviews with palliative and end-of-life care patients in the home setting: A consensus paper *BMJ Supportive & Palliative Care* 0 (1–7). doi:10.1136/bmjspcare-2015-000892.

Spence, A. 2012. Syringe driver/pump management and symptom control in palliative care. In: O'Brien L (ed.) *District Nursing Manual of Clinical Procedures*. Chichester: John Wiley and Sons, 272–302.

Stevens, A.M. 2015. Patient comfort and end-of-life care. In: Dougherty, L. and Lister, S. (eds.) *Royal Marsden Hospital Manual of Clinical Nursing Procedures* Chichester: Wiley-Blackwell, 331–421.

Thomas, K., Armstrong-Wilson, F., Tanner, T. 2016. Evidence that use of GSF helps improve Advance Care Planning Discussions: National GSF Centre. Available from: https://www.goldstandardsframework.org.uk/cd-content/uploads/files/2%20%20%20vs%203%20Evidence%20that%20use%20of%20GSF%20Improves%20ACP%20n%20different%20settings%20vs%203%20(002)%20JAW%20(002)%20(1).pdf (Accessed on 23 June 2021).

Thomas, T. and Barclay, S. 2015. Continuous subcutaneous infusion in palliative care: A review of current practice. *International Journal of Palliative Nursing* 21(2): 60–64. https://doi.org/10.12968/ijpn.2015.21.2.60.

Thomson, R., Geddis-Regan, A., Errington, L. et al. 2021. Enhancing shared and surrogate decision making for people living with dementia: A systematic review of the effectiveness of interventions. *Health Expectations*. 24(1): 19–32.

Twycross R. and Wilcock A. (eds.) 2016. *Introducing Palliative Care*, 5th edn. Nottingham: palliativedrugs.com Ltd.

Walter, C.A. and McCoyd, J.L.M. 2009. *Grief and Loss across the Lifespan: A Biopsychosocial Perspective*. New York: Springer Publishing Company.

Worden, J.W. 1991. *Grief Counselling and Grief Therapy*, 2nd edn. London: Routledge.

World Health Organization. 2020. *WHO Definition of Palliative Care*. Geneva: WHO.

Appendix

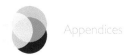

Table A.1: Standards of proficiency for registered nurses

Platform 1. Being an accountable professional	Chapters														
	1	2	3	4	5	6	7	8	9	10	11	12	13	14	15
Act in accordance with the code	✓	✓	✓	✓	✓	✓	✓	✓	✓	✓	✓	✓	✓	✓	✓
Apply relevant legal, regulatory and governance requirements, policies and ethical frameworks	✓	✓	✓		✓		✓	✓	✓	✓	✓	✓	✓	✓	✓
Apply the principles of courage and the duty of candour	✓		✓												
Demonstrate the ability to challenge discriminatory behaviour	✓	✓	✓												
Recognise signs of vulnerability in themselves or their colleagues		✓	✓												
Adopt a healthy lifestyle															
Demonstrate an understanding if research methods, ethics and governance		✓	✓												✓
Demonstrate the knowledge, skills and ability to think critically when applying evidence	✓		✓									✓	✓	✓	✓
Based on all decisions regarding care and interventions on people's needs and preferences	✓	✓	✓			✓	✓			✓	✓	✓	✓	✓	✓
Demonstrate resilience and emotional intelligence		✓													✓
Communicate effectively using a range of skills and strategies	✓	✓	✓	✓		✓	✓	✓		✓	✓	✓	✓	✓	✓

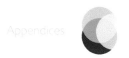

Table A.1: (Continued)

Platform 1. Being an accountable professional	Chapters														
	1	2	3	4	5	6	7	8	9	10	11	12	13	14	15
Demonstrate the skills and abilities required to support people at all stages of life who are emotionally or physically vulnerable	✓	✓	✓			✓	✓			✓		✓	✓	✓	✓
Demonstrate the skills and abilities required to develop, manage and maintain appropriate relationships	✓	✓	✓												✓
Promote non-discriminatory, person-centred and sensitive care at all times	✓	✓	✓				✓			✓					
Demonstrate the numeracy, literacy, digital and technological skills required	✓	✓		✓		✓				✓				✓	
Demonstrate the ability to keep complete, clear, accurate and timely records	✓	✓	✓	✓	✓	✓	✓					✓	✓	✓	✓
Take responsibility for continuous reflection	✓	✓													
Demonstrate the knowledge and confidence to contribute effectively and proactively in an interdisciplinary team		✓	✓			✓				✓	✓		✓		
Act as an ambassador, upholding the reputation of their profession	✓	✓										✓			
Safely demonstrate evidence-based practice	✓	✓	✓	✓	✓	✓	✓	✓	✓	✓	✓	✓	✓	✓	✓

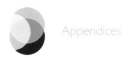

Table A.2: Standards of proficiency for registered nurses

Platform 2. Promoting health and preventing ill health	Chapters														
	1	2	3	4	5	6	7	8	9	10	11	12	13	14	15
Apply the aims and principles of health promotion, protection and improvement	✓												✓		
Demonstrate knowledge of epidemiology, demography and genomics															
Understand the factors that may lead to inequalities in health outcomes			✓												✓
Use all appropriate opportunities, making reasonable adjustments when required		✓	✓												
Promote and improve mental, physical, behavioural and other health-related outcomes		✓	✓	✓		✓	✓		✓		✓	✓	✓	✓	
Understand the importance of early years and childhood experiences			✓												
Understand and explain the contributing of social influences, health literacy, individual circumstance, behaviours and lifestyle choices	✓		✓			✓	✓				✓				✓
Demonstrate the use of up to date approaches to behaviour change		✓	✓												

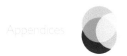

Table A.2: (Continued)

Platform 2. Promoting health and preventing ill health	Chapters														
	1	2	3	4	5	6	7	8	9	10	11	12	13	14	15
Use appropriate communication skills and strength-based approaches to support and enable people to make informed choices	✓	✓	✓		✓	✓	✓	✓	✓		✓	✓	✓	✓	✓
Provide information in accessible ways to help people understand and make decisions about their health, life choices, illness and care	✓	✓	✓			✓		✓	✓			✓	✓		✓
Promote health and prevent ill health	✓	✓	✓			✓	✓				✓	✓	✓	✓	
Protect health through understanding and applying the principles of infection prevention and control						✓							✓		

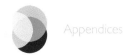

Table A.3: Standards of proficiency for registered nurses

Platform 3. Assessing needs and planning care	Chapters														
	1	2	3	4	5	6	7	8	9	10	11	12	13	14	15
Apply knowledge of human development from conception to death when undertaking full and accurate person-centred nursing assessments		✓	✓		✓										✓
Apply knowledge of body systems and homeostasis, human anatomy and physiology, biology, genomics				✓	✓	✓					✓		✓	✓	✓
Apply knowledge of all commonly encountered mental, physical, behavioural and cognitive health conditions		✓	✓		✓	✓				✓	✓		✓		✓
Apply a person-centred approach to nursing care, demonstrating shared assessment, planning decision making and goal setting	✓	✓	✓		✓	✓	✓	✓	✓	✓	✓	✓	✓	✓	✓
Demonstrate the ability to accurately process all information gathered during the assessment process	✓	✓	✓	✓	✓	✓	✓	✓	✓		✓	✓	✓	✓	✓
Effectively assess a person's capacity to make decisions about their own care and to give or withhold consent	✓	✓	✓		✓	✓				✓				✓	✓
Apply the principles and processes for making reasonable adjustments	✓	✓	✓												✓
Understand and apply the relevant laws about mental capacity	✓	✓	✓		✓										✓
Recognise and assess people at risk of harm and the situations that may put them at risk ensuring prompt action is taken to safeguard those who are vulnerable			✓				✓		✓		✓		✓	✓	
Demonstrate the skills and abilities required to recognise and assess people who show signs of self harm and/or suicidal ideation			✓												

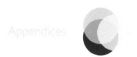

Table A.3: (Continued)

Platform 3. Assessing needs and planning care	1	2	3	4	5	6	7	8	9	10	11	12	13	14	15
Undertake routine investigations, interpreting and sharing findings				✓		✓						✓	✓	✓	✓
Interpret results from routine investigations taking prompt action when required				✓		✓								✓	✓
Demonstrate a understanding of comorbidities and the demands of meeting people's complex nursing and social care needs		✓									✓		✓	✓	✓
Identify and assess the needs to people and families for care at the end of life															✓
Demonstrate the ability to work in partnership with people, families and carers to continuously monitor, evaluate and reassess the effectiveness of agreed nursing care plans and care	✓	✓	✓	✓	✓	✓					✓		✓	✓	✓
Demonstrate knowledge of when and how to refer people safely to other professionals or services for clinical intervention or support	✓		✓					✓		✓				✓	

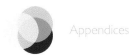

Table A.4: Standards of proficiency for registered nurses

Platform 4. Providing and evaluating care	Chapters														
	1	2	3	4	5	6	7	8	9	10	11	12	13	14	15
Apply an understanding of what is important to people and how to use this knowledge to ensure their needs for safety, dignity, privacy, comfort and sleep can be met	✓		✓			✓	✓	✓	✓		✓	✓	✓	✓	✓
Work in partnership with people to encourage shared decision-making	✓	✓	✓			✓	✓		✓		✓	✓	✓	✓	✓
Demonstrate the knowledge, communication and relationship management skills required	✓	✓	✓					✓	✓			✓	✓	✓	✓
Demonstrate the knowledge and skills required to support people with commonly encountered mental health, behavioural, cognitive and learning challenges, and act as a role model	✓	✓	✓				✓							✓	✓
Support people with commonly encountered physical health conditions, their medication usage and treatments				✓	✓	✓	✓	✓	✓	✓	✓	✓		✓	✓
Act as a role model for others in providing evidence-based nursing care to meet people's needs related to nutrition, hydration and bladder and bowel health					✓	✓						✓			✓
Act as a role model for others in providing evidence-based, person-centred nursing care to meet people's needs related to mobility, hygiene, oral care, wound care and skin integrity					✓	✓	✓				✓	✓	✓		✓
Demonstrate the knowledge and skills required to identify and initiate appropriate interventions to support people with commonly encountered symptoms including anxiety, confusion, discomfort and pain		✓	✓			✓		✓	✓		✓	✓	✓		✓
Prioritise what is important to people and their families when proving evidence-based person-centred nursing care at end of life														✓	
Respond proactively and promptly to signs of deterioration or distress in mental, physical, cognitive and behavioural health and use this knowledge to make sound clinical decisions		✓	✓						✓			✓		✓	✓
Initiate and evaluate appropriate interventions to support people who show signs of self-harm and/or suicidal ideation			✓												

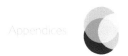

Table A.4: (Continued)

Platform 4. Providing and evaluating care	1	2	3	4	5	6	7	8	9	10	11	12	13	14	15
										Chapters					
Manage commonly encountered devices and confidently carry out related to nursing procedures				✓		✓	✓				✓			✓	✓
Demonstrate the knowledge, skills and confidence to provide first aid procedures and basic life support														✓	
Understand the principles of safe administration and optimisation of medicines					✓	✓		✓	✓	✓	✓	✓	✓	✓	✓
Demonstrate knowledge of pharmacology and the ability to recognise the effects of medicines, allergies, drug sensitivities, side effects, contraindications, incompatibilities, adverse reactions and prescribing errors					✓			✓	✓	✓		✓		✓	✓
Demonstrate knowledge of how prescriptions can be generated										✓					
Apply knowledge of pharmacology to the care of people, demonstrating the ability to progress to a prescribing qualification following registration					✓					✓					
Demonstrate the ability to coordinate and undertake the processes and procedures involved in routing planning and management of safe discharge home or transfer of people between care settings															✓

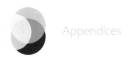
Table A.5: Standards of proficiency for registered nurses

Platform 5. Leading and managing nursing care and working in teams	Chapters														
	1	2	3	4	5	6	7	8	9	10	11	12	13	14	15
Understand the principles of effective leadership, management, group and organisational dynamics and culture	✓	✓													✓
Understand and apply the principles of human factors, environmental factors and strength-based approaches when working in teams		✓	✓												
Understand the principles and application of processes for performance management															
Demonstrate and understanding of the roles, responsibilities and scope of practice for all members of the nursing and interdisciplinary team	✓	✓				✓	✓				✓	✓		✓	✓
Safely lead and manage the nursing care of a group of people	✓														✓
Exhibit leadership potential by demonstrating the ability to guide, support and motivate individuals	✓														✓
Demonstrate the ability to monitor and evaluate the quality of care delivered by others in the team and lay carers	✓														✓
Support and supervise students in the delivery of nursing care	✓														
Challenge and provide constructive feedback about care delivered by others in the team	✓														
Contribute to supervision and team reflection activities to promote improvements in practice and services	✓														
Effectively and responsibly use a range of digital technologies	✓			✓										✓	✓
Understand the mechanisms that can be used to influence organisational change and public policy															✓

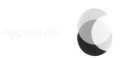

Table A.6: Standards of proficiency for registered nurses

Platform 6. Improving safety and quality of care	Chapters														
	1	2	3	4	5	6	7	8	9	10	11	12	13	14	15
Apply the principles of health and safety legislation and regulations			✓			✓					✓	✓		✓	
Understand the relationship between safe staffing levels, appropriate skills mix, safety and quality of care			✓												✓
Comply with local and national frameworks, legislation and regulations for assessing, managing and reporting risks, ensuring that the appropriate action is taken		✓	✓								✓	✓		✓	
Demonstrate an understanding of the principles of improvement methodologies															
Demonstrate the ability to accurately undertake risk assessments in a range of care settings, using a range of contemporary assessment and improvement tools			✓	✓	✓	✓	✓	✓	✓	✓	✓	✓	✓	✓	✓
Identify the need to make improvements and proactively respond to potential hazards			✓												
Understand how the quality and effectiveness of nursing care can be evaluated in practice	✓														
Demonstrate an understanding of how to identify, report and critically reflect on near misses, critical incidents, major incidents and serious adverse events															
Work with people, their families, carers and colleagues to develop effective improvement strategies for quality and safety	✓										✓				
Apply and understanding of the differences between risk aversion and risk management and how to avoid compromising quality of care and health outcomes			✓												
Acknowledge the need to accept and manage uncertainty														✓	✓
Understand the role of registered nurses and other health and care professionals at different levels of experience and seniority when managing and prioritising actions and care	✓														

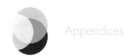

Table A.7: Standards of proficiency for registered nurses

Platform 6. Coordinating care	Chapters														
	1	2	3	4	5	6	7	8	9	10	11	12	13	14	15
Understand and apply the principles of partnership, collaboration and interagency working		✓	✓												✓
Understand health legislation and current health and social care policies	✓	✓	✓								✓				✓
Understand the principles of health economics and their relevance to resource allocation	✓		✓												✓
Identify the implications of current health policy and future policy changes for nursing and other professions	✓	✓	✓												✓
Understand and recognise the need to respond to the challenges of providing safe, effective and person-centred nursing care for people	✓	✓	✓				✓		✓		✓	✓	✓		✓
Demonstrate an understanding of the complexities of providing mental, cognitive, behavioural and physical care services	✓	✓	✓								✓	✓			✓
Understand how to monitor and evaluate the quality of people's experience of complex care			✓					✓	✓		✓	✓			
Understand the principles and processes involved in supporting people and families with a range of care needs	✓	✓	✓			✓			✓						✓
Facilitate equitable access to healthcare for people who are vulnerable or have a disability, demonstrate the ability to advocate on their behalf	✓	✓	✓												✓
Understand the principles and processes of planning and facilitating the safe discharge and transition of people between caseloads, setting and services															✓
Demonstrate the ability to identify and manage risks and take proactive measures to improve the quality of care			✓												
Demonstrate an understanding of the processes involved in developing a basic business case for additional care funding															
Demonstrate an understanding of the importance of exercising political awareness throughout their career															

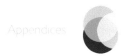

Table B.1: Standards of proficiency for nursing associates

Platform 1. Being an accountable professional	Chapters														
	1	2	3	4	5	6	7	8	9	10	11	12	13	14	15
Act in accordance with the code	✓	✓	✓	✓	✓	✓	✓	✓	✓	✓	✓	✓	✓	✓	✓
Apply relevant legal, regulatory and governance requirements	✓	✓	✓		✓			✓	✓	✓	✓	✓	✓	✓	✓
Apply the duty of candour	✓		✓												
Challenge or report discriminatory behaviour	✓	✓	✓												
Recognise signs of vulnerability in themselves or their colleagues		✓	✓												
Adopt a healthy lifestyle															
Apply evidence-based practice		✓	✓			✓				✓	✓	✓	✓	✓	✓
Demonstrate resilience and emotional intelligence		✓	✓												✓
Communicate effectively	✓		✓	✓		✓	✓	✓		✓	✓	✓	✓	✓	✓
Develop, manage and maintain appropriate relationships	✓	✓													✓
Non-discriminatory, person-centred and sensitive care	✓	✓	✓			✓		✓		✓		✓	✓	✓	✓
Recognise and report any factors that may adversely impact safe and effective care provision	✓	✓								✓					
Demonstrate the numeracy, literacy, digital and technological skills	✓	✓	✓	✓						✓			✓		
Demonstrate the ability to keep complete, clear, accurate and timely records	✓	✓	✓	✓		✓		✓		✓		✓	✓	✓	✓
Take responsibility for continuous self-reflection	✓	✓	✓												
Act as an ambassador for their profession and promote public confidence in health and care services	✓	✓													
Safely demonstrate evidence-based practice in all skills and procedures stated	✓	✓	✓	✓	✓	✓	✓	✓	✓	✓	✓	✓	✓	✓	✓

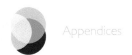

Table B.2: Standards of proficiency for nursing associates

Platform 2. Promoting health and preventing ill health	Chapters														
	1	2	3	4	5	6	7	8	9	10	11	12	13	14	15
Apply the aims and principles of health promotion, protection and improvement	✓						✓	✓	✓			✓	✓	✓	✓
Promote preventative health behaviours			✓	✓		✓					✓	✓	✓		
Principles of epidemiology, demography and genomics															
Understand the factors that may lead to inequalities in health outcomes		✓	✓			✓									
Understand the importance of early years and childhood															
Understand and explain the contribution of social influences, health literacy, individual circumstances, behaviours and lifestyle choices	✓	✓	✓		✓	✓	✓		✓		✓	✓	✓	✓	✓
Explain why health screening is important				✓										✓	
Promote health and prevent ill health		✓	✓	✓		✓	✓		✓		✓	✓	✓	✓	
Principles of infection prevention and control												✓	✓		

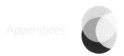

Table B.3:   Standards of proficiency for nursing associates

Platform 3. Provide and monitor care	Chapters														
	1	2	3	4	5	6	7	8	9	10	11	12	13	14	15
Understanding of human development															
Apply knowledge of body systems					✓				✓				✓	✓	
Apply knowledge of commonly encountered mental, physical, behavioural and cognitive health conditions	✓	✓		✓	✓	✓	✓	✓	✓	✓	✓			✓	✓
Knowledge, communication and relationship management skills	✓	✓	✓		✓	✓	✓	✓	✓	✓	✓	✓	✓	✓	✓
Work in partnership with people	✓	✓	✓	✓	✓	✓	✓	✓	✓	✓	✓	✓	✓	✓	✓
Knowledge, skills and ability to perform a range of nursing procedures	✓		✓	✓	✓	✓	✓		✓	✓	✓	✓	✓	✓	✓
How and when to escalate to the appropriate professional	✓		✓	✓	✓			✓	✓				✓	✓	✓
Peoples needs for safety, dignity, privacy, comfort and sleep		✓						✓	✓	✓	✓	✓	✓	✓	✓
Meet people's needs related to nutrition, hydration and bladder and bowel health					✓	✓		✓						✓	✓
Act as required to meet people's needs related to mobility, hygiene, oral care, wound care and skin integrity						✓	✓	✓			✓	✓	✓	✓	✓
Recognise when a person's condition has improved or deteriorated				✓	✓	✓	✓	✓	✓		✓	✓	✓	✓	✓
Knowledge and skills required to support people with commonly encountered symptoms including anxiety, confusion, discomfort and pain		✓	✓			✓			✓		✓	✓	✓	✓	✓
Deliver sensitive and compassionate end-of-life care							✓	✓						✓	✓
Act in line with any end-of-life decisions and orders															✓
Safe and effective administration and optimisation of medicines in accordance with local and national policies					✓	✓		✓	✓	✓	✓	✓	✓	✓	✓

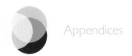
Table B.3: (Continued)

Platform 3. Provide and monitor care	Chapters														
	1	2	3	4	5	6	7	8	9	10	11	12	13	14	15
Recognise the effects of medicines, allergies, drug sensitivity, side effects, contraindications and adverse reactions								✓	✓	✓		✓		✓	✓
Different ways by which medicines can be prescribed								✓		✓				✓	
Monitor the effectiveness of care in partnership with people, families and carers		✓	✓		✓	✓	✓		✓	✓	✓	✓	✓	✓	✓
Understanding of comorbidities and the demands of meeting people's holistic needs			✓		✓	✓			✓	✓				✓	✓
Apply the principles and processes for making reasonable adjustments		✓								✓					✓
Recognise how a person's capacity affects their ability to make decisions about their own care and to give or withhold consent	✓		✓						✓	✓					✓
Recognise when capacity has changed and understand where and how to seek guidance and support	✓		✓							✓					✓
Recognise people at risk of abuse, self-harm and/or suicidal ideation			✓												
Take personal responsibility to ensure that relevant information is shared according to local policy	✓	✓	✓	✓	✓	✓	✓	✓	✓	✓	✓	✓	✓	✓	✓

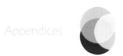

Table B.4: Standards of proficiency for nursing associates

Platform 4. Working in teams	Chapters														
	1	2	3	4	5	6	7	8	9	10	11	12	13	14	15
Awareness of the roles, responsibilities and scope of practice of different members of the nursing and interdisciplinary team	✓	✓	✓	✓	✓	✓	✓	✓	✓	✓	✓	✓	✓	✓	✓
Support and motivate other members of the care team	✓	✓									✓	✓	✓	✓	✓
Apply the principles of human factors and environmental factors when working in teams		✓													
Effectively and responsibly access, input and apply information and data	✓		✓	✓	✓	✓	✓	✓	✓	✓	✓	✓	✓	✓	✓
Prioritise and manage their own workload and recognise where elements of care can safety be delegated to other colleagues	✓			✓			✓	✓	✓		✓	✓		✓	
Monitor and review the quality of care delivered	✓				✓			✓			✓	✓		✓	
Support, supervise and act as role model	✓	✓			✓	✓					✓	✓		✓	✓
Contribute to team reflection activities, to promote improvements in practice and services	✓														
Discuss the influence of policy and political drivers that impact health and care provision															

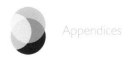

Table B.5: Standards of proficiency for nursing associates

Platform 5. Improving safety and quality of care	Chapters														
	1	2	3	4	5	6	7	8	9	10	11	12	13	14	15
Apply the principles of health and safety legislation and regulations and maintain safe work and care environments	✓		✓	✓	✓	✓	✓	✓	✓	✓	✓	✓	✓	✓	✓
Support audit activity										✓		✓	✓		
Undertake risk assessments, using contemporary assessment tools			✓	✓	✓	✓	✓	✓	✓	✓	✓	✓	✓	✓	✓
Respond to and escalate potential hazards that may affect the safety of people			✓		✓		✓		✓	✓	✓	✓	✓	✓	
Recognise when inadequate staffing levels impact on the ability to provide safe care and escalate concerns appropriately			✓	✓	✓	✓	✓	✓	✓	✓	✓	✓	✓	✓	
Act in line with local and national organisational frameworks, legislation and regulations to report risks and implement actions, following up and escalating as required			✓	✓	✓	✓	✓		✓	✓	✓	✓	✓		
Understand what constitutes a near miss, a serious adverse event, a critical incident and a major incident			✓							✓					
Seek appropriate advice to manage a risk and avoid compromising quality of care and health outcomes			✓						✓	✓		✓			
Recognise uncertainty, and demonstrate an awareness of strategies to develop resilience	✓	✓													✓
Understand their own role and the roles of all other staff in the event of a major incident															

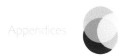

Table B.6: Standards of proficiency for nursing associates

Platform 6. Contributing to integrated care	Chapters														
	1	2	3	4	5	6	7	8	9	10	11	12	13	14	15
Understand the roles of the different providers of health and care	✓	✓	✓	✓	✓	✓	✓	✓	✓	✓	✓	✓	✓	✓	✓
Explore the challenges of providing safe nursing care for people with complex comorbidities and complex care needs			✓		✓			✓	✓	✓			✓	✓	
Understanding of the complexities of providing mental, cognitive, behavioural and physical care needs across a wide range integrated care setting		✓	✓	✓	✓		✓		✓						
Principles and processes involved in supporting people and families with a range of care needs to maintain optimal independence	✓	✓	✓		✓			✓	✓		✓				
Identify when people need help to facilitate equitable access to care, support and escalate concerns appropriately	✓	✓	✓			✓									
Demonstrate an understanding of their own role and contribution when involved in the care of a person who is undergoing discharge or transition of care															

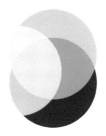

Index

Note: Page numbers followed by "*b*" refer to boxes, by "*f*" refer to figures, and "*t*" denote tables.

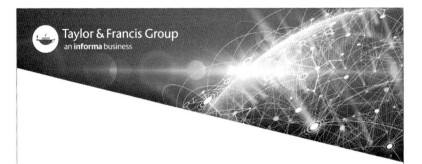